Knowledge and Context in Tibetan Medicine

Brill's Tibetan Studies Library

Edited by

Henk Blezer
Alex McKay
Charles Ramble

VOLUME 43

The titles published in this series are listed at *brill.com/btsl*

Knowledge and Context in Tibetan Medicine

Edited by

William A. McGrath

BRILL

LEIDEN | BOSTON

Cover illustration: The Buddha, Master of Medicine, and the emanated sages, Rikpé Yeshé and Yilekyé. Reproduced with permission from Yuri Parfionovitch, Fernand Meyer, and Gyurme Dorje, eds., *Tibetan Medical Paintings: Illustrations to the Blue Beryl Treatise of Sangye Gyamtso (1635–1705)* (London: Serindia Publications, 1992), vol. 1, p. 124, plate 54.

The Library of Congress Cataloging-in-Publication Data is available online at http://catalog.loc.gov
LC record available at http://lccn.loc.gov/2019015904

Typeface for the Latin, Greek, and Cyrillic scripts: "Brill". See and download: brill.com/brill-typeface.

ISSN 1568-6183
ISBN 978-90-04-40149-5 (hardback)
ISBN 978-90-04-40444-1 (e-book)

This book is printed on acid-free paper and produced in a sustainable manner.

Contents

INTRODUCTION

Navigating the Ocean of Tibetan Medical Literature

William A. McGrath

Approximately ten years ago, a team of scholars published an outline of desiderata in the field of Tibetan medicine. Although the European-language study of Tibetan medicine had already persisted for decades (or even centuries if we consider the pioneering work of Alexander Csoma de Kőrös [1784–1842]),[1] as late as 1988 R. E. Emmerick commented that the *Four Tantras* (*rgyud bzhi*), the seminal work of the Tibetan medical tradition, "was for a long time difficult of access but it is now readily available."[2] Here Emmerick refers to the modern-book edition of the *Four Tantras* that was published in Lhasa in 1982 based on the Degé xylographic edition,[3] as well as two facsimile editions that had been published in Leh in 1975 and 1978.[4] Indeed, without access to such editions, what work could have been done?

Around the same time that new editions of the *Four Tantras* were being published, several encyclopedic volumes introduced the central tenets, instructions, and histories of the Tibetan medical tradition to readers of European languages for the first time. A complete list of such works would be far too long to delineate here, but it would certainly have to include Rechung Rinpoche's *Tibetan Medicine* (1973), Manfred Taube's *Beiträge zur Geschichte der medizinischen Literatur Tibets* (1981), and Fernand Meyer's *Gso-ba rig-pa: Le système médical* (1982), among others. Explanations and translations of the *Four Tantras* and its associated medical *thangka*s have continued to be published down to the present, culminating in relatively comprehensive overviews

1 Alexander Csoma de Kőrös, "Analysis of a Tibetan Medical Work," *Journal of the Asiatic Society* 37 (1835): 1–20.

2 Ronald E. Emmerick, "Tibetan *nor-ra-re*," *Bulletin of the School of Oriental and African Studies* 51, no. 3 (1988): 537.

3 Blo bzang tshe ring, ed. *Bdud rtsi snying po yan lag brgyad pa gsang ba man ngag gi rgyud* (Lhasa: Bod ljongs mi dmangs dpe skrun khang, 1982).

4 *Rgyud bźi: A Reproduction of a Set of Prints from the 18th Century Zuṅ-cu Ze Blocks from the Collections of Raghu Vira*, Smanrtsis Shesrig Spendzod Series, vol. 68 (Leh: S. W. Tashigangpa, 1975); and *Rgyud Bźi: A Reproduction of a Set of Prints from the 1988 Lha-sa Lcags-po-ri Blocks*, Smanrtsis Shesrig Spendzod Series, vol. 87 (Leh: T. S. Tashigangpa, 1978).

of orthodox Tibetan medicine in several European languages,[5] as well as the modern Tibetan, Chinese, Japanese, and Mongolian languages, among others. It is perhaps this abundance, or even excess, of introductory and orthodox materials that caused the aforementioned team of scholars to lament the "lack of detailed analytical (rather than encyclopaedic) knowledge" and the need to "reveal the composite, variegated and dynamic nature of Tibetan medical traditions."[6] The present volume, *Knowledge and Context in Tibetan Medicine*, seeks to answer this call.

Since the early 2000s, a veritable deluge of Tibetan medical resources has been published for the first time. With collections like the Arura Group's "Ancient Literature of Tibetan Medicine Series" (*bod kyi gso ba rig pa'i gna' dpe phyogs bsgrigs dpe tshogs*), currently boasting well over one hundred volumes, and the nearly one thousand unique medical and astrological manuscripts that are held at the Potala Palace,[7] the academic study of Tibetan medicine must now widen its focus to a textual corpus that is much larger than the *Four Tantras* and its exegetical literature. Grappling with such an abundance of literature may feel overwhelming, but we are not the only scholars to have felt this way.

In an apocryphal story the ancestor of the Drangti clan, Gyelnyé Kharbu (*brang ti rgyal mnyes mkhar bu*), is said to have been frustrated by the abundance of medical texts and commentaries that were available during the Tibetan imperial period (ca. 600–850). How could he possibly learn and practice such an excess of instructions, especially without an experienced teacher? Seeing no other alternative, he is said to have supplicated the Tibetan emperor, Jé Tri Dhé Aktsom (*rje khri dhe ag tsom*), also known as Tri Detsuktsen (*khri lde gtsug brtsan*, ca. 704–754): "My Lord, these instructions that we have are profound, but they still require that one seek out a master. Do you have any treasure texts or instructions that do not require a teacher?"[8] After years of effort and service to the emperor, Gyelnyé Kharbu was finally awarded with the

5 For what is perhaps the best single overview of this material, see Yuri Parfionovitch, Fernand Meyer, and Gyurme Dorje, eds., *Tibetan Medical Paintings: Illustrations to the Blue Beryl Treatise of Sangye Gyamtso (1653–1705)* (New York, NY: Harry N. Abrams, 1992).

6 Henk Blezer et al., "Brief Outlook: Desiderata in the Study of the History of Tibetan Medicine," in *Soundings in Tibetan Medicine: Anthropological and Historical Perspectives*, ed. Mona Schrempf (Leiden: Brill, 2007), 428–29.

7 Bod ljongs bod lugs gso rig slob grwa chen mo, ed., *Krung go'i bod lugs gso rig rtsa che'i dpe rnying kun btus: Pho brang po ta la'i gsung rab gter mdzod las btus* (Lhasa: Bod ljongs mi dmangs dpe skrun khang, 2014), 30 vols.

8 *Byang khog dmar byang gsal ba'i sgron me*, Bod kyi gso ba rig pa'i gna' dpe phyogs bsgrigs dpe tshogs, vol. 101 (Beijing: Mi rigs dpe skrun khang, 2014), 205: *des kyang rgyal mnyes kho thag ma chod nas/ rje lags 'di rnams pas kyang zab pa cig bdog ste mchi bas/ 'di rnams la slob dpon*

Lamp That Illuminates the Red Register (*byang khog dmar byang gsal ba'i sgron me*), a work that is both "small in size and great in reasoning" (*bungs su chung la tshigs su che ba*), which "does not require a teacher" (*bla ma mi dgos pa*). Legend holds that this practical manual was transmitted among the Drangti family for half a millennium, until it was redacted at the end of the thirteenth century, and finally published by Arura for the first time in 2014.

In addition to the uncanny familiarity of Gyelnyé Kharbu's frustrations, I also relate this story because it highlights a central tension within medical traditions, Tibetan and otherwise—a tension between complexity and practicality, diversity and centralization, the subaltern and the orthodox. The story of Gyelnyé Kharbu, probably composed in the thirteenth century and projected back to the time of the Tibetan empire, reflects a period of great intercultural exchange. The medical traditions of South, East, and Central Asia were all coming into communication under the aegis of the Yuan dynasty (ca. 1250–1350), and the available methods for the diagnosis and treatment of disease had reached an unprecedented level of diversity and complexity. Was a patient's fever caused by a humoral imbalance or a thermal imbalance? By karmic transgression or spirit possession? Should it be treated by medicinal compounds, external therapies, or ritual interventions? A similar degree of pluralism also characterizes the etiological and therapeutic choices of the present day, reminiscent of the unresolved controversies fossilized in the medical traditions that have been transmitted over the past millennium.

If one goal of this study is to reconcile the dichotomies of unity and diversity, another is to also explore a related dichotomy of disciplinary approaches: philology and ethnography. This divide has helped to organize the academic study of Tibetan medicine down to the present—allowing one group to discuss textual developments and prescriptive instructions, and the other to describe practical methods and lived realities. This divide between history and anthropology even served to bifurcate the panels on Tibetan medicine at the Fourteenth Seminar of the International Association for Tibetan Studies in Bergen (2016), from which the current volume derives.[9] Despite the potential advantages of such a divide, the reification of disciplinary boundaries also sometimes entails unanticipated risks, emphasizing approach at the expense

---

'tshal bar gda' ba/ gter ma lags par gda' ba dang / bla ma mi dgos pa'i man ngag cig bdog ste mchi bas/ de thugs la rtags par zhu byas pas/.

9 The panels focused on Tibetan medicine at IATS 14 were divided into two, Panel 15: "Knowledge and Context in the History of Tibetan Medicine," convened by Olaf Czaja and myself; and Panel 25: "Sowa Rigpa (Tibetan Medicine): Contemporary and Anthropological Studies," convened by Geoffrey Samuel and Mingji Cuomu. Despite this formal separation, most members of each panel attended the presentations of the other.

of context, distinction at the expense of continuity. Indeed, ethnography without philology or archeology is the description of a lived reality that is bereft of history, and philology without ethnography is an isolated truth without obvious relevance for the present day.[10] Challenging the entrenched boundaries of history and anthropology, the present volume focuses upon context—historical and contemporary—in order to explore the vicissitudes of semantics and the complex relationship between medicine and religion in Tibet. By combining both historical and anthropological perspectives, we seek to fuse the horizon of each discipline, allowing meaning and healing to shift across temporal, spatial, and social contexts.

Each part of this volume has been divided into five chapters. Part One, "The Vicissitudes of Meaning in Context," is concerned with both semantic and historical meaning in the Tibetan medical tradition. It begins with Henk W. A. Blezer's chapter on "brown phlegm" in early Tibetan medical sources, focusing on potential intersections with the Greco-Arab notions of black bile and melancholia. In the following chapter, Yang Ga attempts not to define a word, but a person. "Who was Yutok the Elder?" he asks, "And how do we know?" Although he refrains from definitively answering this question, he incontrovertibly challenges naïve interpretations of Yutok's biography. In Chapter Three, Tony Chui analyzes "secret medicine" in the writings of Desi Sanggyé Gyatso (1653–1705), particularly in relation to the healing of life-wind illnesses. By exploring the processes of encryption in secret medicine, Chui effectively brings Tibetan medical literature into the theoretical debates of Tantric studies. Katharina Sabernig also takes up several cryptic terms depicted on the seventeenth-century Tibetan medical paintings, and examines their transformations in later illustrations as they came into contact with biomedical conceptions and anatomical terminology. Finally, Part One concludes with Tawni Tidwell's ambitious exploration of cancer and its correlates in the Tibetan language. Like Sabernig, Tidwell combines philological and biomedical approaches to understanding medical realities, illuminating the purview of each perspective in the process.

Part Two, "Medicine and Religion in Context," takes up yet another disciplinary divide, exploring the relationship between medical and religious healing in Tibet. In Chapter Six, Tsering Samdrup examines the relationship between medical and ritual modes of healing in an early wartime medical manual, the *Nine-fold Magical Cord* (twelfth-century?). In the next chapter Carmen Simioli

10 For further reflections on the future of philology, see the work of Sheldon Pollock, such as his "Philology in Three Dimensions," *Postmedieval: A Journal of Medieval Cultural Studies* 5, no. 4 (2014): 398–413.

similarly juxtaposes empirical and ritual approaches to contagious disease in the medical treasure text cycle, the *Vase of the Amṛta of Immortality*. Like many of the works examined in Part Two, Simioli describes an uneasy compromise between humoral and demonic understandings of disease. My own work follows that of Simioli, examining the historical integration of *prasenā* divination and channel examination in the *Four Tantras* and the Drangti lineage of Tibetan medicine. In Chapter Nine, Susannah Deane relates two tales of spirit possession that she encountered while doing fieldwork in Darjeeling, reconsidering the relationship between textual knowledge and practical application in medically and religiously pluralistic communities. In the final chapter of Part Two, Barbara Gerke represents the transformation of the Tibetan medical tradition in the People's Republic of China through the example of a single precious pill: Jikmé's Old Turquoise-70. Shedding the contexts of demonic etiology, ritual empowerment, and religious integration explored in the other chapters of Part Two, Gerke explores the processes of rebranding Tibetan precious pills for cross-cultural consumption.

Despite differences in temporal context, Chapter One begins and Chapter Ten concludes with the very same subject: the transformation of medical concepts across traditions. As the present age of medical pluralism continues, we need not look further than the historical intersections of diverse medical traditions to find precedents and pathways for present exchanges. Indeed, such is the dual-task of the medical historian, in the words of the Swiss historian of medicine, Henry E. Sigerist (1891–1957): to both "light up the darkness of the past" and "[render] it fruitful for a better future."

> The history of medicine has entered upon a decisive phase. Summoned to cooperation by the living healing art, it will have to show whether it is able to follow this summons, whether it is able to participate in the solution of the great problems which today occupy the physicians' world. But the history of medicine has a Janus-head. One face looks to the future with the eyes of the physician, and the other one is turned backward. With the eyes of the historian it tries to light up the darkness of the past. Here too the history of medicine will have to prove itself. Here too it will have to show whether the rebirth of spirit which today we experience in all spheres has passed it by, whether in purely positivistic fashion it wishes to add facts to facts, or whether it is capable of interpreting the past, of enlivening it, and of rendering it fruitful for a better future.[11]

11 Henry E. Sigerist, *Kyklos: Jahrbuch des Instituts für Geschichte der Medizin an der Universität Leipzig* (Leipzig: Georg Thieme, 1932), vol. 1, 5; cited and translated in Owsei

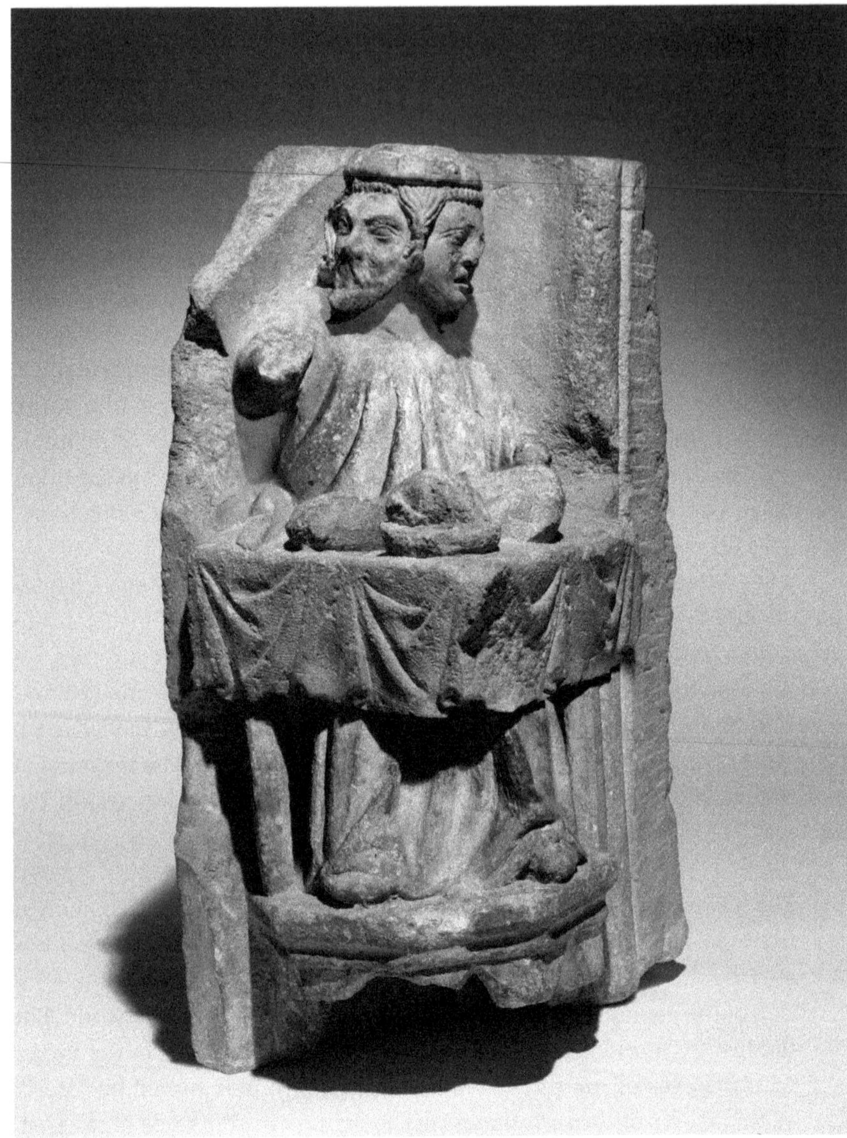

FIGURE 0.1 The double face of Janus (limestone; Burgundy, France; 1250–1275)
USED WITH PERMISSION FROM THE PHILADELPHIA MUSEUM OF ART. PURCHASED WITH MUSEUM FUNDS FROM THE GEORGE GREY BARNARD COLLECTION, 1945 (1945-25-74).

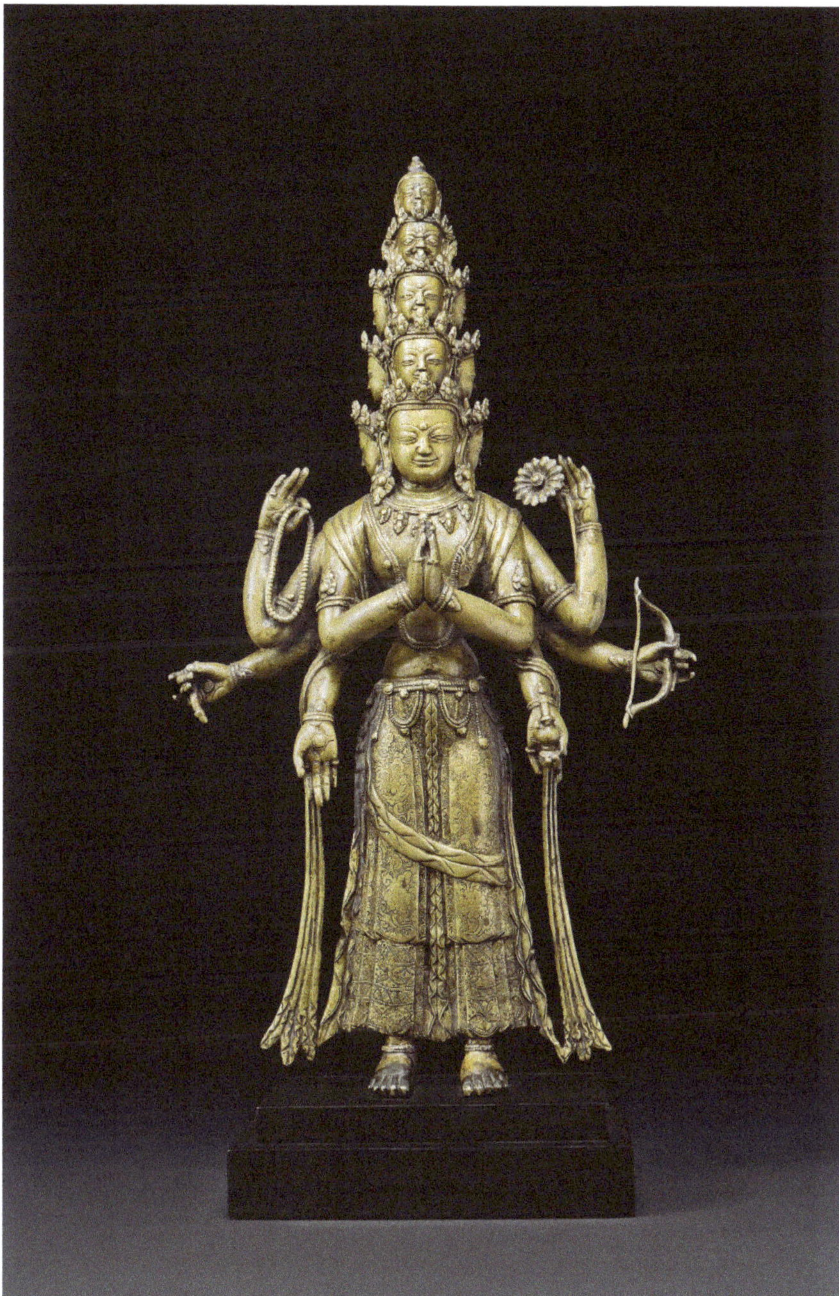

FIGURE 0.2 Avalokiteśvara with eleven faces and eight hands (metal; Tibet; 16th c.)
USED WITH PERMISSION FROM W. ARADER. ARADER COLLECTION (HIMALAYAN ART RESOURCES #66738).

If the task for the biomedical historian is Janus-faced—to light up the singular past for the unified future—then the historian of Asian medicines surely needs all eleven faces of Avalokiteśvara. Even the seemingly unified tradition of Sowa Rigpa and the *Four Tantras* must be understood not only in the contexts of past and future times, but also those of diverse spaces—from Central Tibet to Ngari, Amdo, and Kham, as well as the rest of the PRC, Bhutan, Mongolia, Nepal, India, Europe, the Americas, and beyond—not to mention the countless lineages and schools of Tibetan medicine that are just beginning to be understood. There is still much work that needs to be done.

Despite the overwhelming number of texts and instructions that are now known in the Tibetan medical tradition, reminiscent of the textual diversity lamented by Drangti Gyelnyé Kharbu centuries ago, let us seek to do more than just "add facts to facts." Inspired by Sigerist, let us seek to "participate in the solution of the great problems which today occupy the physicians' world," recognizing that the problems of health and disease, of life and death, will undoubtedly involve a multifaceted (or multifaced!) solution. As indicated one decade ago in the precursor to this volume, it is with the "composite, variegated and dynamic nature of Tibetan medical traditions"—the many contexts of Tibetan medicine—that we may light up the past. By reveling in complexity, looking with many faces, reaching with many hands, and seeing with many eyes, we might continue to render diverse pasts fruitful for better futures.

Bibliography

A ru ra, ed. *Byang khog dmar byang gsal ba'i sgron me*. Bod kyi gso ba rig pa'i gna' dpe phyogs bsgrigs dpe tshogs, vol. 101. Beijing: Mi rigs dpe skrun khang, 2014.

Blezer, Henk, et al. "Brief Outlook: Desiderata in the Study of the History of Tibetan Medicine." In *Soundings in Tibetan Medicine: Anthropological and Historical Perspectives. PIATS 2003: Proceedings of the Tenth Seminar of the International Association for Tibetan Studies, Oxford, 2003*, edited by Mona Schrempf, 427–38. Leiden: Brill, 2007.

Blo bzang tshe ring, ed. *Bdud rtsi snying po yan lag brgyad pa gsang ba man ngag gi rgyud*. Lhasa: Bod ljongs mi dmangs dpe skrun khang, 1982.

Bod ljongs bod lugs gso rig slob grwa chen mo, ed. *Krung go'i bod lugs gso rig rtsa che'i dpe rnying kun btus: Pho brang po ta la'i gsung rab gter mdzod las btus* [Zhongguo yiyao yingyin guji zhenben 中国藏医药影印古籍珍本; China's Traditional Tibetan

Temkin, *The Double Face of Janus and Other Essays in the History of Medicine* (Baltimore, MD: The Johns Hopkins University Press, 1977), 9.

Medical Texts: A Treasury of Scriptures from the Potala Palace]. Lhasa: Bod ljongs mi dmangs dpe skrun khang, 2014.

Csoma de Kőrös, Alexander. "Analysis of a Tibetan Medical Work." *Journal of the Asiatic Society* 37 (1835): 1–20.

Emmerick, Ronald E. "Tibetan *nor-ra-re*." *Bulletin of the School of Oriental and African Studies* 51, no. 3 (1988): 537–39.

Parfionovitch, Yuri, Fernand Meyer, and Gyurme Dorje, eds. *Tibetan Medical Paintings: Illustrations to the Blue Beryl Treatise of Sangye Gyamtso (1653–1705)*. New York, NY: Harry N. Abrams, 1992.

Pollock, Sheldon. "Philology in Three Dimensions." *Postmedieval: A Journal of Medieval Cultural Studies* 5, no. 4 (2014): 398–413.

Rgyud bźi: A Reproduction of a Set of Prints from the 18th Century Zuṅ-cu Ze Blocks from the Collections of Raghu Vira. Smanrtsis Shesrig Spendzod Series, vol. 68. Leh: S. W. Tashigangpa, 1975.

Rgyud Bźi: A Reproduction of a Set of Prints from the 1988 Lha-sa Lcags-po-ri Blocks. Smanrtsis Shesrig Spendzod Series, vol. 87. Leh: T. S. Tashigangpa, 1978.

Sigerist, Henry E. *Kyklos: Jahrbuch des Instituts für Geschichte der Medizin an der Universität Leipzig*. Leipzig: Georg Thieme, 1932.

Temkin, Owsei. *The Double Face of Janus and Other Essays in the History of Medicine*. Baltimore, MD: The Johns Hopkins University Press, 1977.

A Note on Transcription, Transliteration, and Bibliography

For convenience and general legibility, this volume uses a system of phonetic transcription that was developed by David Germano and Nicholas Tournadre, the Tibetan and Himalayan Library's Simplified Phonetic Transcription of Standard Tibetan.[12] The first appearance of a transcribed personal or place name will also include THL Extended Wylie Transliteration in parentheses,[13] which is based on the Wylie transliteration system.[14] Although it is common practice to capitalize the first letter of Tibetan proper nouns in transliteration, in the present volume transliterated Tibetan is not capitalized in order to avoid redundancy and confusion with diacritic letters, which are usually indicated with capital letters in Tibetan transliteration. Tibetan-language text titles and special terms have also been translated into English whenever possible, followed by transliteration in parentheses after the first use. In a volume such as this one there will inevitably be some terms that resist translation, and these terms have been rendered in phonetic transcription, along with English-language explanations, at the discretion of the authors. This volume also follows the conventions of the *Chicago Manual of Style* (the "Notes and Bibliography System"), wherein a full bibliographic record is included in a footnote at the site of the first citation, followed by an abbreviated record for each subsequent citation and a full bibliography at the end of each chapter. These conventions were carefully chosen by the editor in order to ensure that both specialists and non-specialists are able to read and understand this volume, while also retaining and concisely conveying all salient information.

12 David Germano and Nicolas Tournadre, "THL Simplified Phonetic Transcription of Standard Tibetan," *Tibetan and Himalayan Library*, 2003. <http://www.thlib.org/reference/transliteration/#!essay=/thl/phonetics/>.

13 David Germano et al., "THL Extended Wylie Transliteration Scheme," *Tibetan and Himalayan Library*, 2004. <http://www.thlib.org/reference/transliteration/#!essay=/thl/ewts>.

14 Turrell V. Wylie, "A Standard System of Tibetan Transcription," *Harvard Journal of Asiatic Studies* 22 (1959): 261–67.

Figures

Contributors

Henk Blezer

Henk Blezer has been involved in academic research and publication on (Indian and Tibetan) Buddhism and Bön since the early nineties. He teaches Buddhist Studies at Leiden University and presently also lectures on Asian and Religious Studies (in the International Studies program). He also is senior lecturer Buddhist Studies at the Vrije Universiteit Amsterdam.

Tony Chui

Tony Chui is a neurobiologist and a Tibetologist. His multidisciplinary training enables him to conduct research at the fertile edge of pre-industrial and contemporary healing worldviews. Tony obtained his BSc in Human Biology at the University of Toronto, following which he received his MPhil in Neurobiology from the Faculty of Medicine and a Master of Buddhist Studies from the Centre of Buddhist Studies at the University of Hong Kong. Pursuing his research into Tibetan modes of healing "life-wind" illness, he received his PhD from the same University. His current research interests focus on the impact of Tibetan Buddhist ideas on the conceptualization and management of illness.

Susannah Deane

Susannah Deane is a British Academy Postdoctoral Research Fellow in the Centre for Buddhist Studies at the University of Bristol. She completed her PhD at Cardiff University in 2015, on the topic of Tibetan approaches to mental health, illness, and healing within a Tibetan exile community in Darjeeling. Susannah's current research project at the University of Bristol focuses on Tibetan medical and religious understandings of "madness."

Barbara Gerke

Barbara Gerke (M.Sc. Medical Anthropology and D.Phil. Social Anthropology, University of Oxford) completed a DFG (German Research Foundation) principal investigator project on Tibetan mercury practices at Humboldt University of Berlin (2011–2015) and an FWF (Austrian Science Fund) Lise-Meitner senior research fellowship (2015–2018) at the University of Vienna, researching biographies of Tibetan precious pills. She currently leads a three-year FWF-funded project at the University of Vienna (2018–2021) on Tibetan ritual and medical understandings of potency. She is the author of *Long Lives and Untimely Deaths: Life-Span Concepts and Longevity Practices among Tibetans in the Darjeeling Hills, India* (Brill, 2012) and *Taming the Poisonous: Mercury, Toxicity and Safety in Tibetan Medical Practice* (Heidelberg University Publishing, forthcoming).

William A. McGrath

William A. McGrath is a Visiting Assistant Professor of Religious Studies at Manhattan College, where he teaches courses on Asian religions. His research agenda primarily concerns the historical intersections of religious and medical traditions in Tibet and China.

Katharina Sabernig

Katharina Sabernig is a medical doctor and shiatsu practitioner in Vienna, who has studied ethnomedicine and completed her academic education with a doctorate in social and cultural anthropology. She is a lecturer in different fields of Tibetan Medicine, ethnomedicine, and medical terminology at several Universities of Vienna. Beyond her research on the medical murals at Labrang Monastery in Northeastern Tibet (modern Gansu province) her interests focus on medical illustrations, history, terminology, and development of contents in Tibetan medicine, particularly in the field of anatomy and pharmacology.

Personal website: www.katharinasabernig.at Tibetan medical terms website: https://crossasia.org/en/service/crossasia-lab/tibetische-medizin-termini/.

Carmen Simioli

Carmen Simioli is adjunct professor of classical Tibetan at Ca' Foscari, University of Venice. She studied Tibetan language and culture at "L'Orientale" University of Naples, where she completed her PhD in Indological and Tibetological studies in 2015. Her doctoral dissertation focused on the history and literature of Tibetan mercurial alchemy and iatrochemistry. Some results have been published in "Annali dell'Orientale Università di Napoli" (AION), *Asian Medicine: Journal of the International Association for the Study of Traditional Asian Medicine* (ASME) and *Revue d'Etudes Tibétaines* (RET). Her main research interests revolve around the history of medieval and early modern Tibetan medicine, alchemy and ritual magic. She is currently working on a series of Tibetan medico-magical texts that deal with the preparation and consecration of protective amulets for averting diseases-carrier demons. She has been served as interpreter of Tibetan doctors since 2011 and her current studies are closely related to her collaboration with Tibetan physicians.

Tawni Tidwell

Tawni Tidwell is a Tibetan medical doctor and biocultural anthropologist whose research and clinical work focuses on cancer, metabolic, and neurologic disorders as well as the pharmacologic innovations in Tibetan medicine to treat such disorders. She completed her PhD at Emory University in 2017, focusing her doctoral research on the sensory entrainment processes for diagnostics in Tibetan medical education and training.

Tsering Samdrup

Tsering Samdrup is a PhD student at SOAS, University of London. He has a Bachelor of Arts degree from Duke University and a Master of Philosophy degree from the University of Oslo, Norway. His current research focuses on the use of pragmatics in the Tibetan language, as well as the language and culture of Tibet in general and the Amdo region in particular. He also translates both scholarly and non-scholarly works from English into Tibetan and vice versa.

Yang Ga

Yang Ga is a professor and dean of the Tibet University of Tibetan Medicine in Lhasa. In his research he primarily focuses on the early history and instructions of the Tibetan medical tradition.

PART 1

The Vicissitudes of Meaning in Context

CHAPTER 1

A New Sense of (Dark) Humor in Tibet: Brown Phlegm and Black Bile

Henk Blezer

1 Introductory Notes

This is a modest contribution to ongoing investigation of so-called "brown phlegm" (disorders) in Tibet (*bad kan smug po*). The field of engagement and its time depth both are so vast that this cannot but be a provisional engagement. The main hypothesis of this long-term project is that the Tibetan medical category of "brown phlegm," which looks to be a Tibetan innovation, may ultimately be of Greco-Arab ("black bile") origin. This hypothesis was first introduced at the Seventh International Congress on Traditional Asian Medicine (ICTAM VII),[1] as a tangential concern, and was published as such, with the promise to revisit it.[2]

The research logic was laid out at the Ninth International Convention of Asia Scholars (ICAS 9; esp. the Tibetan side of the equation),[3] while I proceeded to discuss a preliminary survey of the Greco-Arab side at the Fourteenth Seminar of the International Association for Tibetan Studies (IATS XIV).[4] The precise historical contact between these medical epistemes has remained elusive, so far. For the most recent ICTAM IX,[5] I therefore looked into possible points of contact between these Greco-Arab and Indo-Tibetan medical epistemes and found an imaginary Byzantine friend and intermediary, Basil. This article, while mostly based on work for the IATS XIV, is a résumé of my explorations so far, with a glance toward the future. There are three main aspects to this endeavor.

---

1 Thimphu, Bhutan, September 2009.

2 See Henk W. A. Blezer, "'Light' on the Human Body: The Coarse Physical Body and its Functions in the Aural Transmission from Zhang zhung on the Six Lamps," *Revue d'Etudes Tibétaines* 23 (2012): 117–68.

3 Adelaide, Australia, July 2015.

4 Bergen, Norway, June 2016.

5 Kiel, Germany, August 2017.

 | DOI:10.1163/9789004404441_002

1.1 *We Need to Take a Closer Look at the History of Ideas of "Brown Phlegm" in Tibet*

Discussion of "brown phlegm" is already extant in early (and even the earliest) grand medical syntheses in Tibet and in some of the former's precursors and satellites as well: e.g., in the *Moon King* (*zla ba'i rgyal po*), the *Jewel Rosary* (*nor bu'i 'phreng ba*), the *Sons' Benefit* (*bu don ma*), the *Small Tantra* (*rgyud chung*), the *Brown Phlegm Résumé of a Thousand* [*Sections*] (*bad kan smug po stong thun*), and of course in the fourfold treatises—the *Fourfold Collection* (*'bum bzhi*) and the *Fourfold Tantra* (*rgyud bzhi*)—the descriptions in the former, mostly earlier sources, often are very close to latter two.

In some later sources, which sit (probably only somewhat later) in the beginning of the second millennium, "brown phlegm" is systematically set apart and explicitly discussed as a "combined disease" (*'dus pa'i nad*); most conspicuously in the fourfold treatises but also in the closely related *Jewel Rosary*. In other sources "brown phlegm" is simply included in the "phlegm" chapter, together with various other types of "phlegm." These may represent stages in its reception history.

1.2 *Locating Greco-Arab Sources*

Greco-Arab sources may have impacted Tibetan epistemes (in)directly. Humoral systems in the area are diverse and unstable: we look for data that we find in Tibet, the types of medical conditions and humoral systems that reception histories may suggest.

1.3 *A Possible Point of Contact*

I should like to consider a common Tibetan narrative on dissemination of Greco-Arab medical lore, which was ultimately attributed to Galen himself: the "Biji" (*bi ji*, *bi ci*, or *be ci*) lineage that starts from a figure called Tsan pa shi la ha (eighth c. CE). While most parse his name in the most plausible Tibetan way as Tsanpa Shilaha, Martin proposes a more convincing caesura: Tsan Pashilaha, deriving from the Byzantine name, Basilius, or Bāsil of Tsan.[6]

According to surviving narratives, Tsan Pashilaha was a doctor of "Turkic" descent (i.e., hailing from "Phrom") who taught and eventually also settled down in Lhasa. His system is said to go back to the famous Galenos or Galen of Pergamum (130–200 CE).[7] Alas, the most significant trace to date of this so-

---

6 Dan P. Martin, "Greek and Islamic Medicines' Historical Contact with Tibet," in *Islam and Tibet: Interactions along the Musk Routes*, ed. Anna Akasoy et al. (Farnham, VT: Ashgate, 2011), 117–43.

7 In some Tibetan sources there is even mention of someone (also) bearing the name Galenos (complete with a correct Tibetan transliteration of the Greek spelling), who presumably was in Tibet a little earlier, in the 7th c. CE, but Beckwith has exposed this as a myth (Christopher

called Biji lineage, *Biji's Yellow-covered Book* (*bi ji'i po ti kha ser*), does not take us very far back in time, due to its seemingly late redaction.

2 Working Hypotheses on Brown Phlegm

- The main hypothesis here is that Greco-Arab and Indian Ayurvedic humoral systems come together in novel Tibetan articulations of "brown phlegm" (*bad kan smug po*) disorders: the category of "brown phlegm" disorders may have been incorporated into Tibetan medical knowledge, directly or indirectly, with knowledge of Greco-Arab "black bile" disorders, in particular those of the *melancholia hypochondriaca* type.[8]
- "Brown phlegm" thus is a good example for Tibetan medicine at the crossroads, particularly in the late first, early second millennium CE: Indian Ayurvedic, Greco-Arab, and East Asian "Chinese" epistemes, and most likely also hybrid cultures, meet in and around Tibet.
- The "brown phlegm" disorder in Tibetan medicine does not appear to be known in antecedent Indian Ayurvedic medicine, or any other system, as far as I can trace.
- The possibility of derivation or mediation through "eccentric" Indic medical traditions outside of what is recorded and reflected in the major extant treatises from before the end of the first millennium has to await viable clues to warrant investment of time.
- More in particular, the possibility of mediation through Unani traditions of medicine, roughly at the turn of the first millennium CE, merits looking into as an intermediary, but due to a lack of access to closely contemporary data, this alternative—or better, additional—hypothesis will not be argued here. As was argued for the previous point, until viable clues emerge, I should leave this for follow-up research.
- At the turn of the first millennium, mainstream Tibetan medical traditions apparently provided a "niche market" for expertise on specific types of digestive disorders of the *melancholia hypochondriaca* type, but, demonstrably, there was no explanatory need in Tibet for its attendant mental

I. Beckwith, "The Introduction of Greek Medicine into Tibet in the 7th and 8th Century," *Journal of the American Oriental Society* 99 [1979]: 297–313).

8 These theses and the meanderings of their heuristics in Bon *rDzogs chen* cosmology have been introduced in previous publication (Blezer, "'Light' on the Human Body") and those introductory remarks shall not be resumed here.

symptoms, which traditionally indeed are covered in Ayurvedic pneumatic (*rlung*) disorders, concepts concerning demonic possession, and the like.[9]

On the Tibetan side of the equation we shall survey major Tibetan medical syntheses:
- The *Fourfold Collection* (*'bum bzhi*)
- The *Fourfold Tantra* (*rgyud bzhi*)
- The *Moon King* (*zla ba'i rgyal po*)

We shall also survey closely related satellites, some of which may preserve earlier stages or redactions:
- *Jewel Rosary* (*nor bu'i 'phreng ba*)
- *Sons' Benefit* (*bu don ma*)
- *Small Tantra* (*rgyud chung*)
- *Brown Phlegm Résumé of a Thousand* [*Sections*] (*bad kan smug po stong thun*)[10]

On the other side of the "divide" (it is probably more like a continuum than a divide proper), we shall survey some major time slices in "Greco-Arab" medical thought:[11]
- Hippocrates of Kos (4th–5th c. BCE)
- Diocles of Carystus (4th c. BCE)
- Rufus of Ephesus (approx. 1st c. CE)
- Galen of Pergamum (130–200 CE)
- Ibn Sīnā, Avicenna (980–1037 CE)

3 What is the "Brown Phlegm" (*bad kan smug po*) Disorder?

Even though "brown phlegm" disorders seem to be fairly common in Tibetan medical practice,[12] there is not yet much to go by in terms of dictionary defini-

9 See, e.g., the *Instructional Tantra* (*man ngag rgyud*) of the *Fourfold Tantra*, esp. chapters 77–79.

10 Many thanks to Bill McGrath for bringing this interesting early source to my attention.

11 While I am keenly aware that more time slices (and more sources) could have been adduced, and that one should also take into account hybrid Indic and Central Asian traditions, my main concern for this paper is to triangulate, roughly, possible points of contact. Covering the great variety and intellectual history of humoral systems, or the initial lack of system in them, in the Greco-Arab world is not one of my objectives.

12 See, e.g., Audrey Prost, "*Sa cha 'Di ma 'Phrod na* ... Displacement and Traditional Tibetan Medicine among Refugees in India," in *Soundings in Tibetan Medicine: Anthropological and Historical Perspectives. PIATS 2003, Tibetan Studies: Proceedings of the International*

tions. Medical and medicinal plant dictionaries for obvious reasons tend to follow or paraphrase the *Fourfold Tantra*,[13] which will be discussed in more detail below. There is a very useful summary of contemporary perceptions of the symptoms of "brown phlegm" disorders in an entry in the cited *Tibetan-English Dictionary of Tibetan Medicine and Astrology*, when discussing a medicinal cure for "brown phlegm" disorders by "The Conqueror of Brown Phlegm" (*smug po g.yul rgyal*):[14]

> A compound which cures heart burn, sour watery vomitus, emesis of blood and bile, pain between 12th vertebra and [the] stomach[-]liver region, descending of blood-*mkhris pa* disorders into [the] stomach, upper backache, expansion, hidden[?] and disturbance of brown phlegm (*bad kan smug po*).[15]

It is interesting to note here that for the intended comparison contemporary elaborations tend to be more informative and helpful with a view on understanding the actual symptoms than the classical Tibetan medical references, which nonetheless are repeated most often.

The Great Tibetan-Chinese Dictionary (*bod rgya tshig mdzod chen mo*) has some useful information, but has its most informative entry not at the "brown phlegm" lemma proper (which discusses the various colours of body fluids),[16] but at the entry for "brown [phlegm] that imposes itself" (*smug po 'gyings pa*): "when brown phlegm imposes itself on the stomach, throwing up and purging from below [evacuating] are not possible: being full and swollen, the stomach hurts."[17]

Association for Tibetan Studies, Oxford 2003, edited by Mona Schrempf (Leiden: Brill, 2007), 45–64; see particularly the tables on pp. 47ff, esp. the entry on *mchin nad* (liver problem) on p. 48, which indicates a fairly common incidence.

13 See, for example, Tsering Trakchoe Drungtso and Tsering Dolma Drungtso, *Bod lugs sman rtsis kyi tshig mdzod bod dbyin shar sbyar* (Dharamsala: Drungtso Publications 2005), 283; and Christa Kletter and Monika Kriechbaum, *Tibetan Medicinal Plants* (Boca Raton, FL: CRC Press/Medpharm, 2001), 340.2ff.

14 Note that the Tibetan of the entry has *g.yus*.

15 Drungtso and Drungtso, *Bod lugs sman rtsis kyi tshig mdzod bod dbyin shar sbyar*, 351.2.

16 Zhang Yisun, *Bod rgya tshig mdzod chen mo* (Beijing: Mi rigs dpe skrun khang, 1996 [repr. 1993]), 1811.2.

17 Zhang, *Bod rgya tshig mdzod chen mo*, 2172.1: *bad kan smug po pho bar 'gyings te yar skyug pa dang / mar bshal ba byed mi thub pa pho ba khengs shing hrem mer na zhig.* John Valby captures the gist of common symptoms of this digestive disorder: "convulsions, choler<a>ic cramps"; Ives Waldo in his rendering captures some of the progressive symptoms: "unable to purge below or vomit"; Waldo's entry is based on the *Bod rgya tshig mdzod chen mo*, quoted above (both entries are from the THL online version at http://dictionary.thlib.org).

3.1 *The* Fourfold Tantra *on Brown Phlegm*

The *Fourfold Tantra*, arguably, is the most influential Tibetan medical treatise. It is called Fourfold "Tantra" (or better: "Treatise") for obvious reasons: it is composed of four main parts:

1. The *Root Tantra* (*rtsa rgyud*);
2. The *Explanatory Tantra* (*bshad rgyud*);
3. The *Instructional Tantra* (*man ngag rgyud*); and
4. The *Subsequent* or *Final Tantra* (*phyi ma'i rgyud*).[18]

We are mostly concerned here with the clinical manual, the *Instructional Tantra*, for this is where we find the main discussion of brown phlegm.

3.1.1 Authorship and Origins of the *Fourfold Tantra* and Working Hypotheses

There are widely diverging opinions on the authorship and (date of) origin of the *Fourfold Tantra*. The formative period of its main ideas may indeed lie in the twelfth or, perhaps, the eleventh century CE, typically close to extant "memory traces" that we find narrativized into traditional histories. Drapa Ngönshé (*grwa pa mngon shes*; 11th c. CE) is said to have unearthed the texts from a Samyé (*bsam yas*) pillar and then passed them on to Üpa Dardrak (*dbus pa dar grags*; 11th c. CE?) and Tötön Könchok Kyap (*stod ston dkon mchog skyabs*; 12th c. CE). Finally, it is said to have reached Yutok Yönten Gönpo (*g.yu thog yon tan mgon po*; 12th c. CE).

Karmay (1989) developed an elegant and plausible alternative thesis, in which Bönpos play a significant role, to start with the treasure revealer (*gter ston*) Khutsa Dawö (*k[h]u ts[h]a zla 'od*; 12th–13th c. CE). According to Shardza Trashi Gyeltsen's (*shar rdza bkra shis rgyal mtshan*; 1859–1934) *Precious Treasury of Good Sayings* (*legs bshad rin po che'i mdzod*), a Bönpo treasure revealer named Khutsa Dawö is supposed to have rediscovered medical texts

18 Yang Ga, *The Sources for the Writing of the Rgyud bzhi, Tibetan Medical Classic* (Cambridge, MA: Doctoral Dissertation at Harvard University, 2010), 2: "The *Rgyud bzhi* is divided into four main separate sections, or 'treatises.' The first section is the *Rtsa rgyud* ('Root Treatise'), which presents an outline of the whole of *Rgyud bzhi*, in six chapters. The second section is the *Bshad rgyud* ('Explanatory Treatise') which presents a basic theory of medicine. It discusses eleven principles (*gnas*), which are discussed over the course of thirty-one chapters. The third section is the *Man ngag rgyud* ('Oral Instruction Treatise'). This is a clinical manual, and has fifteen divisions (*skabs*) that are covered in ninety-two chapters. The last section is the *Phyi ma rgyud* ('Final Treatise') and is a manual of diagnosis, treatment, and production of medicine. It also provides a conclusion to the *Rgyud bzhi*. This part contains four compilations (*mdo*), which are covered in twenty-seven chapters. The total number of chapters in the *Rgyud bzhi* is 156."

(which, alas, always remain unnamed) in the Tiger's Den (*stag tshang*) in Paro (*spa gro*), Bhutan. Both Bönpo and Nyingma traditions take Khutsa Dawö to be identical with Yutokpa.[19] Codification into a text approximately as it is known to us now probably ensued much later, partly in the thirteenth or fourteenth century CE, and may have involved multiple authors and intermediate versions. The best-informed discussion on the formation of the *textus receptus* of the *Fourfold Tantra*, making use of the narrative framing of these and cognate texts, is McGrath.[20]

To facilitate work within this great chronological uncertainty, I have postulated four informed working hypotheses, just to get the investigations started:

1. The Bönpo *Fourfold Collection* contains earlier redactions of medical material very similar to that contained in the *Fourfold Tantra*, as is indeed variously indicated in emic narratives. Text-historically, it therefore makes more sense to compare sources such as the *Compendium of the Essence of the Eight Branches* (*yan lag brgyad pa'i snying po bsdus pa*; Skt. *aṣṭāṅgahṛdayasaṃhitā*) to the *Fourfold Collection* than to the *Fourfold Tantra*.[21]
2. The traditional narrative of the pedigree of the *Fourfold Tantra* (also adopted by Buddhists) seems problematic, to say the least. Alternative derivation through Bönpo medical practitioners is not at all unlikely. For instance, surprisingly many relic-like references to Bön are "still" extant in the *Fourfold Tantra*.[22]
3. The *Fourfold Tantra* is a highly syncretistic and composite text in which many influences are combined into an intellectually coherent system.[23]
4. One or more texts called the *Moon King* may be considered less successful syncretistic precursors of what the *Fourfold Tantra*, from a canonical

19 For a recent résumé, indeed as advertised, much indebted to Karmay, see Yang Ga, *The Sources for the Writing of the Rgyud bzhi*, 3f, and more in detail on 125ff.

20 See William A. McGrath, *Buddhism and Medicine in Tibet: Origins, Ethics, and Tradition* (Charlottesville, VA: Doctoral Dissertation at the University of Virginia, 2017), 94ff and esp. 124ff; more in reference to the *Fourfold Tantra* than to the *Fourfold Collection*.

21 Ronald E. Emmerick, "Sources of the *rGyud-bzhi*," *Zeitschrift der Deutschen Morgenländischen Gesellschaft* 2, no. 3 (1977): 1135–42.

22 Samten G. Karmay, "Vairocana and the *rGyud-bzhi*," *Tibetan Medicine: A Publication for the Study of Tibetan Medicine* 12 (1989): 19–31.

23 Fernand Meyer, "Introduction: The Medical Paintings of Tibet," in *Tibetan Medical Paintings: Illustrations to the Blue Beryl Treatise of Sangye Gyamtso (1653–1705)*, ed. Yuri Parfionovitch et al. (New York, NY: Harry N. Abrams, Inc., 1992), vol. 1, 2–13.

> point of view, more successfully became.[24] "It" (or they) may be the first record, or even the point of entry, of expertise on pulse analysis into the Tibetan medical system.[25]

But there are more closely related precursors and (possibly also) digests of the *Fourfold Tantras*—the *Jewel Rosary, Sons' Benefit*, and *Small Tantra* (which may be a post-hoc résumé rather than a precursor)[26]—that deserve to be looked at in this context, and we will do so shortly. First, we shall turn to the introductory exposition of "brown phlegm" as it appears in the fourfold treatises.

The section on "brown phlegm" in the *Instructional Tantra* of the *Fourfold Tantra*, interestingly, covers the whole of chapter five.[27] The introductory parts are interesting to quote in full;[28] the choice of the base edition has had to be more or less arbitrary at this point and does not indicate a preferred reading.

3.1.2 Introductory Parts of the *Fourfold Tantra*

/de nas yang d[r]ang srong yid las skyes kyis 'di skad ces zhus so/ /kye drang srong chen po rig pa'i ye shes lags/ /rlung mkhris bad kan bcos thabs de ltar na/ /'dus pa'i nad la gso thabs ji [134] *ltar bgyi/ /mtson byed ming dang dbye ba ji ltar lags/ /'tso mdzad sman pa'i rgyal pos bshad du gsol/ /zhes zhus pa las/ ston pas gsungs pa/ /kye drang srong chen po yid las* [G6: *la*] *skyes/*

'dus pa'i nad la gsum gas bcos pa ste/

1) */'on kyang rang bzhin rgyu yis 'dus pa dang* [cf. position in *Fourfold Collection*]*/*
2) */byung tshul dus gyi* [G8, D8, Y13: *kyi*] *sgo nas 'dus pa dang /*
3) */'du ba 'khrugs pa'i sgo nas 'dus pa gsum/*

24 Fernand Meyer, "Programme de l'année 2001–2," *Livret-Annuaire* 17 (2002).

25 Fernand Meyer, "Théorie et pratique de l'examen des pouls dans un chapitre du *rGyud-bzhi*," in *Indo-Tibetan Studies*, ed. Tadeusz Skorupski (Tring: Institute of Buddhist Studies, 1990), 209–56; Henk W. A. Blezer, "Brief Outlook: Desiderata in the Study of the History of Tibetan Medicine," in *Soundings in Tibetan Medicine: Anthropological and Historical Perspectives*, ed. Mona Schrempf (Leiden: Brill Academic Publishers, 2007), 432f.

26 See Barbara Gerke, "The Authorship of the Tibetan Medical Treatise *Cha lag bco brgyad* (Twelfth Century AD) and a Description of its Historical Background," *Traditional South Asian Medicine* 6 (2001): 27–50; and McGrath, *Buddhism and Medicine in Tibet*, 124ff.

27 See Blezer, "'Light' on the Human Body." "Brown phlegm" is indeed considered a very central disorder and generally perceived to be at the root of internal diseases (*Bdud rtsi snying po yan lag brgyad pa gsang ba man ngag gi rgyud ces bya ba bzhugs so* [Lhasa: Bod ljongs mi dmangs dpe skrun khang, 1992], 139.9ff: *khong nad phal cher smug po'i rgyu yis skyed//*).

28 *Bdud rtsi snying po yan lag brgyad pa gsang ba* (Lhasa 1992), 133.16ff, esp. 134.3ff.

/phyi ma ma smin tsha ba dug nad de [cf. position in *Fourfold Collection*]/
ad 1) */dang po mtshon byed bad kan smug por btags/*
/de la rgyu rkyen gnas dus rigs dang rtags/
/bcos pa'i thabs dang rjes bcad brgyad du bshad/
/rgyu ni bad kan khrag mkhris rlung dang bzhi/
/nad kun 'dus phyir 'dus nad rtags bcos dka'/
/de la skyed pa'i rkyen ni tsha grang gnyis/

1) */tsha rkyen 'grams khrag lhag dang mtshon khrag lus/ /de nyid mchin pa'i steng du lhung ba*[ ]*'am/ /tsha skyur zas kyis khrag 'phel mchin pa rgyas/ /de dag zungs su 'gyur du ma 'dod par/ /mchin gnas pho bar babs pas bad kan 'dres/ /khrag dang bad kan rul nas rgyu mar lhung / /mkhris par 'dres pas kha dog dud khur 'gyur/ /de nyid long du 'phyugs pas* [G18: *'chugs pas*] *rlung dang bsdongs* [G18: *sdongs*]/ */de la smug po yas babs zhes su 'dod/*
2) */grang rkyen 'ju dka' mi 'phrod zas bsten pas/ /pho bar ma zhu de yis be snabs 'phel/ /me mnyam rlung dang* [*dang* not in G20] *'ju byed mthu nyams pas/ /dangs snyigs ma phyed mchin pa'i gnas su shor/ /zungs su ma gyur khrag ngan mchin par rgyas/ /kha lud gong bzhin pho bar lhung ba de/ /ma zhus rgyu byas bad kan grang shas che/ /smug po gab pas wa ltar gzha' bar byed/ /de la smug po mas chags zhes byar 'dod/*
/smug po'i gnas la rang gnas gzhan gnas gnyis/ /rang gnas pho mchin rgyu long rnam pa bzhi/
   1) */pho bar gnas pas bad kan nad dang 'dra/*
   2) /[135] *mchin par gnas pas khrag gi nad dang 'dra/*
   3) */rgyu mar gnas pas mkhris pa'i nad dang 'dra/*
   4) */long du lhung bas rlung gi nad dang 'dra/*

/gnas gzhan byer la phyi nang rnam pa gnyis/

1) */phyi gnas shar rgyas lpags gram sa bdag 'dra/ /rtsar byer dug 'dra tshigs la grum bur byed/* [135.3]
2) */nang gnas srog rtsa mchin lam khrag la zhon/ /srog rtsa rdzong la tshigs pa mkhar du 'dod/ /yar la mgo la 'phyur bas mgo nad byed/ /glo la glo nad snying la snying rlung byed/ /mcher par mcher nad mkhal mar mkhal nad byed/*[29]

29 Cf., e.g., edition from Grwa thang, p. 147.7ff. (G: *Grwa thang rgyud bzhi* [Beijing: Mi rigs dpe skrun khang, 2005]); from Sde dge, p. 158.7ff. (D: *Sde dge rgyud bzhi* [Beijing: Mi rigs dpe skrun khang, 2007]); Mtsho sngon (Y: *Yan lag brgyad pa gsang ba man ngag gi rgyud* [Xining: Mtsho sngon mi rigs dpe skrun khang, 2009]), pp. 199.11ff.: all of these show only minor variants; note that the *Instructional Tantra* is not included in the Men-tsee-khang edition (*Bdud rtsi snying po yan lag brgyad pa gsang ba man ngag gi rgyud las/ rtsa ba'i rgyud/ bshad pa'i rgyud/ phyi ma'i rgyud/ kha khong dang bcas pa bzhugs so* [Dharamsala: Men-tsee-khang, 1999]).

3.1.3 Highlights in Paraphrase

By "hot" conditions (or weapons and surgical interventions) excess "blood" residue affects the liver. Likewise, by the intake of pungent and sour food, "blood"

Compare these editions of the *Fourfold Tantra* to the *Fourfold Collection* (*'bum bzhi*). Also consisting of four parts ("collections"):

1. The *Sky Blue "Essential" Collection* (*thugs 'bum mkha' sngon*): cf. the *Root Tantra*
2. The *White "Medicine" Collection* (*sman 'bum dkar po*): cf. the *Subsequent Tantra*
3. The *Multicolored "Diagnosis" Collection* (*dpyad 'bum khra bo*): cf. the *Explanatory Tantra*
4. The *Black "Disease" Collection* (*nad 'bum nag po*): cf. the *Instructional Tantra*

Alternative arrangement in three also exist (such as the Triten Norbutse edition, Delhi 1999), without the *The Sky Blue "Essential" Collection* (*thugs 'bum mkha' sngon*):

1. The *White "Medicine" Collection* (*sman 'bum dkar po*)
2. The *Multicolored "Diagnosis" Collection* (*dpyad 'bum khra bo*) and
3. The *Black "Disease" Collection* (*nad 'bum nag po*)

We are mainly concerned with the *Black "Disease" Collection* here.

/de yang gso ba rig pa rig pa [2nd not in Ak9] *'dzin pa des gsol pa/ ston pa lags/ rtsa ba* [39] *bzhi 'dus nad kyi gso thabs ni/ /bdag cag 'dzin pa'i 'khor la bstan du gsol/ de skad zhus pa* [B^{a}8, B^{b}4, Ak11: *pas*] *ston pas bka' stsal* [B^{b}4 emends: *bstsal*] *pa/*

'/dus pa'i nad la gsum ka bcos dgos ste/

1) *'on kyang gzhir gnas* [B^{b}5f adds: *rang bzhin*] *rgyu* [B^{a}9, B^{b}6: *rgyu'i*] *'dus pa dang /*
2) */byung tshul dus dang rkyen gyis 'dus pa dang /*
3) */'du ba 'khrugs* [Ak13: *'khrug*; B^{a}10: *'khyug*; B^{b}7: *'khyug* but emends: *'khyugs*] *pas 'dus pa gsum yin te/*

ad 1) */dang po rang bzhin rgyu* [Ak13, B^{a}11, B^{b}8: *rgyu'i*] *'dus pa ni* [cf. position in *Fourfold Treatise/*
/'di yi ming ni bad kan smug po btag [B^{b}5f emends: *btags*]—
/ci phyir rtsa ba khrag las tsha grang gnyis kyi rkyen/
/'du ba 'dus pas khrag nad smug po zer/
ad 2) */gnyis pa phyi ma ma smig* [Ak16: *na*] *smin dus kyis 'dus pa dang* [cf. position in *Fourfold Treatise*]/
ad 3) /[add: *gsum pa*] *tsha ba dugs* [B^{b}5f emends: *dug*] *nad 'du ba 'khrugs pas 'dus* [idem]/
/'di la rgyu dang rkyen dang gnas dang dus dang bzhi/
/rigs dang rtags dang bcos thabs rjes gcod brgyad/
/dang po rgyu ni bad kan khrag mkhris rlung /
/de'i nad 'dus brtag thabs bcos pa dka'/
/gnyis pa bskyed pa'i rkyen ni tsha grang gnyis kyi rkyen/ …

/dang pa [B^{a}18, B^{b}14, Ak3: *dang po*] *tsha ba'i rkyen ni 'gram* [B^{b}15 emends: *'grams*] *khrag lhag dang mtshon khrag lus/ /khrag de mchin pa'i thog du* [Ak4: *tu*] *babs pa*[ ]*'am/ /tsha skyung* [B^{a}19, B^{b}16 emends and Ak4: *skyur*] *zas kyis khrag 'phel mchin pa rgyas/ /de bas lus zung* [B^{b}17 emends: *zungs*] *dag tu 'grer* [B^{a}22, B^{b}17, Ak5: *'gror*] *ma 'dod / /mchin pa'i* [B^{b}18 emends: *par*] *rgyud* [B^{b}18 emends: *brgyud*] *nas phor* [B^{b}18 emends, Ak6: *pho*] *bar bsags pas bad kan 'dres/ /khrag dang bad kan kun rdul* [B^{b}19 emends, Ak7: *rul*] *nas rgyu mar babs/ /mkhris pa rgyu mar 'dres pa* [B^{a}22, B^{b}20, Ak7: *pas*] *kha dog dud/ /de nyid long song long ka'i rlung dang sdong / /de'i ming ni smug po yas babs zer/*

increases, the liver gets enlarged, and their vital strength is compromised. This excess "blood" subsequently affects the stomach and gets mixed with "phlegm." "Blood" and putrid "phlegm" then affect the small intestine. Mixing with "bile," it gets its typical smoky color. This enters into the colon and gets further mixed with "wind." Thus, all three "faults" are sequentially combined.

In the cold variety, the intake of food that is hard to digest and unwholesome, in the stomach leads to indigestion and results in large amounts of "phlegm." Because the digestive powers of the patient have diminished, the unrefined food affects the liver. This again affects the vital strength and bad "blood" increases in the liver. Spittle or mucus affects the stomach, as before. Because of the indigestion the cold aspect of "phlegm" increases.

/gnyis pa grang rkyen 'jub ba [B^{a}24 emends *'jub* to *'ju ba*, B^{b}21 emends, Ak9: *'ju* to *'ju ba*] *dkar* [B^{a}24, B^{b}183.1 emends: *dka'*] *ba*[ ]*'am/ /mi 'phrod pa'i zas kyi rkyen pa des/ /pho bar ma zhu bel snabs* [B^{b}2 emends: *'snab* to *snabs*, B^{a}260.1, Ak10: *snab*] *de yis 'phel/ /'ju byed drod mnyams* [B^{a}1: *nyams*] *rlung gi stobs nyams* [B^{a}2, B^{b}3 emends: *nyam* to *nyams*] *pas/ /dangs* [B^{a}2: *dvangs*] *snyigs ma phyed mchin pa'i yul du song / /zungs du* [B^{a}3, B^{b}3, Ak12: *su*] *ma gyur ngan khrag mchin par rgyas/ /khrag gi* [40] *kha lhud* [B^{b}4 emends: *lud*] *phor* [B^{b}4 emends, Ak12: *pho bar*] *babs pa des/ /ma zhu'i rgyu byas bad kan grang shas bskyed/ /smug po babs pa dbyi ltar gzha' bar byed/ /de'i ming ni bad smug mas chags zer/ /gsum pa*[*?*] *smug po'i gnas la rang gnas gzhan gnas gnyis/ /rang gnas pho mchin rgyu long bzhi yin no/*

1) */pho bar gnas pa* [B^{a}7, Ak16: *pas*] *bad kan rang gi nad/*
2) */mchin par gnas pas khrag gi nad* [B^{b}9 emends: *bad* to *nad*] *dang 'dra/*
3) */rgyu mal* [B^{b}9 emends, Ak17: *mar*] *gnas pa'i* [B^{a}8, B^{b}9, Ak17: *pas*] *mkhris pa'i nad dang 'dra/*
4) */long khar gnas pas rlung gi nad dang 'dra/*

/bad kan byer bas gzhan gnas phyi nang gnyis/

2)[!]*/nang gnas srog pa* [B^{a}9: *sa*, B^{b}11 emends: *sa* to *pa*] *rtsa ru zhugs* [B^{a}9, B^{b}12 emends: *zhug* to *zhugs*] *pa des/ /mchin par lam bstod* [B^{b}12 emends: *gtod*] *khrag la zhug* [B^{a}11, B^{b}12 emends, Ak19.2: *zhugs*] *pa des/ /srog rtsa rdzong 'dod mkhris pa mkhar du 'dod / /yar la 'phyur bas mgo'i nang kyang bskyed/ /glo la glo nad snying la snying rlung bskyed*[*/*] */mtsher* [B^{a1}3, B^{b}14 emends: *'tsher* to *mtsher*; Ak4: *'tsher*] *pa mtsher* [B^{a}13, emends: *'tsher*, Ak4: *'tsher*] *nad mkha' dmar* [B^{b}15 emends: *mkhal mar*, Ak4: *mkhal mar*] *mkhar* [B^{a}14 emends: *mkha'*, B^{b}15 no *mkhar*: adds *mkhal*, Ak4: *mkhal*] *nad bskyed/*

1)[!]*/phyi gnas shar* [Ak5: *sha*] *rgyas lpags* [B^{b}16 emends: *pags*] *gram yul bdag 'dra/ /rtsa* [B^{a}15, B^{b}16, Ak5: *rtsar*] *rgyug dug 'dra tshigs zhugs grum bu yin/* [40.11]

See the *Nad 'bum nag po* from the *'Bum bzhi* (*Gso ba rig pa'i bdud rtsi'i bang mdzod 'bum bzhi bzhugs* [New Delhi: Paljor Publications, 1999], vol. 2, 39.2ff). Again, the choice of the base edition has had to be more or less arbitrary at this point and does not indicate a preferred reading. See also Beijing edition A (B^{a}: *Gso rig 'bum bzhi* [Beijing: Mi rigs dpe skrun khang, 2005], 259.8ff); the Beijing Arura edition (B^{b}: *Gso ba rig pa'i bdud rtsi'i bang mdzod 'bum bzhi bzhugs* [Beijing: Mi rigs dpe skrun khang, 2005], 182.5ff.); and the Chengdu Akong edition (Ak: *Gso rig 'bum bzhi zhes bya ba bzhugs so* [Chengdu: Si khron mi rigs dpe skrun khang, 2003], vol. 7, p. 47.11ff). All of these show only minor variants.

In the stomach, "brown phlegm" gives rise to diseases of "phlegm"; in the liver, "blood" diseases; in the small intestine, "bile" diseases; and in the large intestine, "wind" diseases.[30]

The Tibetan editions of the *Fourfold Tantra* and *Fourfold Collection* that have been examined for this article each seem to depend on one main reading, showing only minor editorial interventions. The relevant distinction in this chapter is not between the individual testimonies of each text, but between readings of the *Fourfold Tantra* and *Fourfold Collection*. For a preliminary assessment of some relevant parts of these texts I refer to Blezer;[31] the stemmatic and philological work on these corpora still needs to be done, but promises interesting results.

In the selected passage, the *Fourfold Collection*, in spite of the many spelling errors, occasionally shows readings that seem to be embedded in a context that makes more sense, whether that be *the* (or *an*) original auctorial intent or an intermediary redaction is hard to tell. It confirms my working hypothesis that reconstructions of the origins of the *Fourfold Tantra* will be difficult without recourse to the possibly old variant readings that the *Fourfold Collection* has preserved. But that is for another long-term project and should not detain us here any further.

3.2.1 Sources of the *Fourfold Collection* and *Tantra* Relevant to "Brown Phlegm"

There are several other medical works ascribed to Yutok Yönten Gönpo, or that are closely contemporaneous with these treatises, that seem to inform the later *Fourfold Collection* and *Fourfold Tantra* and that feature extensive sections on "brown phlegm" (*bad kan smug po*) that are quite similar to those in the fourfold treatises. Unfortunately, the scope of this publication does not allow comparing and discussing the contents of the satellites in full; but it would be very illuminating indeed for the reception and early history in Tibet to do so.

30 See the rather free and interpolated rendering by Dash, included in the appendix; this is the only published translation that I am presently aware of. Tibetan medical doctors and scholars at the Dharamsala Men-tsee-khang are working on a five volume translation, the *Root Tantra* and *Explanatory Tantra* were published in one volume, in 2008 (reprint 2011), and the *Subsequent Tantra* came out in 2011; the last of the fourfold treatise to come out is the *Instructional Tantra*, presently still forthcoming, projected in three volumes (http://www.men-tsee-khang.org/dept/doc_pub/translation.htm).

31 Blezer, "'Light' on the Human Body," 143.

- The *Jewel Rosary* (*nor bu'i 'phreng ba*):[32] After comparison, Yang Ga concluded that this medical text is very similar to the *Instructional Tantra* in the *Fourfold Tantra*.[33] He reports that the text was recently discovered by Ludrup Gyatso (*klu sgrub rgya mtsho*), an incarnate lama at Troru (*khro ru*) Monastery.

  The *Jewel Rosary*, like the fourfold treatises, discusses "brown phlegm" in a separate section of combined diseases (*'dus pa'i nad*), after the chapter on phlegm. From all the satellite sources, it features the longest discussion of "brown phlegm." While there is a good deal of similarity, there is less overlap than in the *Brown Phlegm Résumé*. Incidentally, in contrast to the fourfold treatises, the *Sons' Benefit* and the *Small Tantra*, the *Jewel Rosary* distinguishes only two main types of phlegm: white and brown; it does not list the yellow phlegm separately.[34]
- The *Sons' Benefit* (*bu don ma*):[35] According to Yang Ga, there are at least two different manuscripts of this work in Tibet, one in the Lhasa Mentsikhang library and one in the Potala Palace (which he has not seen). The Lhasa Mentsikhang *Sons' Benefit by Master Yutokpa* (*mkhas pa g-yu thog pa'i* [*pas*] *mzdad pa'i bu don*) manuscript was edited and published by the Qinghai Province Tibetan Medical Research Center in 2005, in the said Arura Series (12). The title is explained in the text itself: "the essence of the instruction was composed for [my] son. [You] should keep it secret from all students who are not your own sons." Despite this admonition, the colophon also refers to his students.[36]

  "Brown phlegm" is discussed here as one of the three types of phlegm (white, yellow, and brown),[37] and thus is not set apart in its own chapter as

32 Rokpa Series 9, in 13 chapters (*Yan lag brgyad pa'i gzhung las bsdus pa nor bu'i 'phreng ba* [Chengdu: Si khron mi rigs dpe skrun khang, 2003], 22.12ff).

33 Yang Ga, *The Sources for the Writing of the Rgyud bzhi*, 104.

34 *Yan lag brgyad pa'i gzhung las bsdus pa nor bu'i 'phreng ba*, 19.6ff (Chapter 3: *Bad kan gyi nad bcos pa/*): ... *//gti mug las gyur bad kan nad/ /dbye na skya smug po gnyis su 'dus/ / smug po 'dus pa'i nad yin te/ /skya bo grang ba rkyang pa yin/ /'di la rgyu rkyen dbye ba dang / /mtshan nyid bcos pa'i thabs yin no//....*

35 Arura Series 12, in 85 chapters (*Bu don ma* [Beijing: Mi rigs dpe skrun khang, 2005], 14f, see esp. 15.15ff).

36 Yang Ga, *The Sources for the Writing of the Rgyud bzhi*, 110f; his translation. He refers to his Lhasa Sman rtsis khang edition of the *Bu don ma*: folio 62b: */man ngag gnad kyi ti ka 'di/ / bu'i don du bkod pa yin/ /bu min slob ma kun la gsang /.*

37 *Bu don ma*, 14.2ff (Chapter 3: *Bad kan gyi nad gso ba/*): ... *//gti mug las gyur bad kan nad/ /'di la dbye ba mtshan nyid dang / /bcos pa'i thabs dang rnam gsum las/ /dbye ba skya bo ser po dang / /smug po gsum du bshad pa yin/.*

a combined disease. However, "brown phlegm" is explicitly introduced and labelled as a multiple-disorder condition caused by other factors (*gzhan rgyud*) and not just phlegm-related.

- The so-called *Small Tantra* (*rgyud chung*) is also attributed to Yutokpa,[38] and is included within the *Eighteen Auxiliary Branches* (*cha lag bco brgyad*) collection. The *Eighteen Auxiliary Branches* was published by the Gansu Minority Publishing House in Lanzhou in 1994, and by the Minority Publishing House in Beijing in 2005, in the Arura Series (25). There it bears the title, the *Small Tantra: The Essence of Ambrosia* (*rgyud chung bdud rtsi snying po*), abbreviated to the *Small Tantra*. The work is largely based on the *Compendium of the Essence of the Eight Branches* (Skt. *aṣṭāṅgahṛdayasaṃhitā*; in Tibetan translation), apart, of course, from the sections on urine and pulse diagnosis. The beginning of text states that it was summarized from the *Essence of the Eight Branches*.[39]

  Most of the texts from the *Eighteen Auxiliary Branches*, however, were composed after Yutokpa, and the attribution of the *Small Tantra* to Yutokpa, according to Gerke, most likely is a posthumous honor.[40] This text features brief discussion of white, yellow, and brown phlegm,[41] first its general characteristics and distinction, and later its treatment.

- The *Brown Phlegm Résumé of a Thousand* [*Sections*] (*bad kan smug po'i stong thun*):[42] Another text included in the *Eighteen Auxiliary Branches* also deserves to be mentioned here briefly. Since these "thousand-section résumés" (*stong thun*) represent some of the earliest practical instructions that

---

1. */skya bo rlung gi lo ma yin/*
2. */ser po mkhris pa'i kha lud yin/*
3. */smug po khrag gi lo ma yin//....*

38 Arura Series 25, in 101 chapters (*Bdud rtsi snying po gsang ba man ngag gi rgyud*, in *Cha lag cho brgyad* [Beijing: Mi rigs dpe skrun khang, 2005], 596.11ff, esp. 597.6ff and 599.5ff). According to Yang Ga (*The Sources for the Writing of the Rgyud bzhi*, 112), some more traditionally minded scholars, such as Khro ru tshe rnam (2003) and Bsam gtan (2002), also attribute it to the legendary Yutokpa the Elder.

39 Yang Ga, *The Sources for the Writing of the Rgyud bzhi*, 114.

40 See Gerke ("The Authorship of the Tibetan Medical Treatise *Cha lag bco brgyad*") on its mixed authorship and late (later than Yutokpa) redaction of most (13 out of 18).

41 *Bdud rtsi snying po gsang ba man ngag gi rgyud*, 596.12ff (Chapter 28: *Bad kan gyi nad bcos pa/*): *de nas bad kan bcos pa'i thabs bstan pa/ /dbye ba rtags dang bcos thabs gsum du bstan/ /dbye brag spyi dang bye brag rnam pa gnyis/ /spyi la skya bo ser po smug po gsum/*
1. */bad kan skya bo rlung gi lo ma yin/*
2. */bad kan ser po mkhris pa'i kha lud yin/*
3. */bad kan smug po khrag gi rtsigs ma yin//....*

42 *Bad kan smug po'i stong thun*, in *Cha lag bco brgyad* (Beijing: Mi rigs dpe skrun khang, 2005), 342–46.

were transmitted within the school of Yutokpa, perhaps being arranged by himself, this places them in the beginning in the twelfth century CE. This work deserves to be included among the above-mentioned satellites. The group of eleven résumés of a thousand sections represent teachings of Lharjé Sanggyé Pelrin (*lha rje sangs rgyas dpal rin*) and were included in the *Eighteen Auxiliary Branches* around the turn of the fourteenth century CE.[43] Content-wise, this text is fairly close to the readings in the fourfold treatises and, even though it is more concise, features a similar sequence, occasionally even literal intertextuality. It may be noteworthy that "brown phlegm" here is explicitly labelled a combined disease (*'dus pa'i nad*).[44]

Among the early works that traditionally are attributed to Yutokpa, both the *Sons' Benefit* and the *Jewel Rosary* have detailed descriptions of complex "brown phlegm" disorders, very similar to what is found in the *Fourfold Tantra* chapter on "brown phlegm", but only the *Jewel Rosary* puts them in a separate section of combined disease (*'dus pa'i nad*). The *Small Tantra* also has a brief description of the disorders, which, again, is similar to the *Fourfold Tantra*.[45] The exact nature of these parallels cannot be summarized here.

In conclusion, it seems clear to Yang Ga that the chapter on "brown phlegm" was largely based on (presumably) earlier works attributed to Yutokpa, especially the *Sons' Benefit* and *Jewel Rosary* (as we saw above, whether the *Small Tantra* is in fact earlier is very doubtful, but in any case, it is roughly contemporaneous). So, most parts of this division of the fourfold treatises are very similar to the corresponding parts in the early works that can safely be attributed to Yutokpa and it seems likely that the former depend on the latter. In general, we can find similarities in the "brown phlegm" sections of the fourfold treatises and the materials not only in what Yang Ga labels as "pre-*Aṣṭāṅga*" medical works (but may more cautiously be referred to as not dependent on the "Eight Branches," without suggesting a clear chronology), but also in the *Essence of the Eight Branches* itself: "pre-*Aṣṭāṅga*" medical works therefore might also be indirect sources for the *Instructional Tantra* and the *Black "Disease" Collection*.

43 McGrath, *Buddhism and Medicine in Tibet*, chapter 4 et passim; and, in summary, on p. 254. McGrath (personal communication, August 2017) furthermore adds: "The *Bad kan smug po'i stong thun* can be found as part of the *sKor tshoms stong thun bcu gcig*, included in the *Cha lag bco brgyad*, but these works also circulated separately in the *Krung go'i bod lugs gso rig rtsa che'i dpe rnying kun btus* (the *Skor tshoms stong thun bcu gcig las dang po rtsa'i stong thun*, vol. 3, text 5; *rTsa chu'i stong thun g.yu thog gi bzhed pa*, vol. 3, text 7; *Grang ba'i stong thun*, vol. 3, text 9; *Grang ba'i stong thun*, vol. 14, text 4; *Bad kan smug po'i stong thun*, vol. 14, text 5; *sKor tshoms stong thun bcu gcig*, vol. 14, text 3)."

44 E.g., *Bad kan smug po'i stong thun* (Beijing 2005), 346.5.

45 Yang Ga, *The Sources for the Writing of the Rgyud bzhi*, 187.

Thus, both "pre-*Aṣṭāṅga*" medical works and the *Essence of the Eight Branches* may have served as sources for parts of the *Instructional Tantra* in general,[46] and, of course, the *Black "Disease" Collection.* In the *Essence of the Eight Branches*, generally assumed to be also earlier than the *Fourfold Tantra*, the "brown phlegm" disorder is not described. Even the name of the disorder is absent there.

3.2.2 Résumé of Late Dependencies

So, according to Yang Ga, the *Jewel Rosary, Sons' Benefit*, and *Small Tantra* contain original compositions, but also draw from the *Essence of the Eight Branches* and other works that predate the *Eight Branches* (or do not depend on it).[47] The (*Fourfold Collection* and) *Fourfold Tantra*, in turn, sometimes draw from these intermediary works by Yutokpa, sometimes directly draw from earlier sources. Besides the *Eight Branches*, important earlier sources are the *Lamp that Illuminates the Red Register* (*byang khog dmar byang gsal ba'i sgron me*), *Biji's Yellow-covered Book* (*bi ji'i po ti kha ser*), and the *Medicine of the Moon King* (*sman dpyad zla ba'i rgyal po*). Especially the *Jewel Rosary* and the *Sons' Benefit* contain many passages that were eventually incorporated into chapter five of the *Instructional Tantra* of the *Fourfold Tantra* and the *Black "Disease" Collection* of the *Fourfold Collection*, which concerns our discussion of "brown phlegm." This incidentally suggests that a rough draft of parts of *Instructional Tantra* was already in existence before the composition of the other three parts of the *Fourfold Tantra*. The *Small Tantra* contains passages that went into the (*Fourfold Tantra*) *Explanatory Tantra, Instructional Tantra*, and *Subsequent Tantra*. Apparently, Yutok Yönten Gönpo only gradually developed an overarching treatise on medicine: he did not compose the *Fourfold Tantra* in one go; instead, he, and, according to McGrath,[48] also his students and later authors, seem(s) to have spent his entire life composing "his" *magnum opus*.

3.3 *Early Testimonies: the* Moon King (zla ba'i rgyal po)

The *Medicine of the Moon King*, in relative chronology, seems to precede the *Fourfold Tantra*, and, as said, looks like an earlier attempt at a Tibetan synthesis of various medical materials.[49] Various versions and editions are reported to have existed, which may have varied considerably. Many competing narratives about its origins also are in existence. This tangle has not yet been

46 Yang Ga, *The Sources for the Writing of the Rgyud bzhi*, 187.
47 Yang Ga, *The Sources for the Writing of the Rgyud bzhi*, 380 et passim.
48 McGrath, *Buddhism and Medicine in Tibet.*
49 Meyer, "Programme de l'année 2001–2."

sorted out. Repeated references to China occur and some considerable overlap with sections on pulse diagnosis from the *Inner Classic of the Yellow Emperor* (*Huangdi neijing*) has been demonstrated by McGrath.[50]

According to Yang Ga many chapters of the *Moon King* are similar to corresponding chapters in the *Explanatory Tantra, Instructional Tantra,* and *Subsequent Tantra,* and it therefore seems to be a key source of some parts of the *Fourfold Tantra*.[51] At the time of composing his thesis Yang Ga found no evidence of influence of *Essence of the Eight Branches* on the *Moon King*; he argues that the Tibetan translation of the former postdates the latter. This categorical statement may need more careful philological reflection.

In any case, the *Moon King* possibly is the earliest entry point for pulse diagnosis in Tibetan cultural world: its origins may be pre-tenth century CE, perhaps even Imperial Period (7th to 9th c. CE); the dating is very uncertain. The extant redaction appears to be later (McGrath dates the redaction even as late as the eleventh or twelfth century CE).[52] And, more importantly, for our quest, in history of ideas, it may also be the earliest systematic incorporation of the notion of "brown phlegm."

The *Medicine of the Moon King* distinguishes more types of phlegm than the later sources. It discusses five types and colors of phlegm in five different "locations" or organs (phlegm is white in the stomach; brown in the liver; yellow in the gall bladder; red in the lungs (in the source emended to: kidneys); and black in the spleen, mixed with wind). Note that both brown and black phlegm are distinguished here.[53] But basically it works with a classification of

---

50 William A. McGrath, "Vessel Examination in the *Medicine of the Moon King*," in *Buddhism and Medicine: An Anthology of Premodern Sources*, ed. C. Pierce Salguero (New York, NY: Columbia University Press, 2017), 501–13.

51 Yang Ga, *The Sources for the Writing of the Rgyud bzhi.*

52 McGrath, *Buddhism and Medicine in Tibet*, 12.

53 *Sman dpyad zla ba'i rgyal po* (Dharamsala: Tibetan Medical and Astro Institute, 1994), 36.22ff (Chapter 6: *Nad gzhi ji ltar gnas pa bstan pa/*): "*Bad kan* in the liver is brown." Yang Ga, *The Sources for the Writing of the Rgyud bzhi*, 72: "Chapter six discusses various topics regarding diseases, such as their cause and location. It also talks about the nature of food, tastes, and provides classification of food and medicine that is based on four elements. It gives a detailed interpretation of the digestive process. The chapter also indicates the relationship between the seasons and humors. Finally, it discusses abnormal humors in the organs. It talks about different diseases in the heart, lung, liver, gallbladder, spleen, stomach, kidney and bladder."

... //bad kan dbye na mang yod de//

1. *pho ba la gnas dkar po yin//*
2. *mchin pa la gnas smug po yin//*
3. *ser po mkhris par bsdongs pa'o//*

seven: brown, white, (greenish) yellow, red, black (note that dark varieties such as black phlegm and brown phlegm are distinguished), and finally two varieties of phlegm related to acid reflux/vomiting (*chu skyegs/skyugs*) and some kind of digestive consumption (*'ju skem*), successively.[54] In a section on the powers of meat and grain, the so-called humors (*nyes pa*), or better, "faults" or "noxious substances,"[55] are connected to the elements: blood and bile to fire; "brown phlegm" to earth; wind to the space; phlegm (?) to water. Note that blood is mentioned along with bile and that "brown phlegm" is mentioned along with the other faults, as in some Bön traditions, as discussed below.[56]

---

4. *dmar* [37] *po* (*mkhal ma la gnas pa yin zer*) *glo la gnas pa yin//*
5. *bad kan nag po mcher par te//rlung dang bsdongs pas nag po'o//....*

54 *Sman dpyad zla ba'i rgyal po* (Dharamsala 1994), 87.7ff (Chapter 26: *Bad kan gyi mtshan nyid bstan pa/*). Yang Ga, *The Sources for the Writing of the Rgyud bzhi*, 73: "From chapters twenty-five to fifty-one, the author of the text discusses the causes, conditions, divisions, and symptoms of the following diseases ... phlegm diseases ..."
bad kan dag gi rgyu dag ni//'grangs dang rlan la 'dug pa dang//ma zhu ngal dub bcud can zas//chu'am chang mang 'thungs las byung//dbye na smug po dkar po dang//ser po dang ni dmar po dang//nag po dang ni chu skyags [='khru skyag, diarrhea] *dang//bad kan 'ju skem* [digestive consumption] *dang bdun no//....*
... bad kan smug po rnam lnga ni//mchin pa'i nad dag yin pa ste//
1. *mchin dri yol kar babs pa ste/*
2. *khong tsha mig rus na ba ste//*
3. *lci la byin pa mi theg dang//*
4. *rked pa na dang sgal par 'dril//chu dmar srog rtsa gcu ba dang//*
5. *zas mi 'dod cing rgyun skam mo//*

mchin pa dag la babs pa ni//sna khrag 'dzag cing khrag tu skyug /mchin pa'i kha na klad pa gzer//bkrag nyams mdog ni nag po'o//smug po mchin pa zags pa ni//sha ser gsus pa che ba dang//byin rtsa phyi ru byung ba dang//sha 'bros yan lag phra ba'o//smug po glo mchin 'tshangs pa ni/ khrag rnag lu dang rnag bam lu//ro stod gzer la rkang pa rengs//'gros drags chang mang 'thungs na na/ khrag rtsa skyugs nyam chung mkhal rked zhan//smug po glo la babs pa ni//brang tsha btsos khrag 'dra ba skyug /pho ba dag nas de 'byung ngo//.

55 "Faults" or "noxious gatherings" are a more literal and accurate rendering than the problematic term "humors," derived from (equally debatable) conventions of translation from Greco-Arab epistemes; just consider the presumed wind "humor," humoring translators of Ayurvedic lore. See Blezer, "'Light' on the Human Body."

56 *Sman dpyad zla ba'i rgyal po* (Dharamsala 1994), 252.9ff (Chapter 93: *Zas dang sha'i skor bstan pa/*). Yang Ga, *The Sources for the Writing of the Rgyud bzhi*, 74: "From chapters seventy-nine to ninety-four, the author of [the] text talks about different forms of compounds, various therapies, the powers of medicines and food, and human behaviour. These chapters cover the following different forms of medical compounds: ... Some chapters also talk about diet, behaviour, and medicine.... Chapter ninety-three discusses the powers of grain and meat...." *Khrag dang mkhris pa me dang 'dra ste tsha ba'i rang bzhin yin//bad kan smug po sa dang 'dra ste lci ba'i rang bzhin yin//rlung ni nam mkha'i sprin dang 'dra ste tsha grang gnyis kar 'gyur//bad kan <delete: smug po> chu dang 'dra ste grang*

The extant "early" syntheses labelled as the *Moon King* and *Biji's Yellow-covered Book*, in terms of relative history of ideas, probably are the earliest sources on "brown phlegm" (but note that the received texts may be later than the claimed dates). They briefly describe the symptoms of "brown phlegm" in the different organs, such as in the lung, liver, stomach, and gallbladder; indeed, a typical format in these early sources. These descriptions are similar to passages in the corresponding chapter in the fourfold treatises, but the overall arrangement is different and seems to preserve an earlier stage in the reception history and organization of these materials.

The discussion of "brown phlegm" in the versions of the *Moon King* is very close to what we find in the doctor's *Yellow-covered Book*. This may present an interesting clue for the "reception" history of "black bile" and "brown phlegm" disorders in Tibet. Both sources, in their present form, discuss "brown phlegm" in a structurally different way from what appears in some later accounts, such as we find in the fourfold treatises and the *Jewel Rosary*. The latter explicitly set "brown phlegm" apart as a combined or combination disease (*'dus pa'i nad*). Thus, the editors of these later texts effectively rearrange the lingering implicit clash of two systems of "faults" by rearranging the various factors involved in "brown phlegm" disorders: phlegm (*bad kan*), blood [!] (*khrag*), yellow bile (*mkhris pa*), and wind (*rlung*), by taking "brown phlegm"—the hypothetical correlate of "black bile"—out of harm's way, and setting it apart as a fourth, separate category: combined disease (*'dus pa'i nad*).[57]

In line with the depiction of "brown phlegm" in the *Medicine of the Moon King*,[58] the Bön *Instructions of the Six Lamps* (*sgron ma drug gi gdams pa*) lists "combined disease" as a fourth of the (noxious) gatherings ([*nad*] *'du ba rnams bzhi*).[59] Incidentally, this Bön tradition lists blood as the cause of phlegm and not as an independent factor of disease. Flesh is identified as the causal factor for combined disease.[60] As such, Bön medical instructions are crucial in figuring out the history of ideas and concomitant semantic shifts, often preserving older or eccentric traditions.

---

zhing rlon pa'i rang bzhin no/ /.... The Arura edition (*Sman dpyad zla ba'i rgyal po// bi ji po ti kha ser//* [Beijing: Mi rigs dpe skrun khang, 2005], 253.19ff) is close to identical, also including the extra "*smug po*."

57 See the introductory part of the fourfold treatises above.

58 *Sman dpyad zla ba'i rgyal po* (Dharamsala 1994), 252.9ff (Chapter 93: *Zas dang sha'i skor bstan pa/*); quoted above.

59 Nb. [*nad*] *'du ba*, in Bön idiom, is closely synonymous with *nyes pa*.

60 Blezer, "'Light' on the Human Body."

On the other hand, Bön traditions occasionally also explicitly list blood (*khrag*) as one of the so-called "humors" or noxious substances,[61] or, as here, "nauseating accumulations" (*rlung mkhris bad kan khrag nad 'du ba bzhi*). This appears in a relatively recent quote by Menrampa Pasang Yönten (*sman rams pa pa sangs yon tan*), which he attributes to the *Ziji* (*gzi brjid*).[62] This is again consonant with early sensibilities reflected in the *Medicine of the Moon King*.

3.4 *Résumé of "Brown Phlegm" and Other Types of Phlegm*

In the cluster of Tibetan satellite texts that relates to the fourfold treatises of the *Fourfold Tantra* and *Fourfold Collection*, one commonly, or perhaps even typically, finds a distinction into three types of phlegm: white, yellow, and brown, as quoted from several Tibetan medical sources above (however, as said, the *Jewel Rosary* does not distinguish yellow phlegm separately). They are associated with various so-called "leafs" and factors, and connected to different organs and elements. These Tibetan sources all seem to sit at the beginning of the second millennium: some slightly earlier than the fourfold treatises, some perhaps a little later, maybe even close to touching the start of the Yuan Dynasty (when the distinction into white and yellow phlegm also is in evidence in China).[63] As mentioned, in some of the (probably) later sources "brown phlegm" is, for the first time, explicitly set apart as a combined disease.

As seen above, in the oldest sources one does not finds a distinction into three, but at times into no less than seven types of phlegm, be they not always listed in the same order and with the exact same color.[64] The origins of these earlier sources may sit somewhere at the end of the first millennium, but their dates are notoriously difficult to establish.

---

61 *Sman dpyad zla ba'i rgyal po* (Dharamsala 1994), 252.9ff (Chapter 93: *Zas dang sha'i skor bstan pa/*); quoted above.

62 Martin, "Greek and Islamic Medicines' Historical Contact with Tibet," 132, n. 41.

63 See Natalie Köhle, "A Confluence of Humors: Āyurvedic Conceptions of Digestion and the History of Chinese 'Phlegm' (*tan* 痰)," *Journal of the American Oriental Society* 136, no. 3 (2016): 465–93. Also, based on a personal e-mail communication with Köhle on Aug 1st 2016: "… There is a dis<c>tinction between new and old phlegm (which is of white and yellow color), but that is not prior to the Tibetan. Much rather, I suspect it is of Greco-Arab origin as well, it simply came with the Mongol translations and Mongol doctors during the Yuan dynasty." And on August 4th, 2016: "… As for the Yuan texts' distinction of colours: 'White' phlegm is the phlegm that 'floats on top' and easily comes out when coughing, while 'Yellow' phlegm is that which has been in the body longer, and has coagulated at the bottom, due to the influence of heat. It does not easily come out when coughing…."

64 See *Sman dpyad zla ba'i rgyal po* (Dharamsala 1994), 87.7ff (Chapter 26: *Bad kan gyi mtshan nyid bstan pa/*); quoted above.

The division into three, as far as white and yellow phlegm are concerned, may be fairly close to what Natalie Köhle has observed in Yuan Dynasty "China," except of course, for the third type: "brown phlegm," which on the face of things seems to be absent there.[65] It is not clear at this point whether the distinction into white and yellow arrived there with Mongol translations and Mongol doctors during the Yuan dynasty, or possibly, even was mediated through earlier Tibetan contacts. This may incidentally underline Buell's point that, of course together with the foundational influx of "Islamic" (Greek) medicine, some of the Tibetan systematizations—incidentally also already informed by Greco-Arab traditions—had a significant impact on the formation and outlook of medicine in the Yuan period in these areas.[66] One such instance of possible Tibetan influence on Yuan-era medicine is the convention of using the "three faults" (*nyes pa gsum*) of wind, bile, and phlegm, instead of the more customary schema four "humors" (blood, phlegm, and yellow and black bile), of certain Greco-Arab systems that may have entered the area at the time.[67]

Chinese-language sources of the Yuan dynasty seem to be aware of a "dark" phlegm, phlegm mixed with blood, indeed as in "brown phlegm", which basically also is phlegm mixed with bad blood, and if blood, as mixed with phlegm, newly emerges on the scene at the time,[68] then maybe all three of them are represented after all: white, yellow *and*, be it not yet systematized, "dark" phlegm. In general, "brown phlegm" indeed is much involved with vitiated blood, and so is "black bile"—counter to what Buell, for reasons that elude me, seems to

65 Köhle, "A Confluence of Humors."

66 P. D. Buell, "Tibetans, Mongols and the Fusion of Tibetan Cultures," in *Islam and Tibet: Interactions along the Musk Routes*, ed. Anna Akasoy et al. (Farnham, VT: Ashgate, 2011), 189–208.

67 See McGrath, *Buddhism and Medicine in Tibet*, 143, for another possible example.

68 Personal e-mail communication with Köhle, Aug 4th, 2016: "… there is no 'Brown' phlegm per se, but there is phlegm that is dark and mixed up with blood. Blood comes into play starting from the Yuan dynasty, and that in itself is very telling." More references are to be found in her Harvard Ph.D. thesis: *Phlegm* (tan 痰)*: Toward a History of Humors in Early Chinese Medicine* (Cambridge, MA: Doctoral Dissertation at Harvard University, 2015; at this point is not yet publically available). Discussion on connections between blood and phlegm in the Yuan period will also appear in a forthcoming article, "The Many Colours of Excrement: Phlegm and Coproscopy in Medieval China," which is based on Köhle's paper at a conference on *Histories of Healthy Aging*, Groningen, 21–23 June 2017. It also was featured in a paper on "Islamic Influences in Yuan Chinese Medicine: The Case of Phlegm," presented at a symposium on *The Classical Oriental Medicine across the Border: Dialogue and Interaction*, at the Oriental Institute, Peking University, Beijing PRC, 22–23 September 2018.

believe;[69] in fact, so much so that the world's most famous specialist on "black bile" disorders, Rufus of Ephesus, in his reconstructed two-volume treatise on melancholia, often even seems to be struggling to tell their roles and agency apart (see quotations below).

However, without additional data it will be difficult to figure out the precise causal connections between Tibet and Yuan China. It may also simply be a real-life messy affair, not at all neatly mono-causal. However, this is not my area of expertise and I'd be happy to defer the matter to specialists on Yuan China. In any case, it is not at all unthinkable that Tibetan sensibilities regarding three types of phlegm: white, yellow, and brown, which seem to have been well-established before the Yuan Dynasty, have formatted or systematized extant confusion on white and yellow phlegm and bile in Yuan Mongol areas,[70] simultaneously suggesting the inclusion of another type of "dark" phlegm, mixed with blood.

From my nascent appreciation of "brown phlegm" disorders in Tibetan medical sources, I have always felt that the boundaries between "phlegm" (*bad kan*) and "bile" (*mkhris pa*) must, in the actual practice of medicine, have been much more porous than they are generally made out to be. Descriptions of the actual factors involved in the ailments, as here, often seem to suggest something along this vein—in any case for the "combination" disease, for obvious reasons. This may explain why people have missed—or, when pointed out, have strongly resisted ...—the "brown phlegm" connection to "black bile." Perhaps heavy scholarly investments in the logic of "the" system of "the three faults" (*nyes pa gsum*) can also be an intellectual trap: in theoretical frames of reference, there is a tendency to be too categorical when wielding and interpreting these terms. Yet, overall, I do not see many signs of actual confusion on the matter in Tibet: it seems like Tibetans have employed these categories in a down-to-earth and practical manner.[71]

69 Buell, "Tibetans, Mongols and the Fusion of Tibetan Cultures," 205.

70 Köhle, "A Confluence of Humors." The considerations and speculative propositions outlined above notwithstanding—Köhle's hypothesis on possible confusion between white and yellow phlegm and bile sounds very plausible. It is absolutely fascinating and telling that initially even the same Chinese character was used for both, and that bile was merely distinguished by the added characterization of "yellow." Köhle here states: "Endō et al. further observe that in later periods the character *tan* 痰 often does double duty to represent phlegm *and* bile, as in 'yellow and white *tanyin*' 黃白痰癊 (yellow *tan* 黃痰 = bile; white *tan* 白痰 = phlegm)." The proposed connection to digestion also looks convincing.

71 I believe that is in fact one of the major hurdles for appreciating surviving texts on the matter of (brown) phlegm; we simply do not know what the actual practices looked like. In our fields of study, texts are interestingly entangled artefacts, more often than not also somewhat ideologically involved. They are notoriously hard to translate into social history

Text-historically, it seems significant that only some of the later sources, which sit at the beginning of the second millennium, systematically set "brown phlegm" apart and discuss it separately and explicitly as a "combined disease" (*'dus pa'i nad*): most notably in the fourfold treatises, but also (already) in the closely related *Jewel Rosary*. In contrast, the said "earlier" sources (the *Moon King* and the *Yellow-covered Book*) and some later sources (the *Sons' Benefit* and the *Small Tantra*) discuss "brown phlegm" as a part of phlegm disorders (this is about relative history of ideas, not about compilation dates), together with various other types of phlegm. We may be looking at a relative chronology and developments in systematization in treatment of "brown phlegm." Particularly the dating of the source needs more work in order to make this firmer.

3.5 *Missing Antecedents for "Brown Phlegm"*

As hypothesized above, no evidence has yet come to light for a proper Sanskrit equivalent of "brown phlegm" in Indian Ayurvedic texts,[72] such as in the *Compendium of Caraka* (*carakasaṃhitā*; which is more geared toward internal medicine), the *Compendium of Suśruta* (*suśrutasaṃhitā*; with special expertise on surgical procedures), and the mentioned *Compendium of the Essence of the Eight Branches* (*aṣṭāṅgahṛdayasaṃhitā*; which seems to have been compiled for use of the general physician). This makes the origins of the concept only more interesting. It may be good to reiterate the fact that the *Compendium of Suśruta*, by the nature of this surgical treatise, often refers to blood (Skt. *rakta* = Tib. *khrag*), also as a "fault" or so-called "humor" (Skt. *doṣa* = Tib. *nyes pa*), which may be relevant for the discussion of the factors involved in "brown phlegm" (as we saw, the Bönpos, as usual, tend to preserve slightly eccentric or marginal traditions).

At about this point in my preliminary deliberations several individuals, steeped in Tibetan medicine entered into the fray: a Tibetan medical doctor at the ICTAM VIII, whom I grant the courtesy of anonymity, and a vocal,

---

and practice; certainly of non-elite groups. I sympathise with Kuriyama's ("Forgotten Fear of Excrement," *Journal of Medieval and Early Modern Studies* 38, no. 3 [2008]: 413–42) theses on borders that originally and in actual practice may have been fuzzier, and on "confusion" in the following centuries, possibly due to the hypostases of later, ideologically charged categorizations.

72 Somewhat anachronistically reconstructed by Bhagwan Dash (*Encyclopaedia of Tibetan Medicine* [Delhi: Sri Satguru Publications, 1999]) as *aruṇakapha*, on the mistaken assumption that the fourfold treatises would be in any straightforward sense be translated from a Sanskrit original.

Tibetophile translator, named Malcolm Smith.[73] Unbeknownst to them, they may in fact have shared my initial impression and reservation that "brown phlegm" disorders appear rather far removed from the predominantly mental afflictions that we have come to associate with melancholia, and that the connection cannot but appear spurious.[74] Even though one might perhaps argue about little details in Smith's brief digest, quoted in the footnote above, his exposé still seems fairly accurate, as far as present day understandings of

73 Malcolm Smith [on http://tibetanstudies.forumprod.com, 14 Aug 2012, 16:10]: "Blezer's speculations on *bad kan smug po* are completely off the mark. *Smug po* refers to a condition that often begins with acid reflux (*chu tsha ba*) in its hot expression, gastric ulcers in the middle and ultimately the disruption of colon's ability to eliminate. The disease passes th[r]ough four distinct phases, (varying depending on whether it is hot or cold natured) and is entirely a product of *ma zhu ba*, maldigestion. I saw many patients with mugpo at the Tibetan Medical Hospital in Amdo when I [w]as there for my internship for three months in the summer of 2009."

[15 Aug 2012, 15:44]: "… In general, the reason why *bad kan smug po* is considered a so[-]called combination disease, and given its own chapter, is as Blezer points out, because it involves all three *dośas* [HB: emend: *doṣa*-s], plus blood—however, unlike other dual dośic [idem] and tridośic [idem] conditions, the way in which the three or four *dośas* [idem] are involved here are sequential—starting with maldigestion that is caused by *mkhris pa* (*pitta*) first or *bad kan* (*kapha* first) dependent on whether the condition is hot[-] or cold[-]natured.

In the former case [hot], the condition<s> begins [sic] with *dwangs ma ma shu* [*zhu*] *ba*, which leads first to unhealthy blood forming in the liver i.e. disordered *mkhris pa*, which then leads to gastric ulcers, then disruption of the *myag byed bad kan*, and then finally a disorder of the *thur sel rlung*.

The progression of the cold natured version is that due to a disorder of the *myag byed bad kan*, there is maldigestion that results in impure *dwangs ma* being sent to the liver, this again leads to the formation of unhealthy blood in the liver, the formation of unhealthy blood leads to gastric ulceration and ultimately again, disorder of the *thur sel rlung*…."

74 See the apparent modernist incarnation of melancholia in the category of mood disorders, and more in particular so-called depressive disorders, in contemporary jargon: "Depressive disorders include disruptive mood dysregulation disorder, major depressive disorder (including major depressive episode), persistent depressive disorder (dysthymia), premenstrual dysphoric disorder, substance/medication-induced depressive disorder, depressive disorder due to another medical condition, other specified depressive disorder, and unspecified depressive disorder. Unlike in DSM-IV, this chapter 'Depressive Disorders' has been separated from the previous chapter 'Bipolar and Related Disorders.' The common feature of all of these disorders is the presence of sad, empty, or irritable mood, accompanied by somatic and cognitive changes that significantly affect the individual's capacity to function. What differs among them are issues of duration, timing, or presumed etiology" (American Psychiatric Association, ed., *Diagnostic and Statistical Manual of Mental Disorders* [Arlington, VA: American Psychiatric Publishing, 2013], 155). For the high degree of comorbidity, see ibidem, p. 160.

the disorder go. However, his may be more an emic scholarly than an etic academic argument: he seems to be blissfully unaware of the proximity of his rebuttal to *melancholia hypochondriaca* in Greco-Arab sources, which we shall discuss shortly.

This may be a good point to resume some of the findings so far. There are a great many variant readings in the fourfold treatises and there moreover are multifarious, variegated symptoms connected to an effulgence of "brown phlegm." Those mostly are described in the remaining parts of the "brown phlegm" chapter of the fourfold treatises that could not be presented or paraphrased here. Yet in all that effulgence, the so-called "brown phlegm" disorders, both in their hot and their cold varieties, share a few principal features that are primarily related to indigestion and involve (bad) blood, the liver, and an excess of phlegm from the stomach; "bile" is admixed in the small intestine and "wind" in the large intestine. The ailments are clearly concentrated in what could be styled the hypochondria.[75] Descriptions that appear, somewhat scattered, in those later parts of the chapter (not resumed here), frequently mention belching and eructation or acid reflux (*sgregs pa*), but occasionally also heart burn (*zos/grangs rjes na; pho ba 'tshing*),[76] sour eructation and vomiting ([*chu tshan chu skyur*] *skyugs pa*), gurgling or sloshing noises in the belly (*sbo 'khrog pa, 'ur ba*), flatulence (*lon/thur rlung*), diarrhea (*'khru*), difficulty evacuating and hard stool (*dri ma skam*), and the like. Also, contemporary descriptions of developed stages of "brown phlegm" disorders indeed usually refer to heart burn, gastric ulcers and, technically, to inflammation of the pylorus, and, as a consequence, in the ultimate stages, refer to the inability to evacuate. The same symptoms are frequently mentioned in Greco-Arab sources on *melancholia hypochondriaca*.

See also Malcolm Smith's summary of a typical progression of "brown phlegm" disorders (quoted above in note 73), which he observed during a

75 Here referring to the soft parts of the belly or viscera, below sternal cartilage of the ribs (or diaphragm).

76 *Bdud rtsi snying po yan lag brgyad pa gsang ba* (Lhasa 1992), 139.3. Based on the readings in the *Fourfold Tantra* alone, I am not completely sure about this rendering; is the rare *'tshing ba* somehow cognate to *'tshigs pa*? See the *Blue Beryl 'Mallika'* commentary (*Gso ba rig pa'i bstan bcos sman bla'i dgongs rgyan rgyud bzhi'i gsal byed bai ḍūrya sngon po'i malli ka* [Lhasa: Bod ljongs mi dmangs dpe skrun khang, 1982], 487.11) and Dash (*Encyclopaedia of Tibetan Medicine*, 29). Editions of the Bönpo *Fourfold Collection*, as so often, have helpful variant readings and make the burning sensation explicit by apposition of *tsha*. See, for example, *Gso ba rig pa'i bdud rtsi'i bang mdzod 'bum bzhi bzhugs* (New Delhi 1999), 44.16; *Gso rig 'bum bzhi* (Beijing 2005[a]), 264.5; *Gso ba rig pa'i bdud rtsi'i bang mdzod 'bum bzhi bzhugs* (Beijing 2005[b]), 187.20; and *Gso rig 'bum bzhi zhes bya ba bzhugs so* (Chengdu 2003), 54.2: *pho ba 'tshang* [sic] *tsha*.

three-month internship in a hospital in Amdo. His description may be typical of modern-day accounts of these disorders, such as Drungtso's. Even though this pitch was clearly intended polemically, a comparison of his "off the cuff", résumé with the Greco-Arab sources quoted below, rather to the contrary, forcefully underlines the point he is arguing *against*. It would be useful, in a later stage of these investigations, also to stake stock of contemporary views on the matter, and relate those to various canonical sources and their commentaries.

4 Greco-Arab Sources

I should therefore like to proceed to discuss some important time slices of sources from the Greco-Arab side, to wit, by highlighting translated quotations of:[77]

- Hippocrates of Kos (4th–5th c. BCE)
- Diocles of Carystus (4th c. BCE)
- Rufus of Ephesus (ca. 1st c. CE)
- Galen of Pergamum (130–200 CE)
- Ibn Sīnā, Avicenna (980–1037 CE)

I shall start with the briefest of previews of extant discourse on *melancholia hypochondriaca* in Greco-Arab sources. Galen found that in hypochondriac patients the normal symptoms of melancholia were associated with flatulence and impaired digestion.[78] According to Rufus of Ephesus: the etiology of melancholia is relatively straightforward. It first appears as an overheating of the liver and the stomach.[79] Galen, by contrast, argues for a swelling of the portal vein in the liver. Others seem to have believed that a blockage in the mesenteric veins (in the lower abdomen or the hypochondria) was responsible. But all classical authorities agree that the location of the disease's first manifestation is in the hypochondria. It is worth noting that only very rarely in the ancient sources do we find a form of melancholia with purely psychological

77 In fact, we do not need to go to non-modern Asia or the Middle East to redress the assumption that melancholia mainly pertains to mental disorders; for early modern European discussion of melancholia and dyspepsia or indigestion, see, for example, Thomas Mayo, *An Essay on the Influence of Temperament in Modifying Dyspepsia, or Indigestion* (London: 1831).

78 Stanley Jackson, "Melancholia and the Waning of the Humoral Theory," *Journal of the History of Medicine* 33 (1968): 367–76 (at p. 367); as quoted in Matthew Bell, *Melancholia: The Western Malady* (Cambridge: Cambridge University Press, 2014).

79 Rufus, 31; cited in Bell (based on the reconstructed edition by Pormann of his *On Melancholy*), *Melancholia*. Also see the near-identical descriptions quoted above, from the fourfold treatises.

causes [QED ...]. At around Rufus' or Galen's time, around 1st–2nd c. CE, the disease was believed to develop into three types: general, encephalic, and hypochondriac.

It is indeed the last type mentioned by Rufus of Ephesus that bears the best resemblance to "brown phlegm" (*bad kan smug po*). So, in the Greco-Arab fold we ought to look particularly at the hypochondriac type. In the following, I will present translations of relevant passages (as referenced) with highlights of the parts that have strong resemblance to the descriptions of "brown phlegm" disorders that I have summarized above. I will refrain from commenting on the obvious, I shall however note some matches that appear in the other parts of the chapters on "brown phlegm" in the fourfold treatises, particularly parts that have not been quoted above (and that is by far the majority of the descriptive parts). Salient elements are underlined.

4.1 *Hippocrates of Kos (ca. 460–370 BCE)*

Radden, *The Nature of Melancholy*:

> The following statement is written at the end of [Hippocrates'] sixth book *On epidemic diseases*: ... Those affected by black bile [literally: melancholies] become, as a rule, epileptics after a long [delay] and the epileptics suffer from black bile [literally: become melancholies]. Each of these [conditions] occurs by preference, if weakness befalls one or the other: if weakness [affects] the body, people become epileptics: if it [affects] the mind they become melancholic.[80]

4.2 *Diocles of Carystus, 4th c. BCE*

From *Disease, Cause and Cure*, cited in Radden, *The Nature of Melancholy*:

> ... Another disease arises in the cavity of the stomach, unlike those previously mentioned; some [physicians] call it melancholic [atra-bilious], others gassy. After meals, and especially after food which is difficult to digest and feels hot, this condition is accompanied by much watery spitting, sour eructations, gas and heartburn [literally: burning in the hypochondria], also by splashing noises [in the abdomen][81] which do not occur instantly but after some delay. Sometimes there are severe pains of the [gastric] cavity which in a few persons extend toward the broad

80 Jennifer Radden, ed., *The Nature of Melancholy: From Aristotle to Kristeva* (Oxford: Oxford University Press, 2000), 64.

81 Cf. the gurgling or sloshing noises in the belly (*sbo 'khrog pa, 'ur ba*), mentioned in the *Fourfold Tantra*, referred to above.

of the back.[82] These pains abate by [the use of] well-cooked food but return when the same [heavy] food is eaten again. The pain often becomes annoying during fasting and after the principal meal. Those who suffer from vomiting bring up undigested food and mucus which is not very bitter but hot and so acid that even the teeth become bloody. This befalls mostly young people and quite suddenly. But in whatever form it may start, it can persist in all cases. One should assume that the so-called flatulent persons have more heat than customary in those veins which receive the nutrients from the stomach and that the blood of these patients becomes thick. This shows that these veins are obstructed, since the body does not receive the nutrients, which remain in the stomach, whereas prior to this condition first these pores had absorbed, then discharged most foodstuffs into the lower abdominal organs. Therefore, on the next day these patients vomited foodstuff which was not absorbed into the body. One can well understand that there is more than natural heat because of the fever from which they suffer and of the type of their nourishment. But they seem to obtain relief from cold food which cools this type of heat and quenches the [innate fire]. Some people say that in similar affections the [lower] opening of the stomach which leads to the intestines is inflamed and that because of the inflammation this opening is obstructed and blocked so that transfer of food to the bowels cannot take place during the allotted time. Since under these circumstances the food has to remain in the stomach for a longer period, it provokes swelling, heat and the other [symptoms] already mentioned.[83]

Brief résumé of salient points for comparison:
- Arises in the cavity of the stomach
- Called melancholic or gassy
- Due to food which is difficult to digest and feels hot
- Much watery spitting, sour eructations, gas, and heartburn
- Splashing noises [in the abdomen] which do not occur instantly but after some delay

82 While not referred to in the brief excerpts of the fourfold treatises quoted above, *rgyab na*, *sgal tshigs na*, etc. are often mentioned in relation to symptoms of *bad kan smug po* in later parts of the relevant section (close to half a dozen references). This of course is a much less specific symptom than the ones related to indigestion.

83 Radden, *The Nature of Melancholy*, 66f.

- Severe pains of the gastric cavity which in a few persons extend toward the broad of the back
- Bring up undigested food and mucus
- The lower opening of the stomach that leads to the intestines is inflamed and because of the inflammation this opening is obstructed and blocked so that transfer of food to the bowels cannot take place during the allotted time

The description of Diocles of Carystus, which Galen closely follows and also complements (see below), has a very clear exposition of the major symptoms and already provides a truly spectacular match with various descriptions of "brown phlegm" that are discussed above. See, for instance, the symptoms that are listed in the Drungtso medical dictionary, quoted above: "heart burn, sour watery vomitus, emesis of blood and bile, pain between [the] 12th vertebra and [the] stomach-liver region, descending of blood-*mkhris*[.]*pa* disorders into [the] stomach, upper backache, expansion, hidden[?] and disturbance of brown phlegm (*bad.kan.smug.po*)." The following sources provide equally fine matches, with some minor variants and additions. I will summarize the salient points after each quotation, but try not to repeat myself unnecessarily.

4.3 *Rufus of Ephesus (late 1st c. CE)*

Bell, *Melancholia*:

> Melancholia hypochondriaca gives rise to a litany of digestive complaints. Flatulence and a distended stomach are the key signs of this type, especially after eating foods that are hard to digest (Rufus, 50). Cf. 'edition' by Peter E. Pormann. Indigestion and flatulence are particularly common among the elderly, who are especially prone to melancholia 'since the old are naturally depressed' (Rufus, 39). Melancholia sometimes reveals itself in black bodily discharges, whether vomit, faeces or urine. But this is not the case in every melancholic: 'rather, phlegm appears more frequently' (Rufus, 41). Do not make the patient suspect that he has melancholy. Rather just treat him for indigestion; help him against his excessive belief, terror and joy; and keep him from [too much] thinking' (Rufus, 53).[84]

84 Bell, *Melancholia*, 45ff.

Abou-Aly, *The Medical Writings of Rufus of Ephesus*:

> Rufus, though admitting black bile as a sub-species of bile identifies it as the sediment of blood. Almost the same identification appears in some of his fragments in ar-Razi's *al-Hawi* [Muhammad ibn Zakariyā Rāzī, aka Rhazes or Rasis; 854–925 CE]. Yet Rufus seems to differentiate between the two substances as he expresses the difficulty in identifying the liquid that goes from the liver into the stomach as either blood or black bile. For, as he confesses, "the two are close to each other in nature." It is clear that Rufus admits its presence in the body in health.
>
> Dealing with melancholy in fragment no.70, Rufus clearly states that heat and cold turn blood and phlegm into that humour. Ill-temperament can lead to the same result ….
>
> … There is some evidence that black bile exists all the time in the liver while the spleen's function is to drag it out and hence clean the body. When the spleen fails to function a type of jaundice results that is different from the usual jaundice associated with yellow bile.
>
> We have just alluded to the fact that black bile is linked not only with melancholy but also with jaundice. It is of some importance to recognize that black bile plays a role not only in jaundice and melancholy but also in lethargy and epilepsy ….
>
> … Yet the relief of the patient for melancholy is not only attained by the expulsion of the black bile but also by that of the phlegm and in fact he is more relieved with the expulsion of phlegm. One can conclude that although there is evidence of the role of black bile in this illness, yet this role is shared with phlegm.
>
> While in ar-Razi one can be positive of the existence of the humour by itself without the need of the transformation of another humour to develop black bile, which eventually produces the illness, in fragment no. 70, Rufus maintains that by cooling blood or overheating yellow bile the black bile is produced which creates the illness.
>
> On the other hand he mentions two types of black bile: the one which results from a natural crasis and the other which comes from a bad diet. The second one is worse.
>
> Black bile seems responsible for some symptoms. By cooling the stomach it causes a dyscrasis which, along with the body being full of excrements, leads to continuous indigestion.
>
> The outpouring of such a humour leads to the black coloration of the skin. The excessively burnt yellow bile explains some of the psychic symptoms such as delirium, rashness, passion, and even violence.

In the first and third cases of the *Kranken Journale* where melancholy is the illness Rufus speaks of burnt blood as the cause of the illness. In the first one he does not even mention black bile and it is difficult to identify the burnt blood with black bile. In case no. 3 Rufus begins by saying that it starts from the burning of blood. He again says that studying geometry, attending on nobles, and a sharp temperament lead to black bilious matter which is the cause of the disorder. This black bile then is noxious as it produces an illness. One cannot again decide whether the burnt blood is identical to black bile.

In case no. 2 there is the only reference to the presence of black bile in the body. It is called a surplus of black bile that reached the head and found dry burnt humours in it that changed to black bile. This is further evidence of black bile being both congenital and non-congenital.

In the fourth and the fifth cases there is no mention of the cause but the presence of the black bile is indicated in evacuation only in no. 5.

Black bile in Rufus' writings is both congenital and non-congenital. There is evidence that both of them can produce illness. When the first one is stirred up, then the disease can occur, while the second, which can have both materialistic and non-materialistic causes, leads to the same result. It does not affect the body in only melancholy but also in the form of other disorders. In such disorders phlegm indicates its presence alongside that of black bile.[85]

Brief résumé:

- Melancholia hypochondriaca gives rise to a litany of digestive complaints
- Flatulence and a distended stomach are the key signs of this type, especially after eating foods that are hard to digest
- Indigestion and flatulence are particularly common among the elderly
- Black bodily discharges
- Phlegm appears more frequently
- Black bile is a sub-species of bile identified as the sediment of blood.
- Blood and black bile are close to each other in nature
- Heat and cold turn blood and phlegm into black bile
- Black bile shares a role with phlegm
- Cooling the stomach causes a dyscrasis which, along with the body being full of excrements, leads to continuous indigestion
- Burnt blood as the cause of the illness

---

85 Amal Mohamed Abdullah Abou-Aly, *The Medical Writings of Rufus of Ephesus* (London: Doctoral Dissertation at the University College of London, 1992), 141ff.

- Confusion between burnt blood and black bile, one cannot again decide whether the burnt blood is identical to black bile

Rufus of Ephesus no doubt was the greatest authority on "black bile" disorders in antiquity, who, for example in Europe, held his ground even into early modernity. He addresses many of the points that we also find articulated in Diocles and Galen. Note, however, his references to a profusion of, and "combination" with, phlegm; the stress on bad ("burnt") blood (as in the *Fourfold Treatises*), to the point where it is difficult to tell the latter apart from "black bile"; the body being full of excrement; etc.

4.4 *Galen of Pergamum (130–200 CE)*

Radden, *The Nature of Melancholy*:

> Court physician to the Emperor Marcus Aurelius, Galen of Pergamum (or Pergamos) stands as one of the two most influential Greek physicians of the Roman era. (The other was the [said] Rufus of Ephesus, who lived during the time of Emperor Trajan [98–117].) Galen was born of Greek parents in Pergamum, in Asia Minor, and he is believed to have lived between the years 130 and 200.
>
> From Galen, "Function of Diseases of Brain and Spinal Cord", in *Diseases of the Black Bile*, from *On the Affected Parts* (ca. 165 CE):
>
> … There also exists a third type of melancholia which, as in epilepsy, has its origin in the gastric cavity. Some physicians call this condition a hypochondriac or gassy disease. It is sufficient for me to quote here the related symptoms which Diocles described in the book *Disease, cause and cure* where he wrote in exactly these words: … [quoted above] … Why did Diocles write in his explanation of the causes of other symptoms, but failed to discuss that it is worthwhile to investigate [the conditions] which cause a damage to the intellect? This question is worth asking. He omitted explaining why melancholic symptoms arise when the heat in the gastric veins is excessive, or when the parts around the pylorus are inflamed. It is evident that when the stomach is filled with gassy pneuma the patients are relieved by belching and, above all, by vomiting, as Diocles himself mentioned. But it was difficult to describe the characteristic symptoms of melancholy together with the above-mentioned affection of the stomach. Let us now supplement this with a clear explanation of the diathesis of the stomach in these affections. For it seems that there is an inflammation in the stomach and that the blood contained in the

inflamed part is thicker and more atrabilious. As some kind of sooty and smoke-like evaporation or some sort of heavy vapors are carried up from the stomach to the eyes, equally and for the same reason the symptoms of suffusion occur, when an atrabilious evaporation produces melancholic symptoms of the mind by ascending to the brain like a sooty substance or a smoky vapor.[86]

We certainly observe that headaches most frequently arise from yellow bile contained in the stomach, just as they instantly subside when the bile is eliminated by vomiting. Some pains of this type are biting and corrosive, others are heavy or accompanied by tension or sinking spells.

The best physicians agree that not only these [pains] but also epilepsy start in the stomach but then affect the head. Fear generally befalls the melancholic patients, but the same type of abnormal sensory images do not always present themselves. As for instance, one patient believes that he has been turned into a kind of snail and therefore runs away from everyone he meets lest [its shell] should get crushed; or when another patient sees some crowing cocks flapping their wings to their song, he beats his own arms against his ribs and imitates the voice of the animals. Again, another patient is afraid that Atlas who supports the world will become tired and throw it away and he and all of us will be crushed and pushed together. And there are a thousand other imaginary ideas....

... All of the best physicians and philosophers agree that the humors and actually the whole constitution of the body change the activity of the soul. I demonstrated this in a single commentary, *Why the faculties of the soul correspond to the humoral composition of the body*. Therefore, those who were ignorant of the activity of the humors, like for instance the followers of Erasistratus, did not dare to write anything about melancholy. It is worthwhile here to question the common notions of people and many other beliefs [of Erasistratus] of which quite a few philosophers and physicians are ignorant. All persons call this affection melancholia, indicating by this term the humor responsible for it. If the first symptoms which appear in the stomach become more severe, they are followed by a melancholic affection. When the patient is relieved through bowel movements, vomiting, expulsion of flatus and belching, then we should rather call this illness hypochondriac and flatulent and define despondency and

86 See the description, in chapter five of the *Instructional Tantra* of the *Fourfold Tantra*, of "brown phlegm" rising to the head and causing diseases of the head, e.g., in *Bdud rtsi snying po yan lag brgyad pa gsang ba* (Lhasa 1992), 135.4f: */yar la mgo la 'phyur bas mgo nad byed/*.

> fear as its symptoms. If, however, the symptoms of melancholy become serious but the [gastric] cavity is hardly involved, then we should consider this disease as a primary affection of the brain due to an accumulation of black bile in this organ.
>
> Based on these symptoms one has to distinguish whether this humor is confined only to the brain or [distributed] throughout the entire body, as was mentioned a short time ago. I want to remind you that my pupils saw me achieve a perfect cure of melancholy by [recommending] frequent bathing; a well-balanced and fluid regimen, without other remedies if the damaging humor did not resist evacuation for any length of time. When, however, the illness had become chronic, it required stronger methods of treatment than those previously mentioned. This type of melancholy follows a preceding hot condition of the head which can arise from a burning fever, an inflammatory affection of the head, or phrenitis. It also comes from worry and grief combined with sleeplessness. But this should be enough [discussion] about melancholy.[87]

Brief résumé:
- Has its origin in the gastric cavity
- A hypochondriac or gassy disease
- Heat in the gastric veins is excessive, or when the parts around the pylorus are inflamed
- An inflammation in the stomach

Since Galen, on the relevant points, mostly follows Diocles, the résumé can be relatively brief. He clearly has much invested in theorizing the connection between the digestive nature of the disorders and ubiquitous mental problems. In terms of history of ideas (such as early body and mind distinctions) this is extremely interesting indeed, but it is less relevant for our present comparative exercise. There is some emphasis on inflammation of the stomach and pylorus, which, according to some of the Tibetan traditions outlined above, is responsible for blockage of the digestive tract and the inability to evacuate.

4.5 *Avicenna (980–1037 CE)*

Radden, *The Nature of Melancholy*:

> Avicenna is the Latinized form of the Arabic Ibn Sīnā (Abū ʿAlī al-Husain ibn ʿAbd Allāh ibn Sīnā). He lived from 980 to 1037. He was born near Bukhara and was of Persian origin. Some quotes from the *Canon of*

87 Radden, *The Nature of Melancholy*, 61ff.

Medicine (ca. 1170–87 CE) by Avicenna, "On the Signs of Melancholy's Appearance," in *On Black Bile and Melancholy*.

… The signs of melancholy, however, which are common to the whole body are the body's blackness, its dryness, its retention of that which is emptied out of the spleen and stomach and that which is cleaned out with the periods of the year and months, the multitude of body hair, its powerful blackness, the preceding intake of bad and melancholic foods and such things as we teach in the second book. The sicknesses that melancholy follows are thus temporary and disordered fevers. The signs of melancholy which are derived from the spleen, are a multitude of cravings because of the effusion of black bile to the stomach, a scarcity of digestion because of the coldness of the melancholic condition, a multitude of wrinkles on the left side,[88] and a swelling of the spleen.…

The signs of melancholy that are from the stomach … are an increase of sickness with dry nauseousness and a feeling of uncomfortable fullness accompanying digestion. Very many times pains are felt in the stomach, and these pains continually spread. Then they rest near the digestive tract. If it is hot, however, this leads to inflammation and dryness in the abdomen and consequently the spleen has more melancholy. The signs of melancholy which are in the phlegmatic humor are a heaviness of the phlegm, its attraction to the upper parts of the body, constant nausea, a sickness of the spirit, the disruption of digestion, sour vomit, wet spit, wrinkles, the expulsion of flatulence, swelling, pain in the stomach or pain between both shoulder blades, and the pain spreading especially after eating. He vomits phlegmatic bile. And sour phlegm congeals his teeth. And these things happen due to intake of food, or soon thereafter.

88 It is not entirely clear to me what symptom these wrinkles in the side refer to. Without access to the original sources I am not in a position to check the translation, but one cannot help to be reminded of an equally puzzling translation of *brla sul* in the "brown phlegm" section of the *Fourfold Tantra* in Dash (*Encyclopaedia of Tibetan Medicine*, 23): where *brla sul* is translated as "furrows in the thigh" (cf. the only other occurrence in this chapter, on p. 21, where *brla sul* is translated as "calf region"). The reference occurs when discussing specific diagnostic signs in the kidneys (see *Bdud rtsi snying po yan lag brgyad pa gsang ba*, 137.16f: */mkhal byer rked pa 'khor zhing rkang pa lci/ /brla sul mkhal rtsa 'phrig cing chu mdog dmar/*, and cf. earlier, on 137.11, */mkhal rked brla sul tshigs gzhi byin nywa na/*). My guess is that this apparent semblance is a mere fluke due to inconsistency in translation in Dash; "appearance of furrows in the thigh," probably relates to pain in (the region of) the crevice or fold of the thigh, as suggested in his earlier translation, but I am not sure why Dash shifts from the idiomatic translation "thigh" to "calf" here and reconstructs a different Sanskrit "original" (and of course why he presumes that there would need to be a Sanskrit original in the first place …).

> The phlegmatic bile will be carried away and alleviated on account of the goodness in food eaten, and increased by the decrease of good foods .... Great trembling may be discovered in the abdomen at certain hours. The sickness, however, is increased with the dryness of the nausea and the speed of digestion.
>
> We say above that the black bile makes the disease of melancholy. When black bile is mixed with blood, there is happiness and laughter, and strong sadness does not share in it. If however it is mixed in with phlegm, there is laziness, inertia, and rest. And if it is mixed with or from yellow bile, there are agitation, lesions, some demonic influences, and similar manias. And if it were pure black bile, then there would be a great deal of deliberating, and a reduction of agitation or frenzy; unless it was stirred and upset, or unless there were enmities which could not be forgotten.[89]

Brief résumé:
- Retention of that which is emptied out of the spleen and stomach
- Intake of bad and melancholic foods
- Derived from the spleen, are a multitude of cravings because of the effusion of black bile to the stomach, a scarcity of digestion because of the coldness of the melancholic condition, a multitude of wrinkles on the left side, and a swelling of the spleen
- Uncomfortable fullness accompanying digestion
- Pains are felt in the stomach
- If it is hot this leads to inflammation and dryness in the abdomen
- The signs of melancholy which are in the phlegmatic humor are a heaviness of the phlegm
- Disruption of digestion, sour vomit, wet spit, wrinkles, the expulsion of flatulence, swelling, pain in the stomach or pain between both shoulder blades, and the pain spreading especially after eating
- Due to intake of food, or soon thereafter
- The phlegmatic bile will be carried away and alleviated on account of the goodness in food eaten, and increased by the decrease of good foods
- The sickness increased with the dryness of the nausea and the speed of digestion

Avicenna again provides a very close match, with additional minutiae and also minor variants. The passage quoted from the Drungtso dictionary is close to a paraphrase of his "disruption of digestion, sour vomit, wet spit, wrinkles, the

89 Radden, *The Nature of Melancholy*, 75ff.

expulsion of flatulence, swelling, pain in the stomach or pain between both shoulder blades, and the pain spreading especially after eating."

Most of the matches,[90] highlighted in red, with the array of primarily digestive afflictions associated with "brown phlegm" disorders that were briefly outlined above are rather spectacular and convincing, both in quantitative and qualitative detail. Nonetheless, disorders that involve digestive problems by their very nature tend to have generic and converging characteristics. Also, each of the apparent matches would need to be discussed in greater depth and detail, adducing their proper contextual data, and under closer philological scrutiny of the sources, also those on the Greco-Arab side. However, this would require a monograph-size engagement, rather than a cursory treatment in just one chapter of an edited volume. In any case, there is sufficient overlap between these domains of medical knowledge to recommend pursuing this.

5 My Imaginary Friend Basil: All Roads Lead to Rome

While the patterns of overlap stand out very clearly and have convinced me that *melancholia hypochondriaca* and "brown phlegm" disorders are not just phenotypically but also genetically related, the many steps in between, in terms of historical connections, have to remain elusive. Yet, there are some tantalizing clues extant in the narrativization of Tibetan medical histories. Tibetan narratives on the dissemination of Greco-Arab medical lore, mention a "Biji" (*bi ji*, *bi ci*, or *be ci*) lineage that is attributed to Galen, ultimately. This lineage starts from the figure Tsan Pashilaha (*tsan pa shi la ha*; 8th c. CE), who is also known from other sources.[91] Most studies have parsed his name in a Tibetan manner: Tsenpa Shilaha (thinking of the productive Sanskrit element *śīla* in some names). But Dan Martin has proposed a more convincing *caesura*: Tsan Pashilaha, i.e., Basileos of Tsan.[92]

According to Tibetan narratives, Tsan Pashilaha was a "Turkic" doctor who taught and also "settled down" in Lhasa, where he served Mé Aktsom (*mes ag tshoms; khri lde gtsug brtsan*; r. 712–55 CE). Basileos is generally said to hail from Phrom, which, as indicated, in this case probably refers to present day Trabzon,

90 A few salient points are highlighted for other reasons, such as their centrality to the argument (e.g. in Galen).

91 See an early reference in Mkhas pa lde'u, *rGya bod kyi chos 'byung rgyas pa* (13th c. CE, reference from Martin "Greek and Islamic Medicines' Historical Contact with Tibet").

92 See the Sannoi/Tzannoi (Sanni/Tsanni) near Trebizond (cf. the Gr. Τραπεζοῦς, Trapezous); now Trabzon, Turkey (Martin, "Greek and Islamic Medicines' Historical Contact with Tibet").

in Turkey. His system, most tellingly, is traced back to Galen of Pergamum (130–200 CE). According to Desi Sanggyé Gyatso (*sde srid sangs rgyas rgya mtsho*), he bequeathed *Biji's Yellow-covered Book* to his three students when he left Tibet. Alas, the *Yellow-covered Book*, due to its presumably late redaction, does not take us very far back in time.[93] Beckwith builds an argument for a more significant impact of the Greco-Arab system in this early period.[94] Kongtrül Lodrö Tayé (*kong sprul blo gros mtha' yas*) in his *All-Encompassing Knowledge* (or *Encyclopedia*) *of Knowledge* (*shes bya kun khyab*) suggests Tsan Pashilaha was also involved in compiling the *Somarāja*, indeed, the Sanskrit or Sanskritized name of one of the versions of the *Medicine of the Moon King*, often quoted above. As mentioned there, both the *Moon King* and the *Yellow-covered Book* briefly describe the symptoms of "brown phlegm" in the different organs.

As is well known by now, some Tibetan sources mention a doctor (also) bearing the name "Galenos," who presumably was in Tibet a little earlier, i.e. in the seventh century CE. Beckwith has already exposed this as a myth.[95] Likewise, this reference to a Biji lineage from Phrom may not provide a sound hypothesis on an originary event but a late narrativization of lineage (and authority), even though the person of Tsan Pashilaha may have a better likelihood of being historical than the Tibetan Galenos. What we have before us, in the Tsan Pashilaha narrative, most likely is not a historical account that we can still confidently reconstruct to a real event in space and time, but a reference without a clear historical referent, carefully constructed in accordance with non-modern Tibetan historiographical sensibilities. Indeed, imaginary friends rarely solve real problems. All we can say is that, in general, Tibetans over the centuries have tended to agree with the received wisdom that there is considerable impact from Greco-Arab knowledge systems on various early Tibetan medical compendia, underlined by our particular engagement and assessment of "brown phlegm" and "black bile."

6 Conclusion

The match in the (digestive) disorders of *melancholia hypochondriaca* and "brown phlegm" (*bad kan smug po*) appears more spectacular and convincing than anticipated. They involve many of the same factors, symptoms and organs, so much so that alternative origins have to appear implausible. Indigestion,

93 Yang Ga, *The Sources for the Writing of the Rgyud bzhi*, 54ff.
94 Beckwith, "The Introduction of Greek Medicine into Tibet."
95 Beckwith, "The Introduction of Greek Medicine into Tibet."

bad blood, and an abundance of phlegm, and an array of problems in the hypochondria are ubiquitous in all of the descriptions. Black bile itself, which, as a "humor," is known to be the most problematic of the later system of four, appears to be "combined" in much the same way as "brown phlegm" is eventually construed in Tibet (i.e., as a "combined disease" or *'dus pa'i nad*). There may, in fact, be good reasons to recommend, retrospectively, introducing a category of "combined disease," also in Greco-Arab systems.

However, in spite of the apparent match the connection still has to be argued in detail, also based on the original Greco-Arab sources and on painstaking philological work on the four treatises and their cognates, and on earlier sources in Tibet. For such a monograph-size, future endeavor, it would be of immense help indeed if the historical window of possible contact could be rendered more narrow and more clear than it is now.

What still remains unclear, however, is precisely the concrete interface of exchange. The initial hypothesis that the origins of the new Tibetan medical category of "brown phlegm," which, with the hindsight of this argument, perhaps is not entirely unprecedented after all ..., lies in *some* Greco-Arab episteme, after this brief comparison, may indeed still stand strong. Except for a tantalizing memory trace in relatively late Tibetan historical narrativizations, however, possible referents of the Biji narratives have to remain somewhat elusive (for now): in order to move this argument further along, the "where and when" require in-depth research. To be continued ...

Tibetan Sources

rGyud bzhi (*The Fourfold Tantra*), Satellites and Commentaries

Bad kan smug po'i stong thun. In *Cha lag bco brgyad*, 342–46. Beijing: Mi rigs dpe skrun khang, 2005.

Bad kan smug po'i stong thun. In the *Krung go'i bod lugs gso rig rtsa che'i dpe rnying kun btus*, vol. 14, text 5. Lhasa: Bod ljongs mi dmangs dpe skrun khang, 2014.

Bdud rtsi snying po gsang ba man ngag gi rgyud. In *Cha lag cho brgyad*. Bod kyi gso ba rig pa'i gna' dpe phyogs bsgrigs dpe tshogs, vol. 25. Beijing: Mi rigs dpe skrun khang, 2005.

Bdud rtsi snying po yan lag brgyad pa gsang ba man ngag gi rgyud ces bya ba bzhugs so. Lhasa: Bod ljongs mi dmangs dpe skrun khang, 1992 [repr. 1982].[96]

96 I gratefully acknowledge the use of an ITTM e-text, which was kindly provided by Barbara Gerke.

Bdud rtsi snying po yan lag brgyad pa gsang ba man ngag gi rgyud las/ rtsa ba'i rgyud/ bshad pa'i rgyud/ phyi ma'i rgyud/ kha khong dang bcas pa bzhugs so. Dharamsala: Men-tsee-khang, 1999.

Bu don ma. Bod kyi gso ba rig pa'i gna' dpe phyogs bsgrigs dpe tshogs, vol. 12. Beijing: Mi rigs dpe skrun khang, 2005.

Cha lag cho brgyad. Bod kyi gso ba rig pa'i gna' dpe phyogs bsgrigs dpe tshogs, vol. 25. Beijing: Mi rigs dpe skrun khang, 2005.

Grwa thang rgyud bzhi. Bod kyi gso ba rig pa'i gna' dpe phyogs bsgrigs dpe tshogs, vol. 20. Beijing: Mi rigs dpe skrun khang, 2005.

Gso ba rig pa'i bstan bcos sman bla'i dgongs rgyan rgyud bzhi'i gsal byed bai ḍūrya sngon po'i malli ka, two volumes. Lhasa: Bod ljongs mi dmangs dpe skrun khang, 1982.

G.yu thog cha lag bco brgyad. Sarnath, UP: 1967.

Rgyud bzhi'i 'grel pa mes po'i zhal lung. Bod kyi gso ba rig pa'i gna' dpe phyogs bsgrigs dpe tshogs, vol. 19, two parts. Beijing: Mi rigs dpe skrun khang, 2005.

Rgyud bzhi'i gsal byed bai ḍūrya sngon po. Bod kyi gso ba rig pa'i gna' dpe phyogs bsgrigs dpe tshogs, vol. 18, two parts. Beijing: Mi rigs dpe skrun khang, 2005.

Sde dge rgyud bzhi. Bod kyi gso ba rig pa'i gna' dpe phyogs bsgrigs dpe tshogs, vol. 57. Beijing: Mi rigs dpe skrun khang, 2007.

Yan lag brgyad pa gsang ba man ngag gi rgyud. In *Sman dpe rtsa chen phyogs bsgrigs*, vol. 1. Xining: Mtsho sngon mi rigs dpe skrun khang, 2009.

Yan lag brgyad pa'i gzhung las bsdus pa nor bu'i 'phreng ba. Bod kyi gso rig dpe rnying phyogs bsgrigs gangs ri dkar po'i phreng ba, vol. 9. Chengdu: Si khron mi rigs dpe skrun khang, 2003.

'Bum bzhi (*The Fourfold Collection*)

Gso ba rig pa'i bdud rtsi'i bang mdzod 'bum bzhi bzhugs [The Four Collections of Nectar Treasures of Medicine Science]. New Delhi: Paljor Publications, 1999.

Gso rig 'bum bzhi. Beijing: Mi rigs dpe skrun khang, 2005[a].

Gso ba rig pa'i bdud rtsi'i bang mdzod 'bum bzhi bzhugs. Bod kyi gso ba rig pa'i gna' dpe phyogs bsgrigs dpe tshogs, vol. 36. Beijing: Mi rigs dpe skrun khang, 2005[b].

Gso rig 'bum bzhi zhes bya ba bzhugs so. Bod kyi gso rig dpe rnying phyogs sgrigs gangs ri dkar po'i phreng ba, vol. 6. Chengdu: Si khron mi rigs dpe skrun khang, 2003.

Zla ba'i rgyal po (*The Moon King*)

Sman dpyad zla ba'i rgyal po. Dharamsala: Tibetan Medical and Astro Institute, 1994.[97]

Sman dpyad zla ba'i rgyal po// bi ji po ti kha ser//. Bod kyi gso ba rig pa'i gna' dpe phyogs bsgrigs dpe tshogs, vol. 33. Beijing: Mi rigs dpe skrun khang, 2005.

97 I gratefully acknowledge the use of an ITTM e-text, which was kindly provided by Barbara Gerke.

Secondary References

Abou-Aly, Amal Mohamed Abdullah. *The Medical Writings of Rufus of Ephesus*. London: Doctoral Dissertation at the University College of London, 1992.

American Psychiatric Association, ed. *Diagnostic and Statistical Manual of Mental Disorders*. Arlington, VA: American Psychiatric Publishing, 2013.

Avicenna. *Leerdicht der Geneeskunst*. Introduced and translated by M. M. J. Reyners. Meppel: Boom, 1991.

Avicenna. *The Metaphysics of The Healing*. Islamic Translation Series, translated by Michael E. Marmura. Provo, UT: Brigham Young University Press, 2005.

Avicenna. *The Physics of the Healing: A Parallel English-Arabic Text in Two Volumes*. Islamic Translation Series, translated by Jon McGinnis, two vols. Provo, UT: Brigham Young University Press, 2009.

Beckwith, Christopher I. "The Introduction of Greek Medicine into Tibet in the 7th and 8th Century." *Journal of the American Oriental Society* 99 (1979): 297–313.

Bell, Matthew. *Melancholia: The Western Malady*. Cambridge: Cambridge University Press, 2014.

Blezer, Henk W. A. "Brief Outlook: Desiderata in the Study of the History of Tibetan Medicine." In *Soundings in Tibetan Medicine: Anthropological and Historical Perspectives. PIATS 2003, Tibetan Studies: Proceedings of the International Association for Tibetan Studies*, Oxford 2003, edited by Mona Schrempf, 427–38. Leiden: Brill Academic Publishers, 2007.

Blezer, Henk W. A. "'Light' on the Human Body: The Coarse Physical Body and its Functions in the Aural Transmission from Zhang zhung on the Six Lamps." Paper at the ICTAM VII conference on "Asian Medicine: Cultivating Traditions and the Challenges Of Globalisation." Institute of Traditional Medicine Services, Thimphu, Bhutan, Sept. 7–11th, 2009. In *Revue d'Etudes Tibétaines* 23 (2012): 117–68.

Brown, George W., and Tirril O. Harris. *Social Origins of Depression: A Study of Psychiatric Disorder in Women*. New York, NY: Free Press, 1978.

Buell, P. D. "Tibetans, Mongols and the Fusion of Tibetan Cultures." In *Islam and Tibet: Interactions along the Musk Routes*, edited by Anna Akasoy, Charles Burnett, and Ronit Yoeli-Tlalim, 189–208. Farnham, VT: Ashgate, 2011.

Burton, Robert. *The Anatomy of Melancholy* [full title: *The Anatomy of Melancholy, What it is: With all the Kinds, Causes, Symptomes, Prognostickes, and Several Cures of it. In Three Maine Partitions with their several Sections, Members, and Subsections. Philosophically, Medicinally, Historically, Opened and Cut Up*]. 1621.

Chishti, Hakim G. M. *The Traditional Healer's Handbook: A Classic Guide to the Medicine of Avicenna*. Rochester, VT: Healing Arts Press, 1988.

Clark, Barry, trans. *The Quintessence Tantras of Tibetan Medicine*. Ithaca, NY: Snow Lion Publishers, 1995.

Clifford, Terry. *Tibetan Buddhist Medicine and Psychiatry: The Diamond Healing*. Delhi: Motilal Banarsidass Publishers, 1994 [repr. 1984].

Dash, Vaidya Bhagwan. *Encyclopaedia of Tibetan Medicine: Being the Tibetan Text of rGyud bzhi and Sanskrit Restauration of Amṛta Hṛdaya Aṣṭāṅga Guhyopadeśa Tantra and Expository Translation in English*, 7 vols. Delhi: Sri Satguru Publications, 1995–2001.

Dell'Angelo, Enrico. "Notes on the History of Tibetan Medicine." *Tibetan Medicine* 8 (1984): 3–14.

Drungtso, Tsering Trakchoe, and Tsering Dolma Drungtso. *Bod lugs sman rtsis kyi tshig mdzod bo dbyin shar sbyar* [Tibetan-English Dictionary of Tibetan Medicine and Astrology]. Dharamsala: Drungtso Publications, 2005 [repr. 1999].

Emmerick, Ronald E. "A Chapter from the Rgyud-bzhi." *Asia Major* 19, no. 2 (1975): 141–62.

Emmerick, Ronald E. "Sources of the rGyud-bzhi." In *Zeitschrift der Deutschen Morgenlandischen Gesellschaft* 2, no. 3 (1977): 1135–42.

Emmerick, Ronald E. *Vāgbhaṭa's Aṣṭāṅgahṛdayasaṃhitā: The Romanised Text Accompanied by Line and Words Indexes, comp. and ed. by Rahul Peter Das & Ronald Eric Emmerick*. Groningen: Forsten, 1998.

Fenner, T. "The Origin of the rGyud bzhi: A Tibetan Medical Tantra." In *Tibetan Literature: Studies in Genre*, edited by José I. Cabezón and Roger R. Jackson, 458–69. Ithaca, NY: Snow Lion, 1996.

Flatley, Jonathan. *Affective Mapping, Melancholia and the Politics of Modernism*. Cambridge, MA: Harvard University Press, 2008.

Foucault, Michel. *Folie et déraison: Histoire de la folie à l'âge Classique*. Paris: Gallimard, 1972 [repr. 1961]. [Later published in abbreviated form in the Union générale d'éditions 10/18 series in 1964, as *Histoire de la folie à l'âge classique*, this was later translated as: *Madness and Civilization: A History of Insanity in the Age of Reason* (New York, NY: Random House, 1965); and later translated in full as: *History of Madness* (New York, NY: Routledge, 2006). Cf. also earlier drafts, such as, *Maladie mentale et personnalité* (1954), later revised as *Maladie mentale et psychologie* (1962)—*Mental Illness and Psychology* (1967).]

Foucault, Michel. *Les Mots et Les Choses*. Paris: Gallimard, 1966. [Translated as: *The Order of Things*. New York, NY: Vintage, 1994.]

Foucault, Michel. *L'Archéologie du savoir*. Paris: Gallimard, 1969. [Translated as *The Archaeology of Knowledge*. New York, NY: Routledge, 2002.]

Gaines, Atwood D. *Ethnopsychiatry, The Cultural Construction of Professional and Folk Psychiatries*. SUNY Series in Medical Anthropology. Albany, NY: SUNY Press, 1992.

Gerke, Barbara. "On the History of the Two Tibetan Medical Schools: Janglug and Zurlug." In *AyurVijnana* 6 (1999).

Gerke, Barbara. "The Authorship of the Tibetan Medical Treatise *Cha lag bco brgyad* (Twelfth Century AD) and a Description of its Historical Background." *Traditional South Asian Medicine* 6 (2001): 27–50.

Gyatso, Janet. *Being Human in a Buddhist World: An Intellectual History of Medicine in Early Modern Tibet*. New York, NY: Columbia University Press, 2015.

Horstmanshoff, Manfred, and Cornelis van Tilburg. *Hippocrates and Medical Education: Selected papers read at the XIIth international Hippocrates Colloquium Universiteit Leiden, 24–26 August 2005*. Leiden: Brill, 2010.

Horstmanshoff, Manfred, Helen King, and Claus Zittel. *Blood, Sweat and Tears: The Changing Concepts of Physiology from Antiquity into Early Modern Europe*. Leiden: Brill, 2012.

Karmay, Samten G., "The Appearance of the Little Black-headed Man." In *The Arrow and the Spindle: Studies in History, Myths, Rituals and Beliefs in Tibet*, 245–81. Kathmandu: Mandala Book Point, 1998[b] [repr. 1986]. [First appeared as "L'apparition du petit home tète-noire." *Journal Asiatique* 274, nos. 1–2 (1986): 79–138.]

Karmay, Samten G. *A Catalogue of Bonpo Publications*. Tokyo: Toyo Bunko, 1977.

Karmay, Samten G. *The Little Luminous Boy*. Bangkok: White Orchid Press, 1998[a].

Karmay, Samten G. *The Treasury of Good Sayings: A Tibetan History of Bon*. London Oriental Series, vol. 26. Delhi: Motilal Banarsidass 2001 [repr. 1972].

Karmay, Samten G. "Vairocana and the *rGyud-bzhi*." *Tibetan Medicine: A Publication for the Study of Tibetan Medicine* 12 (1989): 19–31.

Kleinman, Arthur, and Byron Good, eds. *Culture and Depression: Studies in the Anthropology and Cross-cultural Psychiatry of Affect and Disorder*. Berkeley, CA: University of California Press, 1985.

Kletter, Christa, and Monika Kriechbaum. *Tibetan Medicinal Plants*. Boca Raton, FL: CRC Press/Medpharm, 2001.

Klibansky, Raymond, Erwin Panofsky, and Fritz Saxl. *Saturn and Melancholy: Studies in the History of Natural Philosophy, Religion and Art*. Nendeln: Kraus Reprint, 1979 [repr. 1964].

Köhle, Natalie. "A Confluence of Humors: Āyurvedic Conceptions of Digestion and the History of Chinese 'Phlegm' (*tan* 痰)." *Journal of the American Oriental Society* 136, no. 3 (2016): 465–93.

Köhle, Natalie. *Phlegm* (tan 痰)*: Toward a History of Humors in Early Chinese Medicine*. Cambridge, MA: Doctoral Dissertation at Harvard University, 2015.

Komito, David. "Tibetan Buddhism and Psychotherapy: Conversations with the Dalai Lama." *Journal of Transpersonal Psychology* 15, no. 1 (1983): 10.

Kottow, Michael H. "A Medical Definition of Disease." *Medical Hypotheses* 6, no. 2 (1980): 209–13.

Kuriyama, Shigehisa. *The Expressiveness of the Body and the Divergences of Greek and Chinese Medicine*. New York, NY: Zone Books, 2002.

Kuriyama, Shigehisa. "Forgotten Fear of Excrement." *Journal of Medieval and Early Modern Studies* 38, no. 3 (2008): 413–42.

Kuriyama, Shigehisa. "When Money Became a Humour." In *The Body in Balance: Humoral Medicines in Practice*, edited by Peregrine Horden and Elisabeth Hsu, 69–85. New York, NY: Berghahn Books, 2013.

Kværne, Per. "The Canon of the Bonpos." *Indo-Iranian Journal* 16 (1975): 18–56 [Pt. I: "Introduction"], 96–144 [Pt. II: "Index of the Canon"].

Kværne, Per. "A Chronological Table of the Bon po the bsTan rtsis of Ñi ma bstan 'jin." *Acta Orientalia* 33 (1971): 203–82.

Lund, Mary Ann. *Melancholy, Medicine and Religion in Early Modern England: Reading The Anatomy of Melancholy*. Cambridge: Cambridge University Press, 2010.

Martin, Dan P. "An Early Tibetan History of Indian Medicine." In *Soundings in Tibetan Medicine: Anthropological and Historical Perspectives. PIATS 2003, Tibetan Studies: Proceedings of the International Association for Tibetan Studies*, Oxford 2003, edited by Mona Schrempf, 305–26. Leiden: Brill, 2007.

Martin, Dan P. "Greek and Islamic Medicines' Historical Contact with Tibet." In *Islam and Tibet: Interactions along the Musk Routes*, edited by Anna Akasoy, Charles Burnett, and Ronit Yoeli-Tlalim, 117–43. Farnham, VT: Ashgate, 2011.

Martin, Dan P. *Tibetan Histories: A Bibliography of Tibetan-Language Historical Works*. London: Serindia Publications, 1997.

Martin, Dan P., Yasuhiko Nagano, and Per Kværne, eds. *A Catalogue of the Bon Kanjur*. Bon Studies, vol. 8. Senri Ethnological Reports, vol. 40. Osaka: The National Museum of Ethnology, 2003.

Mayo, Thomas. *An Essay on the Influence of Temperament in Modifying Dyspepsia, or Indigestion*. London: 1831.

McGrath, William A. *Buddhism and Medicine in Tibet: Origins, Ethics, and Tradition*. Charlottesville, VA: Doctoral Dissertation at the University of Virginia, 2017.

McGrath, William A. "Early Developments in Tibetan Sphygmology: The Yellow Emperor and the Moon King." Presented at the XIIIth Seminar for the International Association of Tibetan Studies, Ulaanbaatar, July 22, 2013.

McGrath, William A. "Vessel Examination in the *Medicine of the Moon King*." In *Buddhism and Medicine: An Anthology of Premodern Sources*, edited by C. Pierce Salguero, pp. 501–513. New York, NY: Columbia University Press, 2017.

Meulenbeld, G. J., and Dominik Wujastyk. *Studies on Indian Medical History: Papers Presented at the International Workshop on the Study of Indian Medicine Held at the Wellcome Institute for the History of Medicine, 2–4 September 1985*. Groningen: Forsten, 1987.

Meulenbeld, G. J. *A History of Indian Medical Literature*, five volumes. Groningen: Forsten, 1999–2002.

Meyer, Fernand. *Gso-ba rig-pa: Le système médical tibétain*. Paris: Presses du CNRS, 1988.

Meyer, Fernand. "Introduction à l'étude d'une série de peintures médicales créée à Lhasa au XVIIe siècle." In *Tibet, Civilisation et Société*, edited by Fernand Meyer, 29–58. Paris: Editions de la Fondation Singer-Polignac et de la Maison des Sciences de l'Homme, 1990[a].

Meyer, Fernand. "Introduction: The Medical Paintings of Tibet." In *Tibetan Medical Paintings: Illustrations to the Blue Beryl Treatise of Sangye Gyamtso (1653–1705)*, edited by Yuri Parfionovitch et al., vol. 1, 2–13. New York, NY: Harry N. Abrams, Inc., 1992.

Meyer, Fernand. "Programme de l'année 2001–2." In *Livret-Annuaire* 17. Paris: EPHE, 2002.

Meyer, Fernand. "Theory and Practice of Tibetan Medicine." In *Oriental Medicine*, edited by J. V. Alphen and A. Aris, 109–43. London: Serindia, 1995.

Meyer, Fernand. "Théorie et pratique de l'examen des pouls dans un chapitre du *rGyud-bzhi*." In *Indo-Tibetan Studies: Papers in Honour and Appreciation of Professor David L. Snellgrove's Contribution to Indo-Tibetan Studies*, edited by Tadeusz Skorupski, 209–56. Tring: Institute of Buddhist Studies, 1990[b].

Nagano, Yasuhiko. *A Survey of Bonpo Monasteries and Temples in Tibet and the Himalaya*. Bon Studies, vol. 7. Senri Ethnological Reports, vol. 38. Osaka: The National Museum of Ethnology, 2003.

Nagano, Yasuhiko, and Samten G. Karmay. *A Catalogue of the New Collection of Bonpo Katen Texts*. Bon Studies, vols. 3–4. Senri Ethnological Reports, vols. 24–25, two volumes. Osaka: The National Museum of Ethnology, 2001.

Obeyesekere, Gananath. "Depression, Buddhism, and the Work of Culture in Sri Lanka." In *Culture and Depression: Studies in the Anthropology and Cross-cultural Psychiatry of Affect and Disorder*, edited by Arthur Kleinman and Byron Good, 134–52. Berkeley, CA: University of California Press, 1985.

Parker, Gordon, and Dusan Hadzi-Pavlovic, ed. *Melancholia: A Disorder of Movement and Mood: A Phenomenological and Neurobiological Review*. Cambridge: Cambridge University Press, 1996.

Parfionovitch, Yuri, Fernand Meyer, and Gyurme Dorje, eds. *Tibetan Medical Paintings: Illustrations to the Blue Beryl Treatise of Sangye Gyamtso (1653–1705)*. New York, NY: Harry N. Abrams, Inc. Publishers, 1992.

Pormann, Peter E., ed. *Ruphus of Ephesus, On Melancholy*. Scripta Antiquitatis Posterioris ad Ethicam Religionemque pertinentia, vol. 12. Tübingen: Mohr Siebeck, 2008.

Prost, Audrey. "*Sa cha 'Di ma 'Phrod na* ... Displacement and Traditional Tibetan Medicine among Refugees in India." In *Soundings in Tibetan Medicine: Anthropological and Historical Perspectives. PIATS 2003, Tibetan Studies: Proceedings of the*

International Association for Tibetan Studies, Oxford 2003, edited by Mona Schrempf, 45–64. Leiden: Brill, 2007.

Radden, Jennifer, ed. *The Nature of Melancholy, From Aristotle to Kristeva*. Oxford: Oxford University Press, 2000.

Samuel, Geoffrey. "Tibetan Medicine in Contemporary India: Theory and Practice." In *Healing Powers and Modernity: Traditional Medicine, Shamanism, and Science in Asian Societies*, edited by L. Connor and G. Samuel, 247–74. London: Bergin and Garvey, 2001.

Savage-Smith, Emilie. "Were the Four Humours Fundamental to Medieval Islamic Medical Practice?" In *The Body in Balance: Humoral Medicines in Practice*, edited by Peregrine Horden and Elisabeth Hsu, 89–106. New York, NY: Berghahn Books, 2013.

Schmidt, Jeremy. *Melancholy and the Care of the Soul: Religion, Moral Philosophy and Madness in Early Modern England*. Burlington, VT: Ashgate Publishing, 2007.

Shorter, Edward, and Max Fink. *Endocrine Psychiatry: Solving the Riddle of Melancholia*. Oxford: Oxford University Press, 2010.

Solomon, Andrew. *The Noonday Demon: An Atlas of Depression*. NewYork, NY: Scribner, 2015.

Sournia, Jean-Charles, Jacques Poulet, and Marcel Martiny. *Illustrierte Geschichte der Medizin. Geschichte der Medizin, der Pharmazie, der Zahnheilkunde und der Tierheilkunde*. Translated by Michael Hesse, 9 vols. Salzburg: Andreas und Andreas, 1980–1984.

Stewart, Keith Andrew. *What Factors Influence Galen's Development of a Theory of Black Bile for His Explanation of Health and Disease in the Body?* Exeter: Doctoral Dissertation at the University of Exeter, 2016.

Taube, Manfred. *Beitrage zur Geschichte der Medizinischen Literatur Tibets*. Sankt Augustin: VGH Wissenschaftsverlag, 1981.

Taylor, Michael A., and Max Fink. *Melancholia, The Diagnosis, Pathophysiology, and Treatment of Depressive Illness*. Cambridge: Cambridge University Press, 2006.

Toohey, Peter. *Melancholy, Love, and Time: Boundaries of the Self in Ancient Literature*. Ann Arbor, MI: University of Michigan Press, 2004.

Unschuld, Paul U. *Medicine in China: A History of Ideas*. Berkeley, CA: University of California Press, 1985.

Vogel, Claus, trans. *Vāgbhaṭa's Aṣṭāṅgahṛdayasaṃhitā: The First Five Chapters of its Tibetan Version*. Abhandlungen fur die Kunde des Morgenlandes. Wiesbaden: Deutsche Morgenländische Gesellschaft, Komissionsverlag Franz Steiner GMBH, 1965.

Webb, James. *Flight from Reason*. London: The Book Service Ltd., 1971. [Cf. *The Occult Underground*. Chicago, IL: Open Court Publishing, 1974.]

Winder, Marianne. "Tibetan Medicine Compared with Ancient and Mediaeval Western Medicine." *Bulletin of Tibetology* 1 (1981): 5–22.

Yang Ga. *The Sources for the Writing of the Rgyud bzhi, Tibetan Medical Classic.* Cambridge, MA: Doctoral Dissertation at Harvard University, 2010.

Yonten, Pasang. "A History of the Tibetan Medical System." *Tibetan Medicine* 12 (1989): 32–51.

Zhang, Yisun. *Bod rgya tshig mdzod chen mo*. Beijing: Mi rigs dpe skrun khang, 1996 [repr. 1993].

Appendix 1—*sMan dpyad zla ba'i rgyal po*—Dharamsala 1994[98]

p. 12.18f. (1. *lus bskyed pa dang nus pa rdzogs pa bstan pa/*; embryology, week forty-three; Yang Ga: "The first chapter of the work discusses embryology"**):**

... / /bdun phrag bzhi bcu rtsa gsum na/ /las kyi dbang gis skye bar
byed (nyis brgya go lnga na pho mo gang yin skye ba ste)/ /mkhris pa shas che myur du skye (mdog
'gyur dang tsha ba dang rma bur 'gyur byed dang rigs bzhi la)/ /rlung yang myur du skye ba ste
(ldog pa'i rlung dang khyab pa'i rlung bskyod pa dang yang 'pho ba dang)/ /bad kan sha rgyas bul
ba'o (smug po dang ni ser po dang / skya bo dang ni nag po bzhi)/ / ...

pp. 27.19ff. (5. *ldang ba dang lus kyi tshad bstan pa/*; Yang Ga: "The fifth chapter describes the site and quantity of bodily organs, bodily constituents and humors. It discusses the locations and functions of the five subdivisions of wind bile and phlegm. It also indicates three abnormal humors and their anatomical mapping"**):**

bad kan lhag pa nad yin te/ /mkhal mar bad kan zhugs pa na/ /grang dang
mkhal tshil skran du'o/ /snod ni lgang phugs nad du 'gro /rde'u dag dang chu
sdoms pa'o/ /de nas yang lhag bsam se'u dang / /long du song bas long
skran dang / /mngal skran dang ni grang rlung ngo / /srog rtsar chu ser dkar por
'gro/ /mchin par song na khrag 'khrugs dang / /grang bar song na grang skran
[#028] *dang / /mchin par chu lud grang bar ro/ /bad rlung 'khrugs pas snying nad de/ /*
bad kan smug po dag yin no/ /rlung zhi bad kan khrag ror 'gro /rlung dang
bad kan mkhris par song / /rim ste rlung zhi bad kan sel/ /bad kan zhi nas
tshad rnying du'o/ /rlung dang bad kan glor song na/ /glo 'khrugs bad kan zhi ba
'o/ tshad rnying zhi bas bad kan 'tshangs/ /mcher par bad kan song ba na/ /

98 I gratefully acknowledge the use of the ITTM e-text, which is based on this edition and was kindly provided by Barbara Gerke. Notes appear in parenthesis; key references in underline.

nag po rlung dang bsdongs pa'o/ /mkhris pa'i gnas (cha shas che dang drod dang gzi mdangs cha/ de la me drod che) su mkhris pa< pa>'o/ / ...

pp. 36.22ff (6. *nad gzhi ji ltar gnas pa bstan pa/*; *bad kan* in the liver is brown; Yang Ga: "Chapter six discusses various topics regarding diseases, such as their cause and location. It also talks about the nature of food, tastes, and provides classification of food and medicine that is based on four elements. It gives a detailed interpretation of the digestive process. The chapter also indicates the relationship between the seasons and humors. Finally, it discusses abnormal humors in the organs. It talks about different diseases in the heart, lung, liver, gallbladder, spleen, stomach, kidney and bladder"**):**

... / /bad kan dbye na mang yod de/ /pho ba la gnas dkar po yin/ / mchin pa la gnas smug po yin/ /ser po mkhris par bsdongs pa'o/ / dmar [#037] *po (mkhal ma la gnas pa yin zer) glo la gnas pa yin/ /bad kan nag po mcher par te/ /rlung dang bsdongs pas nag po'o/ / ...*

p. 44.13 (10. *lta ba chu'i dpyad las drang srong dang bstun pa/*; urine diagnosis, color urine; Yang Ga: "Chapters ten to fourteen contain extensive description of urine diagnosis [*chu la brtag pa*]"**):**

... / smug po bad kan smug po rgyas/ /dmar smug sla ba rlung dang grang ba'o/ kham smug bad kan skya bo rgyas/ /dkar smug bad kan ma zhu rlung / / mdog nag chad pa bad kan nag /chu ser nag dang rlung bsdongs pa'o/ ...

p. 45.11f (10. *lta ba chu'i dpyad las drang srong dang bstun pa/*; urine diagnosis, color bubbles; Yang Ga: "Chapters ten to fourteen contain extensive description of urine diagnosis [*chu la brtag pa*]"**):**

... / /smug pa bad kan smug po'o/ / ...

p. 57.11f (14. *tha skar la bstan pa'i ling tshe dgu pa/*; Yang Ga: "Chapters ten to fourteen contain extensive description of urine diagnosis [*chu la brtag pa*]"**):**

... /rlung ni kha dog sngon po ste/ /mkhris pa ser te gser bzhin ni/ /bad kan smug po snyigs ma dkar/ / ...

p. 63.14ff (16. *snying rtsa bstan pa/*; pulse of the heart; Yang Ga: "Chapters fifteen to twenty-four contain very detailed description of pulse diagnosis [*rtsa la brtag pa*]"**):**

... / /g.yas g.yon mtho dman byed pa ni/ /g.yab mo g.yob pa dgra yi rtsa/ /grang la mang nyung bsngor ma btub/ /'khrugs shing mi gsal mya ngan rtsa/ /ya zur zhan la ma zur drag / g-yas pa pha sa g.yon pa dag /ma sa yin par shes par bya/ /stod mtho smad zhan smad mtho zhing / /stod zhan dag kyang 'dre sdod yin/ /'dar zhing mkhrang ba bad smug po/ /yang na bying ba bad kan smug po'o/ / ...

p. 65.3 (19. *glo rtsa bstan pa/*; pulse of the lung; Yang Ga: "Chapters fifteen to twenty-four contain very detailed description of pulse diagnosis [*rtsa la brtag pa*]"):

... de nas g.yas pa'i tshon la ni/ /glo rtsa dag ni blta ba ste/ /gsum pa snyoms la dang po stong / /glo ba rlung ni zhugs pa ste/ /gsum pa khong grims tshon rtsa ni/ /grims pa bad kan ('bur na khrag) smug po'o/ / ...

p. 66.14ff (20. *mcher rtsa bstan pa/*; pulse of the spleen; Yang Ga: "Chapters fifteen to twenty-four contain very detailed description of pulse diagnosis [*rtsa la brtag pa*]"):

... / /kan rtsa nyam chung pho mcher rgud/ /kan rtsa mdud pa thum por 'phar/ /bad kan nag po yin te skyug /kan rtsa dal la gang bar 'phar/ / bad kan rgyas pa'i nad yin no/ /kan rtsa phra la grims pa ni/ /bad kan ser po dag gi nad/ /rtsa gsum bying la grims pa na/ /bad kan smug po dag yin no/ / ...

pp. 87.7ff (26. *bad kan gyi mtshan nyid bstan pa/*; Yang Ga: "From chapters twenty-five to fifty-one, the author of the text discusses the causes, conditions, divisions, and symptoms of the following diseases ... phlegm diseases ..."):

bad kan dag gi rgyu dag ni/ /'grangs dang rlan la 'dug pa dang / /ma zhu ngal dub bcud can zas/ /chu'am chang mang 'thungs las byung / /dbye na smug po dkar po dang / /ser po dang ni dmar po dang / /nag po dang ni chu skyags dang / /bad kan 'ju skem dang bdun no/ /bad kan smug po rnam lnga ni/ / mchin pa'i nad dag yin pa ste/ /mchin dri yol kar babs pa ste/ khong tsha mig rus na ba ste/ /lci la byin pa mi theg dang / /rked pa na dang sgal par 'dril/ /chu dmar srog rtsa gcu ba dang / /zas mi 'dod cing rgyun skam mo/ / mchin pa dag la babs pa ni/ /sna khrag 'dzag cing khrag tu skyug /mchin pa'i kha na klad pa gzer/ /bkrag nyams mdog ni nag po'o/ /smug po mchin pa zags pa ni/ /sha ser gsus pa che ba dang / /byin rtsa phyi ru byung ba dang / /sha 'bros yan lag phra ba'o/ /smug po glo mchin 'tshangs pa ni/ khrag rnag lu dang rnag bam lu/ /ro stod gzer la rkang pa rengs/ /'gros drags chang mang 'thungs na na/ khrag rtsa skyugs nyam chung mkhal rked zhan/ /smug po glo la babs pa ni/ /brang tsha btsos khrag 'dra ba skyug /pho ba dag nas de 'byung ngo/ /bad kan dkar po rnams gsum ni/ /dkar po glo rtsa la babs pa ni/ /lhen sna na zhing brang tsha ste/ /stod brgyangs kha kha klad pa 'khor/ /dkar po pho bar babs pa [#088] *ni/ /brang tsha chu tshan skyug pa'o/ /bad kan grum bu dkar po ni/ /lhen snar dregs chags brang tsha zhing / /gang na cha med zas mi zhim/ /nyva bzhi dang ni mig rus brtse/ /dog pa bcangs pa 'dra ba'i srin/ /bar 'ga' 'khru skyug mig mi gsal/ /ser po mkhris pa las gyur te/ /de las rnam pa gnyis dag go / ser po pho bar babs pa ni/ /mdog ser ba dang tsha ba dang / /zas ni mi 'ju mi 'phrod cing / /sgyid skyur shed nyam chung ba dang / /zas ches pas ni na ba'o/ / grang ba dag dang 'thab pa'o/ /ser po long du lhung ba ni/ khong sbos 'khrog cing long mi bde/ /zas kyang phan gnod mi shes te/ /long chu ser po skyugs pa dang / khong nyam chung zhing mkhal rked na/ -khong dbugs 'byung zhing rnga pas thebs/ /bad kan nag po pho mcher la/ /babs pas gnyid che bying ba yin/ / nyva bzhi na zhing sgyid pa skyur/ khong sbos byed cing 'gro mi nus/ /grang ba'i mdog gam khrag nag 'khru/ /bad kan dmar po mkhal rtsa'am/ /srog rtsa rked pa dag la babs/ /dpyi dang rked pa 'khril zhing na/ /chu sri rdul dag 'ong ba 'o/ /sha chung nyam chung 'khru ba dmar/ /chu yang khrag tu 'ong ba'o/ /bad kan chu skyags dag gis ni/ /sgregs shing lbu ba can du skyug /nar nur skyug cing dang ga zhan/ /rgyu ba ngan pa sbyin dag go /'ju skems nyam chung sgyid pa skyur/ /sha chung gsus che byin pa 'dar/ /zas ci zos kyang 'grangs pa med/ /so ma rā dza las bad kan gyi mtshan nyid bstan pa'i le'u ste nyer drug pa'o// //.*

p. 100.9ff (34. *pho ba'i nad kyi mtshan nyid bstan pa/*; falls on stomach: *smug po*: brown blood from the liver; Yang Ga: "From chapters twenty-five to fifty-one, the author of the text discusses the causes, conditions, divisions, and symptoms of the following diseases ... stomachic diseases ..."**):**

... / /bad kan dag la lhen dang ni/ smug dang ser dang dkar po dang / / bad kan lcags dreg grang ba'i skran/ /lhen ni ma zhu dag la ste/ /be snabs dag gis gang bas so/ /<u>smug po mchin khrag</u> pho bar lhung / /gam 'khrugs rnyongs pa dag las byung / /mtshan nyid ngo snum dud ka skyug /dang ga mi bde lus lci'o/ / ser po ...

p. 112.9 (45. *dug brtag pa'i mtshan nyid bstan pa/*; Yang Ga: "From chapters twenty-five to fifty-one, the author of the text discusses the causes, conditions, divisions, and symptoms of the following diseases ... poisoning ..."**):**

... / /zas dug zas dang spyod lam mo/ /bad kan smug po can la ni/ /chang dang 'o ma 'dres pas dug /mar dang sbrang rtsi 'dres pa dag /'khar ba'i snod du zhag bdun (bzhag pa) dug /gro chang mar rnying 'dres pa dug /de rnams bad kan smug po la/ /yun ring na ba'i shul du ni/ /bud med dag dang lhan cig nyal/ /yun ring na ba'i mal shul nyal/ mchin pa rnyong bu'i dug tu'o/ / ...

pp. 147.21ff (57. *bad kan bcos thabs bstan pa/*; Yang Ga: "From chapters fifty-five to seventy-eight, the author discusses the following diseases ... phlegm diseases ..."**):**

de nas bad kan bcos pa ni/ /zas rtsub pa dang drod chen dang / /zas la thag yod snum nag nas/ /snum bag bcud can rul sungs spang / /bad kan [#148] *smug po bcos pa ni/ /sha ba'i tsho khu ma nu dang / /'u su kaṇṭa kā ri dang / / sle tres ma nu dag dang ni/ /ra mnye ba dang nye shing ba/ /mchog tu bsngags pa yin par gsung / /rtse'u cung ru thung snod rtsa gdab/ /shin tu skyugs na gson khrag gtang / /ma nu'i bshal ni mchog tu bsngags/ /a ru ra dang skyu ru ra/ /rgyam tshva ma nu'i thang gtang ngo- / /bzang drug gtang zhing chu grang blud/ /*

'bras bu gsum gyi thang bshal gtang / /chu blud chu bskol gtang bar bya/ / smug po 'thab na 'chi bar 'gyur/ /mchin pa zags pa de bzhin no/ /brag zhun kha ru tshva dag dang / /pi pi ling dang sbyar la gtang / /glo mig 'tshangs na star bu dang / /dzā ti cu gang sug smel dang / /sbrang rtsi'i lde gu gtang bar bya/ /glo rtsa dag kyang gtang bar bya/ /ma nu kaṇṭa kā ri dang / /a ru ra yi thang dang ni/ /bca' lga'i bzhi thang gtang bar bya/ /ma nu'i drod bshal gtang bar bya/ /rtsa grims lus lci ngo snum dang / /bad kan smug po dag tu'o/ / long du lhung na lte ba na/ /rgod zho mdzo zho shin tu bsngags/ /tshva chang bsrung zhing yan la gtad/ /bad mkhris 'doms rtsa gtar bar bya/ /gla ba dgo ba skom sha gtang / /lug sha gsar dang chang yang gtang / /rtsa ni shin tu zhan 'gyur na/ /skyug cing dang ga mi bde zhing / kha bsngal lce skya skam pa ni/ /ma nu'i bshal thang gtang bar bya/ /cung zad tsam ni skyug tu gzhug /shu mo za yi sman mar gtang / /bad kan smug po pho bar babs/ /ma nu'i bshal gtang snod bzhi gtar/ /bad kan mchin pa la song na/ /rdo bzhin 'ong zhing mig sprin nag /dang ga mi bde lus shed chung / /de ni 'chi bas spang bar bya/ /glo rtsa'i sbugs su song ba na/ /rtsa ba brgyad pa'i bshal bya'o/ /pho bar bu ram kha ru tshva/ /bca' lga cung tsam a ru ra/ /yang na se'u 'bru'i phye ma gtang / / bad kan dkar po glor song na/ /glo gsang bsreg cing zas drod gtang / /a [#149] *ru ra yi phye ma'am/ /yang na dzā ti sug smel dang / /cu gang shing mngar shing tshva dang / /sbrang rtsi'i lde gu gtang bar bya/ /dkar po pho bar babs pa na/ / sle tres kaṇṭa kā ri dang / /ma nu dong ga chang dang sbyar/ /ma nu'i bshal ni gtang bar bya/ /zas ni drod la bsten par bya/ /pho ba dag la de bzhin no/ / bad kan skran ni thur mang gis/ /bcos pa dag tu shes par bya/ /bad kan grum bu bcos pa ni/ /pi pi ling dang rgyam tshwa dang / /byi tang ka dang ru rta dang / /sug smel gla rtsi phye ma gtang / /pho ba'i rdzings dang long gsang bsreg- /bad kan ser po bcos pa ni/ /pho ba dag la babs pa na/ /rgyam tshva'i thang dang phye ma gtang / /long du babs pa bcos pa ni/ /'bras bu gsum gyi thang dag gtang / tig ta dag gi 'jam rtsi gtang / /mcher par babs pa bad kan nag kha ru tshva yi thang dag gtang / /'bras bu gsum dang kha ru tshva/ /bu ram dag dang sbyar la gtang / /bad kan glo la babs pas dmar/ / dmar po gsum* (*skag btsod 'bri mog*) *gyi thang bshal gtang / /bad kan mkhal mar babs pa la/ /rtsa ba lnga dang da byid sha/ /sman mar gze ma'i chang dag gtang / /chu skyags dag la phan pa ni/ /drag po'i las ni shin tu shis/ yang ba'i zas dang rtsub pa gtang / /tshva ni shin tu bsngags pa ste/ /yang na so cha dag gis bya/ /bsku mnye dugs kyis shin tu bsngags/ /'ju skem dag la skyugs phan te/ /sbrang rgod skyugs ni shin tu bsngags/ /yang na so cha dag gis bya/ / yang na dkar po* (*'bri rta sa 'dzin*) *gcig skyugs gtang / /bca' lga kha ru tshva dag dang / /a ru ra dang skyu ru ra'i/ /phye ma bu ram dag dang sbyar/ /bad kan pho bar babs pa ni/ /bsregs pas 'gal bar mi 'gyur ro/ /so ma rā dza las bad kan bcos pa'i le'u ste nga bdun pa'o// //.*

p. 153.19f (60. *glo nad bcos thabs bstan pa/*: *bad kan smug po* gathers in the gall bladder; Yang Ga: "From chapters fifty-five to seventy-eight, the author discusses the following diseases ... lung diseases ..."):

... / / byad ser skya la rbab pa dang / /rtsa grims chu mdog gur gum 'dra/ /'bras bu gsum gyi thang gshal gtang / /rtse'u chung gdab la sman yang gtang / /tshva dang rul sungs bsrung bar bya/ /bad kan smug po mkhris par bsdongs/ /glo yi rtsa dang mkhris rtsa gtar/ / ...

p. 231.10 (87. *sna bshal gyi skor bstan pa/*; Yang Ga: "From chapters seventy-nine to ninety-four, the author of [the] text talks about different forms of compounds, various therapies, the powers of medicines and food, and human behaviour. These chapters cover the following different forms of medical compounds: ... They also cover the following therapies: ... nasal cleansing ..."):

... / /bad kan smug po skyugs pa dang / / ...

p. 249.13ff (92. *darya kan gyi skor bstan pa/*; Yang Ga: "From chapters seventy-nine to ninety-four, the author of [the] text talks about different forms of compounds, various therapies, the powers of medicines and food, and human behaviour. These chapters cover the following different forms of medical compounds: ... Some chapters also talk about diet, behaviour, and medicine.... Chapter ninety-one discusses the powers of medicine and some recipes ...."):

... / /tshva rnams khrag mkhris kun la gnod/ /rgyam tshva kha ru tshvas ni bad rlung sel/ /rgyam tshva lce myang tshvas ni nus pa 'dra/ /tsabs ru tshvas ni pho ba'i ma zhu sel / -kha ru tshvas ni grang nad rlung nad dang / /tshad pa rnying pa rlung gi mi 'byang sel/ /bad kan smug po'i nad la 'di rnams phan/ /rgyam tshvas skyugs pa dag kyang gcod/ /'khru dang skyugs pa dag kyang 'byed/ /rgya tshwas ...

p. 252.9ff (93. *zas dang sha'i skor bstan pa/*; Yang Ga: "From chapters seventy-nine to ninety-four, the author of [the] text talks about different forms of compounds, various therapies, the powers of medicines and food, and human behaviour. These chapters cover the following different forms of medical compounds: ... Some chapters also talk about diet, behaviour, and medicine .... Chapter ninety-three discusses the powers of grain and meat...."):

khrag dang mkhris pa me dang 'dra ste tsha ba'i rang bzhin yin/ /bad kan smug po sa dang 'dra ste lci ba'i rang bzhin yin/ /rlung ni nam mkha'i sprin dang 'dra ste tsha grang gnyis kar 'gyur/ /bad kan smug po chu dang 'dra ste grang zhing rlon pa'i rang bzhin no/ / ...

Appendix II

Transl. Vaidya Bhagwan Dash (1999:1–7):

Chapter V
(*Of Man Ṅag Rgyud or Upadeśa Tantra*)
Treatment of 'Dus Bad-kan Smug-Po or
Sannipātika Aruṇa-Kapha

Prologue

Thereafter, the sage Yid-las-skyes (Manasija) solicited as follows:

O! Great Sage Rig-pa'i Ye-des (Vidyājñāna), earlier you have explained the method of treatment for the diseases caused by *rluṅ* (*vāyu*), *mkhris-pa* (*pitta*) and *bad-kan* (*kapha*). O! Giver of Life and King amongst the Physicians, I pray you to let us know the method of treatment of ailments caused by the combination of *doṣas* (*sannipāta*) along with their examples, names and classification.

Preceptor's Reply

Thereafter, the Preceptor replied as follows:

O! Great Sage Yid-las-skyes (Manasija), as per the treatment of the ailment caused by the combination of all the three *nad-pas* (*doṣas*), such an event takes place in three different ways, as follows:

(1) Combination of the *nad-pas* (*doṣas*) because of their own causative factors;
(2) Combination of *nad-pas* (*doṣas*) by the way of their time of manifestation; and
(3) By the way of simultaneous aggravation of these three *nad-pas* (*doṣas*). Afterwards they get manifested in the uncooked (*ma-smin* = *āma*) form which is hot and poisonous ailment (*āma-viṣa*).

Bad-kan Smug-po (*Aruṇa-kapha*)

To begin with, as an illustration, *Bad-kan Smug-po* (*Aruṇa-kapha*) will be described with reference to its eight different aspects as follows:

(I) *Rgyu* (*viprakṛṣṭa-hetu*) or distant cause;
(II) *Rkyen* (*sannikṛṣṭa-hetu*) or immediate cause;
(III) *Gnas* (*sthāna*) or location;
(IV) *Dus* (*kāla*) or time of provocation;
(V) *Rigs* (*kula*) or varieties
(VI) *Rtags* (*lakṣaṇa*) or signs including method of examination
(VII) *Bcos-pa'i thabs* (*cikitsā-vidhi*) or line of treatment; and
(VIII) *Rjes-bcad* (*uttarakāla-cheda*) or the treatment of the residual morbidity.

I Rgyu (Viprakṛṣṭa-Hetu) or Distant Cause

As per *the rgyu* (*viprakṛṣṭa-hetu*) or distant cause, [this ailment *bad-kan smug-po*] is caused by the aggravation or vitiation of four elements, viz., *bad-kan* (*kapha*), *khrag* (*rakta*) or blood, *mkhris-pa* (*pitta*), and *rlung* (*vāyu*).

Since the ailment is caused by the combination of all the *nad-pas* (*doṣas*), signs of all these *nad-pas* are manifested because of which it is difficult to cure.

II *Rkyen* (*Sannikṛṣṭa-Hetu*) or Immediate Cause

As per the *rkyen* (*sannikṛṣṭa-hetu*) or immediate cause, which is responsible for the manifestation of this ailment, it is of two types, as follows:

II(A) *Tsha* (*uṣṇa*) or hot; and
II(B) *Graṅ* (śīta) or cold.

II(A) Etiology and Pathogenesis of Bad-kan Smug-po Caused by Hot Ingredients

Because of the heating causative factors, the blood becomes excessively vitiated. Blood may also get vitiated because of surgical interventions. This vitiated blood falls on the liver which is the natural habitat of blood.

Alternatively, because of the intake of pungent and sour food, blood gets vitiated, and the liver gets enlarged. This causes malnourishment of the tissue elements. It becomes located in the liver, and falls upon the stomach to get mixed up with *bad-kan* (*kapha*). The putrefied *khrag* (*rakta*) or blood and *bad-kan* (*kapha*), thereafter, fall on, the small intestine. Being mixed with bile, it becomes smoky (*dud-khu*) in colour. This morbid matter, then, enters into the colon and gets associated with *rluṅ* (*vāyu*). The ailment, thus, manifested is called [*Bad-kan*] *Smug-po* (*Aruṇa-kapha*).

II(B) Etiology and Pathogenesis of Bad-kan Smug-po Caused by Cooling Ingredients

Manifestation of the *bad-kan smug-po* (*aruṇa-kapha*) by the cooling causative factors takes place as follows:

Because of the intake of undigestible and unwholesome ingredients, the food does not get digested in the stomach resulting in the formation of *be-snabs* (mucus = *āma*) in large quantity. As a result of this, the *mñam-rluṅ* (*samāna-vāyu*) and *'ju-byed* (*pācaka-pitta*) become less active. This mucous material, not being separated from (or by getting mixed with) the *daṅs* (*rasa*) or nutrient fluid, enters into the liver. As a result of this, the tissue elements do not get nourishment, the blood gets vitiated, and the liver gets enlarged. Like the exudation from a bolus, this morbid material falls on the stomach. Because of the circulation of this uncooked material, the *bad-kan* (*kapha*) which is cold in nature gets excessively aggravated.

This type of *bad-kan smug-po* remains hidden like a jackal. It is called *mas-chags* (upward rising) type of *bad-kan smug-po* (*ūrdhvaga aruṇa-kapha*).

III *Gnas (Sthāna) or Location of Bad-kan Smug-po*

Locations of *bad-kan smug-po* (*aruṇa-kapha*) are of two types as follows:

III(A) *Raṅ-gnas* (*sva-sthāna*) or own habitat; and

III(B) *Gźan-gnas* (*apara-sthāna*) or the habitat of others.

III(A) Own Habitat

Bad-kan smug-po (*aruṇa-kapha*) gets manifested in its own habitats which are four in number, as follows:

IIIA(a) *Pho* (*āmāśaya*) or stomach;

IIIA(b) *Mchin* (*yakṛt*) or liver;

IIIA(c) *Rgyu* (*kṣudrāntra*) or small intestine; and

IIIA(d) *Loṅ* (*pakvāśaya*) or large intestine.

IIIA(a) *Location in Stomach*

When located in the stomach, *bad-kan smug-po* gives rise to signs like the diseases of *bad-kan* (*kapha*).

IIIA(b) *Location in Liver*

When located in the liver, *bad-kan smug-po* gives rise to signs like those of blood diseases (*khrag-gi nad*).

IIIA(c) *Location in Small Intestine*

When located in the small intestine, *bad-kan smug-po* gives rise to signs like those of the diseases of *mkhris-pa* (*pitta*).

IIIA(d) *Location in Large Intestine*

When located in the large intestine, *bad-kan smug-po* gives rise to signs like those of the diseases caused by *rluṅ* (*vāyu*).

III(B) Location of Bad-kan Smug-po in Other's Habitats

Other's habitats in which *bad-kan smug-po* gets located (manifested) are of two types, as follows:

IIIB(a) *Phyi* (*bāhya*) or exterior of the body; and

IIIB(b) *Naṅ* (*ābhyantara*) or the interior of the body.

IIIB(a) *Location of Bad-kan Smug-po in the Exterior of Body*

If the *bad-kan smug-po* is located in the exterior of the body, then the following signs and symptoms are manifested:

(1) Growth of [tumours in] the muscles;

(2) Cold feeling in the skin;

(3) The skin appears like mud;

(4) If the vessels are afflicted, they appear as if poisoned; and
(5) Swelling in the joints.

IIIB(b) *Location of Bad-kan Smug-po in the Interior of Body*

When the *bad-kan smug-po* gets located in the interior of the body, it passes through the vital channels (*prāṇa-nāḍī*) and liver (*yakṛt*) to be mounted in the blood.

When it afflicts the vital channels, then the joints become stiff.

When it rises up to the head in the upper part of the body, it causes the diseases of the head.

When it approaches the lungs, it causes the diseases of the lungs.

When it reaches the heart, then the heart is afflicted with *rluṅ* (*vāyu*). When it reaches the spleen, it causes splenic disorders.

When it reaches the kidneys, then it causes the diseases of the kidneys.

CHAPTER 2

A Preliminary Study on the Biography of Yutok Yönten Gönpo the Elder: Reflections on the Origins of Tibetan Medicine

Yang Ga

1 Introduction

Today the question of Yutok Yönten Gönpo the Elder (*g.yu thog rnying ma yon tan mgon po*) is a very sensitive topic in the Tibetan areas of China, and it is the source of heated debates among Tibetan scholars and physicians. One group of scholars has attempted to prove that Yutok Yönten Gönpo the Elder is the most important Tibetan physician in Tibetan history, the one who composed the *Four Tantras* (*rgyud bzhi*).[1] Another group rejects this thesis and believes that the Elder Yutok is not the author of the *Four Tantras*, doubting whether he even was a historical figure.[2]

The life story of Yutok Yönten Gönpo the Elder that is commonly told today is based on a biography of the Elder Yutok, which will be introduced below.[3] Because of its later popularity, it is very important to understand the nature of this biography, including the questions of its authorship, reliability, and so on. According to the printer's colophon, Darmo Menrampa Lozang Chödrak (*dar mo sman rams pa blo bzang chos grags*), the personal physician of the Fifth Dalai Lama, edited and carved the biography in Lhasa in the seventeenth century. In 1982, the biography of the Elder Yutok was published by the Minzu Publishing House in Beijing.[4] Since then, the text has been available to Tibetan-reading scholars and physicians, including medical students in the Tibetan regions. The life story of the Elder Yutok became very popular in Tibetan intellectual circles, and the Elder Yutok biography was published again

1 Go 'jo dbang 'dus, *Rje btsun g.yu thog yon tan mgon po dang dpal ldan rgyud bzhi'i skor gleng ba* (unpublished paper, 2013).

2 Thub bstan phun tshogs, *G.yu thog rnying ma'i mtha' dpyad rgyal ba dgyes pa'i mchod sprin* (unpublished paper, 2014).

3 Jo bo lhun grub bkra shis and Dar mo sman rams pa blo bzang chos grags, *G.yu thog gsar rnying gi rnam thar* (Beijing: Mi rigs dpe skrun khang, 1982).

4 Jo bo lhun grub bkra shis, *G.yu thog gsar rnying gi rnam thar*.

 | DOI:10.1163/9789004404441_003

by the same press in 2005.[5] Rechung Rinpoche Jampal Kunzang translated the biography of the Elder Yutok into English in 1976.[6] Then the English version of the Elder Yutok biography was translated into Chinese in 1986.[7] Thus, by the late 1980s the history of the Elder Yutok had become well known to both English- and Chinese-reading audiences.

In following section, I will discuss the views of traditional Tibetan scholars, modern scholars in the PRC, as well as modern scholars in Europe and America. I also try to analyze the author, the time of composition, and the contents of the biography. I will point out the controversial accounts in the biography that contradict reliable Tibetan medical histories, as well as the standard sources for Tibetan political and religious history. Our knowledge of the history of Tibetan medicine, as well as the history of Yutok's lineage and the *Four Tantras*, is mainly based on the biography of the Elder Yutok. Because the reliability of these biographies is questionable, I am concerned that our present knowledge of the history of Tibetan medicine may not be as correct as we might hope or expect.

2 The Views of Traditional Tibetan Scholars

In his presentation of the biography of the Elder Yutok, Desi Sanggyé Gyatso (*sde srid sangs rgyas rgya mtsho*, 1653–1705) contradicts himself. On the one hand, he states that the Elder Yutok biography is not reliable, for it contradicts Buddhist doctrine in general and the *Four Tantras* in particular. He states that some of the concepts in the Elder Yutok biography are based on the Bön religion and Vedas.[8] On the other hand, the Desi's own account of the Elder Yutok is very similar to the Elder Yutok biography that was published by Darmo

5 Kong po bde rgyal and Dar mo sman rams pa blo bzang chos grags, *G.yu thog gsar rnying gi rnam thar* (Beijing: Mi rigs dpe skrun khang, 2005).

6 Rechung Rinpoche Jampal Kunzang, *Tibetan Medicine: Illustrated in Original Texts* (Berkeley, CA: University of California Press, 1976).

7 Riqiong Renpoqie Jiabai Gunsang, *Xizang yixue* (Lhasa: Xizang Renmin Chubanshe, 1986).

8 Sde srid sangs rgyas rgya mtsho, *Sde srid sman gyi khog 'bubs* (Beijing: Mi rigs dpe skrun khang, 2004), 154: ལོ་རྒྱུས་འདི་དག་ལ་དམ་པ་ཧོག་དཀར་མི་ཡུལ་དུ་ཐེབས་པ་དང་སངས་རྒྱས་གསེར་ཐུབ་ཀྱི་དུས་ནས་བོད་ཡུལ་ཆགས་ཟིན་པ་དང་། སྔོན་པོའི་རྒྱལ་པོར་མགོ་ཉི་ཤུ་རྩ་གཅིག་ཡོད་པ་སོགས་གསུང་རབ་སྤྱི་དང་མི་མཐུན་ཅིང་། རྡོ་རྗེ་གདན་ནས་དཔག་ཚད་གཅིག་དང་རྒྱང་གྲགས་གཅིག་གི་སར་གྲོང་ཁྱེར་ལྟ་ན་སྡུག་རི་བོ་སྤོས་ངད་ལྡན་དང་ཐུག་པ་དང་། ཕྱོགས་བཞིའི་རི་རྣམས་དཔག་ཚད་ལྔ་བརྒྱ་ཙམ་གྱི་ཕ་རོལ་ན་ཡོད་པའང་གསོ་དཔྱད་རྩ་རྒྱུད་དང་འགལ་ལ། ལྷ་མིའི་རྒྱུད་ལམ་ལ་ལྷའི་སྐུ་ཐབ་ཡོད་པ་གཡུང་དྲུང་བོན་གྱི་ཟེར་སྒྲོས་དང་། ཅི་འདོད་འགྲུབ་པའི་འཁོར་ལོ་སོགས་རིག་བྱེད་ཀྱི་གཏམ་རྒྱུད་ལྟ་བུ་ལས་ཡིད་བརྟན་དུ་རུང་བ་དཀའ་ནའང་།

Menrampa.[9] It seems clear that the Desi's own description of the Elder Yutok was based on the Elder Yutok biography published by Darmo Menrampa.

The Desi's medical history (*khog 'bubs*) was composed at the beginning of the eighteenth century. Most scholars of Tibetan medicine have accepted this work as providing an authentic history of Tibetan medicine. Thus, the Desi's narrative of the Elder Yutok, based in turn on the Elder Yutok biography published by Darmo Menrampa, became a kind of classical and orthodox interpretation for the life of the Elder Yutok, widely quoted in Tibetan medical literature. In Central Tibet, physicians and scholars never challenged this narrative regarding the Elder Yutok, but it is odd that nobody has heretofore paid attention to the Desi's criticisms of the Elder Yutok biography published by Darmo Menrampa.

Some Tibetan scholars from Eastern Tibet, however, did come to question the story about the Elder Yutok in the biography published by Darmo Menrampa and the Desi's medical history. For example, the eighteenth-century Tibetan scholar, Belo Tsewang Künkhyap (*'be lo tshe dbang kun khyab*, b. 1718), the disciple of Situ Panchen Chökyi Jungné (*si tu paṇ chen chos kyi 'byung gnas*, 1700–1774), vehemently rejected the biography of the Elder Yutok as unreliable. We find the following statement in his medical history:

> As mentioned previously in [Zurkhar] Lodrö Gyelpo's *Questions and Answers*, the biography of the so-called "Elder Yutok" must have been composed by Doctor Künlek because he lost [the debate]. Because of Darmowa's insistence, the Great Fifth gave permission to print the biography. Even though the Desi doubted the biography, his medical history and other works correspond with it. The reason is that he thought it was good for the "Buddha Word" thesis.[10] Regardless, this [biography] is a disaster for Tibetan medicine.[11]

---

9 Sde srid sangs rgyas rgya mtsho, *Sde srid sman gyi khog 'bubs*, 149–62.

10 Some Tibetan scholars have claimed that the *Four Tantras* (*rgyud bzhi*) is the "Word of the Buddha" (*sangs rgyas kyi bka'* = Skt. *buddhavacana*). They have tried to prove that the text was taught by an emanation of the Medicine Buddha or the Medicine Buddha himself. The position can be summarized as the "Buddha Word" (*bka' sgrub*) thesis.

11 'Be lo tshe dbang kun khyab, *'Be lo tshe dbang kun khyab kyi gsung thor bu'i skor* (Lhasa: Bod ljongs bod yig dpe rnying dpe skrun khang, 2013), 171: གཡུ་ཐོག་རྙིང་མ་ཟེར་བའི་རྣམ་ཐར་དེ་བློ་གྲོས་རྒྱལ་པོའི་དྲི་བ་དང་དྲིས་ལན་སྔར་བཤད་པ་ལྟར་ཨེམ་ཆི་ཀུན་ལེགས་པའི་མཚང་ལ་ཐོག་ནས་དེས་བྱས་པ་ལས་མ་འདས་ཀྱང་། དར་མོ་བས་དབང་ཡོད་ཀྱིས་རྗེ་ལྔ་པ་ཆེན་པོ་ལ་ཞུས་ནས་པར་དུ་གནང་བ་དང་། སྡེ་སྲིད་ནས་ཀྱང་ཐུགས་མ་ཆེས་བཞིན་དུ་རྒྱུད་བཞི་བཀའ་སྒྲུབ་ལ་ཕན་འདུག་དགོངས་ནས་སྤྱི་དོན་ཁོག་དབུབ་སོགས་དེ་དང་བསྟུན་པ་ནི་སྨན་དཔྱད་ཀྱི་ཆག་སློ་ཆེན་པོ་སྟེ།

He continues:

> To conclude, [the biography of Yutok the Elder] contradicts both the Canon of Translated Scriptures (Kangyur) and the Canon of Translated Treatises (Tengyur). It also contradicts all historical texts and the names of places and periods. If intelligent scholars read it once, they can easily notice that the biography is fake.[12]

Finally, Belo goes on to state that Zurkhar Lodrö Gyelpo sent many letters to the physicians of the different regions of Tibet, including a Doctor Künlek.[13] In Künlek's response to Zurkhar, he states that there were nine royal physicians during the reign of Tri Songdetsen (*khri srong lde btsan*, r. 755–ca. 800), including Yutok and Drangti. In the letter Künlek also tries to prove that the *Four Tantras* belongs to both the "continuous transmission" (*bka' ma*) and "treasure" (*gter ma*) traditions. Zurkhar Lodrö Gyelpo then composed several works in order to reject his thesis and answer his questions.[14] In these works, Zurkhar demonstrates that (1.) the name Yutok did not exist before the life of Drejé Gyagar Vajra (*'dre rje rgya gar badzra*); (2.) over two hundred years passed from the eighth-century reign of Tri Songdetsen to the life of Yutok Yönten Gönpo; and (3.) the name of the *Four Tantras* did not appear before Yutok Yönten Gönpo's lifetime. Belo asserts that Künlek secretly made a biography of the Elder Yutok in order to "prove" his existence to Zurkhar. Belo asserts that there is no record of two distinct Yutoks—namely, the Elder and the Younger—before that time.[15]

---

12 'Be lo tshe dbang kun khyab, *'Be lo tshe dbang kun khyab kyi gsung thor bu'i skor*, 171–72: མདོར་ན་ཚིག་དོན་ཐམས་ཅད་བཀའ་བསྟན་གྱི་དང་འགལ་བ། ལོ་རྒྱུས་ཀུན་དང་འགལ་བ་ཡུལ་དང་དུས་དང་འགལ་བ་སོགས་དཔྱོད་ལྡན་དག་གིས་ལན་གཅིག་མཐོང་བས་རྫུན་དུ་རྟོགས་ཤིན་ཏུ་སླ་བ་ཞིག་འདུག་གོ།

13 'Be lo tshe dbang kun khyab, *'Be lo tshe dbang kun khyab kyi gsung thor bu'i skor*, 141. According Belo's medical history, people also called Künlek by the name Panam Tsojé (*pa rnam 'tsho byed*).

14 Most these works have not found yet. Only one letter, namely, *'Tsho byed kun legs pa'i dris lan zla ba'i thig pa*, is preserved in the Degé Tibetan Medical Hospital of Ganzi Tibetan Autonomous Prefecture. The letter was published by the Lhasa Mentsikhang in 2016. See Zur mkhar ba blo gros rgyal po, *'Tsho byed kun legs pa'i dris lan zla ba'i thig pa*, in *Gangs ljongs sman rtsis rig mdzod chen mo* (Beijing: Krung go'i bod rig pa dpe skrun khang, 2016), vol. 40, 211–16.

15 'Be lo tshe dbang kun khyab, *'Be lo tshe dbang kun khyab kyi gsung thor bu'i skor*, 141–42: ཟུར་མཁར་བློ་གྲོས་རྒྱལ་པོས་ཕྱོགས་ཕྱོགས་ཀྱི་སྨན་པ་རྣམས་ལ་དྲི་ཡིག་མང་དུ་བྱས་ཏེ། སྟོད་ལུང་གི་ཨེམ་ཆི་ཀུན་ལེགས་ཟེར་བ་ཕྱིས་སུ་པ་རྣམ་འཚོ་བྱེད་དུ་འབོད་པ་ལ་འདང་དྲི་བ་བྱས་པའི་དྲིས་ལན་དུ། རྒྱལ་པོ་ཁྲི་སྲོང་ལྡེའུ་བཙན་གྱི་བླ་སྨན་དགུ་ནི་སྟོད་ན་ཆེར་རྗེ། ཨུག་པ། བི་ཇི་གསུམ།བར་ན་གཡུ་ཐོག་བྲང་ཏི། མི་ཉག་གསུམ།སྨད་ན་གཉའ་པ། མཐའ་བཞི། སྟོང་པ་གསུམ་སྟེ་དགུ་རུ་འདོད་པ་དང་། རྒྱུད་བཞི་བཀའ་གཏེར་ཡིན་པའི་སྒྲུབ་བྱེད་བཀོད་པ་སོགས་བྱུང་བར། ཟུར་མཁར་བས་སླར་ཡང་དྲིས་ལན་ལེགས་བཤད་རྒྱུགས་པ། ཟླ་ཐིགས། ཉིན་བྱེད་འོད་མཆོ། དབྱར་སྐྱེས་ཛ་གསང་རྣམས་བྱས་སྟེ། འདི་

The original copy of the medical history by Belo is written in a "headless" cursive script (*dbu med*), which is quite clear and legible. As far as I know, the text was never produced as a block print. Before the text was published in 2013, it was not available to most Tibetan physicians and scholars.[16] Thus, in recent years Tibetan physicians, scholars, and even ordinary Tibetan people have been shocked by Belo's comments and criticisms of the Elder Yutok biography. Some physicians and scholars have come to worry that Belo's comments might damage the reputation and integrity of Tibetan medicine as a whole.

3 The Views of Modern Scholars in the PRC

Under the guidance of the Ministry of Health of the People's Republic of China, the editorial committee of *China's Medical Encyclopedia: Tibetan Medicine* (*krung go'i gso rig kun 'dus las bod kyi gso ba rig pa*) was established at the Lhasa Mentsikhang in 1979. Many great Tibetan physicians and scholars, such as Khenpo Troru Tsenam (*mkhan po khro ru tshe rnam*, 1926–2004), Tupten Tsering (*thub bstan tshe ring*, 1908–1990), and Jampa Trinlé (*byams pa 'phrin las*, 1928–2011), were involved in composing this medical encyclopedia. Tupten Tsering and Jampa Trinlé were editors of the chapter entitled the "History of Tibetan Medicine" (*bod kyi gso ba rig pa'i lo rgyus*).[17] This is the first Tibetan-language scholarly work published in China to discuss the history of Tibetan medicine since the political turmoil of 1959. While composing the history, they used the biography of the Elder Yutok as the most important source for interpreting the early history of Tibetan medicine. They considered the Elder Yutok biography as an authentic and reliable source for Tibetan medical history. In addition, they assert that the Elder Yutok is the primary author of the *Four Tantras*.[18] Professor Jampa Trinlé repeated this thesis again in his own book on history of Tibetan medicine, called *China's Tibetan Medicine*

ཇེ་རྒྱ་གར་བརྡའི་གོང་ཡན་ལ་གཡུ་ཐོག་ཅེས་ཐ་སྙད་མེད་ཚུལ། ཆོས་རྒྱལ་དང་ཡོན་ཏན་མགོན་པོའི་བར་ལ་མི་ལོ་ཉིས་བརྒྱ་ཙམ་གྱི་སྔ་ཕྱི་ཡོད་ཚུལ། རྒྱུད་བཞི་གཡུ་ཐོག་མགོན་པོའི་གོང་ཡན་སུ་ལ་འང་མ་གྲགས་པའི་ཚུལ་སོགས་ལུང་རིག་རྡོ་རྗེ་ཟེགས་མས་ཚར་བཅད་དེ་སྣ་ཐུ་མེད་པར་བྱས་པ་ན། ཕྱི་རྗེས་རང་གི་སྨན་ཆོག་གི་ལོ་རྒྱུས་སྒྲུབ་བྱེད་དུ་གཡུ་ཐོག་མགོན་པོ་རྙིང་མ་ཞིག་ཡོད་ཚུལ་རྣམ་ཐར་དེ་ཁོ་པས་ཁྲོག་ཏུ་བྱས་པ་སྟེ། དེ་ཡན་ཆད་མཁས་སྨན་སུ་ལའང་གཡུ་ཐོག་མགོན་པོ་ཡབ་སྲས་གསར་རྙིང་གཉིས་ཡོད་པའི་སྒྲོས་གཏན་ནས་མེད་པའི་ཕྱིར་རོ།

16 'Be lo tshe dbang kun khyab, *'Be lo tshe dbang kun khyab kyi gsung thor bu'i skor*.

17 Byams pa 'phrin las and Thub bstan tshe ring, *Bod kyi gso ba rig pa'i lo rgyus*, in *Krung go'i gso rig kun 'dus las bod kyi gso ba rig pa* (Lhasa: Bod ljongs mi dmangs dpe skrun khang, 1990), vol. 1, 1–53.

18 Byams pa 'phrin las and Thub bstan tshe ring, *Bod kyi gso ba rig pa'i lo rgyus*, 12.

(*krung go'i bod kyi gso ba rig pa*).[19] Since then, this thesis has been widely used in Tibetan medical literature, such as the *History of Tibetan Medicine* (*gso rig lo rgyus*), the standard textbook for Tibetan medical schools in the PRC. They also maintain that the Elder Yutok is the primary author of the *Four Tantras*.[20] Interestingly, the thesis is not indicated in the biography of the Elder Yutok itself.

4 The Views of Modern Scholars in Europe and America

Since Rechung Rinpoche translated the biography of the Elder Yutok into English in 1973, the life story of the Elder Yutok has become popular among Western audiences. Many serious Western scholars, such as Ronald E. Emmerick and Christopher I. Bechwith, used this Elder Yutok biography as a reliable source in their works.[21]

Samten Karmay has asserted that Yutok Yönten Gönpo the Elder is a fictitious character and a transposition of Yutok Yönten Gönpo the Younger. He also believes that the *Four Tantras* was composed by Yutok Yönten Gönpo the Younger.[22] It seems to me that Karmay does not think that the biography of the Elder is a reliable source.

Marianne Winder disagrees with such sentiments, however, for she believes that we cannot deny the existence of the Elder Yutok just because that are legendary materials in his biography.[23] Before we assess these positions, let us first consider the provenance and contents of the biography of the Elder Yutok.

---

19 Byams pa 'phrin las, *Krung go'i bod kyi gso ba rig pa* (Beijing: Krung go'i bod kyi shes rig dpe skrun khang, 1996), 8.

20 Byams pa 'phrin las, *Gso rig lo rgyus* (Beijing: Mi rigs dpe skrun khang, 2004), 58–62.

21 Christopher I. Beckwith, "The Introduction of Greek Medicine into Tibet in the Seventh and Eighth Centuries," *Journal of the American Oriental Society* 99, no. 2 (1979): 297–313.

22 Samten G. Karmay, "The Four Tibetan Medical Tantras and Their Critics," in *The Arrow and the Spindle: Studies in History, Myths, Rituals and Beliefs in Tibet*, (Kathmandu: Mandala Book Point, 1998), 230: "The other interesting aspect of the *rNam thar bka' rgya can* is that it is totally silent with regard to the question of g.Yu-thog the first, who is said to have lived in the eight century. He is in all probability a transposition of g.Yu-thog Yon-tan mgon-po the second, who certainly lived around the twelfth century."

23 Rechung Rinpoche, *Tibetan Medicine*, 4: "While there is, of course, some legendary material in all mediaeval biographies, East and West, it seems absurd to deny altogether the existence of the famous hero of such a biography."

5 Who is the Author of the Elder Yutok Biography?

In the printer's colophon of the Elder Yutok biography, Darmo Menrampa claims that he found a copy of the biography of Yutok Yönten Gönpo the Elder from his descendant.[24] The biography of the Elder Yutok itself states that the Elder Yutok gave a prophecy that Penden Lhündrup (*dpal ldan lhun grub*) would compile his biography.[25] Although the Elder Yutok biography claims that Penden Lhündrup was a descendant of Yutok Yönten Gönpo, we can find information about such a person in neither the Tibetan medical histories (*khog dbub*) nor the standard Tibetan political and religious historical genres (*rgyal rabs* and *chos 'byung*). Putting this information together, it seems to me that Darmo Menrampa tried to suggest that the author of the Elder Yutok biography is Penden Lhündrup, but he himself edited and carved the seventeenth-century edition.

According to the Desi's *Mirror of Beryl*, Larawa Lozang Dönden (*la ra ba blo bzang don ldan*) edited the biography of Yutok Yönten Gönpo the Elder at the order of the Fifth Dalai Lama.[26] As we have seen, Belo Tsewang Künkhyap asserts that the Elder Yutok biography was composed by the Tibetan physician Künlek (16th century) after he had debated with Zurkhar Lodrö Gyelpo in the sixteenth century.

Based on these assertions, it is hard to determine the primary author of the Elder Yutok biography. Regardless, it seems clear that Darmo Menrampa or Larawa Lozang Dönden made the biography of the Elder Yutok known to the public with the support of the Fifth Dalai Lama in the seventeenth century.

6 The Time of Composition of the Elder Yutok Biography

In the biography of Yutok the Elder, we can find many names of physicians and medical works, and these are important sources of information for dating the composition of the Elder Yutok biography. For example, the biography discusses the *Golden Measuring Dish* (*gser bre*), a medical text compiled by Drangti Penden Gyeltsen (*brang ti dpal ldan rgyal mtshan*) in the fourteenth century. This evidence suggests that the original biography of the Elder Yutok was composed after the fourteenth century.

---

24 Jo bo lhun grub bkra shis, *G.yu thog gsar rnying gi rnam thar*, 312.

25 Jo bo lhun grub bkra shis, *G.yu thog gsar rnying gi rnam thar*, 127.

26 Sde srid sangs rgyas rgya mtsho, *Sde srid sman gyi khog 'bubs*, 269.

7 The Contents of the Elder Yutok Biography

There are four parts in the Elder Yutok biography. The first part explains why the life story of the Elder Yutok is reliable. The second part discusses how the Elder Yutok's ancestor came to Tibet from India. The third part describes how the Elder Yutok went to India from Tibet. The last part introduces how the Elder Yutok spread the teachings of medicine in Tibet.[27]

At beginning of the first part, the biography describes how Kongpo Degyel asked the Elder Yutok to tell his life story, along with the suggestion of eight beautiful ladies. The Elder Yutok refuses to tell his life story, however. The first part also describes Kongpo Degyel's dream, in which he goes to the Beautiful Medical City where the King of Medicine tells him that he is the person who is responsible for asking the life story of the Elder Yutok. Under the Kongpo Degyel's insistence, the Elder Yutok starts to tell his life story.[28] In the following section, I will discuss various controversial accounts that are recorded in the last three parts of the Elder Yutok biography.

8 Controversial Accounts in the Elder Yutok Biography

In the Elder Yutok biography, we can find various questionable narratives which have heretofore been ignored by most Tibetan and western scholars. Today, most Tibetan scholars consider the biography of the Elder Yutok as the most important source for interpreting the early history of Tibetan medicine. However, we can find that many descriptions in the biography contradict the standard Tibetan political and religious histories in general and the history of the Tibetan medicine in particular. I am afraid that this description in the biography may come from the author's imagination, and it is an unreliable historical document. In addition, the author of biography may not have had sufficient knowledge regarding the early history of Tibet. I am worried that the biography may not provide an authentic history Tibetan medicine in general, as well as the history of Yutok's lineage and the *Four Tantras* in particular. In the following section, I will identify and analyze twelve controversial accounts from the biography.

8.1 *The Legendary Homeland of the Elder Yutok's Ancestor*

It is said that there was a great land (*yul chen po*) called the "Land of Lotus Flowers," which consisted of nine districts, and each district had fifty-six

27 Jo bo lhun grub bkra shis, *G.yu thog gsar rnying gi rnam thar*, 4.
28 Jo bo lhun grub bkra shis, *G.yu thog gsar rnying gi rnam thar*, 4–11.

thousand cities. Śvetaketu (*dam pa tog dkar po*), the son of the gods, came down from heaven into the central district called the "Essence of Lotus Flowers." If the so-called "Land of Lotus Flowers" truly did have 504,000 cities, some information about the land should have been recorded in reliable sources, such as the *Great Tang Records on the Western Regions* by Tang Xuanzang (602–664),[29] or the biography of Chak Lotsawa Chöjé Pel (*chag lo tsā ba chos rje dpal*, 1197–1264).[30] Unfortunately, I have not found any information about a so-called "Land of Lotus Flowers" in India in these sources. I am afraid that this description may come from the author's imagination.

8.2 *The Legend of the Elder Yutok's Ancestor*

According to the Yutok biography, the Elder Yutok claims that his ancestry on his father's side is the same as the Buddha Śākyamuni.[31] It also states that the Elder Yutok's ancestry derives from heaven, however. The story can be summarized as follows:

Śvetaketu came down from heaven to earth and fell in love with a Brahmin woman. They had two sons. The son of the gods then went back to heaven two times. During his second journey, the evil husband of the Brahmin woman cut off his celestial rope (*rmu thag*), which connected the gods and humans. The husband of the Brahmin woman did this because he was jealous of the gods. Since then the connection between the gods and human has been broken.[32]

Here the author of biography says that the son of the gods could travel between heaven and earth through a rope called a *mutak* in Tibetan, which means "celestial rope." The concept of the celestial rope can be found in Tibetan legend. According to some Tibetan historical accounts, the first seven Tibetan kings went back to heaven through celestial ropes when their sons grew up.[33] The Desi believed that the concept of the celestial rope is a notion from the Bön religion. He writes that various controversial statements like these are difficult to accept.[34] Thus, the author of the Elder Yutok biography

29 Dong Zhiqiao, *Datang xiyuji* (Beijing: Zhonghua shuju, 2016).

30 Blo bzang dpal 'byor, *Bla ma chag lo tsā ba chos rje dpal ba'i rnam par thar pa bla ma'i gsung dri ma med bar sgrigs pa*, in *Lo chen rin chen bzang po dang/ chag lo tsā ba chos rje dpal/ rngo lo tsā ba blo ldan shes rab gsum gyi rnam thar* (Lhasa: Ser gtsug nang bstan dpe rnying 'tshol bsdu phyogs sgrig khang), 108–236.

31 Jo bo lhun grub bkra shis, *G.yu thog gsar rnying gi rnam thar*, 11; Rechung Rinpoche, *Tibetan Medicine*, 152.

32 Jo bo lhun grub bkra shis, *G.yu thog gsar rnying gi rnam thar*, 12–13; Rechung Rinpoche, *Tibetan Medicine*, 153.

33 Dpa' bo gtsug lag phreng ba, *Chos 'byung mkhas pa'i dga' ston* (Beijing: Mi rigs dpe skrun khang, 1986), 160.

34 Sde srid sangs rgyas rgya mtsho, *Sde srid sman gyi khog 'bubs*, 154.

used a Tibetan legend to tell a story that supposedly happened in the land of India. It seems to me that the author did not know whether the concept of the celestial rope originated in India or Tibet.

8.3 *The Origin of Sowa Rigpa*

The author of the Elder Yutok biography indicates that the Elder Yutok introduced Sowa Rigpa, the "science of medicine," to a Sogdian doctor according to his request. The following is summarized from Yutok's narrative: in India, there was a Brahmin called Hala Mikyang (*ha la mig yang*) and his wife. The wife was sick, so she asked her husband to treat her disease. Hala Mikyang went to search for medical teachings, and he met a naked rishi in the jungle. The Brahmin bowed before the rishi and gave a piece of gold, telling him all about his wife's illness. The rishi chanted a mantra and pointed to sky. The Medicine Buddha appeared in the sky, talked to the Brahmin, and then several medical tantras fell from sky. Hala Mikyang, the Brahmin, brought those texts and returned back to his hometown. Hala Mikyang gave those texts to Jowo Banu and, through several physicians, the texts were finally received by Biji Gajé, who transmitted the texts to the Dunggi Thorchok Chen. Finally, the Yutok lineage received those very same texts.[35]

As far as I know, such a legendary narrative regarding the origins of Sowa Rigpa cannot be found in any major Tibetan medical histories. It was included in neither Drangti's *Elucidation of Knowledge* (*shes bya rab gsal*), Zurkhar's *History of General Knowledge* (*shes bya spyi'i khog dbub*), nor the Desi's *Mirror of Beryl* (*baidurya'i me long*). A detailed analysis of the origin of Tibetan Medicine can be found in the following section.

8.4 *The Introduction of Indian Medicine into Tibet*

The Elder Yutok biography states that the brother and sister duo, Biji Gajé and Bilha Gazé, traveled to Tibet according to the prophecy of Tārā during the reign of Tibetan king, Lha Totori Nyenshel (5th century). When they arrived in Tibet, they saw a young lady carrying an old woman as she left her house. Then a very strange conversation ensues between the two Indian physicians and the Tibetan young lady. The two physicians ask her: "Why did you take this lady out of the house?" She replies: "She is my mother and she is sick." The physicians reply: "If she is your mother and particularly if she is sick now, please do not take her outdoors and let her stay in your home." The Young lady then says: "Even if she is my mother, the smell of disease might reach us, and the deities of the house will not be pleased. This is our Tibetan custom." After few lines,

35 Jo bo lhun grub bkra shis, *G.yu thog gsar rnying gi rnam thar*, 103–106.

there is another conversation between the physicians and the young lady. The physicians ask: "According to Tibetan custom, are all sick people taken outdoors?" She replies: "If children and grandchildren are sick, their parents will not take them out. If parents are sick, their children will turn them out."[36]

In the medical history of Drangti Penden Tsojé (ca. 1372),[37] he states that medical theory, such as the benefits and harms of certain diets and the methods for stopping bleeding from fresh wounds using melted butter, began to appear during the reign of the Tibetan king Lha Totori Nyenshel.[38] Thus, it is indeed possible that Tibetan medicine was founded during the reign of this Tibetan king. Drangti says again that King Tri Detsukten invited two Indian physicians, Biji and Bilha, to Tibet. The history records that the two physicians translated texts on medicine, divination, and astronomy into the Tibetan language. Among the corpus of medical literature that they translated, there are said to have been two texts called the *Root Text* and the *Commentary on the Explicit Treatise*.[39]

Zurkhar Lodrö Gyelpo rejects Drangti's position, for he states that numerous kinds of medical knowledge based on Bön religion already existed in Tibet before the reign of King Lha Totori Nyenshel. He further asserts that Shenrap Miwoché, the putative founder of Bön, was born as early as Śākyamuni, suggesting that it is improper to say that Tibetan medicine was founded during the reign of King Lha Totori Nyenshel. Drangti and Zurkhar never talk about the conversation between the two Indian physicians and the Tibetan young lady that is mentioned above. In *A Feast for Scholars* (*mkhas pa'i dga' ston*), Pawo Tsuklak Trengwa also does not mention the journey of two Indian physicians to Tibet at all.

8.5 *How the Name of Yutok Began to Be Used for Their Family*

The name Yutok literally means "turquoise roof" in Tibetan. The author of the Elder Yutok biography indicates that name Yutok was first used during the

36 Jo bo lhun grub bkra shis, *G.yu thog gsar rnying gi rnam thar*, 60–63; Rechung Rinpoche, *Tibetan Medicine*, 179–81.

37 William A. McGrath, *Buddhism and Medicine in Tibet: Origins, Ethics, and Tradition* (Charlottesville, VA: Doctoral Dissertation at the University of Virginia, 2017), 141.

38 Brang ti dpal ldan 'tsho byed, *Bdud rtsi snying po yan lag brgyad pa gsang ba man ngag gi rgyud kyi spyi don shes bya rab gsal rgyas pa* (Beijing: Manuscript, n.d.), 27a: ཆོས་རྒྱལ་མེས་དབོན་གྱི་སྐུ་དྲིན་ལས། སངས་རྒྱས་བསྟན་པ་བཞིན་དུ་གསོ་སྤྱད་ཀྱང་བྱུང་སྟེ། བྱང་ཆུབ་སེམས་དཔའ་ཀུན་ཏུ་བཟང་པོའི་རྣམ་འཕྲུལ་ལྷ་ཐོ་ཐོ་རི་སྙན་ཤལ་གྱི་རིང་ལ། ན་ལུགས་ལ་ཟས་ཀྱི་ཕན་གནོད་དང་། རྨ་གསར་པ་ལ་མར་གསར་བཞུ་བ་བཏང་སྟེ་ཁྲ་ཁ་བསྡམས་པ་ཞེས་ཙམ་བྱུང་སྟེ། སྨན་སྤྱད་དབུ་བརྙེས།

39 Brang ti dpal ldan 'tsho byed, *Shes bya rab gsal rgyas pa*, 28a; Zur mkhar ba blo gros rgyal po, *Sman pa rnams kyis mi shes su mi rung ba'i shes bya spyi'i khog dbubs* (Chengdu: Si khron mi rigs dpe skrun khang, 2001), 255.

life of Drejé Gyagar Vajra, the grandfather of Yutok Yönten Gönpo the Elder. It is said that Gyagar Vajra treated a serpent demon (*klu bdud*) who had been wounded near his hometown, called Tölung Kyina (*stod lung skyid sna*). The next day, in return for his treatment, Gyagar Vajra received a female corpse that was covered by gold and turquoise in the river. Gyagar Vajra kept the ornaments and left the corpse in the river. He put the gold and turquoise on the roof of his house to let them dry. A shepherd saw them and said: "the Lord of the Beneficent Presence has a turquoise roof!" Since then, he came to be called Yutokpa, the "One with a Turquoise Roof."[40] Darmo Menrampa repeats this story again in his biography of Yutok the Younger.[41] The only difference is that the latter story purportedly took place in Gozhi Retang, a place in Tsang.

Pawo Tsuklak Trengwa and Zurkhar Lodrö Gyelpo assert that the name of Yutok has been in use since the lifetime of Gyagar Vajra.[42] As mentioned above, Belo's medical history shows that Zurkhar Lodrö Gyelpo believed that the name of Yutok was never used for their family before Gyagar Vajra's life time.[43] If the name of Yutok was already used in the lifetime of the Elder Yutok's grandfather, and if the Elder Yutok and the Younger Yutok belong to the same family lineage, there is no reason to give such a name again to a Gyagar Vajra, the grandfather of the Younger Yutok. It is likely that the story in the Elder Yutok's biography was borrowed from the biography of Yutok the Younger.

8.6 *The Lineage of the Elder Yutok*

The following lineage of the Elder Yutok is a summary from the Elder Yutok biography itself. It is said that Biji Gajé married Lhacham Yikyi Rölcha. They had a son called Dunggi Torchok Chen (*dung gi thor cog can*) who later became the court physician of King Lha Totori Nyenshel and King Tri Nyensungtsen (*khri snyan gzungs btsan*). Since then, the physicians from his family had served as the court physicians of Tibetan kings (see Fig. 2.1).

Yutok Jampa Tukjé's son was Könchok Delek (*dkon mchog bde legs*) and his son was Jampa Delek (*byams pa bde legs*). Before Jampa Delek, the lineage is labeled as the Elder Yutok's lineage.[44]

---

40 Jo bo lhun grub bkra shis, *G.yu thog gsar rnying gi rnam thar*, 67–71.

41 Jo bo lhun grub bkra shis, *G.yu thog gsar rnying gi rnam thar*, 323.

42 Dpa' bo gtsug lag phreng ba, *Chos 'byung mkhas pa'i dga' ston*, 1521; Zur mkhar ba blo gros rgyal po, *Sman pa rnams kyis mi shes su mi rung ba'i shes bya spyi'i khog dbubs*, 313–14. In the medical histories of Pawo, Zurkhar, and Belo, Gyagar Vajra only is the grandfather of Younger Yutok.

43 'Be lo tshe dbang kun khyab, *'Be lo tshe dbang kun khyab kyi gsung thor bu'i skor*, 142.

44 Jo bo lhun grub bkra shis, *G.yu thog gsar rnying gi rnam thar*, 65–67.

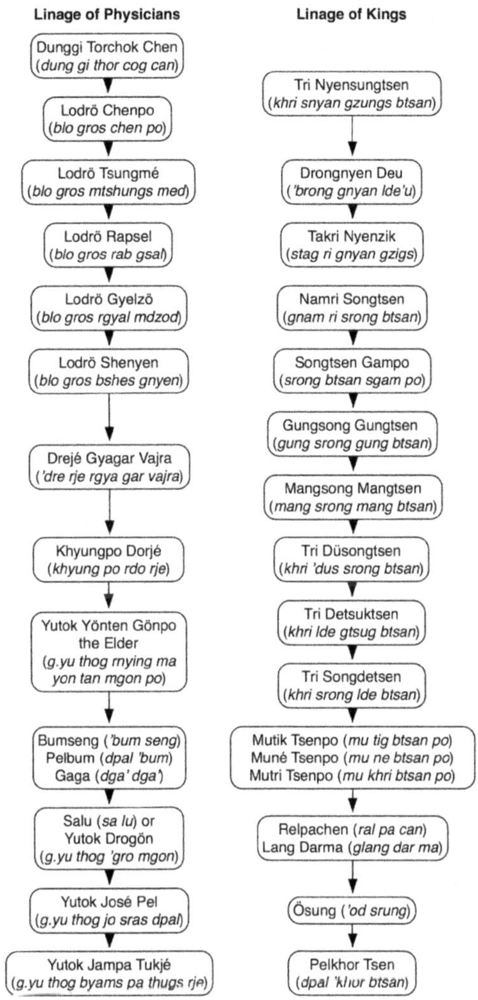

FIGURE 2.1
The corresponding lineages of physicians and kings according to the Elder Yutok biography

The Desi may have worried about the reliability of the Elder Yutok biography, but he still used this description of the lineage of the Elder Yutok in his medical history, the *Mirror of Beryl*.[45] The "History of Tibetan Medicine" in *China's Medical Encyclopedia* also uses the same narrative regarding to the lineage of the Elder Yutok.[46] Interestingly, such accounts of lineages can be found in

45 Sde srid sangs rgyas rgya mtsho, *Sde srid sman gyi khog 'bubs*, 153–54.
46 Byams pa 'phrin las and Thub bstan tshe ring, *Bod kyi gso ba rig pa'i lo rgyus*, vol. 1, 5.

neither Tibetan medical histories (such as *khog dbub*) nor the standard Tibetan political and religious histories that predate the seventeenth century.

8.7 *The Relationship between the Lineage of the Elder Yutok and the Younger Yutok*

It has been said that the lineage of the Younger Yutok emerged from the Elder Yutok's lineage.[47] The Elder Yutok biography states that from Jowo Banu down to Jampa Pel (*byams pa dpal*), the lineage is called the Elder Yutok's lineage. It seems to me that Jampa Pel and Jampa Delek refer to the same person. As for the Younger Yutok's lineage, on the one hand, the biography states that after Drejé Gyagar Vajra, the grandfather of the Younger Yutok, it is called the Younger Yutok's lineage.[48] On the other hand, the biography records that from Pema Özer (*padma 'od zer*) down to the end of the lineage is called the Younger Yutok's lineage.[49] Even if the author's narrative about the division between the Elder and Younger lineages is not very clear, it still seems that the Younger lineage connects to the Elder lineage in the Elder Yutok biography. In the Elder Yutok biography, it is said that Yutok Khyungpo Dorjé prophesied that Yutok Yönten Gönpo the Younger would be born in Yutok's lineage after thirteen generations, starting from Yutok Yönten Gönpo the Elder.[50] The Desi also repeated this account again in his medical history.[51]

Many reliable historical documents, such as Pawo's *Feast for Scholars* and Zurkhar's *Medical History*, indicate that the "Yutok" lineage was actually called Dré (*'bre* or *'dre*) in Tibetan before Drejé Gyagar Vajra, the grandfather of the Younger Yutok, gained the name of Yutok for his clan.[52] In fact, we can find the name of the Dré clan before founding Tibetan Empire. A document found at Dunhuang states: "In the place of Nyangro Shampo, there are King Lo Ngam Gyidrom and two Ministers, namely Ngapnyi and Dré."[53] Another Dunhuang document also mentions that Dré was the minister of King Lo Ngam or Long

47 Jo bo lhun grub bkra shis, *G.yu thog gsar rnying gi rnam thar*, 67, 124–30.

48 Jo bo lhun grub bkra shis, *G.yu thog gsar rnying gi rnam thar*, 125.

49 Jo bo lhun grub bkra shis, *G.yu thog gsar rnying gi rnam thar*, 125.

50 Jo bo lhun grub bkra shis, *G.yu thog gsar rnying gi rnam thar*, 80.

51 Sde srid sangs rgyas rgya mtsho, *Sde srid sman gyi khog 'bubs*, 162.

52 Dpa' bo gtsug lag phreng ba, *Chos 'byung mkhas pa'i dga' ston*, 1521; Zur mkhar ba blo gros rgyal po, *Sman pa rnams kyis mi shes su mi rung ba'i shes bya spyi'i khog dbubs*, 313–14.

53 Stobs ldan and Kha sgang bkra shis tshe ring, *Pha ran sir nyar ba'i tun hong yig rnying gi bshus yig phyogs bsgrigs* (Lhasa: Bod ljongs mi dmangs dpe skrun khang, 2017), vol. 11, 375. 'Bri gung skabs mgon che tshang, *Tun hong bod kyi yig rnying las byung ba: bod btsan po'i rgyal rabs* (Dehradun: Sangtsen Library, 2010), 33–36. PT 1286, 0010: ཡུལ་ཉང་རོ་འི་ཤམ་པོ་ན། རྗེ་ལོ་ངམ་གྱི་བྲོམ་ཆེ། བློན་པོ་ངབ་སྙི་དང་འབྲེ་གཉིས། །

Ngam. It seems clear that the Dré clan was an important noble family in the Upper Nyangchu River Valley during the period of fragmentation.[54]

During the reign of Songtsen Gampo, Dré was one of thousands of households (*stong sde*) in the Tibetan Empire. There was a famous commander called Dré Gyel Tori Trilö (*'dre rgyal to ri khri lod*) from this same clan.[55] In addition, Pawo Tsuklak Trengwa states that the land of Nyangro and Drompa once belonged to the Dré (*'bre*) and Ché (*lce*) clans.[56] The *Dharma History of Nyang* also asserts that the Upper Nyangchu River Valley was occupied by the Dré and Khyung clans.[57]

The Nyangchu River runs from the Nojin Gangzang Mountain, then it passes by the town of Zhikatsé before it enters the Brahmaputra. The Nyangchu River Valley is located in the place where the river runs. The valley can be divided into three parts: the Upper Nyangchu River Valley (*myang stod*), the Middle Nyangchu River Valley (*myang bar*), and the Lower Nyangchu River Valley (*myang smad*).

The Upper Nyangchu River Valley is the place between Rinang Pangkhar (*ri nang spang khar*) and the Nine-peaked Mount Shampo (*sham bu rtse dgu*).[58] The term of Nyangro (*myang ro*) may refer to the Nyangchu River Valley. It has

---

54 'Bri gung skabs mgon che tshang, *Tun hong bod kyi yig rnying las byung ba*, 39. PT 1060, 0085–86: མཁར་སྙྱང་རོ་ཤམ་པོ་དགུ་རྩིགས་ལང་ཡིང་གི་ནང་ནའ། རྒྱལ་པོ་ [0086] སོང་ངམ་རྗེ་དང། ངམ་ཙ་ཕྱི་བྲོམ་དཀར་པོ། བློན་པོ་ངབ་སྦྱི་དང་འབྲེ་གས།

55 Gu ru o rgyan gling pa, *Bka' thang sde lnga* (Beijing: Mi rigs dpe skrun khang, 1986), 438: རུ་ལག་སྣད་ཀྱི་སྟོང་སྡེ་བཞི། །ཉང་རོ་འདྲེ་ཡི་སྟོང་སྡེ་ཡིན། །ཁྲི་ཐ་ཁྱུང་པོའི་སྟོང་སྡེ་ཡིན། །གད་བཀྲམ་འགོས་ཀྱི་སྟོང་སྡེ་ཡིན། །མཁར་པ་ཤུ་གུའི་སྟོང་སྡེ་ཡིན། །འཚོང་མ་སྟོང་བུ་ཆུང་སྒྲོའི་སྟོང་སྡེ་ཡིན། །རུ་ལག་སྣད་ཀྱི་དམག་དཔོན་ནི། །ཡིན། །རུ་རྙ་ངང་པ་ཏོག་ནག་ཡིན། །རུ་དར་དར་དཀར་ཐང་འགེབས་ཡིན། །རུ་སྣབ་ཁྱུང་པོ་སྤྱུ་སྣ་ཟུང་། །ཡིག་ཚངས་གཡུ་ཡི་ཡི་གེ་ཡིན། །དམག་བཞེད་ཐང་ལ་སེར་བ་བབ་པ་འདྲ། །དེ་ཡང་སུམ་འབུམ་དྲུག་ཁྲི་སྟེ། །སྟོད་སྨད་གཉིས་ཀའི་མགོ་གྲངས་ནི། །བདུན་འབུམ་ཉི་ཁྲི་ཡོད་དོ་སྐད། །

56 Dpa' bo gtsug lag phreng ba, *Chos 'byung mkhas pa'i dga' ston*, 187: དེ་རྣམས་ལ་ཡུལ་གྱི་དབང་རིས་ནི། དབུ་རུ་ཤོད་ཆེན་བཙན་པོ་མངའ་བདག་ཡུལ། །ཕོ་བྲང་སྐྱི་ཆེ་བཙན་པོ་རྒྱལ་འབངས་ཡུལ། །ཡར་ལུང་སོགས་ཁ་ཁུ་དང་གཉགས་ཀྱི་ཡུལ། །ཡ་འབྲོག་གངས་ཁྱིམ་ཀུ་རིངས་སྣེ་ལྦའི་ཡུལ། །འཆིང་དང་འཆིང་ཡུལ་མགོས་དང་སྣུབས་ཀྱི་ཡུལ། །བྱ་ཝུག་ས་ཚོགས་ཧུར་རྗེ་ཕ་ལྦའི་ཡུལ། །བྲད་དང་ཞོང་པ་སྣ་ནམ་ཡུལ་དུ་བཅད། །བྲག་རུམ་སྟོད་སྨད་ཆེ་སྤོང་ཡུལ་དུ་བྱས། །གཙང་སྟོད་གཙང་སྨད་འབྲོ་དང་ཁྱུང་པོའི་ཡུལ། །ཀླུངས་ཤོད་ནམ་པོ་འདྲུ་དང་ཞུགས་མཚམས་ཡུལ། །འཕན་ཡུལ་སྟོང་སྡེ་སྒྲོ་དང་རྨ་ཡི་ཡུལ། །ཉང་རོ་གྲོམ་པ་འབྲེ་དང་ལྕེ་ཡི་ཡུལ། །ཤངས་དང་གླེ་ཕྱི་རི་དང་གླེ་ཡི་ཡུལ། །ཡུང་བ་ཆེ་ཆུང་བྲན་ཀའི་ཡུལ་དུ་བཅད། །ཞ་གད་སྡེ་གསུམ་བློན་པོ་སྦས་ཀྱི་ཡུལ། །ནམ་ར་ཆག་གོང་འཕྲིན་དང་ཆག་གི་ཡུལ། །འདམ་ཤོད་དཀར་མོ་ཕྱུ་དང་རྔ་ཡི་ཡུལ། །མདོ་ཁམས་མདོ་ཆེན་ཆོད་སྟོང་སྡེ་བརྒྱད་ཡུལ། །ཞེས་བཅོ་བརྒྱད་དུ་ཕྱེའོ། །

57 Jo nang tā ra na tha, *Myang yul stod smad bar gsum gyi ngo mtshar gtam gyi legs bshad mkhas pa'i 'jug ngogs* (Lhasa: Bod ljongs mi dmangs dpe skrun khang, 1983), 7–8: སྨྱང་སྟོད་འདྲེ་དང་ཁྱུང་གིས་འཛིན། །སྨྱང་བར་རྒྱད་པོ་འབྲུས་འཛིན། །སྨྱང་སྨད་ལྕེ་དང་དཔྱལ་གྱིས་འཛིན། །

58 Jo nang tā ra na tha, *Myang yul stod smad bar gsum gyi ngo mtshar gtam gyi legs bshad mkhas pa'i 'jug ngogs*, 8: སྨྱང་སྟོད་སྨད་བར་གསུམ་དུ་བཤད་པའི་སྟོད་ཀྱི་ཡུལ་ནི་ཕུ་རི་ནང་སྤང་ཁར་ལ་གཏད། མདའ་གཤམ་བུ་རྩེ་དགུ་ལ་གཏད་པ་འདི་ལ་ཚོང་འདུས་ཆེན་པོ་གཅིག མི་རིགས་མ་གཅིག་པ་གཉིས། འབྲོག་སྡེ་ཆེན་པོ་གསུམ། ཐོང་སྐྱ་མི་གཅིག་པ་གསུམ་ཡོད་ལགས།

been said that Mt. Shampo is one of the thirteen evil signs of the mountains in the Upper Nyangchu River Valley.[59] The mountain is located in the Tsechen Township in Gyantsé County of the Tibetan Autonomous Region.

As Zurkhar Lodrö Gyelpo once pointed out, the eighth-century Dré Gyelwé Lodrö (*'bre rgyal ba'i blo gros*) and the twelfth-century Dré Sherap Bar (*'bre shes rab 'bar*) also belonged to the Dré clan. Also, as I mentioned above, before the lifetime of Drejé Gyagar Vajra, there was no Yutok family distinct from the Dré clan. Thus, we cannot find any evidence to prove that the lineage of the Younger Yutok was connected to the lineage of the Elder Yutok.

8.8 *Drejé Gyagar Vajra's Journey to India*

The Elder Yutok biography said that Drejé Gyagar Vajra made a trip to India in order to retrieve two texts, namely, *Turning Medicine into Nectar* (*bdud rtsi sman sgrub*) and the *Essence of the Explanation of Measuring the Head* (*mgo thig rin chen gnad 'grel*). He received a teaching of the *Essence of the Explanation of Measuring the Head* from Nāgārjuna and a teaching of *Turning Medicine into Nectar* from the Medical Buddha, the Eight Medical Goddesses, the Three Sage Brothers, and Kumāra Jīvaka (*'tsho byed gzhon nu*). He also met Biji Gajé in India.[60]

As we know, Kumāra Jīvaka was the legendary physician of Gautama Buddha, who probably lived in 6th century BCE. Nāgārjuna is widely considered to have been one of the most important Buddhist philosophers who lived between 150 and 250 CE. The biography of the Elder Yutok asserts that Biji Gajé visited Tibet during the reign of King Lha Totori Nyenshel, and modern scholars have asserted that King Lha Totori Nyenshel lived in the fifth century.[61] According to the biography, Drejé Gyagar Vajra is supposed to have lived in the seventh century. How could these people who lived in different centuries have met together in one place and time? It seems to me that the biography only can be considered a work of fiction. There is no good reason to believe that this is a reliable historical document.

8.9 *The Elder Yutok's Connection with the Tibetan Royal Family*

It has been said that both the Elder Yutok and Tri Songdetsen were born in the male earth-monkey year. Under the invitation of King Tri Detsuktsen,

---

59 Jo nang tā ra na tha, *Myang yul stod smad bar gsum gyi ngo mtshar gtam gyi legs bshad mkhas pa'i 'jug ngogs*, 6: མྱང་སྟོད་ལ་ལྟས་ངན་གྱི་རི་བཅུ་གསུམ་ཡོད། །འབྲོང་རྩེའི་རི་འདི་འབྲོང་པོ་རབ་རྫར་བ་འདྲ། །དྲན་མའི་རི་འདི་གཅེས་ཕྲུག་ཐང་ལ་བསྐྱུར་བ་འདྲ། །སྤྲུལ་གདོང་གི་རི་འདི་ཛ་མོང་ག་པ་རྒྱ་འཕྱང་བ་འདྲ། ཤམ་བུ་རྩེ་དགུའི་རི་འདི་སྒྲོ་བ་རྒྱབ་ཤལ་བ་འདྲ། །

60 Jo bo lhun grub bkra shis, *G.yu thog gsar rnying gi rnam thar*, 71, 142–53.

61 Alex McKay, ed., *The History of Tibet* (London: RoutledgeCurzon, 2003), vol. 1, 159.

the ten-year-old Elder Yutok visited the main temple of Samyé Monastery (*bsam yas dbu rtse rigs gsum*), where he debated with Drangti Gyelnyé Kharpuk (*brang ti rgyal mnyes mkhar phug*) and other Tibetan doctors.[62] Then King Tri Detsuktsen and his son Tri Songdetsen had great faith in the Elder Yutok. He was appointed as the court physician of Tri Songdetsen.[63] The biography states that King Tri Detsuktsen and his son had invited Śāntarakṣita (*zhi ba 'tsho*, 725–788) and Padmasambhava (*padma 'byung gnas*, 8th century) to Tibet. They laid the foundations for Samyé monastery when Tri Songdetsen was five years old, and the construction of monastery was completed when Tri Songdetsen was fifteen years old.[64]

According to the *Old Book of Tang* and the *New Book of Tang*, Tri Songdetsen became the emperor of Tibet between 755 and 797 CE.[65] A document found at Dunhuang indicates that Tri Songdetsen was born in a horse year (742 CE).[66] A copy of Tri Desongtsen's decree that was kept in Samyé Monastery states that Tri Songdetsen built Samyé Monastery.[67] There are different dates for the building the monastery in Tibetan historical works: from a hare year to a sheep year,[68] from one hare year to the next hare year,[69] from a female fire-hare year to a female earth-hare year,[70] or from an iron-hare year (751) to a water-hare year (763).[71]

Tibetan historical works also give various ages of Tri Songdetsen when the foundation of Samyé monastery was laid: thirteen years old,[72] twenty-two

---

62 Jo bo lhun grub bkra shis, *G.yu thog gsar rnying gi rnam thar*, 86–87.

63 Jo bo lhun grub bkra shis, *G.yu thog gsar rnying gi rnam thar*, 87.

64 Jo bo lhun grub bkra shis, *G.yu thog gsar rnying gi rnam thar*, 111.

65 Luo Guangwu, *Liang tangshu tubozhuan yizhu* (Beijing: Zhongguo zangxue chubanshe, 2014), 56, 230.

66 'Bri gung skabs mgon che tshang, *Tun hong bod kyi yig rnying lus byung ba*, 372: རྟ་ཡི་ལོ་ལ། བཙན་པོའི་ཕོ་བྲང་དབྱར་ད་མཚར་བུ་སྣ་ན་བཞུགས། རྒྱལ་ཕྱི་ཕོ་ཇ་ཨན་ད་ཡང་དང་། སྣ་ནག་པོའི་ཕོ་ཇ་ལ་ཕྲི་སྤྱག་འཚལད། ཀློར་ཤུད་པུ་ཁོང་བྲུང་དང་། ལང་གྲོ་ཁོང་རྩན་གཉིས། འབྲུང་འཇུག་གི་ཕྱིས་བགྱིསྟེ། ཐང་ཁྲམ་བཏབ། ཁུ་ཆེ་མོན་གདང་སྣོན་མང་པོ་རྗེས་འཞག་གི་འཕོས་བགྱིས། བཙན་པོ་སྲོང་ལྡེ་བརྩན་བྲག་མར་དུར་བལྟམས། ཡུམ་མང་མོ་རྗེ་ནོངས་པར་ལོ་གཅིག

67 Dpa' bo gtsug lag phreng ba, *Chos 'byung mkhas pa'i dga' ston*, 409: ཡབ་ཁྲི་སྲོང་ལྡེ་བཙན་གྱིས། ཆོས་རྒྱ་ཆེར་ཐུགས་སུ་ཆུད་ནས། བསམ་ཡས་ལྷུན་གྱིས་གྲུབ་པ་ལ་སོགས་སྟེ། བོད་ཁམས་སུ་གཙུག་ལག་ཁང་མང་པོ་བརྩིགས་པ་དང་།

68 Dba' gsal snang, *Dba' bzhed* (Lhasa: Bod ljongs bod yig dpe rnying dpe skrun khang, 2011), 28, 33; 'Gos lo gzhon nu dpal, *Deb ther sngon po* (Chengdu: Si khron mi rigs dpe skrun khang, 1985), 69–70.

69 Dba' gsal snang, *Dba' bzhed*, 106, 124, 190, 197, 209.

70 Bu ston rin chen grub, *Bu ston chos 'byung* (Beijing: Krung go'i bod kyi shes rig dpe skrun khang, 1988), 186.

71 Dpa' bo gtsug lag phreng ba, *Chos 'byung mkhas pa'i dga' ston*, 352.

72 Dba' gsal snang, *Dba' bzhed*, 106, 197.

years old,[73] or twenty-one years old.[74] In any case, as I have shown above, I have not found any reliable sources that indicate that King Tri Detsuktsen made any contributions to building Samyé monastery. In addition, there is no evidence to prove that Samyé monastery was already constructed when Tri Songdetsen was ten years old. As far as I know, there is no strong evidence to prove that the Elder Yutok was the court physician of Tri Songdetsen. Thus, it seems to me that the statement in Elder Yutok's biography contradicts the more reliable sources of Tibetan history, as well as the Elder Yutok biography itself. I am concerned that the author of the biography may not have had sufficient knowledge regarding the early history of Tibet.

8.10 *The Origin and Transmission of the Four Tantras*

The *Four Tantras*, known as the *Gyüzhi* (*rgyud bzhi*) in Tibetan, is the classical text for Tibetan medicine. There are different accounts of its origins. The author of the Elder Yutok biography states that the great Tibetan translator Vairocana received the *Four Tantras*, its instructions, and its supplements from Paṇḍita Candradeva in India. Candradeva asked Vairocana to pass the text to the Tibetan king and the Elder Yutok. When the Elder Yutok met Vairocana on the border between Nepal and India, he instructed Vairocana to keep the *Four Tantras* as a hidden treasure in Samyé Monastery. Thus, Vairocana and the King did as the Elder Yutok had directed. Then the Elder Yutok went to visit Candradeva in India, and the Paṇḍita gave him the supplementary instructions for the *Four Tantras*, as well as great number of different instructions on medicine and other topics. During another one of Yutok's trips to India, it is said that he got a text called the *Notes for Explanations of the Hidden Meanings in the Four Tantras* (*dpal ldan rgyud bzhi'i gab pa gsal byed tho byang*).[75] The biography records that the Elder Yutok unearthed the *Four Tantras* from the monastery when he was forty-five years old.[76]

The origin of the *Four Tantras* has been an important subject of debate among Tibetan scholars for many centuries. The debate has mainly focused on the question of whether the text is a teaching of the Buddha or if it is a later composition by a Tibetan scholar. In the *Sealed Account of Transmission of Tibetan Medical Four Tantras' Master* (*gso rig rgyud bzhi'i bla ma brgyud pa'i rnam thar bka' rgya ma*), the twelfth-century Tibetan physician Sumtön Yeshé Zung, a direct disciple of Yutok Yönten Gönpo the Younger, claimed that the *Four*

---

73 Dpa' bo gtsug lag phreng ba, *Chos 'byung mkhas pa'i dga' ston*, 352.

74 Dpal 'byor bzang po, *Rgya bod yig tshang chen mo* (Chengdu: Si khron mi rigs dpe skrun khang, 1985), 180.

75 Jo bo lhun grub bkra shis, *G.yu thog gsar rnying gi rnam thar*, 112–13.

76 Jo bo lhun grub bkra shis, *G.yu thog gsar rnying gi rnam thar*, 267.

Tantras was based on the teachings of an emanation of the Medicine Buddha. According to Sumtön's account, the *Four Tantras* was taught by Vidyājñāna (*rig pa'i ye shes*) in Oḍḍiyāna. The teaching of the text was transmitted through two lineages: a Buddhist lineage and a non-Buddhist lineage. Candrananda of Kashmir received the text through the Buddhist lineage. In the eighth century, Vairocana got the text from Candrananda. Vairocana then went to Tibet and offered the text to the Tibetan emperor Tri Songdetsen, who concealed it inside a pillar at Samyé Monastery. After three hundred years, in the eleventh century, Drapa Ngönshé took it from the pillar, and through Upa Dardrak and Totön Könchok Kyap, the text finally came into the hands of Yutok Yönten Gönpo the Younger.[77]

Most works of Tibetan medical history that consider the *Four Tantras* to be the teachings of the Buddha repeat this account. Interestingly, this Tibetan medical history, which was composed before the Desi's *Mirror of Beryl*, never mentions the Elder Yutok's connection with the transmission of the *Four Tantras*. Therefore, we have good reason to believe that the *Four Tantras* was a composition of Yutok Yönten Gönpo the Younger. The detailed discussion about this issue can be found in my early works.[78]

8.11 *Medical Schools, Courses, and Degrees*

Between the ages of fifty-five and sixty-five, the Elder Yutok was teaching the *Four Tantras*, its appendix, and its supplement to three hundred students in Kongpo (*kong po*). He is said to have granted four levels of degrees for his students. It is said that about fifty students received Bumram degrees (*'bum rams*), fifty students got Rapjam degrees (*rab 'byams*), and about one hundred students received Kachu degrees (*bka' bcu*). The teaching materials for the Bumram degree include the *Four Tantras*, its commentary, its appendix, and its supplement, as well as medical works by the Nine Tibetan Learned Physicians, the *Somaraja* by Nāgārjuna, *Vase of Nectar* (*bdud rtsi bum pa*) by Padmasambhava, the *Oral Instructions of the Rishi* (*drang srong snyan brgyud*) by Rishi Penden Trengwa, the *Compendium of the Essence of the Eight Branches* (Skt. *aṣṭāṅgahṛdayasaṃhitā* = *yan lag brgyad pa'i snying po bsdus pa*) by

77 Sum ston ye shes gzungs, *Gso rig rgyud bzhi'i bla ma brgyud pa'i rnam thar bka' rgya ma gtsang ru mtshams sum pa jha na rda ra'i gsung 'phros gyim phyogs 'tsho byed gzhon nu la gdams pa*, in *Gangs ljongs sman rtsis rig mdzod chen mo* (Beijing: Krung go'i bod rig pa dpe skrun khang, 2016), vol. 38, 401–11.

78 Yang Ga, "The Origin of the *Four Tantras* and an Account of Its Author, Yuthog Yonten Gonpo," in *Bodies in Balance: The Art of Tibetan Medicine*, ed. Theresia Hofer (Seattle, WA: University of Washington Press, 2014), 154–77; Yang Ga, *The Sources for the Writing of the Rgyud bzhi: Tibetan Medical Classic* (Cambridge, MA: Doctoral Dissertation at Harvard University, 2010).

Vāgbhaṭa, and the *Moon Beams Commentary* (Skt. *padārthacandrikā* = *tshig don zla zer*) by Candranandana.[79]

As I have already indicated in my doctoral dissertation, under the financial support of the ruler of the Gugé kingdom and the four native physicians, Lochen Rinchen Zangpo (958–1055) and the Paṇḍita Janārdana translated the *Essence of the Eight Branches* and its *Moon Beams* commentary into Tibetan in the early eleventh century. We have several sources that prove that the *Four Tantras* was composed after the translation of these two Āyurvedic treatises. It is impossible, then, that the works of Vāgbhaṭa and Candranandana were taught in eight-century Tibet.[80]

8.12 *The Issue of Nine Tibetan Physicians*

According to the Elder Yutok biography, the Elder Yutok prophesied that the Nine Tibetan Physicians (*bod kyi sman pa mi dgu*) would come one after another and that they would not live in the same period. Those nine physicians were Biji Lekgön, Ukpa Chözang, Cherjé Zhikpo, Minyak Rongjé, Yutok Gönpo, Drangti Gyelzang, Nyapa Chözang, Tömen Drakgyel, and Tapzhi Darpo. The Desi believes that these physicians, which he called as the "Nine Learned Tibetan Physicians" (*bod sman mkhas pa mi dgu*), were trained during the reign of King Tri Songdetsen.[81] As far as I know, Drangti Jampel Zangpo (*brang ti 'jam dpal bzang po*) was one of earliest Tibetan physicians to address the notion that "Nine Learned Physicians" (*mkhas pa mi dgu*) lived during the reign of King Tri Songdetsen. Among them, he believes that the so-called Yutok was Drejé Gyagar Vajra. He also thought that the son of Gyagar Vajra was Khyungpo Dorjé, who in turn was the father of Yutok Yönten Gönpo the Younger.[82] According this account, if Drejé Gyagar Vajra truly flourished during the Tibetan empire and also acted as the grandfather of Yutok the Younger, he would have lived for approximately three hundred years, from the eighth century to the eleventh.

---

79 Jo bo lhun grub bkra shis, *G.yu thog gsar rnying gi rnam thar*, 267–68.

80 Yang Ga, *The Sources for the Writing of the Rgyud bzhi.*

81 Sde srid sangs rgyas rgya mtsho, *Sde srid sman gyi khog 'bubs*, 125–26.

82 Brang ti 'jam dpal bzang po, *Lag len gyi snying po pod chung gi 'grel pa bzhugs so* (Manuscript, n.d.), 1a–2a: བོད་ཀྱི་རྒྱལ་པོ་ཁྲི་སྲོང་ལྡེ་བཙན་མངའ་(ཐང་)དར་བའི་དུས་སུ། ལྷ་རྗེ་ལ་སྟུ་བ། མཁས་པ་མི་དགུ་བྱུ་བ་བྱུང་སྟེ། དེ་ཡང་སྔོན་ན་ཆེར་རྗེ་ཨུག་པ་བི་ཛི་གསུམ། བར་མི་ཉག་དང་གཡུ་ཐོག་བྲང་ཏི་གསུམ། སྨད་ན་སྟོང་དང་། མཐའ་བཞི། སྔ་དང་གསུམ་བྱ་བར་གྲགས་པའི་ནང་ནས་གཡུ་ཐོག་ཅེས་གྲགས་པའི་འབྲེ་རྗེ་མཁས་པ་རྒྱ་གར་བཛྲ་ཡིན། དེའི་སྲས་ཁྱུང་པོ་རྡོ་རྗེ། དེའི་སྲས་ཡོན་ཏན་མགོན་པོ་ཡིན། མཁས་པ་དེས་གསོ་སྤྱད་མང་དུ་བརྩམས། ཁྱད་པར་དུ་ཚིག་འདུས་ལ་དོན་ཆེ་བ་ལག་ལེན་པོད་ཆུང་བྱ་བ་འདི་བརྩམས། དེས་བགྲེས་ཁའི་སྲས་དཔོན་འབུམ་སེང་ལ་གནང། དེས་སྲང་མང་དུ་ཡོད་པའི་བརྒྱུད་ཀྱི་རྒྱུད་བ་སློབ་དཔོན་འཇམ་དཔལ་ལ་གནང་། དེའི་སྲས་འཚོ་བྱེད་ཡབ་སྲས་གཉིས་ལ། བདག་བྲང་ཏི་འཇམ་དཔལ་བཟང་པོས་ལུང་ཐོབ་བོ།

In addition to the fact that it would be difficult to convincingly argue that the Elder Yutok prophesied the nine Tibetan physicians in the eighth century, I am also concerned about the reliability of the "Nine Learned Tibetan Physicians" as told by other Tibetan scholars, such as Drangti and the Desi. The reason is that many serious Tibetan scholars, including Pawo Tsuklak Trengwa, Zurkhar Lodrö Gyelpo, Belo Tsewang Künkhyap, and Kongtrül Yönten Gyatso, have stated that those nine physicians came in different periods. They do not think that all of them lived during the Tibetan Empire. In addition, there is not anything about an Elder Yutok acting as a royal physician in the writings of either Yutok Yönten Gönpo or Sumtön Yeshé Zung. For instance, Sumtön talks about the classification of physicians in the *Small Commentary Collection* (*'bum chung*) and the *Black Commentary Collection* (*'bum nag*), both of which are commentaries on the second part of the *Four Tantras*. He does not treat Yutok as part of a lineage of royal physicians that traces back to the Tibetan emperor. Instead, Yutok is counted as a physician who studied medicine under the lineage of royal physicians of Tibetan emperor. This seems to suggest that Yutok was not the royal physician of a Tibetan king, and a more detailed discussion about this issue can be found in my previous works.[83]

9 Comparing the Elder Yutok Biography with Other Biographies of Yutok Yönten Gönpo

Professor Wangdü (*dbang 'dus*) has claimed to hold another biography of the Elder Yutok that was purportedly composed by Lungmar Gönpo Rinchen, a descendant of Yutok Yönten Gönpo. Unfortunately, I have not had a chance to access this work. Thus, I have no grounds to evaluate its reliability.

Recently, two other biographies of Yutok Yönten Gönpo were published. The title of first biography is the *Great Lotus Garden-Jewel Garland Biography of the Scholar Yutok Gönpo* (*mkhas pa g.yu thog mgon po'i rnam thar pad tshal rgyas pa nor bu'i 'phreng ba*). Since the biography is incomplete, we cannot find the name of the author in the colophon at end of the text. The Desi wrote a note on the first folio of the biography with red ink and he believed that the author of the biography was Yutok Kharak Lharjé (*g.yu thog kha rag lha rje*).[84] The Desi

83 Yang Ga, "Study on the Origin of Yutok Family," *Journal of Tibet University* 66, no. 2 (2015): 122–29.

84 G.yu thog kha rag lha rje, *Mkhas pa g.yu thog mgon po'i rnam thar pad tshal brgyas pa nor bu'i 'phreng ba*, in *Krung go'i bod lugs gso rig rtsa che'i dpe rnying kun btus* (Lhasa: Bod ljongs mi dmangs dpe skrun khang, 2013), vol. 15, 193–209.

also mentions the biography in his medical history.[85] The biography claims that Yutok Yönten Gönpo served as a royal physician for Tri Songdetsen under the king's request.[86] It also states that Yutok Yönten Gönpo received the teaching of the *Four Tantras* from Totön Könchok Kyap.[87] The biography also records that Yutok Yönten Gönpo went to heaven and became the personal physician of Indra, the king of the gods in Hindu mythology. It also asserts that Yutok married a goddess and had two sons, namely, Lungmar Yutok Gönpo (*lung dmar g.yu thog mgon po*) and Yutok Bumseng (*g.yu thog 'bum seng.*)[88] Because the reign of Tri Songdetsen was in the eighth century and Totön Könchok Kyap was a twelfth-century scholar, if this biography were accurate, Yutok Yönten Gönpo would have lived nearly four hundred years, from the eighth to twelfth century. Like the biography of the Elder Yutok, this biography also contains a legendary description about the figure. In addition, it also provides contradicting dates for the figure. It is hard to know which Yutok, the Elder or the Younger, the author of biography is describing. It seems clear that this is not a reliable source.

A second biography was published in the *Journal of Tibetan Medicine and Astro-science* in 2017. The editor of the journal stated that the biography was based on two handwritten copies in the Lhasa Mentsikhang. According to the introduction, the Mentsikhang made two handwritten copies from a manuscript that was found in the Potala Palace in 1983. It is not clear who the author of the biography was. The short biography was written in verse, and its main contents and structure are very similar to those of the Elder Yutok biography.[89] It seems to me that this alternative biography is a very important source for the composition of the biography of the Elder Yutok. Interestingly, the author of the biography never uses the term "Elder Yutok" (*g.yu thog rnying ma*) or "Yutok Yönten Gönpo the Elder" (*g.yu thog rnying ma Yon tan mgon po*) at all.

The Desi mentions another biography of Yutok by Kongpo Degyel in his medical history.[90] In addition, Sokdokpa Lodrö Gyeltsen also talks about Kongpo

85 Sde srid sangs rgyas rgya mtsho, *Sde srid sman gyi khog 'bubs*, 211.

86 G.yu thog kha rag lha rje, *Mkhas pa g.yu thog mgon po'i rnam thar pad tshal brgyas pa nor bu'i 'phreng ba*, 202–203.

87 G.yu thog kha rag lha rje, *Mkhas pa g.yu thog mgon po'i rnam thar pad tshal brgyas pa nor bu'i 'phreng ba*, 203.

88 G.yu thog kha rag lha rje, *Mkhas pa g.yu thog mgon po'i rnam thar pad tshal brgyas pa nor bu'i 'phreng ba*, 205–206.

89 Anonymous, "The Biography of Yutok Yönten Gonpo," *Journal of Tibetan Medicine and Astro-science* 34, no. 4 (2017): 1–4.

90 Sde srid sangs rgyas rgya mtsho, *Sde srid sman gyi khog 'bubs*, 211.

Degyel's dream about the Beautiful Medical City in the biography of Yutok.[91] Since the biography is not available to us, there is no way to compare this biography with the biography of the Elder Yutok. As I pointed out earlier, Kongpo Degyal played a very important role in the formation of the biography of the Elder Yutok, and the biography of Yutok by Kongpo Degyal might be another source for the Elder Yutok's biography. Furthermore, as Franz-Karl Ehrhard has observed, there are numerous overlaps and similar elements between the biographies of the Elder and Younger Yutoks.[92] The biography of the Younger Yutok might be another available source for the Elder Yutok's biography.

10 Conclusion

The description of the Nine Learned Tibetan Physicians of the Tibetan Empire can first be found in the historical works of the late thirteenth century.[93] This seems to suggest that, around thirteenth century, some Tibetan scholars might have believed that Yutok was a physician who lived during Tibetan Empire.

From thirteenth to sixteenth centuries, several biographies of Yutok appear to have been produced. However, the term "Yutok the Elder" or "Yutok Yönten Gönpo the Elder" did not appear in those biographies. In addition, we cannot find any information about the biography and the name of the Elder Yutok in Tibetan general histories and medical histories before the sixteenth century.

In sixteenth century, some Tibetan physicians and scholars debated about the issue of the Elder Yutok. One of biographies of the Elder Yutok may have been produced during this time. Ever since the seventeenth century—after Darmo Menrampa edited and carved the biography of the Elder Yutok—the life story of the Elder Yutok has been widely quoted by Tibetan scholars. It seems clear that our knowledge of the Elder Yutok is mainly based on this biography of the Elder Yutok and historical works that were composed after the seventeenth-century publishing of this biography.

A few years after the Elder Yutok biography was published, the Desi also provided a similar account of the Elder Yutok in his medical history, the *Beryl Mirror*, as well as in the *Blue Beryl*, his commentary on the *Four Tantras*. Since

---

91 Sog bzlog pa blo gros rgyal mtshan, *Rgyud bzhi'i bka' bsgrub nges don snying po*, in *Collected Writings of Sog-bzlog-pa Blo-gros-rgyal-mtshan* (New Delhi: Sangje Dorji, 1975), vol. 2, 224.

92 Franz-Karl Ehrhard, "A Short History of the *g.Yu thog snying thig*," in *Indica et Tibetica: Festschrift für Michael Hahn*, ed. Konrad Klaus and Jens-Uwe Hartmann (Wien: Arbeitskreis für Tibetische und Buddhistische Studien Universität Wien, 2007), 151–70.

93 Brang ti 'jam dpal bzang po, *Lag len gyi snying po pod chung gi 'grel pa bzhugs so*, 1a–2a.

then, the Elder Yutok and his biography have been very popular among Tibetan intellectuals.

After reading the biography carefully, I have found many narratives that contradict reliable Tibetan medical histories, as well as the standard sources for Tibetan political and religious history. Thus, I am not convinced that the biography of Yutok Yönten Gönpo the Elder is a reliable historical document. Furthermore, I believe that the biography can provide an authentic history for neither Tibetan medicine in general, nor the history of Yutok's lineage and the *Four Tantras* in particular. Thus, I am confused as to whether the Elder Yutok was an actual, historical figure. The biography of the Elder Yutok may have been composed in the sixteenth century or later, on the basis of several biographies of Yutok the Younger. The reliability of these biographies is questionable.

We also cannot find any strong evidence that proves Yutok was the royal physician of a Tibetan king. There is no evidence to prove that the Younger Yutok was the reincarnation and direct descendant of the Elder Yutok. In addition, there is no good reason to believe that the Elder Yutok was the primary author of the *Four Tantras*. Thus, I would suggest that there is no way to correctly understand the history of Tibetan medicine in general, and the history of Yutok's lineage and the *Four Tantras* in particular, if we do not reevaluate the reliability of the historical works and biographies, including the biography of the Elder Yutok.

Bibliography

Anonymous. "The Biography of Yutok Yönten Gonpo." *Journal of Tibetan Medicine and Astro-science* 34, no. 4 (2017): 1–4.

'Be lo tshe dbang kun khyab. *'Be lo tshe dbang kun khyab kyi gsung thor bu'i skor*. Lhasa: Bod ljongs bod yig dpe rnying dpe skrun khang, 2013.

Beckwith, Christopher I. "The Introduction of Greek Medicine into Tibet in the Seventh and Eighth Centuries." *Journal of the American Oriental Society* 99, no. 2 (1979): 297–313.

Blo bzang dpal 'byor. *Bla ma chag lo tsā ba chos rje dpal ba'i rnam par thar pa bla ma'i gsung dri ma med bar sgrigs pa*. In *Lo chen rin chen bzang po dang/ chag lo tsā ba chos rje dpal/ rngo lo tsā ba blo ldan shes rab gsum gyi rnam thar*, 108–236. Lhasa: Ser gtsug nang bstan dpe rnying 'tshol bsdu phyogs sgrig khang.

Brang ti dpal ldan 'tsho byed. *Bdud rtsi snying po yan lag brgyad pa gsang ba man ngag gi rgyud kyi spyi don shes bya rab gsal rgyas pa*. The Library of the Cultural Palace of Minorities in Beijing: Manuscript, n.d.

Brang ti 'jam dpal bzang po. *Lag len gyi snying po pod chung gi 'grel pa bzhugs so*. Manuscript, n.d.

'Bri gung skabs mgon che tshang. *Tun hong bod kyi yig rnying las byung ba: bod btsan po'i rgyal rabs*. Dehradun: Sangtsen Library, 2010.

Bu ston rin chen grub. *Bu ston chos 'byung*. Beijing: Krung go'i bod kyi shes rig dpe skrun khang, 1988.

Byams pa 'phrin las. *Gso rig lo rgyus*. Beijing: Mi rigs dpe skrun khang, 2004.

Byams pa 'phrin las. *Krung go'i bod kyi gso ba rig pa*. Beijing: Krung go'i bod kyi shes rig dpe skrun khang, 1996.

Byams pa 'phrin las and Thub bstan tshe ring. *Bod kyi gso ba rig pa'i lo rgyus*. In *Krung go'i gso rig kun 'dus las bod kyi gso ba rig pa*, vol. 1, 1–53. Lhasa: Bod ljongs mi dmangs dpe skrun khang, 1990.

Dba' gsal snang. *Dba' bzhed*. Lhasa: Bod ljongs bod yig dpe rnying dpe skrun khang, 2011.

Dong Zhiqiao. *Datang xiyuji*. Beijing: Zhonghua shuju, 2016.

Dpa' bo gtsug lag phreng ba. *Chos 'byung mkhas pa'i dga' ston*. Beijing: Mi rigs dpe skrun khang, 1986.

Dpal 'byor bzang po. *Rgya bod yig tshang chen mo*. Chengdu: Si khron mi rigs dpe skrun khang, 1985.

Dung dkar blo bzang 'phrin las. *Dung dkar blo bzang 'phrin las kyi gsung rtsom phyogs bsgrigs*. Beijing: Krung go'i bod kyi shes rig dpe skrun khang, 1997.

Ehrhard, Franz-Karl. "A Short History of the *g.Yu thog snying thig*." In *Indica et Tibetica: Festschrift für Michael Hahn*, edited by Konrad Klaus and Jens-Uwe Hartmann, 151–70. Wien: Arbeitskreis für Tibetische und Buddhistische Studien Universität Wien, 2007.

Go 'jo dbang 'dus. *Rje btsun g.yu thog yon tan mgon po dang dpal ldan rgyud bzhi'i skor gleng ba*. Unpublished paper, 2013.

'Gos lo gzhon nu dpal. *Deb ther sngon po*. Chengdu: Si khron mi rigs dpe skrun khang, 1985.

Gu ru o rgyan gling pa. *Bka' thang sde lnga*. Beijing: Mi rigs dpe skrun khang, 1986.

G.yu thog kha rag lha rje. *Mkhas pa g.yu thog mgon po'i rnam thar pad tshal brgyas pa nur bu'i 'phreng ba*. In *Krung go'i bod lugs gso rig rtsa che'i dpe rnying kun btus*, vol. 15, 193–209. Lhasa: Bod ljongs mi dmangs dpe skrun khang, 2013.

Jo bo lhun grub bkra shis and Dar mo sman rams pa blo bzang chos grags. *G.yu thog gsar rnying gi rnam thar.* Beijing: Mi rigs dpe skrun khang, 1982.

Jo nang tā ra na tha. *Myang yul stod smad bar gsum gyi ngo mtshar gtam gyi legs bshad mkhas pa'i 'jug ngogs*. Lhasa: Bod ljongs mi dmangs dpe skrun khang, 1983.

Karmay, Samten G. "The Four Tibetan Medical Tantras and Their Critics." In *The Arrow and the Spindle: Studies in History, Myths, Rituals and Beliefs in Tibet*, 228–37. Kathmandu: Mandala Book Point, 1998.

Khang dkar tshul khrim skal bzang. *Khang dkar tshul khrim skal bzang mchog gi gsung 'bum pod bcu pa*. Chengdu: Si khron mi rigs dpe skrun khang, 2013.

Kong po bde rgyal and Dar mo sman rams pa blo bzang chos grags. *G.yu thog gsar rnying gi rnam thar*. Beijing: Mi rigs dpe skrun khang, 2005.

Luo Guangwu. *Liang tangshu tubozhuan yizhu*. Beijing: Zhongguo zangxue chubanshe, 2014.

McKay, Alex, ed. *The History of Tibet*, vol. 1. London: RoutledgeCurzon, 2003.

McGrath, William A. *Buddhism and Medicine in Tibet: Origins, Ethics, and Tradition*. Charlottesville, VA: Doctoral Dissertation at the University of Virginia, 2017.

Rechung Rinpoche Jampal Kunzang. *Tibetan Medicine: Illustrated in Original Texts*. Berkeley, CA: University of California Press, 1976 [repr. Delhi: Sri Satguru Publications, 2001].

Riqiong renpoqie jiabai gunsang. *Xizang yixue*. Lhasa: Xizang renmin chubanshe, 1986.

Sde srid sangs rgyas rgya mtsho. *Sde srid sman gyi khog 'bubs*. Beijing: Mi rigs dpe skrun khang, 2004.

Sog bzlog pa blo gros rgyal mtshan. *Rgyud bzhi'i bka' bsgrub nges don snying po*. In *Collected Writings of Sog-bzlog-pa Blo-gros-rgyal-mtshan: Reproduced from a Unique but Incomplete Dbu-can Manuscript from the Library of the Ven. Bdud-'joms Rin-po-che*, vol. 2, 213–42. New Delhi: Sangje Dorji, 1975.

Stobs ldan and Kha sgang bkra shis tshe ring. *Pha ran sir nyar ba'i tun hong yig rnying gi bshus yig phyogs bsgrigs*, vol. 11. Lhasa: Bod ljongs mi dmangs dpe skrun khang, 2017.

Sum ston ye shes gzungs. *Gso rig rgyud bzhi'i bla ma brgyud pa'i rnam thar bka' rgya ma gtsang ru mtshams sum pa jha na rda ra'i gsung 'phros gyim phyogs 'tsho byed gzhon nu la gdams pa*. In *Gangs ljongs sman rtsis rig mdzod chen mo*, vol. 38, 401–11. Beijing: Krung go'i bod rig pa dpe skrun khang, 2016.

Thub bstan phun tshogs. *G.yu thog rnying ma'i mtha' dpyad rgyal ba dgyes pa'i mchod sprin*. Unpublished paper, 2014.

Zur mkhar ba blo gros rgyal po. *Sman pa rnams kyis mi shes su mi rung ba'i shes bya spyi'i khog dbubs*. Chengdu: Si khron mi rigs dpe skrun khang, 2001.

Zur mkhar ba blo gros rgyal po. *'Tsho byed kun legs pa'i dris lan zla ba'i thig pa*. In *Gangs ljongs sman rtsis rig mdzod chen mo*, vol. 40, 211–16. Beijing: Krung go'i bod rig pa dpe skrun khang, 2016.

Yang Ga. "The Origin of the *Four Tantras* and an Account of Its Author, Yuthog Yonten Gonpo." In *Bodies in Balance: The Art of Tibetan Medicine*, edited by Theresia Hofer, 154–77. Seattle, WA: University of Washington Press, 2014.

Yang Ga. *The Sources for the Writing of the Rgyud bzhi: Tibetan Medical Classic*. Cambridge, MA: Doctoral Dissertation at Harvard University, 2010.

Yang Ga. "Study on the Origin of Yutok Family." *Journal of Tibet University* 66, no. 2 (2015): 122–29.

CHAPTER 3

"Secret Medicine" in the Writings of Sanggyé Gyatso: the Encoded Esoteric Material of Therapeutics

Tony Chui

1 Introduction

The *Four Tantras* (*rgyud bzhi*) is the intellectual foundation of the Tibetan medical tradition. According to traditional accounts, its origin can be traced back to the eighth century of the Common Era,[1] and throughout the development of Tibetan medicine, various therapeutic methods have been adopted and developed. Commentaries and supplementary works were also composed to make up for the practical shortcomings of the *Four Tantras*. In the seventeenth century, for example, during the reign of the Fifth Dalai Lama Ngawang Lozang Gyatso (*ngag dbang blo bzang rgya mtsho*, 1617–1682), a remarkable body of medical instructions augmented the Tibetan medical genre. Together with his regent (*sde srid*) Sanggyé Gyatso, the Fifth Dalai Lama established the leading school of medicine and astrology known as the Chakpori Rikjé Dropen Ling (*lcag po ri rig byed 'gro phan gling*), named after the Iron Mountain (*lcag po ri*), near the Potala Palace in Lhasa.[2] Under this establishment, the Tibetan medical tradition was systematized and institutionalized,[3] and the Chakpori remained an authority of medical education until the 1950s.[4]

In addition to being the regent of the Fifth Dalai Lama, Sanggyé Gyatso was also an eminent medical scholar. During his fairly short lifespan of fifty-two years, he was a prolific writer, composing a number of significant treatises that strongly influenced the Tibetan medical tradition. Among them, three works

1 Yang Ga, *The Sources for the Writing of the Rgyud Bzhi, Tibetan Medical Classic* (Cambridge, MA: PhD dissertation, Harvard University, 2010), 21–22.

2 Janet Gyatso, *Being Human in a Buddhist World: An Intellectual History of Medicine in Early Modern Tibet* (New York, NY: Columbia University Press, 2015), 115.

3 Kurtis R. Schaeffer, "Textual Scholarship, Medical Tradition, and Mahāyāna Buddhist Ideals in Tibet," *Journal of Indian Philosophy* 31, no. 5 (2003): 622.

4 Fernand Meyer "The Golden Century of Tibet Medicine," in *Lhasa in the Seventeenth Century: The Capital of the Dalai Lamas*, ed. Françoise Pommaret (Leiden: Brill, 2003), 117.

 | DOI:10.1163/9789004404441_004

have had momentous impact.[5] Two of them—the *Blue Beryl* (*baiḍūrya sngon po*), a commentary on the *Four Tantras*, and the *Mirror of Beryl* (*baiḍūrya me long*), which delivers a comprehensive account of the history of Tibetan medicine—set out Sanggyé Gyatso's approach to the learning and practice of medicine. Both the *Blue Beryl* and the *Mirror of Beryl* stress the importance of medical scholarship and the Mahāyāna ideal of being a virtuous medical practitioner. Through these two great works, Sanggyé Gyatso shaped and imposed medical professionalism upon Tibetan medical practitioners, prescribing the moral and behavioural standards that every talented practitioner should uphold in accordance with the Chakpori school of medical practice.

The third major text by Sanggyé Gyatso is the "extended commentary" (*lhan thabs*) on the *Instructional Tantra* (*man ngag rgyud*) of the *Four Tantras*: the *Man ngag lhan thabs* (hereafter referred to as the *Extended Commentary*).[6] In the *Extended Commentary*, peculiar esoteric ingredients rarely mentioned in the other two works can frequently be found. To identify these ingredients as literal or figurative is crucial in the study of both Tibetan medicine and Buddhist Tantra. In our case, the way of interpreting these ingredients in the *Extended Commentary* is decisive in the effectiveness of the medicinal recipes. Furthermore, as a study of the *Extended Commentary* reveals, "secret" (*gsang*) terms are scattered throughout the manuscript. These "secret" terms seem to render parts of the *Extended Commentary* incomprehensible to anyone lacking the decrypting key. "Secret" terms are not restricted to medical texts, but also noticeable in other Tantric writings, such as the autobibliography *Visions and Their Significance* (*mthong ba don ldan*) of the Fifth Dalai Lama. As this "encryption" retains the confidentiality of the esoteric tradition, exploration of how these "secret" terms are encoded promises a better understanding of Tantric literature.

In the *Blue Beryl*, Sanggyé Gyatso opines that reading medical texts alone will not lead to sufficient medical training, and that it is necessary to have the guidance of a skilled teacher.[7] Apart from the "medical professionalism" that he advocates, does he mean that some materials are not covered in the ordinary medical texts, and that a "skilled" teacher who holds the keys to these texts is the determining factor in "sufficient" medical training? What do the "secret" encryptions mean and why were they kept secret? In the following

5 Schaeffer, "Textual Scholarship," 624.

6 Full title in Tibetan: *Man ngag yon tan rgyud kyi lhan thabs zug rngu'i tsha gdung sel ba'i katpū ra dus min 'chi zhags gcod pa'i ral gri* (Xining: Mtsho sngon mi rigs dpe skrun khang, 1991).

7 Sangs rgyas rgya mtsho, *Gso ba rig pa'i bstan bcos sman bla'i dgongs rgyan rgyud bzhi'i gsal byed bai durya sngon po'i malli ka* (Leh: D. L. Tashigang, 1981), 494.

section, I will explore Sanggyé Gyatso's *Extended Commentary* on the healing of life-wind illness and discuss the necessity for the encryption of "secret" material. In addition, I will attempt to decrypt and unveil the "secret" terms specified in the text.

2 The *Extended Commentary*

Not only did the *Extended Commentary* help Sanggyé Gyatso demonstrate his talent, but it was also used to epitomize "Tibetan medicine" itself—or the Chakpori school of Tibetan medicine, to be exact. The *Extended Commentary* is one of the most important works in the Tibetan medical tradition, after the *Four Tantras* and its commentaries, such as the *Blue Beryl*. According to Janet Gyatso, the Desi made the *Blue Beryl* and the *Extended Commentary* the core curriculum of medical training in the Chakpori.[8] Likewise, as described by Olaf Czaja, "they are the most important textual sources for the training of Tibetan doctors, past and present, and the medical ideas and concepts contained in them constituted the core Tibetan medical thinking."[9] In sum, Sanggyé Gyatso's *Extended Commentary* has endured to become an important text which is still appreciated in the present day.

The genre of the "extended commentary" (*lhan thabs*) has played an important role in the development of the Tibetan medical tradition. Extended commentaries contain novel information on the diagnosis and treatment of disease, which reflects the perspectives of medical practices within their social, cultural, and political contexts. In other words, they not only provide information on the treatment methods that were transmitted during their historical period, but also provide clues on how the medical "industry" was organized. As noted by Frances Garrett, in conjunction with the flourishing of esoteric practices of the thirteenth century, medical literature written after that time often mentioned the use of esoteric materials.[10] Paradoxically, in the *Blue Beryl* and the *Mirror of Beryl*, substances related to esoteric practices are rarely mentioned. Yet, in the *Extended Commentary*, medicinal substances which are esoteric in nature can be found. Therefore, in terms of novel treatment methods, the *Extended Commentary* reflects the "drugs of choice" and

8 Gyatso, *Being Human in a Buddhist World*, 115 (therein called the *Practical Manual*).

9 Olaf Czaja, "The Four Tantras and the Global Market," in *Medicine between Science and Religion*, ed. Vincanne Adams, Mona Schrempf, and Sienna R Craig (New York, NY: Berghahn Books, 2011), 283, n. 3.

10 Frances Garrett, "Tapping the Body's Nectar: Gastronomy and Incorporation in Tibetan Literature," *History of Religions* 49, no. 3 (2010): 302.

"tantric" conceptualizations of illness and healing held by Sanggyé Gyatso during his time.

In the *Extended Commentary*, for example, illnesses that are difficult to treat are generally classified as magico-religious in nature, and elements such as demons are considered to be the contributory causes of disease.[11] In handling "illness caused by demons" (*gdon nad*), the *Extended Commentary* employs a collection of ritualistic and peculiar medicines that are seldom found in the root text of the *Four Tantras*.[12] A point to note here is that a majority of diseases and disorders can be treated by using mantras and other magical formulae, which exemplifies the tantric healing characteristics of the Tibetan medical tradition of that period.[13] With all of this in mind, let us now explore Sanggyé Gyatso's *Extended Commentary* on the healing of life-wind illness.

3 The Text

"The Healing of Life-wind Illness": Chapter Three of the *Extended Commentary on the Instructional Tantra of the Four Tantras* by Sanggyé Gyatso

> There are the four aspects of life-wind illness: distant causes, immediate causes, symptoms, and treatment.
>
> While the distant causes of wind-illness are alike,[14] the immediate causes include: grief, worry, lack of sleep, harsh diet, inhibition and forceful voiding of stools, gossiping, disturbance by noises, anxiety, and body exhaustion. In conjunction with demons of various kinds,[15] as well as *gyelpo* spirits,[16] the influences of demons and spirits are noticeable by abnormalities in the urine and pulse.[17]

11 Czaja, "The Four Tantras and the Global Market," 269–70.

12 Gyatso, *Being Human in a Buddhist World*, 393.

13 Olaf Czaja, "The Making of the Blue Beryl: Some Remarks on the Textual Sources of the Famous Commentary of Sangye Gyatsho (1653–1705)," in *Soundings in Tibetan Medicine: Anthropological and Historical Perspectives*, ed. Mona Schrempf (Leiden: Brill, 2007), 357.

14 Although it is not elaborated here, in the root text, a distant cause of wind-illness is "desire" (*'dod chags*) resulting from "ignorance" (*ma rig pa*).

15 *Gdon spyi* has the meaning of all kinds of demons in general.

16 *Rgyal po* is a form of mischievous earth spirit.

17 There is no mentioning of demons or spirits in the root text.

Symptoms of life-wind illness include: distress, panic, obscure dreams, shallow sleep, body shivers, over-perspiration, wavering awareness, confusion, and difficulty breathing and swallowing.[18]

The treatment of this illness falls into four categories: medication, external treatment, diet, and lifestyle.[19] Apply the following medicinal recipes as appropriate:

Prepare ginger, nutmeg, fennel, black salt, cumin seed, clove, and pepper. Boil and reduce the above with the essence of three bones[20] and *chang* beer,[21] drink it early in the morning, and after that take the medical preparation Agar-8.[22] Add clove, human flesh, and fennel [to Agar-8] to form the medical preparation of Sokdzin-11,[23] if it is complicated by chest, heart, liver ailment, or insanity.

If life-wind illness is accompanied by heart pain, prescribe [the following recipe consisting of] sword bean, areca nut, black myrobalan, nutmeg, clove, costus, lapsi fruit, aconite,[24] yak fat, ginger, the three peppers, black salt, Wallich milk parsley, and seeds of the wallflower. Mix the above with the heart of a parrot killed by a knife,[25] as well as the hearts of a vulture, a wild yak, a dog, and a pig. Gather the above hearts and the other ingredients and roll them up into pea-sized pills with brown molasses. Take five to seven pills in accordance with the age of the patient, with

18 Further description of the symptoms can be found in the root text. Sanggyé Gyatso may have assumed that the reader would have fully studied the root text before reading the *Extended Commentary*.

19 As with the symptoms, Sanggyé Gyatso does not further elaborate on the treatment regarding diet and lifestyle.

20 The essence of three kinds of bones: ankle, scapula, and sacrum; preferably those of a sheep (Thinley Gyatso and Chris Hakim, *Essentials of Tibetan Traditional Medicine* [Berkeley, CA: North Atlantic Books, 2010], 23).

21 An alcoholic drink made from barley.

22 On *A gar brgyad pa*, see Bhagwan Dash, *Pharmacopoeia of Tibetan Medicine* (Delhi: Sri Satguru Publications, 1994), 220, recipe number 200. Dash lists Agar-8 as a recipe for heart disease, insanity, and pain in chest and liver.

23 On *Srog 'dzin bcu gcig pa*, see Dash, *Pharmacopoeia of Tibetan Medicine*, 203, recipe number 186. There he lists Sokdzin-11 as a recipe for insanity, heart disease, and liver disorder.

24 *Sman chen: Aconitum richardsonianum Lauener var. crispulum* (*bong nga nag po*) and *'bri tshil: Aconitum kongboense Lauener* (*bong nag rigs ser po*). *Sman chen 'bril tshil* may indicate a single plant of *Aconitum sp.*, which is poisonous (Pasang Yonten Arya, *Dictionary of Tibetan Materia Medica* [Delhi: Motilal Banarsidass, 1998], 171, 189).

25 The heart of parrot killed by knife (*gri snying ne tso*) can protect one against *gyelpo* spirits and speechlessness due to mental disorders, and also alleviates heart pain (Pasang Yonten Arya, *Dictionary of Tibetan Materia Medica*, 122).

three-bone-essence or four-animal-essence soup for a duration of five weeks.

Life-wind illness is an agonizing disease, especially if it is accompanied by an unhappy mind, and thus [the following recipe] is recommended. The four types of myrobalan[26] with their pits removed, with equal amounts of sweet flag and long pepper. Together with clove, snow lotus, black salt, and an equal amount of aconite. Add these together with nutmeg fruit and equal amount of the "main secret medicine of eight years,"[27] grind into powder, and bind into a purple pill with the urine [of an eight-year-old boy], gesso, and molasses. Do not overdose; use only appropriate amount for treating life-wind illness.

This [recipe] is effective for all kinds of heart and wind-channel diseases, and is particularly recommended for insanity. Alternately, add to the above preparation processed mercury (one *zho*),[28] powdered sulfur[29] (half *zho*), and the hearts of a wild yak and a parrot. At the end, combine them together with three medicinal fruits,[30] the juice of lapsi fruit, and coriander.[31] Take a small portion (a mouthful) early in the morning. The efficacy is the same as the previous recipe.

Another recipe is to use three hundred lapsi fruits (if this amount is not available, use fifty), with three *dré*[32] of water boiled down to one *dré*, stirred and strained through a satin cloth. Add these together with a handful amount of dri[33] milk and seven *sang* of dri butter. Mix the various ingredients with a handful of bone-essence and nine *sang* of molasses to the thickness similar to that of yogurt and add the following

26 The four types of myrobalan are: *a ru 'jigs med, sha mthug, skem po*, and *sul mang*. Another fruit belonging to the same family is *a ru rnam rgyal*, which is exclusively found in heaven (Pasang Yonten Arya, *Dictionary of Tibetan Materia Medica*, 305).

27 The literal translation from *gsang sman gtso bo ljid mnyam lo brgyad*.

28 Mercury (*dngul chu*) can cure all types of diseases of evil spirit origin (Pasang Yonten Arya, *Dictionary of Tibetan Materia Medica*, 54), which has to be detoxified before use. *Zho* is a Tibetan unit of weight equivalent to 3.75 grams, and 10 *zho* equal 1 *sang*, which corresponds to the Chinese unit of weight, *liang*.

29 It is a common practice to use powdered sulfur with mercury. The amount used has to be precise to avoid poisoning.

30 The "three fruits" (*'bras bu gsum*): *a ru* (*Terminalia chebula*), *ba ru* (*Terminalia bellerica*), and *skyu ru* (*Emblica officinalis*). See Pasang Yonten Arya, *Dictionary of Tibetan Materia Medica*, 170.

31 *Rta bya* refers to either mineral marcasite (*gser rdo*) or *Coriandrum sativum* (*'u su*). See Pasang Yonten Arya, *Dictionary of Tibetan Materia Medica*, 84.

32 *Dré* is a Tibetan unit of volume equivalent to 1 litre.

33 Female yak (*'bri*).

ingredients: frankincense, snow lotus, and burnt garlic[34] (these three have the strength to overcome all fevers that are due to winds); fennel, Wallich milk parsley, and hot salt (these three overcome all kinds of disorders due to winds); aconite, adult heart, and blue hoppy (these three can alleviate the severe pain of any disease); myrobalan,[35] juniper,[36] and strychnine[37] (these three suppress the wind of the upper body); long pepper, black pepper, and ginger (these three kindle the heat of the flame); cumin seed, sugar, and honey (these three bring out the potency of the medicine to eliminate the disease); "the two secret medicines,"[38] and *Pterocephalus hookeri*[39] (these three overcome severe insanity). Take a teaspoonful of this "twenty-one-medicines" mixture at dawn to treat life-wind illness. This is a recipe of the Northern Lhünding tradition.

The above preparation can cure all kinds of life-wind illness. When life-wind illness is attributed to a powerful evil spirit, which is hard to eliminate, prescribe the above recipe along with the secret medicine preparation, "Fierce Wild Garuḍa,"[40] with equal amounts of the "main secret medicine of eight years" and the "main secret medicine of two wheels,"[41] together with a generous amount of nutmeg and clove. The proper dosage should induce a slight adverse reaction (such as tongue-numbness). Subsequently, prescribe Sokdzin-11 together with areca nut and the "minor secret medicine."[42]

For external treatment, perform moxibustion on the sixth and seventh vertebra points, the middle-chest point, the raven-eye point, and the great-vertebra point. Alternatively, cupping can be done on the front and

34 *Sgog* here may be an abbreviation of *sgog skya, Allium sativum*, which can cure wind diseases caused by evil spirits (Pasang Yonten Arya, *Dictionary of Tibetan Materia Medica*, 51).

35 *Dang po'i dbyangs las skyes pa*, a synonym for *a ru ra* (*Terminalia chebula*). See Pasang Yonten Arya, *Dictionary of Tibetan Materia Medica*, 97.

36 Abbreviated term for *shug pa ther can* (*Juniperus formosana*). See Pasang Yonten Arya, *Dictionary of Tibetan Materia Medica*, 267.

37 *Ko bil la, Strychnos nuxvomica* (Pasang Yonten Arya, *Dictionary of Tibetan Materia Medica*, 8).

38 The literal translation from *gsang sman gnyis*.

39 *Spang rtsi do bo*, there is no common name available. According to Gyatso and Hakim (*Essentials of Tibetan Traditional Medicine*, 199), "it seems to be clinically and morphologically similar to dandelion."

40 The literal translation from *khyung rgod drag po*.

41 The literal translation from *gsang sman gtso bo'khor gnyis*.

42 The literal translation from *gsang sman kha tshar*.

back of the body. Bloodletting is also beneficial to patients complicated with blood-bile disease.

Prescribe Sédru-8[43] during the recovery period. If dizziness occurs, apply nasal drops consist of saffron, sugar, and butter. Furthermore, carry out moxibustion on the three meeting-door points, and cauterize the points on the anterior and posterior fontanelles. If there are other symptoms, additional treatment may be utilized.

The diet and lifestyle of the patients should follow the treatment of common wind-illness.

Such is "The Healing of Life-wind Illness," Chapter Three of the *Extended Commentary on Instructional Tantra of the Four Tantras.*

4 Decrypting "Secret Medicine"

From the above translated text, one can see that the standard recipes of medicines are quite similar to those in the *Four Tantras* and the *Blue Beryl*. For example, aloeswood, nutmeg, clove, and pepper are the main ingredients for the treatment of life-wind illness even in modern Tibetan medicine. With respect to the cause and symptoms, the *Extended Commentary* can be taken as a brief summary of its root text. Nonetheless, unexplainable terms, such as the "main secret medicine of eight years" (*gsang sman gtso bo ljid mnyim lo brgyad*) and the "main secret medicine of two wheels" (*gsang sman gtso bo'khor gnyis*) are not found in any part of the *Four Tantras.*[44] One hypothesis is that the encryptions in the *Extended Commentary* were used in order to conceal important or sensitive information from outsiders. These terms in this chapter make it impossible for the reader to fully prepare the medicine in accordance with the recipes, especially for life-wind illness caused by powerful spirits. Throughout the *Extended Commentary*, one can find similar encryptions, and thus these "secret medicines" (*gsang sman*) were intentionally hidden by the author, and keys for their decryption do indeed exist.

I found the keys to these "secret medicines" dispersed in two separate texts. Each one provides a partial solution to the encryption and both must be consulted in order to fully utilize the medicinal recipes in the text. One text—attributed to Ngawang Sanggyé Pelzang (*ngag dbang sangs rgyas dpal bzang*), a

43 On *Se 'bru padma 'dab brgyad*, see Dash, *Pharmacopoeia of Tibetan Medicine*, 192, recipe number 176.

44 An experienced Tibetan medical practitioner, Dr. Dawa, was unable to comprehend the meaning of the *gsang sman* mentioned in the text.

student of Sanggyé Gyatso—is the *Single Lineage of Secret Medicine: The Golden Key for Decoding the Knot of the Extended Commentary on the Instructional Tantra* (*gsang sman chig brgyud/ lhan thabs kyi rgya mdud bkrol ba'i rin chen gser gyi lde mig*).[45] In the introduction to this text, Ngawang Sanggyé Pelzang highlights the fact that the knowledge of secret medicine is to be orally transmitted, and that only those who are capable and have paid respect to their teacher will receive the key. He also adds that since these secret medicines are of great importance in treating diseases, practitioners should receive proper teachings and blessings from their teacher before practicing.[46] Ngawang Sanggyé Pelzang also stresses that the key to the secret medicines should be kept exclusively within a single lineage.

The second text disclosing the key to the secret medicines mentioned in the *Extended Commentary* is the *Writing on the Single Lineage of Secret Medicine* (*gsang sman chig brgyud kyi shog dril skor*) by Darmo Menrampa Lozang Chödrak (*dar mo sman rams pa blo bzang chos grags*, 1638–1710). Darmo Menrampa apparently did not agree with the notion of keeping this secret knowledge within a single lineage, however. Instead, he argues that keeping the secret medicines to oneself (that is, in a single lineage) would lead to the loss of this knowledge. Since these secret medicines are a vital part of medical treatment, it is better to disclose them for the sake of all sentient beings.[47] Darmo Menrampa once served as a teacher in the medical teaching college at Sharchen Chok (*shar chen lcog*) at the Potala Palace, where he was an elder colleague of Sanggyé Gyatso, having established several medical initiatives during the time of the Fifth Dalai Lama.[48] He also made numerous contributions to a range of instructional, anatomical, pharmaceutical, and therapeutic genres.[49] As one of the court physicians (*bla sman*) of the Fifth Dalai Lama, Darmo Menrampa was probably related to Sanggyé Gyatso personally.[50] Their close relationship can be noted in an incident where Darmo Menrampa together

45 According to Meyer ("The Golden Century of Tibet Medicine," in *Lhasa in the Seventeenth Century: The Capital of the Dalai Lamas*, ed. Françoise Pommaret [Leiden: Brill, 2003], 111), Sanggyé Gyatso appointed Ngawang Sanggyé Pelzang as one of his students in charge of medical teaching at the Chakpori.

46 Ngag dbang sangs rgyas dpal bzang, *Gsang sman chig brgyud, lhan thabs kyi rgya mdud bkrol ba'i rin chen gser gyi lde mig*, in *Man ngag lhan thabs dang lde mig* (Beijing: Mi rigs dpe skrun khang, 2005), 461.

47 Blo bzang chos grags, *Gsang sman chig brgyud kyi shog dril skor*, in *Man ngag lhan thabs dang lde mig* (Beijing: Mi rigs dpe skrun khang, 2005), 434.

48 Gyatso, *Being Human in a Buddhist World*, 193.

49 Dkon mchog rin chen, *Bod kyi gso rig chos 'byung baiḍūrya'i 'phreng ba* (Lanzhou: Kan su'u mi rigs dpe skrun khang, 1994), 107–115.

50 Czaja, "The Making of the Blue Beryl," 348.

with the "choir master" (*dbu mdzad*), Lozang Yönten (*blo bzang yon tan*); the "chief sacristan" (*mchod dpon*), Jamyang Drakpa (*'jam dbyang grags pa*); and the "tantrist" (*sngags 'chang*), Agur Zhika Sharpa (*a gur gzhis ka shar pa*); collaborated with Sanggyé Gyatso to maintain the secret of the death of the Fifth Dalai Lama.[51]

Coming back to the decryption key, in the text by Ngawang Sanggyé Pelzang, the undisclosed formula "Fierce Wild Garuḍa," is described as follows:

> Regarding life-wind illness in Chapter 3, the formula "Fierce Wild Garuḍa" is: Four *zho* of fine heart flesh, one [*zho*] of bone, two-thirds [*zho*] of tendons, combined with one-third [*zho*] of blood. Mix together vigorously into a paste. This is the proper composition of the secret formula.[52]

In Darmo Menrampa's text, terms defining the ingredients for the "secret medicines" can be found as follows:

> The "main secret medicine of eight years" is a panacea that consists of three parts: the heart of an adult who experienced sudden death killed by knife, together with the "two secret medicines." The "two secret medicines" are the womb (menstrual) blood of a mourning widow and flesh of a bastard child (or child of incestuous union). For the "main secret medicine of two wheels," [there are two components]: the "main" is the blood, heart, and flesh of a brave man killed by an enemy's knife or the blood and heart of a wild yak, whichever is available. In addition, the "two wheels" means the womb blood [menses] of a mourning widow and bastard flesh, [if not obtainable], use fennel and black salt. Moreover, the "minor secret medicine" is rabbit heart.[53]

The quantities of some medicinal substances to be used are missing from the *Extended Commentary*, and the exact weights of the ingredients to be used cannot be found in any of the three above texts. This information seems to have been kept by another party under the encrypting scheme.

---

51 Samten Gyaltsen Karmay, *Secret Visions of the Fifth Dalai Lama: The Gold Manuscript in the Fournier Collection, Musée Guimet, Paris*, ed. Samten Gyaltsen Karmay and Lionel Fournier (London: Serindia Publications, 1998), 8.

52 Ngag dbang sangs rgyas dpal bzang, *Rin chen gser gyi lde mig*, 473.

53 Blo bzang chos grags, *Gsang sman chig brgyud kyi shog dril skor*, 434–35.

5 Hermeneutics of Secret Medicine

The literal translations, such as for the "heart of an adult killed by a knife" (*dar ma'i gri snying*), and the "womb blood [menses] of a widow and the flesh of a bastard child" (*yug za'i [yugs sa'i] mngal khrag dang nal bu'i sha*),[54] are relatively straightforward and can be translated without much ambiguity. The next question we need to address is what the author meant by these terms.

There has been a long debate on whether the use of ritualistic elements such as human by-products is to be applied literally or merely symbolically. These two interpretations have led to two contrasting scholastic views in tantric literature: literalism and figurativism. The literalists, such as David Snellgrove, assert that tantric techniques are to be interpreted literally;[55] whereas the figurativists, such as Anthony Warder, indicate that the Tantras were merely symbolic.[56] Christian Wedemeyer has suggested a third approach, in which he basically states that the significance lies in the function of an object in a cultural sense but not the object in its literal sense, and thus the notion of using the product itself is irrelevant.[57]

Nonetheless, the literalist's view is not without reason. Frances Garrett opines that the actual use of these products was necessary and of important efficacy.[58] Moreover, illustrations of the literal use of human flesh, menses, and even the bones of a man killed by a knife can be found in the pedagogical paintings of the *Blue Beryl* by Sanggyé Gyatso.[59] If we examine the medical

54 According to a Tibetan medical dictionary (Dbang 'dus, *Gso ba rig pa'i tshig mdzod g.yu thog dgongs rgyan* [Beijing: Mi rigs dpe skrun khang, 1983], 294), the term *nal bu* has the meaning of a child born from: an incestuous couple, parents outside of matrimony, or the sexual union of fathers' kinsman (*rigs rgyud gcig pa'i pho mo 'khrig pa las byung ba'i phru gu'i ming la bzhed dang/ pha ma sogs kyi zhal bsgos ltar 'jig rten lugs mthun gyi gnyen sgrig byas pa ma yin par lkog tu nyal po spyod pa las byung ba'i pha ngos bzung med pa'i phru gu'i ming la bzhed pa zhig dang gnyis mchis te/ sa sku ngag dbang kun dga' bsog nams kyis mdzad pa'i 'jig rten gyi tshul lugs rnam par bzhag pa las/ nal bu ni pha rus gcig pa'i pho mo gnyis bshos pa las byung ba'o/*).

55 David Snellgrove, *Indo-Tibetan Buddhism: Indian Buddhists and Their Tibetan Successors* (Boston, MA: Shambhala, 1987), 160.

56 Anthony Kennedy Warder, *Indian Buddhism* (Delhi: Motilal Banarsidass Publishers, 2000), 475.

57 Christian Wedemeyer, "Beef, Dog, and Other Mythologies: Connotative Semiotics in Mahāyoga Tantra Ritual and Scripture," *Journal of the American Academy of Religion* 75, no. 2 (2007): 390–91.

58 Garrett, "Tapping the Body's Nectar," 317.

59 Yuri Parfionovitch, Fernand Meyer, and Gyurme Dorje, *Tibetan Medical Paintings: Illustrations to the Blue Beryl Treatise of Sangye Gyamtso (1653–1705)* (London: Serindia Publications, 1992), 72, 78.

texts that make further commentaries on the *Extended Commentary*, we find the descriptions to be literal as well. For example, the encrypted information of the *Extended Commentary* was elaborated a century later by the Mongolian physician Sokpo Lungrik Tendar (*sog po lung rigs bstan dar*) in the *Garland of Golden Myrobalan* (*a ru rnam rgyal gser mdog phreng ba*).[60] There he further explains what Sanggyé Gyatso meant by "secret medicine":

> Regarding the heart of a young man who died a sudden death caused by a knife, as indicated, it is not a gentle death. The name "sudden death" as mentioned in the [*Extended Commentary* on the] *Instructional Tantra* is a death caused by a "knife"; which also includes horse-knife, water-knife, thunder-knife, and cliff-knife.[61] These are the "knives" for sudden deaths.[62]
>
> While the "two secret medicines" [*gsang sman gnyis*] are the menses of a widow and the flesh of a bastard child. The latter [i.e. flesh of a bastard child] can also be the flesh of a child [i.e. fetus] who was lost during pregnancy [stillborn].[63]

Thus, according to Sokpo Lungrik Tendar, the substances mentioned by Sanggyé Gyatso were to be understood literally. Nonetheless, there seems to be a shift taking the original meaning of the terms in a more humane direction. Sokpo Lungrik Tendar's examples of the "knives" suggest the possibility of accidental deaths, as does his alternative explanation for bastard flesh as the flesh of a stillborn fetus rather than that of a living child. Whether Sokpo Lungrik Tendar misinterpreted Sanggyé Gyatso's *Extended Commentary* or simply preferred to use these more humane-sounding substances is a question that cannot be conclusively answered here. One point worth mentioning here is that the "sudden death by cliff-knife" was explicitly illustrated in Sanggyé Gyatso's medical paintings. In the *Supplementary Materia Medica* painting, an illustration depicts a man falling off a cliff, resulting in a skeleton lying on the ground.

---

60 Sog po lung rigs bstan dar, *A ru rnam rgyal gser mdog phreng ba*, in *Man ngag lhan thabs dang lde mig* (Beijing: Mi rigs dpe skrun khang, 2005), 559–61.

61 Knife here has the metaphoric meaning for different types of accidental or sudden death. A horse-knife (*rta gri*) refers to death caused by a horse-riding accident; water-knife (*chu dri*) refers to death caused by drowning; rock-knife (*rbab gri*) refers to death caused by a falling rock; and cliff-knife (*gyang gri*) refers to death caused by falling off a cliff.

62 Sog po lung rigs bstan dar, *A ru rnam rgyal gser mdog phreng ba*, 560: *mi na tsho dar la babs pa glo bur shi ba'i snying/ 'dir grir shi zhes 'byung ba mtshon gyis shi ba'i ming min par glo bur shi ba'i ming yin te/ man rgyud du/ rta gri chu gri rbab gri gyang gri dang/ zhes pa'i gri glo bur shi ba'i ming yin pa ltar ro//.*

63 Sog po lung rigs bstan dar, *A ru rnam rgyal gser mdog phreng ba*, 560: *gsang sman gnyis ni/ yugs ma'i mngal khrag/ nal bu'i sha/phyi ma 'di phrug gu shor ba'i 'o//.*

The inscription for this medical substance is the "body of one [suddenly killed by] a knife" (*gri lus*).

In the following section, although not comprehensive, I attempt to provide some background information on the substances that are used in this text.

5.1 *The Heart of a Man That Has Been Killed by Knife*

It is interesting to note that even in a modern-day Tibetan dictionary, the "flesh of a man killed by a knife" (*gri sha*) has the following meaning:

> The flesh of a healthy man that was suddenly killed by a knife. The property of this flesh is sweet and warm. It is effective in treating epidemics, life-wind illness, and diseases caused by *gyelpo* spirits.[64]

Similar terms—such as the "brain of a man killed by a knife" (*gri klad*), the "blood of a man killed by a knife" (*gri khrag*), and the "body of a man killed by a knife" (*gri lus*)—can also be found and used as "offering material" (*mchod rdzas*).[65] Based on these observations, it seems that the idea behind employing body parts of a person that has been "suddenly killed by a knife" (*glo bur du gri shi*) is that the more violent the death, the more powerful its products will be. The flesh of a man who has died a sudden death will have a potent effect. Another pertinent notion is that potent flesh cannot come from a diseased body or just be taken from any cadaver; the product must be obtained from someone who was "healthy" (*nad med*). The "heart" (*snying*), in Tibetan tradition, is believed to be the centre of the mind, and acts as a vessel for holding the "life force" (*srog rtsa*). In its center, it also holds the indestructible "drop" (*thig le*). Channels at the heart conduct all kinds of consciousness.[66] Based on the belief that symptoms of life-wind illness arise from the heart center, if one were to consume a heart according to esoteric understandings, it would benefit the activation of the corresponding drops, channels, and winds.[67]

5.2 *The Menses of a Widow*

Different forms of blood were frequently used in Tibetan magical ceremonies. Blood and body parts from various kinds of animals were mentioned in the

64 Zhang Yisun, *Bod rgya tsig mdzod chen mo* (Beijing: Mi rigs dpe skrun kang, 2013), 399: *mi dar ma nad med glo bur du grir shi ba'i sha ste/ ro mngar/ zhu rjes drod/ nus pas gnyan nad dang/ srog rlung/ rgyal gdon bcas la phan/.*

65 Zhang Yisun, *Bod rgya tsig mdzod chen mo*, 398.

66 Gyatso, *Being Human in a Buddhist World*, 270.

67 Robert Beer, *The Handbook of Tibetan Buddhist Symbols* (Boston, MA: Shambhala, 2003), 165–66.

text above, but the most peculiar type of blood used in "secret medicine" is perhaps that of humans. As noted by de Nebesky-Wojkowitz, the blood used in magical rites was not a red liquid that symbolized blood, but blood itself:

> Tibetan works give detailed information about the kind of blood one should apply. As regards human blood, the blood taken from a corpse or the blood of people suffering from a dangerous, contagious disease, especially of leprosy, further the menstruation-blood of a widow or that of a prostitute are said to be especially efficacious.[68]

The use of menstrual blood was prized and believed to be of commanding power. Its uses range from commanding deities in tantric rituals to ordinary magic rituals, but most regularly in black magic.[69] Under the reign of the Fifth Dalai Lama, four Indian physicians residing at the court translated texts from Sanskrit to Tibetan that involved various new therapeutic techniques.[70] The tantric notion of menses can be traced back to medieval Indian tantric literature, which lists a spectrum of menses from different sources. One such list can be found in the *Kulacūḍāmaṇi Tantra*,[71] which can be dated back to the ninth or tenth century.[72] The specific use of the menses of a widow can also be found in the medieval *Samayacāra Tantra*, in which it was termed as "generated from the ball" (*golodbhava*).[73] The use of the menstrual blood of a widow is not only found in the writing of Sanggyé Gyatso or Tibetan traditional medicine, but can be traced to Indian tantrism.

Widows were considered one of the least auspicious groups in Indic culture,[74] while according to the tantric interpretation, their menses has the

68 René de Nebesky-Wojkowitz, *Oracles and Demons of Tibet: The Cult and Iconography of the Tibetan Protective Deities* (Delhi: Book Faith India, 1993), 343–44.

69 Serinity Young, *Courtesans and Tantric Consorts: Sexualities in Buddhist Narrative, Iconography, and Ritual* (New York, NY: Routledge, 2004), 180.

70 Meyer, "The Golden Century of Tibet Medicine," 104. One of these techniques was cataract surgery performed by Darmo Menrampa on the Great Fifth.

71 David Gordon White, *Kiss of the Yoginī: "Tantric Sex" in its South Asian Contexts* (Chicago, IL: University of Chicago Press, 2003), 78. According to the *Kulacūḍāmaṇi Tantra, kuṇḍa* refers to the first menses after marriage; *gola* is the first menses after the death of her father; *varjrapuṣpa* is the first menses after sexual violence; *svayambhū* refers to the first menses of any woman; *bhavapuṣpa*, a woman's regular menses; and *gopīcandana* refers to a mixture of semen and menstrual blood (Louise Finn, *The Kulacudamani Tantra and the Vamakesvara Tantra with the Jayaratha Commentary* [Wiesbaden: Harrassowitz, 1986]).

72 Finn, *The Kulacudamani Tantra*, 21.

73 Narendra Nath Bhattacharyya, *Indian Puberty Rites* (Delhi: Munshiram Manoharlal, 1980), 17.

74 Young, *Courtesans and Tantric Consorts*, 24.

property of "hot" and "fiery" characteristics.[75] These characteristics could be linked to the heating characteristics of other life-wind medicinal preparations. Up to the present, there is no literature on whether the efficacy of a widow's menses in curing life-wind illness rests on empirical experience or results from tantric rituals. Whether a literal or symbolic notion should be applied to the use of menses is still debatable. Further studies are needed on the detailed mechanism of the menses in relation to the tantric physiology of the Tibetan medical tradition. Nonetheless, the use of specific menses in the *Extended Commentary* exemplifies the assimilation of Indian tantric elements in healing in seventeenth-century Tibet.

5.3 *The Flesh of a Bastard Child*

Human flesh is stated to be an important medical ingredient in the *Four Tantras* and it also has a special position in the history of the Tibetan tradition, where it is known as the "great meat" (*sha chen*). Soup made from human flesh was used in the treatment of wind illness.[76] The source of the flesh is also an important consideration. For instance, a striking ingredient in the "secret medicine" list is the flesh of a bastard child. It is also noted in magical ritual texts as the "flesh of a child which has been born out of an incestuous union."[77] Human products vary in their potency relative to the source, which is categorized by social status. As noted by Robert Beer, the "skull of a Brahmin, or a victim of murder or execution being considered the most effective medium for wrathful practice. The skull of a child who died during the onset of puberty also has great potency, as does the 'misbegotten skull' (*nal thod*) of a seven or eight-years-old child born from an incestuous union."[78] A skull cup (*kapala*) made from this kind of child was highly prized in rituals. For example, in the *Ritual Cycle of Penden Lhamo* by the Fifth Dalai Lama, the heart of a bastard child (*nal bu'i snying*) is used,[79] which suggests that a child from an illegitimate or incestuous union held significant value in tantric practice. Nonetheless, the idea of how the social status of the "medicinal source" could have an effect on the potency is poorly understood and further study is needed. The stillborn fetus previously mentioned by Sokpo Lungrik Tendar might have been used as an alternative, *contra* Sanggyé Gyatso.

75 White, *Kiss of the Yoginī*, 68.
76 Khams smyon dharma seng ge, *G.yu thog snying thig gi yig chos skor* (Leh: D. L. Tashigang, 1981), 199.
77 de Nebesky-Wojkowitz, *Oracles and Demons of Tibet*, 344–45.
78 Beer, *The Handbook of Tibetan Buddhist Symbols*, 111.
79 Karmay, *Secret Visions of the Fifth Dalai Lama*, 95.

6 Why are These Medicines Kept Secret?

The term "secrecy" has two connotations. It can imply the transmission of esoteric and occult insights which are mysterious in nature and revealed only to the so-called "chosen ones" or, on the other hand, it can also refer to specific technical knowledge, such as craft or trade secrets, confined only to a group of individuals as shared knowledge.[80] While we may never know for certain, the secrecy discussed here in this paper can take on both senses of the word. With respect to the former notion, tantric substances are believed to exhibit their full strength when used in a hidden way—in other words, the need for secrecy is to uphold the "potency" of the medicine. As opined by the Tibetan master Jikmé Püntsok, the practice of Vajrayāna had to be kept secret by the practitioner, otherwise the effects would be reduced or even nullified. In addition to spiritual practice:

> even some medical treatments require secrecy or they will not have a significant effect. For instance, in the Tibetan medical system there is a type of medicine that treats lung diseases ... [b]ut the name of this medicine must be kept secret.

Secrecy was required to indicate therapeutic potency. To further elaborate on the effect of secrecy on medicinal substance, Jikmé Püntsok made the following explanation:

> In the past Desi Sangye Gyatso was a well-known medical expert throughout Tibet. He recorded a superb collection of 'secret medicines' in one medical text and used secret codes to represent the uses of some types of Tibetan medicine.[81]

The medical text that Jikmé Püntsok mentions here is probably the *Extended Commentary*. According to him, the motivation for Sanggyé Gyatso's secrecy was to ensure medicinal potency.

As with other tantric teachings, keeping potentially dangerous tantric substances from the uninitiated was the responsibility of the author. A healing paradigm of this kind often involves higher esoteric teachings, which might impose danger to both the unguided practitioner and the patient. Some

80 Leong and Rankin, "Introduction: Secrets and Knowledge," 7–8.

81 Jigme Phuntsok, *Always Present: The Luminous Wisdom of Jigme Phuntsok*, trans. Emyo Yun Jia Wang (Boston, MA: Snow Lion, 2015), 90–91.

substances mentioned in the *Extended Commentary* were also recorded in the secret auto-bibliography *Visions and Their Significance* (*mthong ba don ldan*) of the Fifth Dalai Lama. As mentioned above, the "heart of a bastard" (*nal bu'i snying*) was used in a ritual of the deity Penden Lhamo (*dpal ldan lha mo*).[82] Coincidentally, similar to the encryption used in the *Extended Commentary*, the text which further explains the illustrations and ritual origins of the *Visions and Their Significance* is either missing or has been kept separately. It was not until 1992 that the missing explanatory texts under the titles *Seizure of Mind of the Ocean Heavens* (*zhing khams rgya mtsho'i yid 'phrog*) and *Seizure of the Pride of Illusions* (*sgyu ma'i khengs 'phrogs*) were found.[83] Keeping such explanatory texts separate from encrypted texts seems to indicate the intention of the Fifth Dalai Lama to conceal the important secrets of tantric practices. As explained by the Fourteenth Dalai Lama in the preface to the *Visions and Their Significance*, the misuse of secret teachings might result in personal harm.[84] For this reason, texts involving higher tantric teachings should be hidden from the uninitiated for their own safety.

Apart from these mystical standpoints, another seemingly obvious purpose of applying encryption to the medicinal formulae is to shield the peculiar ingredients from the scrutiny of others in the medical practice of the seventeenth century under the Buddhist hegemony. As already stated, Sanggyé Gyatso dedicated his writings to the praise of the Fifth Dalai Lama, the Ganden Government, and the Gelukpa School.[85] Compassion and non-violence are important Buddhist ideals, with which the use of the "heart of a man killed by a knife" does not sound compatible, especially in a medical work sanctioned by the Fifth Dalai Lama, a Buddhist leader who was venerated as morally superior to the common people. The ingredients might be misread as relating to black magic in nature, and the consumption of human products, such as the "flesh of a human violently killed," might contradict Buddhist ethics. To resolve this tension, Sanggyé Gyatso might have concealed the "secret medicines" to avoid condemnation for inhumanity.

Nonetheless, this explanation can be challenged if we consider the popularity and acceptance of prescribing peculiar substances during that time. Although they are no longer used in modern Tibetan medicine, medical instructions for cannibalism can be observed in the *Four Tantras* and its

82 Karmay, *Secret Visions of the Fifth Dalai Lama*, 95.

83 Karmay, *Secret Visions of the Fifth Dalai Lama, xiii.*

84 Karmay, *Secret Visions of the Fifth Dalai Lama, xi.*

85 Kurtis R. Schaeffer, "Ritual, Festival and Authority under the Fifth Dalai Lama," in *Power, Politics, and the Reinvention of Tradition*, ed. Bryan J. Cuevas and Kurtis R. Schaeffer (Leiden: Brill, 2006), 188.

commentaries. In addition to medical literature, the actual consumption of human by-products was also well recorded in other tantric literature: "they are prescribed in recipes for compound preparations—pills, decoctions, edible charms, and the like—that treat illnesses of all sorts and give one supernormal power, or siddhi."[86] Previously, such products were well known for their use in healing and occult rituals in the Tibetan tradition. For instance, the "five nectars" (*bdud rtsi lnga*) are vital elements used in the Indian and Tibetan tantric rituals. The five nectars include "human feces" (*dri chen*), "urine" (*dri chu*), "menstrual blood" (*rak ta*),[87] "semen" (*khu ba*),[88] and "marrow" (*rkang mar*). They were widely used together with the "five meats" (*sha lnga*): the flesh of a cow, dog, horse, elephant, and human.[89]

The use of peculiar human products such as the menstrual blood of a widow, the flesh of a bastard child, and the heart of a violently killed man were not only described by Sanggyé Gyatso in treating life-wind illness, but in fact, can be found in earlier writings. For instance, similar substances were hailed by Longchenpa (1308–1364) of the Nyingma lineage in his collected works as the "seven powerful secret medicines" (*bdun gsang ba'i sman mchog*), namely the heart of a person killed by knife (*gri snying*), the flesh of a person killed by knife (*'gri sha*), the menses of a widow (*yugs sa'i mngal khrag*), the flesh of bastard child (*nal bu sha*), "skunk" (*te lo*),[90] "hoopoe" (*pu shud*),[91] and "weasel" (*sre mong sha*).[92] These suggest that, rather than inventing these peculiar human products, Sanggyé Gyatso might have assimilated their use from other traditions. As noted by Gyatso, these rare ingredients were used to produce medicinal pills based on an esoteric system from the schools of Zur and Drigung.[93] For example, the heart of an adult killed by a knife (*dar ma'i gri snying*) can be found in the earlier medical text of Chögyi Drakpa (*chos gyi grags pa*, 1626–1659) from the Drigung Kagyü lineage.[94] The use of a widow's

86 Garrett, "Tapping the Body's Nectar," 302.

87 Also known as red bodhicitta (*byang sems dmar po*).

88 Also known as white bodhicitta (*byang sems dkar po*).

89 Garrett, "Tapping the Body's Nectar," 301.

90 *Mephitis mephitis*, effective for demonic disease and "yellow water" disease (*chu ser*).

91 Abbreviated form of *pu pu khu shud*. *Upupa epops*, a bird of striking appearance notable for its unique crown of feathers.

92 *Mustela sibirica*, effective in treating demonic disease and poisoning. See Dri med 'od zer, *Gsung 'bum* (Beijing: Krung go'i bod rig pa dpe skrun khang, 2009), 241.

93 Gyatso, *Being Human in a Buddhist World*, 118; Dkon mchog rin chen, *Bod kyi gso rig chos 'byung baiḍūrya'i 'phreng ba*, 102–104.

94 Chos kyi grags pa, *'Bri gung sman rtsis phyogs bsgrigs* (Beijing: Mi rigs dpe skrun khang, 2008), 224, 237, 364.

menses is also mentioned in another section of the same text.[95] Thus, since the use of these materials was popular in medical circles, it was not necessary for Sanggyé Gyatso to hide them for moral purposes. Furthermore, these peculiar substances can be substituted by other common medicines. In secret medicine the "two wheels," for example, fennel and black salt can be used in place of the widow's menses and, as Lungrik Tendar recommended, a stillborn fetus can be used in place of "bastard flesh." As previously stated, someone "killed by a knife" can be interpreted as a sudden or accidental death due to horse-riding, drowning, being hit by rocks, or falling off a cliff. Thus, during the time of the Fifth Dalai Lama, secrecy was not necessarily implemented solely to conceal the cruelty of the medicinal practice.

With the Fifth Dalai Lama as the leader of the Buddhist Ganden Podrang Government in the seventeenth century, the Gelukpa consolidated its political control over central Tibet.[96] "Buddhist doctrine" (*chos*) and "political power" (*srid*), referred to as the "assembly of doctrine and politics" (*chos srid gnyis 'brel*), came together to comprise a "dual governance" (*lugs gnyis*) of theocratic sovereignty.[97] Through their immense literary, architectural, political, and institutional force, the Gelukpa's hegemony influenced and utterly controlled not only the cultural life of the Tibetan Plateau,[98] but also its medical knowledge. In addition to retaining medicinal potency and escaping moral condemnation, the use of secrecy in the *Extended Commentary* can also exemplify a "craft secret" known only to personnel of the Chakpori medical lineage. Holding knowledge in such a setting would safeguard the lineage of transmission. At the same time, exclusive secret medicinal recipes would place Chakpori in a prominent position and enhance its competitiveness among Tibetan medical schools.

Led by Sanggyé Gyatso, the school at Chakpori was the central institution with authority on Tibetan medicine. Sanggyé Gyatso sought to assert control not only in medical knowledge, but in other areas of religious and

---

95 Chos kyi grags pa, *'Bri gung sman rtsis phyogs bsgrigs*, 258.

96 Tsyrempilov ("Dge Lugs Pa Divided," in *Power, Politics, and the Reinvention of Tradition*, ed. Bryan J. Cuevas and Kurtis R. Schaeffer [Leiden: Brill, 2006], 51–52) noticed that while sharing his authority with the Mongolian military leader Gushri Khan (1582–1655), the Fifth Dalai Lama "occupied a key position in the structure of the country"; as the Dalai Lamas were believed to be Avalokiteśvara, the destined divine protector of the country.

97 Georgios Halkias, "Pure-lands and Other Visions in Seventeeth-century Tibet: A Gnam Chos Sadhana for the Pure-land Sukhavati Revealed in 1658 by Gnam Chos Mi 'Gyur Rdo Rje (1645–1667)," in *Power, Politics, and the Reinvention of Tradition*, ed. Bryan J. Cuevas and Kurtis R. Schaeffer (Leiden: Brill, 2006), 103.

98 Kurtis R. Schaeffer, "The Fifth Dalai Lama," in *The Tibetan History Reader*, ed. Gray Tuttle and Kurtis R. Schaeffer (New York, NY: Columbia University Press, 2013), 348.

intellectual life.[99] The Fifth Dalai Lama's campaign at Chakpori successfully standardized and homogenised Tibetan medicine. Nevertheless, some preference among schools can be seen during the redaction of medical literatures. For instance, although Sanggyé Gyatso did not claim any favorites among different preceding medical lineages, a favoring of the Zur over the Jang school was evident.[100]

The concealment of "secret medicines" within the circle of Chakpori could have been part of a strategy to dominate medical education at that time. The use of secrecy in the medicinal formulae concealed what the Chakpori school believed to be precious healing methods of their lineage tradition from those outside the lineage, particularly their medical competitors. A remarkable point worth noting here is that "secret medicines" do not appear in every chapter of the *Extended Commentary*, but only in sections related to diseases that are difficult to treat. For instance, there is no "secret medicine" to be found in Chapter 28 on "measles" (*beg ge*), which is a disease known to heal without intervention. In Chapter 27 on "infectious small pox" (*'brum pa'i rims*), a hard-to-treat disease even in the modern world,[101] a list of "secret medicines" is presented.

In direct contrast to the use of secrecy as a means to exclude outsiders from reading, the Chakpori circle also managed to boast of holding "secret panacea," which uplifted the school to a more prominent position, where it stood out among other medical lineages. Instead of encrypting secret medicines in a bunch of incomprehensible words, Sanggyé Gyatso used the eye-catching term "secret medicine" (*gsang sman*) to precede each secret term, thus insinuating to the outsider that the Chakpori school did possess something particularly noteworthy. In this way, the possession of "secret" knowledge held an "advertising" function, as noted by Hugh Urban:

> the claim to possess very precious, rare, and valuable knowledge while partially revealing and largely concealing it. For a secret is only worth anything if someone knows that an individual has a secret.[102]

Sanggyé Gyatso's rendering of "secret medicine" amplified the perceived value and authority of the formulae. Under this notion, "secret medicine" was thus a

99 Schaeffer, "Ritual, Festival and Authority under the Fifth Dalai Lama," 187.
100 Meyer, "The Golden Century of Tibet Medicine," 103.
101 The World Health Organization declared the global eradication of smallpox in 1980.
102 Hugh Urban, *The Economics of Ecstasy: Tantra, Secrecy, and Power in Colonial Bengal* (Oxford: Oxford University Press, 2001), 101.

privileged and exclusive knowledge of the Chakpori medical lineage. As different medical lineages were based on the *Four Tantras*, the *Extended Commentary* contains extra "secret" materials when compared to the *Four Tantras*. This simply implies that Chakpori's medicine was more extensive than the conventional medical practice gained from following the *Four Tantras* only. The secrecy endorsed not only the reputation of the Chakpori college, but also that of their graduates; as they possessed extraordinary "secret recipes."

7 Concluding Remarks

According to the anthropological and historical studies of Tibetan medical tradition covered in this paper, it is obvious that the Gelukpa theocracy of the Fifth Dalai Lama not only had great influence on the political and religious aspects of Tibet, but also on the transmission of the Tibetan medical tradition. By examining the cipher of the *Extended Commentary*, I surmise that the intention of Sanggyé Gyatso's secrecy was multi-faceted. Although this present study is neither comprehensive nor definitive, the implementation of secrecy demonstrates a strategic approach when confronting the safety, morality, and authority of Tibetan medicine under the control of the Ganden Government in the seventeenth century. The secret materials not only preclude esoteric knowledge, but also imply that the possession of such medicinal recipes empowers the holder with a potentially valuable asset. Under the Fifth Dalai Lama, Chakpori became the dominant lineage in the medical tradition, synonymous with "orthodox Tibetan medicine" even today. Secrecy could have been one of the necessary factors to contributing to that status.

8 Original Texts in Wylie

8.1 *Chapter 3 of the* Extended Commentary on the Instructional Tantra of the Four Tantras *by Sanggyé Gyatso*[103]

srog rlung nad la rgyu rkyen rtags bcos bzhi// rgyu ni rlung nad kun dang 'dra ba la// de rkyen mya ngan sems las mtshan gnyid med// zas rtsub smyung dang shugs bkag btsir ba dang// mi 'dod gtam dang sgra thos zhogs 'ur sogs// 'jigs skrag drag shul gyur pa'i las kyis bskyed// khyad par 'byung gdon spyi dang rgyal pos byed// rtags ni rtsa chu shas cher rlung spyi mthun// 'ga' zhig nges med rtags kyang 'byung ba srid// yid mi bde zhing 'jigs skrag sems la 'char//

103 Sangs rgyas rgya mtsho, *Man ngag lhan thabs*, 21–24.

rmi lam za zi mang la gnyid chung zhing// lus 'dar rngul mang shes pa 'phyos pa dang// mgo 'khor dbugs sdud dka'i zhing mid mi thub// bcos pa'i thabs la sman dpyad zas spyod bzhi// de yang dang po sman gyis bcos pa ni// sga dang dzā ti shing kun kha ru tsha// go snyod li shi drod sman rus bcud gsum// gar chang bsdus thang tho rangs bsus te btang// de nas phyi rgyud a gar brgyad pa'i steng// li shi sha chen shing kun bsnan pa la// srog 'dzin bcu gcig pa zhes nu mchin dang// snying srog gzer dang smyo lkugs nad la bsngags// yang na mkhal ma go yu ar nag dang// dzā ti li shi ru rta snying zho sha// sman chen 'bri tshil sga dang pi pho gsum// kha ru tsha dang tang kun sgong thog 'bru// de steng dar ma'i gri snying ne tso dang// bya rgod 'brong snying 'di yan gtong khyi phag ma yin pa'i// snying sna gang 'dzom kha tshar btab pa rnams// bur smug ril bur bsgril ba sran ma tsam// lnga bdun la sogs na tshod dang sbyar ba// rus bcud gsum mam bcud bzhi'i thang gis dbul// rlung gi gzer nad kun dang khyad par du// srog rlung snying mi bde ba'i nad la bsngags// a ru sha chen bzhi yi tshi gu spang// de dang ljid mnyam shu dag pi pi ling// li shi ru rta kha ru tsha bcas pa// kun dang mnyam pa'i bi ṣa'i rtsa ba dang// de kun dang mnyam dzā ti pha la dang// gsang sman gtso bo ljid mnyam lo brgyad kyi// dri chus 'dam btags bur smug ril bur bsgril// sman nad med tsam rlung dus bsten pa na// snying dang srog rtsa'i nad kyi rigs kun dang// khyad par smyo 'bog nad la bsngags pa yin// yang na de steng dngul chu zho gang dang// mu zi dul ma zho phyed 'brong ne tso'i// snying dang bcas pa 'bras gsum mar la bsres// snying zho sha yi khu bas rta byas la// tho rangs dus su kham [khem] bu re re bsten// de yang nus pa bshad ma thag dang 'dra// yang na snying zho sha brgya phrag gsum dag gam// ma 'byor lnga bcu chu bre gsum la gdus// bre gang tsam 'dus [gdus] dar la btsags pa de// 'bri 'o phul do mar srang bdun dang ni// rus sna bsdus khu phul gang bu ram srang// dgu btab dkrugs pa gar sla zho tsam dus// spos dkar ru rta sgog bsregs thal ba gsum spyor tshad 'di nad khams dang bstun zhib pa ngag las bslab// de gsum rlung tshad rigs rnams 'joms pa'i gyad// shing kun tang kun kha ru tsha dang gsum// de gsum srog rlung 'joms pa'i gyad gsum yin// bi ṣa dar ma'i gri snying tsher sngon gsum// de gsum gzer rigs gcog pa'i gyad gsum mo// dbang po lag pa shug tsher ko byil gsum// stod du rlung 'tshangs gnon pa'i gyad gsum ste// pi pi ling dang pho ris bca' sga gsum// drod kyi me dpung sbar byed gyad gsum yin// go snyod ka ra sbrang rtsi rnam pa gsum// sman nus rtsar khrid nad sprod gyad gsum mo// gsang sman gnyis dang dkar po chig thub gsum// smyo 'bog gnyan nad sel ba'i gyad gsum ste// de ltar gyad rigs nyi shu rtsa gcig po// gong dang sbyar bsres tho rangs khyem re bsten// srog rlung nad la slebs chog byang lhun sman lugs// gzhan yang rlung tshad srog rlung rlung gzer dang// stod 'tshangs grang rlung la sogs rlung rigs kun// gyad sbyor 'di yis mi sel gang yang med// khyad par gdon rtags che bas sel dka' na// khyung rgod drag po tshad bzhin sbyar ba la// gsang sman gtso bo 'khor gnyis bcas pa'am// gtso bo dzā ti li shi dang bcas pa'i// kha tshar bsnan pa sman nad thon nges btang// rjes la gong gi srog 'dzin bcu gcig pa// go yu'i sbyor ba gang yin steng nyid du// gsang sman kha tshar bsnan pa bsten par bya// dpyad drug bdun dkar nag mtshams dang bya rog mig// yan stong dang po la sogs rlung gsang bsreg// yang na rgyab mdun me bum tshad ldan bya// khrag mkhris rtags yod snod ka gtar ba'ng bshad// rjes la phyi rgyud se 'bru brgyad pa sbyar// mgo bo 'khor tshabs che na le dzā dang// gur kum ka ra zhun mar sna sman btang// 'dus so gsum bsreg sdud sgor snum dugs bya// nad gzhan 'dres na de yi kha 'dzin gces// zas spyod gnyis po rlung nad spyi dang sbyor// zhes bdud rtsi snying po yan lag brgyad pa gsang ba man nag yon tan rgyud kyi lhan thabs zug rngu'i tsha gdung sel ba'i katpū ra dus min 'chi zhags gcod pa'i ral gri zhes pa las rlung nad gdug pa srog rlung bcos pa'i le'u ste gsum pa'o//

8.2 Writing on the Single Lineage of Secret Medicine *by Darmo Menrampa*[104]

gsang sman gtso bo ljid mnyam lo brgyad kyi// zhes pa ni dar ma'i gri snying/ yang gsang sman gnyis dang dkar bo chig thub gsum// zhes pa'i gsang sman gnyis ni/ yug za'i [yugs sa'i] mngal khrag dang nal bu'i sha gnyis so// gsang sman gtso bo 'khor gnyis bcas pa'am// zhes pa'i gtso bo ni/ dpa' bo dgra yul du bsad pa'i gri khrag ces pa ltar phan tshun dpa' rtsal gyis grir shi ba'i snying dang sha chen nas/ 'brong gi snying khrag gang rigs/ 'khor gnyis ni shing kun kha ru tsha'o// yang na/ yug za'i [yugs sa'i] mngal khrag dang nal bu'i sha'o// gsang sman kha tshar bsnan pa bsten par bya// zhes pa'i gsang sman kha tshar ni ri bong gi snying ngo// 'di'i gong gsal gsang sman rnams ni srogs rlung rkyang ba'i gsang no//

8.3 Single Lineage of Secret Medicine: The Golden Key to Decode the Knot of the Extended Commentary on the Instructional Tantra *by Ngawang Sanggyé Pelzang*[105]

gsum pa srog rlung skabs/ khyung rgod drag po ni/ sha snying bzang po zho bzhi mnyam// rus gcig rgyus pa gsum cha gnyis// khrag ni gsum cha gcig sbyar ba// mnyam sbyor drag rgod khyung lnga'o// zhes pa ltar tshad ldan sbyar ba'i khyung lnga mnyam sbyor gyi steng du gsang sman cha bskyed dgos//

104 Blo bzang chos grags, *Gsang sman chig brgyud*, 434–35.

105 Ngag dbang sangs rgyas dpal bzang, *Rin chen gser gyi lde mig*, 473.

Bibliography

Tibetan Sources

Blo bzang chos grags. *Gsang sman chig brgyud kyi shog dril skor*. In *Man ngag lhan thabs dang lde mig*, 431–457. Beijing: Mi rigs dpe skrun khang, 2005.

Chos kyi grags pa. *'Bri gung sman rtsis phyogs bsgrigs*. Beijing: Mi rigs dpe skrun khang, 2008.

Dbang 'dus. *Gso ba rig pa'i tshig mdzod g.yu thog dgongs rgyan*. Beijing: Mi rigs dpe skrun khang, 1983.

Dkon mchog rin chen. *Bod kyi gso rig chos 'byung baiḍūrya'i 'phreng ba*. Lan zhou: Kan su'u mi rigs dpe skrun khang, 1994.

Dri med 'od zer. *Gsung 'bum, Dri med 'od zer/ dpal brtsegs/ mes po'i shul bzhag*. Beijing: Krung go'i bod rig pa dpe skrun khang, 2009.

Khams smyon dharma seng ge. *G.yu thog snying thig gi yig chos skor*. Leh: D. L. Tashigang, 1981.

Ngag dbang sangs rgyas dpal bzang. *Gsang sman chig brgyud, lhan thabs kyi rgya mdud bkrol ba'i rin chen gser gyi lde mig*. In *Man ngag lhan thabs dang lde mig*, 457–536. Beijing: Mi rigs dpe skrun khang, 2005.

Sangs rgyas rgya mtsho. *Gso ba rig pa'i bstan bcos sman bla'i dgongs rgyan rgyud bzhi'i gsal byed bai dura sngon po'i malli ka*. Leh: D. L. Tashigang, 1981.

Sangs rgyas rgya mtsho. *Man ngag lhan thabs bzhugs so*. Zi ling: Mtsho mi rigs dpe skrun khang, 1991.

Sog po lung rigs bstan dar. *A ru rnam rgyal gser mdog phreng ba*. In *Man ngag lhan thabs dang lde mig*, 538–719. Beijing: Mi rigs dpe skrun khang, 2005.

Zhang Yisun. *Bod rgya tsig mdzod chen mo*. Beijing: Mi rigs dpe skrun kang, 2013.

Other Sources

Beer, Robert. *The Handbook of Tibetan Buddhist Symbols*. Boston: Shambhala, 2003.

Bhattacharyya, Narendra Nath. *Indian Puberty Rites*. Delhi: Munshiram Manoharlal, 1980.

Czaja, Olaf. "The Four Tantras and the Global Market." In *Medicine between Science and Religion*, edited by Vincanne Adams, Mona Schrempf and Sienna R Craig, 265–95. New York: Berghahn Books, 2011.

Czaja, Olaf. "The Making of the Blue Beryl: Some Remarks on the Textual Sources of the Famous Commentary of Sangye Gyatsho (1653–1705)." In *Soundings in Tibetan Medicine: Anthropological and Historical Perspectives*, edited by Mona Schrempf, 345–71. Leiden: Brill, 2007.

Dash, Bhagwan. *Pharmacopoeia of Tibetan Medicine*. Indian Medical Science series. Delhi: Sri Satguru Publications, 1994.

Finn, Louise. *The Kulacudamani Tantra and the Vamakesvara Tantra with the Jayaratha Commentary: Introduced, Translated, and Annotated by Louise M. Finn*. Wiesbaden: Harrassowitz, 1986.

Garrett, Frances. "Tapping the Body's Nectar: Gastronomy and Incorporation in Tibetan Literature." *History of Religions* 49, no. 3 (2010): 300–26.

Gyatso, Janet. *Being Human in a Buddhist World: An Intellectual History of Medicine in Early Modern Tibet*. New York, NY: Columbia University Press, 2015.

Gyatso, Thinley, and Chris Hakim. *Essentials of Tibetan Traditional Medicine*. Berkeley, CA: North Atlantic Books, 2010.

Halkias, Georgios. "Pure-lands and Other Visions in Seventeeth-century Tibet: A Gnam Chos Sadhana for the Pure-land Sukhavati Revealed in 1658 by Gnam Chos Mi 'Gyur Rdo Rje (1645–1667)." In *Power, Politics, and the Reinvention of Tradition: Tibet in the Seventeenth and Eighteenth Centuries: PIATS 2003: Tibetan Studies: Proceedings of the Tenth Seminar of the International Association for Tibetan Studies, Oxford, 2003*, edited by Bryan J. Cuevas and Kurtis R. Schaeffer, 103–28. Leiden: Brill, 2006.

Jigme Phuntsok. *Always Present: The Luminous Wisdom of Jigme Phuntsok*. Translated by Emyo Yun Jia Wang. Boston, MA: Snow Lion, 2015.

Karmay, Samten Gyaltsen. *Secret Visions of the Fifth Dalai Lama: The Gold Manuscript in the Fournier Collection, Musée Guimet, Paris*, edited by Samten Gyaltsen Karmay and Lionel Fournier. London: Serindia Publications, 1998.

Leong, Elaine, and Alisha Rankin. "Introduction: Secrets and Knowledge." In *Secrets and Knowledge in Medicine and Science, 1500–1800*, edited by Elaine Leong and Alisha Rankin, 1–20. Burlington, VT: Ashgate, 2011.

Meyer, Fernand. "The Golden Century of Tibet Medicine." In *Lhasa in the Seventeenth Century: the Capital of the Dalai Lamas*, edited by Françoise Pommaret, 99–117. Leiden: Brill, 2003.

Nebesky-Wojkowitz, René de. *Oracles and Demons of Tibet: The Cult and Iconography of the Tibetan Protective Deities*. Delhi: Book Faith India, 1993.

Parfionovitch, Yuri, Fernand Meyer, and Gyurme Dorje. *Tibetan Medical Paintings: Illustrations to the Blue Beryl Treatise of Sangye Gyamtso (1653–1705)*. London: Serindia Publications, 1992.

Pasang Yonten Arya. *Dictionary of Tibetan Materia Medica*. Delhi: Motilal Banarsidass, 1998.

Schaeffer, Kurtis R. "The Fifth Dalai Lama." In *The Tibetan History Reader*, edited by Gray Tuttle and Kurtis R. Schaeffer, 348–62. New York, NY: Columbia University Press, 2013.

Schaeffer, Kurtis R. "Ritual, Festival and Authority under the Fifth Dalai Lama." In *Power, Politics, and the Reinvention of Tradition: Tibet in the Seventeenth and Eighteenth Centuries: PIATS 2003: Tibetan Studies: Proceedings of the Tenth Seminar of the International Association for Tibetan Studies, Oxford, 2003*, edited by Bryan J. Cuevas and Kurtis R. Schaeffer. Leiden: Brill, 2006.

Schaeffer, Kurtis R. "Textual Scholarship, Medical Tradition, and Mahāyāna Buddhist Ideals in Tibet." *Journal of Indian Philosophy* 31, no. 5 (2003): 621–41.

Snellgrove, David. *Indo-Tibetan Buddhism: Indian Buddhists and Their Tibetan Successors*. Boston, MA: Shambhala, 1987.

Tsyrempilov, Nicolay. "Dge Lugs Pa Divided." In *Power, Politics, and the Reinvention of Tradition: Tibet in the Seventeenth and Eighteenth centuries: PIATS 2003: Tibetan studies: Proceedings of the Tenth Seminar of the International Association for Tibetan Studies, Oxford, 2003*, edited by Bryan J. Cuevas and Kurtis R. Schaeffer. Leiden: Brill, 2006.

Urban, Hugh. *The Economics of Ecstasy: Tantra, Secrecy, and Power in Colonial Bengal*. Oxford: Oxford University Press, 2001.

Warder, Anthony Kennedy. *Indian Buddhism*. Delhi: Motilal Banarsidass Publishers, 2000.

Wedemeyer, Christian. "Beef, Dog, and Other Mythologies: Connotative Semiotics in Mahāyoga Tantra Ritual and Scripture." *Journal of the American Academy of Religion* 75, no. 2 (2007): 383–417.

White, David Gordon. *Kiss of the Yoginī: "Tantric Sex" in its South Asian Contexts*. Chicago, IL: University of Chicago Press, 2003.

Yang Ga. *The Sources for the Writing of the Rgyud Bzhi, Tibetan Medical Classic*. Cambridge, MA: Doctoral Dissertation at Harvard University, 2010.

Young, Serinity. *Courtesans and Tantric Consorts: Sexualities in Buddhist Narrative, Iconography, and Ritual*. New York, NY: Routledge, 2004.

CHAPTER 4

Visceral Anatomy as Depicted in Tibetan Medicine

Katharina Sabernig

1 Introduction: The Details of the Internal Organs

In the following[1] I compare examples of anatomical nomenclature of depictions in the thangka paintings of the *Illustrations to the Blue Beryl*, medical paintings from Atsagat Monastery, as well as modern publications, with the latter being examined due to the booming of Tibetan medical and anatomical book production in recent years.[2] An introduction to all available sources on anatomical terminology in Tibet is not within the scope of this paper,[3] nor is a discussion of the challenges involved in the identification and translation of traditional terms, as these problems have already been explained in detail by other authors.[4] In sum, the scholarly world is skeptical that decontextualized

1 This paper is based on a longer abstract included in the "Book of Abstracts" of the "100th Anniversary Celebrations of the Men-Tsee-Khang & the Second Annual Conference of the Tibetan Medicine Committee of the World Federation of Chinese Medicine Societies" held in Lhasa 2016 (Katharina Sabernig, "Description and Depiction of Inner Organs in Classical and Modern Works," in *Lha ldan sman rtsis khang bgu brnyes nas lo ngo brgya 'khor ba'i rgyal spyi'i rig gzhung gros tshogs* [Lhasa: 2016]). The evaluation of the development of coining modern anatomical terms is part of my previous project supported by the Austrian Science Fund: P 26129-G21. In this project I created a database on Tibetan medical terms which was the topic of my presentation at the IATS conference hosted by the University of Bergen in June 2016. The database is already online: https://crossasia.org/en/service/crossasia-lab/tibetische-medizin-termini/.

2 For an overview of medical publications in the Tibetan language, see Michael Balk, "A Bibliographical Survey of Medical Literature in Tibetan Language Based on the Post-war Holdings of the State Library in Berlin: A Strand of Pearls to Enlighten Researchers," *Curare* 39, no. 1 (2016): 88–94.

3 A longer survey on Tibetan medical dictionaries and anatomical literature is included in my article, "Vulnerable Parts: Locating and Defining Vital Areas of the Body in Tibetan Medicine," in which questionable structures of the circulatory system are discussed, see Katharina Sabernig, "Vulnerable Parts: Locating and Defining Vital Areas of the Body in Tibetan Medicine," *Asian Medicine* 12, nos. 1–2 (2017): 86–118.

4 Vincanne Adams, "Complications in the Study of Efficacy of Tibetan Medicine within the Biomedical Context," in *Anthology of 2000 International Academic Conference on Tibetan Medicine*, ed. Apei Awang Jinmei [Ngag dbang 'jigs med] (unpublished), 928–34; or Florian Ploberger, "Anatomical Terms of the 27 Chapters of the *Subsequent Tantra* (*Phyi ma'i rgyud*)," *Curare* 39, no. 1 (2016): 33–41; are just examples of this vivid discussion.

 | DOI:10.1163/9789004404441_005

translations of historical terms into a modern scientific language is possible without running the risk that the meaning is distorted. I emphasize these reservations, but I also believe that examining what could have been meant is a worthwhile endeavor. Instead of theoretical caveats, in this paper I demonstrate the development of anatomical depictions and nomenclatures of internal organs in the Tibetan cultural area based on works produced during the period from the late seventeenth century to the present.

Before I introduce the three Tibetan groups of anatomical depictions that I will compare, a few general aspects on anatomical depiction and nomenclature should be outlined. The original meaning of the term "anatomy" was derived from the Greek for "cutting" (*tomo*) "up" (*ana*) the body. Today it is understood as the study of the structure of living organisms.[5] As macroanatomical structures are perceivable by human senses, the science of anatomy is empirical and it is quite predictable what the anatomist will observe during dissection. Nevertheless, although scientific in their approach, anatomical depictions never present "reality," they always show more or less abstract structures, in most cases aestheticized, highlighting certain structures while others are omitted. Even the photographical *Atlas* by Walter Thiel presents the human body elaborately prepared.[6] The history of anatomical depiction is replete with attempts to aestheticize the human corpse.[7] Early modern anatomical depictions, such as the "Vesalian paintings,"[8] present the dead dissected body in vivid poses embedded in lovely landscapes or edifying architecture. Nevertheless, in somewhat simplified terms, I would like to state that European historical images of the human body are borne by the aesthetics of morbidity, while Tibetan anatomical paintings may be characterized as colorful, with components of playful ease and a sense humor to distract from the dreadfulness of death.[9] Even the skeletons appear to smile. In the context of

5 William Casselman, *A Dictionary of Medical Derivations: The Real Meaning of Medical Terms* (New York, NY: The Pantheon Publishing Group, 1998), 340.

6 Walter Thiel, *Photographischer Atlas der Praktischen Anatomie* (Berlin: Springer, 1996–1999).

7 T. V. N. Persaud, Marios Loukas, and R. Shane Tubbs, *A History of Human Anatomy* (Springfield, IL: Charles C. Thomas, 2014).

8 Andreas Vesalius, *De humani corporis fabrica* (Budapest, 1968 [repr. 1543]).

9 See Janet Gyatso, "Introduction," in *Body and Spirit: Tibetan Medical Paintings*. ed. by Laila Williamson and Serinity Young, Medical Tangkas painted by Romio Shrestha and Atelier (American Museum of Natural History, New York; Seattle and London: University of Washington Press. 2009), p. 3–13; Janet Gyatso, *Being Human in a Buddhist World: An Intellectual History of Medicine in Early Modern Tibet* (New York, NY: Columbia University Press, 2015), 25–62; Sabernig, "Vulnerable Parts," 86–118.

the disgust, sensory perception, and the materiality that anatomical research may evoke, Marieke Hendriksen refers to the concept of "aesthesis."[10]

The visual representation of bodily structures is more easily imagined than descriptions made in prose. Unfortunately, there are no images on the anatomical achievements of Galen of Pergamon available, but his writings were translated from Greek into Syriac, Arabic, Hebrew, and Armenian.[11] Although we know that a representative of the Byzantine medical tradition called "Galen" (*ga le nos*) influenced early medical knowledge in Tibet,[12] we do not know how much anatomical knowledge was transferred from Eastern Mediterranean regions to Tibet in the first millennium. With regard to descriptive anatomical knowledge in the *Four Tantras*, the fourth chapter of the *Explanatory Tantra* (*bshad rgyud*) and its commentaries give concise information on the "condition of the body" (*lus kyi gnas lugs*), or anatomy.[13]

Most of the named anatomical structures in the *Four Tantras* form part of the locomotor, circulatory, and nervous systems, but there are only a few terms regarding the actual substructures of major internal organs.[14] The majority of the anatomical terms listed in the *Four Tantras* and its commentaries are given in the section on the vulnerable body parts, but their clinical relevance is explained in the *Instructional Tantra*. Unfortunately, a translation of the most substantial part of the *Four Tantras* is still not completely available, but in his Harvard dissertation Yang Ga impressively demonstrates the sources of the *Four*

---

10 Marieke M. A. Hendriksen, *Elegant Anatomy: The Eighteenth-Century Leiden Anatomical Collections* (Leiden: Brill, 2015), 10–35.

11 Vivian Nutton, ed., *The Unknown Galen* (London: Institute of Classical Studies, 2002), *vii*.

12 Yang Ga, *The Sources for the Writing of the Rgyud bzhi, Tibetan Medical Classic* (Cambridge, MA: Doctoral Dissertation at Harvard University, 2010), 38; Manfred Taube, *Beiträge zur Geschichte der medizinischen Literatur Tibets* (Sankt Augustin: VGH Wissenschaftsverlag, 1981), 10. See also Henk Blezer, "A New Sense of (Dark) Humor in Tibet: Brown Phlegm and Black Bile," in this volume.

13 The *Explanatory Tantra* describes mainly preclinical knowledge of Tibetan medicine, and it is the second part of the *Four Tantras* (*Rgyud bzhi*). For a critical edition, see Bstan 'dzin don grub, ed., *Dpal ldan rgyud bzhi dpe bsdur ma* (Beijing: Krung go'i bod rig pa dpe skrun khang, 2005–2008).

14 My previous research focused on anatomical findings of the personal physician of the Fifth Dalai Lama, the teacher, anatomist, and surgeon, Blo bzang chos grags [Dar mo sman rams pa], *Legs bshad gser gyi thur ma* (Beijing: Mi rigs dpe skrun khang, 2005). I have also compared his findings with earlier commentaries and later texts in order to analyze if his statements were integrated by subsequent scholars into their own works (e.g.: Ye shes bzang po [Gtsang sman], *Bshad pa'i rgyud kyi gnas lugs le'u'i 'grel bshad rag tho dam pa snga ma'i zhal rgyud*, in *Gtsang sman pa'i sman yig phyogs bsgrigs* [Beijing: Mi rigs dpe skrun khang, 2007], 155–81); cf.: Sabernig, "Anatomical Structures and the Structure of Anatomy in Tibetan Medicine"; and Sabernig, "Vulnerable Parts."

Tantras, including the broad spectrum of anatomical knowledge necessary for the management of wounds, which makes up twenty percent of the third tantra.[15] Only a minor part of the written information included in the *Instructional Tantra* is depicted in the *Illustrations to the Blue Beryl*. Nevertheless, they form a treasure in the history of Asian medical art, revealing many anatomical terms through their labelling and they do not only present medical knowledge, but also aspects of the everyday life in Lhasa on the eve of modernity.[16] As this paper deals mainly with depicted anatomical information it is not in the scope to analyze commentaries to the respective chapters in the *Instructional Tantra*. Even though the anatomical chapter of the *Explanatory Tantra* is not suitable to evaluate the broad spectrum of Tibetan anatomical knowledge, I use terms of visceral structures listed in the section of vulnerable organs in two texts to this chapter as a starting point: The sixteenth-century *Commentary to the Four Treatises: A Treasure of Benefits for Others* by Pema Karpo (*pad ma dkar po*; 1527–92) lists thirteen such visceral structures.[17] Although the importance of this scholar is his religious authority his section on vulnerable visceral structures is even more informative than those later commentaries. The second text was written by the personal physician of the Fifth Dalai Lama, the teacher, anatomist, and surgeon, Darmo Menrampa Lozang Chödrak (*dar mo sman rams pa blo bzang chos grags*; 1638–1710?), entitled the *Unfolded Trees of the Explanatory Treatise* with its short title, *Golden Spoon of Eloquent Sayings*.[18] Both texts structure medical content with the help of a hierarchic arboreal metaphor.[19]

Tibetan anatomical paintings became famous due to the seventeenth-century *Illustrations to the Blue Beryl*, the most important commentary to the *Four Tantras*. It seems that some of these illustrations are based on earlier precursors, such as the drawings of Namgyel Dorjé (*rnam rgyal rdo rje*), but these documents are not explicitly mentioned and have not been preserved for posterity.[20] The almost complete copy of *Illustrations to the Blue Beryl* found its way to

15 Yang Ga, *The Sources for the Writing of the Rgyud bzhi*.

16 Gyatso, *Being Human in a Buddhist World*, 48.

17 Pad ma dkar po [Blo gsal dbang po], *Rgyud bzhi'i 'grel ba gzhan la phan pa'i gter* (Beijing: Mi rigs dpe skrun khang, 2007), 230/11–14.

18 Blo bzang chos grags, *Legs bshad gser gyi thur ma*.

19 Katharina Sabernig, "The Tree of Nosology," in *Cultural Systems of Classification: Sickness, Health and Local Epistemologies*, ed. Ulrike Steinert, forthcoming.

20 Fernand Meyer, "Introduction: The Medical Paintings of Tibet," in *Tibetan Medical Paintings: Illustrations to the 'Blue Beryl' Treatise of Sangs rgyas Rgya mtsho (1653–1705)*, ed. Yuri Parfionovitch et al. (London: Serindia Publications, 1992), vol. 1, 2–13. See also Gyatso, *Being Human in a Buddhist World*.

Buryatia in Russia at the beginning of tcs the "Ulan-Ude set,"[21] whereas another set, commonly called the "Lhasa set," remained in central Tibet.[22] Although the latter set includes two more anatomical paintings, they contain no relevant information on the inner organs, as they deal with superficial blood vessels. Cached in an orthodox church during the Stalin Purges, the "Ulan-Ude set" was later kept in the Museum for the History of Buryatia.[23] Already in the late 1920s, even before Stalin's "Great Terror" began, copies of many of the "Ulan-Ude set" were drawn and new paintings where created, authorized by the director of the Medical College at Atsagat Monastery, the Buryat lama and physician, Dondub Endonov (ca. 1870–1938?). His father's name was Yönten (*yon tan*), which forms the basis of Dondub's commonly used surname, Endonov.[24] The high-ranking Gelukpa dignitary was the director of the committee of the Buryat umbrella organization, the "United School of Tibetan Medicine of all Colleges," and he was committed to reform the monastic education in Tibetan medicine.[25] His status in Buryatia is comparable with the role that the Tibetan physician Khyenrap Norbu (*mkhyen rab nor bu*, 1883–1962) played in the first half of the twentieth century for the development of Tibetan medicine in Central Tibet. As Endonov was interested in modern medicine in general and anatomy in particular, his own paintings (or those which were authorized by Endonov) show some interesting modern anatomical features. Fortunate circumstances and the kind informal cooperation with Natalia Bolsokhoeva made it possible for me to take a closer look at these images, which I call in this paper the "Atsagat paintings." The whole series comprises sixty-five paintings stored in the Museum for the History of Buryatia, most of them unpublished

21 Paintings of the "Ulan-Ude set" numbered 6–8, 10, and 14 to the *Explanatory Tantra*; nos. 38, 39, and 47–49 to the *Instructional Tantra*; and nos. 71–73 to the *Subsequent Tantra* depict internal organs or their topographical relations.

22 Byams pa phrin las and Wang Lei, *Tibetan Medical Thangka of the Four Medical Tantras* [Bod lugs gso rig rgyud bzhi'i nang don bris cha ngo mtshar mthong ba don ldan], trans. Cai Jingfeng (Lhasa: Bod ljongs mi dmangs dpe skrun khang, 1994).

23 Meyer, "Introduction"; Natalia Bolsokhoyeva, "Tibetan Medical Illustrations from the History Museum of Buryatia, Ulan Ude," *Asian Medicine* 3 (2007): 347–67; Natalia Bolsokhoyeva and Kseniya Gerasimova, "The Atlas of Tibetan Medicine: Treasures from The History Museum of Buryatia," in *The Buddha's Art of Healing: Tibetan Paintings Rediscovered*, ed. John Avedon (New York, NY: Rizzoli, 1998), 33–60.

24 See V. A. Shaglakhaev and N. D. Bolsokhoeva, *Atlas tibetskoj mediciny v kul'turnom prostranstve Central'noj Azii* (Ulan-Ude: Izd.—vo GUZ ZCMP MZ RB, 2010); Natalia Bolsokhoyeva, "Tibetan Medical Illustrations from Atsagat Medical College and Other Anatomical Achievements of the Buryat Lama and Physician D. Endonov," *Curare* 39, no. 1 (2016): 6–21.

25 Bolsokhoyeva, "Tibetan Medical Illustrations from Atsagat Medical College," 14.

so far. Only eleven of them where published in a book and four of them in the *Curare* issue *The Human Body in Asian Texts and Images.*[26]

In recent years a series of atlases on modern anatomy in Tibetan language have been published.[27] Before the publication of these anatomical atlases in Tibetan or both Tibetan and Chinese, Tibetan scholars who were interested in modern "biomedical" anatomy found in Chinese anatomical atlases. In the late 1990s I met a Tibetan monk-physician who proudly presented me a Chinese translation of Werner Platzer's *Color Atlas and Textbook of Human Anatomy* (1991), which was the official guidebook to my dissection classes at the University of Vienna. Although the *Nomina Anatomica*, created in 1955 and followed by various editions until it was replaced by *Terminologia Anatomica* in 1998, was the international standard on anatomical terminology, I became used to various forms of synonyms. The peroneus muscles of the lower leg were synonymously called fibularis muscles, for example, and the atrioventricular node (Latin: *nodus atrioventricularis*), as an important part of the electrical conduction system of the heart, was also called the "AV node" or the "Aschoff-Tawara node," named according the discoverers. I will come back to the modern anatomical names of respective structures of the heart later on.

Despite the widespread use of such synonyms, currently there is a tendency to use fewer eponyms and metonyms. Similar to deviations and synonyms in former biomedical atlases, different Tibetan publications have used different terms when translating modern anatomical terms. With the publication of the trilingual dictionary entitled the *Chinese-Tibetan-English Modern Medicine Dictionary*,[28] which is normative in its approach, a Tibetan standard for modern biomedical terms is more or less fixed today. As far as I could observe, the atlas edited by Pema Rapten (*pad ma rab brtan*) and his younger brother Sanggyé Bum (*sangs rgyas 'bum*) mainly use the suggested vocabulary of the trilingual dictionary published in Xining, too. I call these terms *Terminologia*

26 Shaglakhaev and Bolsokhoeva, *Atlas tibetskoj mediciny v kul'turnom prostranstve Central'noj Azii*; Bolsokhoyeva, "Tibetan Medical Illustrations from Atsagat Medical College."

27 The most important ones are: Ting 'dzin, *Gso rig rgyud bzhi'i dka' gnad thor bu la dpyad pa'i gtam brgyad cu rtsa bzhi ba dang lus kyi gnas lugs grub cha'i dpe ris* (Chengdu: Si khron mi rigs dpe skrun khang, 2007); Pad ma rab brtan and Sangs rgyas 'bum, *Gso ba rig pa'i ro bkra'i dpe ris kun gsal me long* (Xining: Mtsho sngon mi rigs dpe skrun khang, 2011); Nyi ma tshe ring and Mig dmar, *Rgya bod shan sbyar tshon khra can gyi ro bkra'i dpe ris mthong ba don gsal* (Lhasa: Bod ljongs mi dmangs dpe skrun khang, 2012); or Mkhas grub, *Gso bya lus kyi tha snyad mdzod* (Chengdu: Si khron mi rigs dpe skrun khang, 2012). For a longer introduction to these publications, see Sabernig, "Vulnerable Parts."

28 *Rgya bod dbyin gsum shan sbyar deng rabs gso rig ming mdzod* (Beijing: Mi rigs dpe skrun khang, 2011).

Anatomica Tibetana.[29] Both physicians are affiliated with the Qinghai Tibetan Medicine Hospital in Xining, whereas their education in Tibetan medicine also included biomedical anatomical knowledge.

In my examination of Tibetan anatomical terms, I have examined the vocabulary used in at least four atlases. My preliminary examination revealed that the atlas edited by Nyima Tsering (*nyi ma tshe ring*) and Mikmar (*mig dmar*) in Lhasa uses more metaphorical terms to name the respective structures. Both atlases are illustrated with conventional anatomical depictions, with international standard color coding such as blue veins, red arteries, and yellow nerves. Yet another atlas by Khedrup (*mkhas grub*) published in Sichuan includes "ultrarealistic" images gained through photography during dissection.[30] All three atlases are bilingual, Chinese and Tibetan, and they clearly aim to present modern empirical anatomy. Completely different is the approach of Tindzin (*ting 'dzin*). His publication in the Tibetan language includes anatomical as well as therapeutic drawings to stabilize joints or broken bones. The introduction presents images of the author wearing traditional clothes while studying real skulls and bones to compare them with descriptions in classical texts. Somewhat similar to the "Vesalian paintings," several images appear to be photomontages, where the dissecting anatomist and his material are transferred into a nice room with plants and furniture. The paintings depict features of modern anatomical knowledge as well as of classic Tibetan texts, and they show not only anatomical aspects but also physiological functions, such as defecation and urination, human functions that we often find on the *Illustrations to the Blue Beryl*.[31] From an artistic and historico-cultural point of view this atlas is my favorite one, even if the other three ones are more useful in regard to anatomical accuracy.

To present a broad spectrum of the manner of depicting and naming structures of internal organs over time, I have chosen three major regions of the human trunk: organs in the thoracic cavity, digestive viscera, and the urogenital system. Modern anatomy divides three major cavities: thoracic, abdominal, and pelvic cavity. Another, more morphological, spatial classification organizes organs below the diaphragm with regard to their relation to the peritoneum, a serous membrane. Simply stated, most parts of the gastrointestinal tract are located intraperitoneal as they are wrapped with peritoneum. The urogenital tract is located retroperitoneal (e.g. kidneys) or infraperitoneal (e.g. bladder,

29 The atlas is based on the nomenclature used in the *Rgya bod dbyin gsum shan sbyar deng rabs gso rig ming mdzod*. See Sabernig, "Vulnerable Parts."

30 Due to these images, this atlas might be disquieting for viewers not used to such kind of images. See Sabernig, "Vulnerable Parts."

31 Ting 'dzin, *Gso rig rgyud bzhi'i dka' gnad thor bu la dpyad pa*, 47.

reproductive organs), as they are located behind or below the membrane. In traditional Chinese medicine we find a similar organization of the viscera, although it is meant more as a representation of function rather than material reality.[32] The concept of the "triple burner" (*sanjiao* 三焦) divides the body in three regions, the "upper burner" is located above the diaphragm, the "middle burner" between the diaphragm and the navel, and the "lower burner" is the region below the navel.[33] Although the assignment of the individual organs varies, Kuryiama mentions the same tripartite body scheme in the context of Chinese pulse diagnostics.[34] The same scheme can be found in channel examination chapters of the early Tibetan medical scripture, the *Medicine of the Moon King* (*sman dpyad zla ba'i rgyal po*).[35]

2 Organs in the Thoracic Cavity

According to the Tibetan medical tradition, the most important organs of the chest cavity or above the diaphragm are the heart (*snying*) and the lungs (*glo ba*). In the metaphorical language of Tibetan medicine, the heart is compared with an "enthroned king" (*rgyal po gdan la shugs pa*), while the five posterior or maternal lobes of the lungs (*glo ba ma lnga*) are regarded as "home ministers" (*nang gi blon po*), and the five anterior or filial lobes (*glo ba bu lnga*) are compared with princes and princesses (*rgyal po'i sras mo*).[36] Despite the extraordinary importance of the heart as the "core organ," we know comparatively little about the names of the respective substructures. Janet Gyatso has highlighted the wide-ranging debate among premodern Tibetan scholars on the incompatibility between theoretical and empirical anatomical knowledge about this organ, the gender specific position of the tip of the heart (*snying gi rtse*), and the position of a "hole" (*bu ga*) as a "mind-entrance opening."[37] Nevertheless, the respective paintings of and commentaries to the chapter on the "condition of the body" give only little insight into the heart-related nomenclature. Pema

---

32 Wung-Seok Cha and Hyuk-Sang Jung, "Body Perception in East Asian Culture," *Curare* 39, no.1 (2016): 75–87.

33 See Giovanni Maciocia, *Die Grundlagen der Chinesischen Medizin: Ein Lehrbuch für Akupunkteure und Arzneimitteltherapeuten* (Kötzting: Verlag für Traditionelle Chinesische Medizin), 126–129.

34 Shigehisa Kuriyama, *The Expressiveness of the Body and the Divergence of Greek and Chinese Medicine* (New York, NY: Zone Books, 1999), 39.

35 William A. McGrath, "Vessel Examination in the *Medicine of the Moon King*," in *Buddhism and Medicine*, ed. C. Pierce Salguero (New York, NY: Columbia University Press, 2017), 501–13.

36 See Parfionovitch et al., *Tibetan Medical Paintings*, 183, nos. 24–26.

37 Gyatso, *Being Human in a Buddhist World*, 251–64, 452, n. 25.

Karpo mentions a "black heart" (*snying nag po*), which could be the cardiac muscle because muscular aspects are often described as black.[38]

The *Instructional Tantra* and its commentaries, especially the chapters on wounds, contain more information on particular organ parts. Painting 49 of the *Illustrations to the Blue Beryl* refers to chapter 85 on wounds of the upper and lower trunk, depicting human organs as they are observed during dissection. This painting was labeled as "observed" (*bltas pa*) by Tendzin Norbuchen of Lhodrak (*lho brag bstan 'dzin nor bu can*), indicating that they were painted with an empirical approach to be naturalist or "real,"[39] in contrast to idealized images. However, as mentioned above, a two-dimensional drawing is only an image of perceived reality and not reality itself. In Tibetan medical paintings it is common knowledge that the heart is depicted as an idealized form: the tip of the heart points upwards like a lotus flower,[40] as it is the case in the central image of thangka nos. 10, 11, 14, 38, 47, 49, 50, 71, and 72. On the left side of thangka 49, organs are presented as "observed," and in this case the tip of the heart points to the lower left side of the thoracic cavity instead of the traditional way of depiction. Therefore, it is empirical in its approach. The central image of the painting depicts the tip of the heart in upward position without being labelled as "observed." Rather idealized geometrical relations between the lobes of the lung and the heart in the form of different triangles. The shape of the lungs is compared with the shape of pigeons, and the five anterior and the five posterior lobes are labeled with individual metaphorical names, such as "enemy's tongue" (*dgra lce*) or

38 The vulnerable points of muscles are not listed in the *Explanatory Tantra* but in the commentaries and some of them are depicted on Thangka no. 15. Darmo Menrampa Lozang Chödrak, for example lists "black neck muscles" (*gnya' sha nag po*) or white and black parts of muscles at the armpit (*bzhag sha dkar nag*; Blo bzang chos grags, *Legs bshad gser gyi thur ma*, 23/ 23–24). In contemporary literature the first one is identified with the trapezius muscle the second one describes of parts latissimus dorsi (*mchan bzhag nag po*; Pad ma rab brtan and Sangs rgyas 'bum, *Gso ba rig pa'i ro bkra'i dpe ris kun gsal me long*, 207). The Thangka presents the cervical part the trapezius as *phung pa'i thal gong gnya' sha* without reference to the black feature, but the "latissimus dorsi" is named *bzhag sha nag* (Parfionovitch et al., *Tibetan Medical Paintings*, 201, nos. 25 and 39). Darmo Menrampa Lozang Chödrak and Pema Karpo also mention a muscle called *bshul sha nag po* (Blo bzang chos grags, *Legs bshad gser gyi thur ma*, 23/22; Pad ma dkar po, *Rgyud bzhi'i 'grel ba gzhan la phan pa'i gter*, 229/17) identified by Samten as parts of the autochthonous back muscles specified as *sgal 'dabs bshul sha* (Bsam gtan, *Gso rig snying bsdus skya rengs gsar pa*, plate 21). The Thangka just mentions *bshul sha phyi*, translated as "outer muscles of the small of the back," identified as "lower trapezius," but the black characteristic is not included again (Parfionovitch et al., *Tibetan Medical Paintings*, 201, no. 48). Probably because of this ambiguous situation modern, anatomical atlases do not use these classical terms to name biomedically specified muscles.

39 Meyer, "Introduction," 8.

40 Meyer, "Introduction," 9.

"tiger's head" (*stag mgo*). Although the geometrical patterns do not allow the identification of material bodily structures, the image reveals that representatives of the classical Tibetan medical tradition already had a clear concept on important relations within the thoracic cavity in general and the mediastinum in particular.[41]

The central image in the version of the "Atsagat paintings" is very similar to the Ulan-Ude image in regard to the ornamentation and body proportions, but the position of the heart is not idealized, but is painted as observable in situ. Additionally, the locations of the nipples (*nu ma*) are indicated, as they are mentioned as a point of orientation in the *Four Tantras*.[42] Another painting drawn by Endonov, which has no direct equivalent in the thangka set, is a painting with labels that are mainly in classical Mongolian (with only smaller parts in Tibetan). It depicts the location of the same triangle but includes even more biomedical features. A closer look reveals the depiction of the five lobes of the lung and allusions of lilac pulmonary tissue consisting of myriads of air sacs, clearly an influence from biomedical thinking. Also, another Atsagat painting presents the five anterior and posterior lobes of the lungs separated from other organs, relatively small, but clearly with lilac pulmonary air sacs, a color which is often utilized in modern anatomical atlases.[43] The Atsagat paintings are characterized by the desire to match both the traditional painting style and scientific knowledge.

In recent years Tibetan scholars of modern anatomy have created and coined new words for the substructures of the heart. Therefore, the anatomical publications mentioned above have integrated various synonyms, metonyms, and eponyms into Tibetan medical terminology. Below I will demonstrate a few examples with regard to the heart: physiologically the heart involves four major valves. The modern topographical name of the valves between the atrium (*snying khang*) and the ventricle (*snying shag*) are called atrioventricular heart valves (a topographical name in the neighborhood to the atrioventricular node). The left one has two biomedically-established metaphorical names (metonyms): *valva mitralis* as well as *valva bicuspidalis*, two synonyms. The former is called the *valva mitralis* because it looks like a "mitre," a bishop's cap, which derives from the notion of the joining of the two peaks of the folded cap. The second name, *valva bicuspidalis*, derives from "two sails."[44] In modern

41 For more details on the anatomy of the torso in this chapter, see also Yang Ga, *The Sources for the Writing of the Rgyud bzhi*, 286, 405.

42 See Yang Ga, *The Sources for the Writing of the Rgyud bzhi*, 286.

43 Bolsokhoeva, "Tibetan Medical Illustrations from Atsagat Medical College," 19.

44 Casselman, *A Dictionary of Medical Derivations*, 354.

Tibetan anatomical publications the *valve* is called either the "two-peaked heart leaf" (*snying 'dab rtse gnyis*),[45] the "two-peaked leaf" (*rtse gnyis 'dab ma*),[46] or the "leaf with two peaks" (*'dab lo rtse gnyis*).[47] These various terms are loosely similar in meaning to the Latin terms, as they involve "two peaks" (*rtse gnyis*) of a "leaf" (*'dab lo*), hence likewise representing a metaphorical way of designating these valves.[48] Modern authors have also created terms for smaller structures according to biomedical models: the cord-like tendons (*chordae tendineae*) that connect the mitral valve with the papillary muscles (*nu 'bur sha*; lit. "nipple flesh") are translated word by word as "tendinous chords" (*rgyus thag*).[49]

The words for the different parts of the cardiac conduction system show some interesting aspects of coining anatomical terms too. Pema Rapten and Sanggyé Bum have topographically labeled the sinoatrial node as *kong bu'i khang mdud*—using *kong bu* for sinus,[50] *khang* for atrium, and *mdud* for a node—and Nyima Tsering and Mikmar named it metaphorically as the "navel of the heartbeat" (*snying 'phar lte ba*).[51] Both editors use the same Chinese term (*dou fang jie* 窦房结). As a logical consequence of the topographical naming, the atrioventricular node is translated literally as *khang shag mdud* by Pema Rapten and Sanggyé Bum.[52] The Tibetan name for the Purkinje fibers, the final part of the cardiac conduction system, is *Phur khin je tshi sna*.[53] Here we have an eponym whereby *tshi sna* is the word for fiber, and *phur khin je* is

45 Pad ma rab brtan and Sangs rgyas 'bum, *Gso ba rig pa'i ro bkra'i dpe ris kun gsal me long*, 116.

46 Nyi ma tshe ring and Mig dmar, *Rgya bod shan sbyar tshon khra can gyi ro bkra'i dpe ris*, 113.

47 Bsam gtan, *Gso rig snying bsdus skya rengs gsar pa* (Lhasa: Bod ljongs mi dmangs dpe skrun khang, 1997), plate 27.

48 See Katharina Sabernig, "On a New Database of Tibetan Pharmacological and Anatomical Terms," in *The Proceedings of the Establishing Meeting for the Specialty Committee of Tibetan Medicine of the World Federation of Chinese Medicine Societies and First Annual Conference* (Xining: 'Dzam gling krung mthun bod gso mthun tshogs gsar 'dzugs. 2015), 679.

49 Pad ma rab brtan and Sangs rgyas 'bum, *Gso ba rig pa'i ro bkra'i dpe ris kun gsal me long*, 115.

50 *Kong bu* is also used to name the Sinus coronarius (*prog dbyibs kong bu*), literally translated as a sinus in the shape of a crown. See Pad ma rab brtan and Sangs rgyas 'bum, *Gso ba rig pa'i ro bkra'i dpe ris kun gsal me long*, 117.

51 Nyi ma tshe ring and Mig dmar, *Rgya bod shan sbyar tshon khra can gyi ro bkra'i dpe ris*, 114.

52 Pad ma rab brtan and Sangs rgyas 'bum, *Gso ba rig pa'i ro bkra'i dpe ris kun gsal me long*, 117.

53 Pad ma rab brtan and Sangs rgyas 'bum, *Gso ba rig pa'i ro bkra'i dpe ris kun gsal me long*, 117.

the Tibetan phonetic for the surname of Jan Evangelista Purkyně (1787–1869), a famous Czech anatomist and physiologist.

A similar development is observable with regard to the lungs: the (biomedical) anatomical atlas by Nyima Tsering and Mikmar integrate classical Tibetan terms with metaphorical descriptions for the different lobes of the lungs by using "tiger's head of the lung" (*glo ba'i stag mgo*) for the upper lobe, "base of the lung" (*glo ba'i gsham*) for the medium lobe of the right lung, and "dripping tip of the lung" (*glo ba'i zags sna*) for the inferior lobe.[54] This kind of mapping demonstrates the approach to include traditional Tibetan medical terms into modern anatomical terminology, but may be somewhat confusing with regard to biomedical designations. The pulmological nomenclature used in the atlas by Pema Rapten and Sanggyé Bum is organized topographically, however, corresponding to modern standards as applied for example in *Gray's Anatomy*,[55] as the "upper lobe" is called literally *gong 'dab*, the "medium lobe" is called *bar 'dab* and the inferior lobe is called *'og 'dab*, respectively. Metaphorical names are only used if the biomedical language is metaphoric in itself, such as in the case of the apex of the lung, which is called *glo rtse*, or the *lingula pulmonis sinistri*, with its accurate translation "small tongue of the left lung" (*glo ba g.yon pa'i lce chung*).[56] Although the wording chosen by the "Chinese-Tibetan-English Modern Medicine Dictionary Work Team" used by Pema Rapten and Sanggyé Bum appears to be less charming with regard to a connection to Tibetan medical tradition, with regard to explicitness and clinical applicability, and therefore patient safety, it is a great contribution in the Tibetan language.

3 The Digestive Viscera

In the case of the intestinal tract the situation is a little different from the organs in the thoracic cavity, as there are quite a few traditional terms for respective parts of the bowels, and many of them found their way into modern Tibetan anatomical publications. In classical texts and their respective illustrations, we find various names for different parts of the gut. In conventional Tibetan-English dictionaries these terms can hardly be found, and in many cases the mentioned terms are often described rather vaguely or even wrongly.

---

54 Nyi ma tshe ring and Mig dmar, *Rgya bod shan sbyar tshon khra can gyi ro bkra'i dpe ris*, 83.

55 Susan Strandring, *Gray's Anatomy: The Anatomical Basis of Clinical Practice* (London: Elsevier, 2008), 995.

56 Pad ma rab brtan and Sangs rgyas 'bum, *Gso ba rig pa'i ro bkra'i dpe ris kun gsal me long*, 117.

Let us take the example of the term *long ka*,[57] which is often translated as the "large intestine" in medical literature.[58] Conventional dictionaries offer rather vague meanings, such as intestines, entrails, guts.[59] On the other hand, Jäschke specifies about *long ka* that, "strictly taken it is said to denote only the blind gut (?),"[60] referring to the verb *long ba*, meaning "to be blind." Yet, it must be mentioned that there is some connection between the Tibetan word *long* and the *caecum*, which derives from the Latin *caecus* or Greek *typhlos* for being blind, but traditional Tibetan medical sources distinguish between different parts of the large intestine. In painting no. 49, for example, the right side of the colon is literally translated as "blood-colon" (*khrag long*), the center as "urine (?)-intestine" ([*r*]*tsam long*), and at the left side of the abdomen as "parasitic colon" (*srin long*).[61] Nowadays many of these terms found their way into modern anatomical terminology or were specified by further attributes. The "blind gut" was given a suitable metaphorical name due to its shape: the "fore colon, the head of a sheep" (*long stod lug gi mgo*),[62] or the "colon head" (*long mgo*).[63] Modern authors identify the classical term "blood-colon" as the *colon ascendens*, the "urine (?)-intestine" as the *colon transversum*, the "parasitic colon" as *colon descendens*, followed by the *colon sigmoideum* (*gnye ma*).[64]

Pema Karpo also mentions the sigmoid part of the colon in his commentary.[65] Another structure, often translated as the "upper and lower parts of the rectum" (*tshil shubs dkar nag*), is listed, literally the term means "white and black fat sheath," but no thangka gives a clear hint where to locate the respective structures. In painting no. 14, the "black and white part of the rectum" is

57 Synonyms are *long kha, long ga*, or just *long*.

58 Parfionovitch et al., *Tibetan Medical Paintings*, 185, no. 17; and 269, nos. 19–21.

59 Heinrich August Jäschke, *A Tibetan-English Dictionary* (Richmond: Curzon Press, 2003 [repr. 1881]), 553; Yuri Nikolayovitch Roerich, *Tibetsko-russko-angliiskii slovar* [Tibetan-Russian-English Dictionary] (Moskva: Izdat. Nauka, 1987), vol. 9, 214.

60 Jäschke, *A Tibetan-English Dictionary*, 553.

61 Parfionovitch et al., *Tibetan Medical Paintings*, 269, nos. 19–21.

62 Usually *stod* is translated with upper, but in the case of the caecum this does not make sense: It is the first part of the large intestine, located physiologically at the lower left side of the abdomen and is followed by the ascending part of the large intestine.

63 Mkhas grub, *Gso bya lus kyi tha snyad mdzod*, 156.

64 Nyi ma tshe ring and Mig dmar, *Rgya bod shan sbyar tshon khra can gyi ro bkra'i dpe ris*, 124; Pad ma rab brtan and Sangs rgyas 'bum, *Gso ba rig pa'i ro bkra'i dpe ris kun gsal me long*, 220; Bod rang skyong ljongs sman rtsis khang, ed., *Bod lugs gso rig tshig mdzod chen mo* (Beijing: Mi rigs dpe skrun khang, 2006), plate 23.

65 Pad ma dkar po, *Rgyud bzhi'i 'grel ba gzhan la phan pa'i gter*, 230/11–14. Only Goldstein (*The New Tibetan-English Dictionary of Modern Tibetan* [Berkeley, CA: University of California Press, 2001], 427) translates this structure as pancreas; all other publications refer to this coiled part of the large intestine.

depicted somewhere between the kidneys and the liver,[66] therefore its location remains doubtful. In this case, either the painter did not know where to locate it or, the translation of "rectum" for *tsilshup* (*tshil shubs*) is wrong.[67] The literal meaning of "fat sheath" and its location in the upper abdomen in painting no. 14 brought me to the idea that it could be a name for the *omentum majus*, an apron like fold of the peritoneum hanging from the stomach and covering the bowels. The structure is covered with fat, in veterinary medicine it is called caul fat, and is the first observable structure when the abdominal cavity is opened by dissection. However, there is no proof for my consideration, and the variety of modern Tibetan terms related to the structure have the same Chinese name (*da wang mo* 大网膜), which ranges from "great intestinal fat" (*rgyu tshil che ba*),[68] to "peritoneum" (*grod skyi*),[69] to "net-shaped skin" (*dra dbyibs skyi mo*).[70]

Apart from the complicated question of the location of "fat sheath," a more precise depiction of the colon can be found in one of the Atsagat paintings mentioned above. The painting, still classical in terms of painting style, shows adaptions with regard to the typical biomedical characteristics of the large intestine: the *vermiform appendix*, as well as the *teania coli*, and the *appendices epiploicae* are clearly depicted. However, Endonov did not add new Tibetan terms to what he painted, but obviously included structures which can be clearly identified anatomically. This gap, so to speak, is abundantly filled in modern Tibetan anatomical publications, which seem to be quite inventive when it comes to finding proper names complying with the Tibetan language for these structures: the *vermiform appendix* is commonly named the "appendix"

66 Parfionovitch et al., *Tibetan Medical Paintings*, 199, no. 105.

67 Jäschke, *A Tibetan-English Dictionary*, 448. I found it only translated as upper and lower parts of the rectum: Parfionovitch et al., *Tibetan Medical Paintings*, 199, no. 105; and Tshe ring thag gcod drung 'tsho and Tshe ring sgrol ma drung 'tsho, *Bod lugs sman rtsis kyi tshig mdzod bod dbyin shan sbyar* [Tibetan-English Dictionary of Tibetan Medicine and Astrology] (Dharamsala: Drungtso Publications, 2005), 374. The *Bod lugs gso rig tshig mdzod chen mo* regards the two as synonyms to *gzhang dkar nag* and depicts *gzhang dkar po* as lower part of the rectum and *gzhang nag po* as the upper part (Bod rang skyong ljongs sman rtsis khang, ed., *Bod lugs gso rig tshig mdzod chen mo* [Beijing: Mi rigs dpe skrun khang, 2006], 722, chart 23). Nyima Tsering and Mikmar locate the term undistinguished at the rectum (Nyi ma tshe ring and Mig dmar, *Rgya bod shan sbyar tshon khra can gyi ro bkra'i dpe ris*, 105, no. 22; 62, no. 13). In the atlas by Pema Rapten and Sanggyé Bum, the rectum is simply called *gzhang* (Pad ma rab brtan and Sangs rgyas 'bum, *Gso ba rig pa'i ro bkra'i dpe ris kun gsal me long*, 221).

68 Nyi ma tshe ring and Mig dmar, *Rgya bod shan sbyar tshon khra can gyi ro bkra'i dpe ris*, 102, no. 13.

69 Mkhas grub, *Gso bya lus kyi tha snyad mdzod*, 99.

70 Pad ma rab brtan and Sangs rgyas 'bum, *Gso ba rig pa'i ro bkra'i dpe ris kun gsal me long*, 69.

(*rgyu lhag*);[71] the *teania coli*—three longitudinal ribbons of smooth muscle tissue along the large intestine—are called the "long large intestinal cord" (*long thig ring ba*),[72] or "long rope" (*rkyang thag*);[73] and the *appendices epiploicae*—small pouches filled with fat along the large intestine—found their Tibetan equivalents in "suspended intestinal fat" (*rgyu tshil 'phyang*),[74] or "suspending fat of the large intestine" (*long gi dpyang tshil*).[75]

The small intestine, five meters in length, is usually called *rgyu ma* in classical texts. Rarely—not in the *Explanatory Tantra*, but in the commentaries to chapter 85 of the *Instructional Tantra* and in paintings no. 49 and 50 on wounds of the trunk—one can also find a division into "upper intestine" (*rgyu stod*) and "lower intestine" (*rgyu smad*).[76] The classical Tibetan terms "upper intestine" and "lower intestine" are still in use: the jejunum is called "upper intestine" and the ileum refers to the "lower intestine." In addition to the "upper" and "lower intestine," modern Tibetan anatomical publications present a third structure, namely the duodenum, which is called "intestine of twelve fingers" (*rgyu sor bcu gnyis*), which—though certainly adapted from Chinese anatomical vocabulary where it is called *shier zhichang* 十二指腸—looks like a splendid loan translation of *intestinum duodenum digitorum*, as the full medieval Latin term has it. What is indicated is that this part of the small intestine has the length of the breadth of twelve fingers. As it happened, the Latin terms is in itself a loan translation via the Arabic language from a very old Greek term, "twelve fingers long outgrowth" (*ekphysis dōdekadaktylon*).[77]

Accordingly, modern Tibetan authors call the respective arteries "jejunal arteries" (*rgyu stod 'phar rtsa*) and "ileal arteries" (*rgyu smad 'phar rtsa*). All these blood vessels are branches of the superior mesenteric artery, and are called the "upper pulsating channel of the intestinal silk" (*rgyu dar sgang gi 'phar rtsa*).[78]

---

71 Pad ma rab brtan and Sangs rgyas 'bum, *Gso ba rig pa'i ro bkra'i dpe ris kun gsal me long*, 72; Nyi ma tshe ring and Mig dmar, *Rgya bod shan sbyar tshon khra can gyi ro bkra'i dpe ris*, 62, no. 13; Mkhas grub, *Gso bya lus kyi tha snyad mdzod*, 87.

72 Pad ma rab brtan and Sangs rgyas 'bum, *Gso ba rig pa'i ro bkra'i dpe ris kun gsal me long*, 71.

73 Nyi ma tshe ring and Mig dmar, *Rgya bod shan sbyar tshon khra can gyi ro bkra'i dpe ris*, 72, no. 13.

74 Pad ma rab brtan and Sangs rgyas 'bum, *Gso ba rig pa'i ro bkra'i dpe ris kun gsal me long*, 71.

75 Nyi ma tshe ring and Mig dmar, *Rgya bod shan sbyar tshon khra can gyi ro bkra'i dpe ris*, 72, no. 22.

76 Parfionovitch et al., *Tibetan Medical Paintings*, 269–72; Zur mkhar blo gros rgyal po, *Rgyud bzhi'i 'grel pa mes po'i zhal lung* (Beijing: Mi rigs dpe skrun khang, 2005), 560/16.

77 Michler and Benedum, *Einführung in die Medizinische Fachsprache*, 165.

78 Nyi ma tshe ring and Mig dmar, *Rgya bod shan sbyar tshon khra can gyi ro bkra'i dpe ris*, 90, no. 18.

To express the idea of "mesentery," another fold of the peritoneal membrane to keep the viscera in their position with "intestinal silk" (*rgyu dar*) is a nice coinage indeed, the nomenclature by Pema Rapten and Sanggyé Bum for the mesentery is "binding skin of the intestine" (*rgyu ma'i sgrog skyi*).[79] The suspension of the mesentery, *radix mesenterii*, has the accurate metaphorical indication, the "root of the intestinal silk" (*rgyu dar gyi rtsa ba*),[80] or the "root of the binding skin of the intestine" (*rgyu ma'i sgrog skyi'i rtsa ba*).[81] This is only one out of numerous examples of modern Tibetan anatomical nomenclature.

Thangka painting 49 depicts the intestinal tract not only with regard to proportional ideals but also as it is observed (*bltas pa*). In this case the whole intestinal bundle is depicted roughly, only labelled as *rgyu ma*, with the stomach (*pho ba*) a bit segregated. Although it is possible to identify the beginning of large intestine with a little imagination, the terminal part of the intestinal tract is not shown. Therefore, the location of the "black and white rectum" cannot be identified, and instead a connection of the small intestine with the urinary bladder is depicted. What does this portend, especially in case of a depiction purportedly indicating "what is observed?" One could leave the matter as a difficulty of the painter to understand the medical function of what is seen during the unpleasant and unaccustomed situation of dissection without proper preservation technique, but one of the Atsagat paintings reveals again some structure which makes it more likely that the painter tried to depict a functional connection between the small intestine and the urinary system.[82] This Atsagat painting does not correspond to any of the thangkas and depicts all of the internal organs, including some of the vascular connections, such as the nine channels between the stomach and the liver, which are already mentioned in the *Four Tantras*.[83] Next to the ureter conducting urine from the kidney to the urinary bladder, a second channel is depicted connecting the small intestine with the kidney. From a biomedical point of view, the existence of such a connection is never physiological, but can be found pathologically in form of a vesicointestinal fistula,[84] as an unpleasant result of various dis-

79 Pad ma rab brtan and Sangs rgyas 'bum, *Gso ba rig pa'i ro bkra'i dpe ris kun gsal me long*, 221.

80 Nyi ma tshe ring and Mig dmar, *Rgya bod shan sbyar tshon khra can gyi ro bkra'i dpe ris*, 105, no. 6.

81 Pad ma rab brtan and Sangs rgyas 'bum, *Gso ba rig pa'i ro bkra'i dpe ris kun gsal me long*, 107.

82 Published in Bolsokhoyeva, "Tibetan Medical Illustrations from Atsagat Medical College," 19.

83 See Bolsokhoyeva, "Tibetan Medical Illustrations from Atsagat Medical College," 19.

84 According to the international classification of diseases published by the WHO it is classified as ICD 10: N32.1.

eases. In the case of Tibetan and Atsagat medical paintings the painter probably wanted to demonstrate the tight functional connection between the small intestine and the urinary system, which can be found in various Asian medical traditions. Again, this Atsagat painting is a document for the effort of Buryat scholars to combine tradition with modern knowledge on a visual basis at the beginning of the twentieth century.

4 The Urogenital System

Aside from the disputable visceral connection between the intestines and the urinary tract, classical Tibetan medical knowledge has some unclear particularities with regard to the urogenital system. Conversely, its precise comprehension is complicated due to the fact that the thangka paintings usually depict either solid viscera (*don*) or hollow viscera (*snod*). None of the thangkas present the connection between the kidneys and the urinary bladder, and no name for the ureter can be found. Even Tashi Tsering did not include it into his dictionary. This lack of information is accentuated in the atlas of Tindzin which depicts traditional anatomical knowledge through the lens of modern anatomical insights, but in the case of the ureter, it is either only presented rudimentarily or not labeled at all.[85] Only one image depicting the womb presents a vascular triple comprising the artery, the vein of the uterus, and the ureter, called the "water channel" (*chu rtsa*).[86] I will come back to this vascular triple at the end of my article. If one is aware of this uncertainty, it is not surprising that different modern authors created different names: Pema Rapten and Sanggyé Bum use "hollow urine drain" (*gcin 'dren sbu gu*),[87] while earlier publications use another term for the ureter—which is almost impossible to translate literally—which is designated as *rgyu grog rtsa*.[88] Once more Nyima Tsering and Mikmar have

85 Ting 'dzin, *Gso rig rgyud bzhi'i dka' gnad thor bu la dpyad pa*, 39, 44.

86 Ting 'dzin, *Gso rig rgyud bzhi'i dka' gnad thor bu la dpyad pa*, 41. Ureter would be at least the third meaning for the term *chu rtsa*, which is usually associated with tendons or nerves (Gyatso, *Being Human in a Buddhist World*, 202; Sabernig "Anatomical Structures and the Structure of Anatomy in Tibetan Medicine," 26).

87 Pad ma rab brtan and Sangs rgyas 'bum, *Gso ba rig pa'i ro bkra'i dpe ris kun gsal me long*, 90–94. Tindzin labels the urethra with *gcin vdren sbu gu* (Ting 'dzin, *Gso rig rgyud bzhi'i dka' gnad thor bu la dpyad pa*, 40)

88 Dbang 'dus, *G.yu thog dgongs rgyan* (Beijing: Mi rigs dpe skrun khang, 1983); Bod rang skyong ljongs sman rtsis khang, ed., *Bod lugs gso rig tshig mdzod chen mo*, plate 34. Khedrup eliminated *rgyu* and labels the ureter as *chu grog rtsa* (Mkhas grub, *Gso bya lus kyi tha snyad mdzod*, 133).

chosen a more metaphorical name: "little bird channel" (*rtsa bye'u*).[89] In the case of the urethra the situation is clearer: colloquially it is called the "water passageway" (*chu lam*),[90] a metonym corresponding to the metaphorical description of the urinary tract, which is compared with drainage gutters in chapter 3 of the *Explanatory Tantra* and depicted vividly in thangka number six of *Illustrations to the Blue Beryl*.[91] Nowadays Tibetan medical language is more precise. All recent specialized anatomical publications and medical dictionaries call it accurately the "urine passageway" (*gcin lam*),[92] similar to the meaning of the Greek *ourethra*, the "passage for urine," coined by Hippocrates.[93]

Aside these "urinary passageways" classical Tibetan language has quite a few designations for smaller anatomical structures of the urogenital system. The sixteenth-century scholar, Pema Karpo, mentioned a structure called the "mouth of the urinary bladder" (*lgang ba'i kha*). Although there is no further explanation, it should be located at the trigone of the urinary bladder where three openings are located; according to Pema Rapten and Sanggyé Bum it is the internal urethral orifice (*meatus urethrae internus*),[94] while Nyima Tsering and Mikmar specify it as the two ureteric orifices.[95] Nowadays, the external urethral orifice is called *chu so*,[96] whereas in former days *chu so*, literally "water tooth," or more appropriate, "water edge," was obviously used in a broader context, as Jäschke describes it as the external and internal urinary organs.[97]

89 Nyi ma tshe ring and Mig dmar, *Rgya bod shan sbyar tshon khra can gyi ro bkra'i dpe ris*, 92, no. 11.

90 Goldstein, *The New Tibetan-English Dictionary of Modern Tibetan*, 367.

91 Parfionovitch et al., *Tibetan Medical Paintings*, 183, no. 35.

92 Dbang 'dus, *G.yu thog dgongs rgyan*, plate 21; Bod rang skyong ljongs sman rtsis khang, ed., *Bod lugs gso rig tshig mdzod chen mo*, plate 34; Bsam gtan, *Gso rig snying bsdus skya rengs gsar pa*, plate 21; Bod rang skyong ljongs sman rtsis khang, ed., *Bod lugs gso rig tshig mdzod chen mo*, plate 34; Pad ma rab brtan and Sangs rgyas 'bum, *Gso ba rig pa'i ro bkra'i dpe ris kun gsal me long*, 95, 98; Nyi ma tshe ring and Mig dmar, *Rgya bod shan sbyar tshon khra can gyi ro bkra'i dpe ris*, 89, no. 6; Tshe ring thag gcod drung 'tsho and Tshe ring sgrol ma drung 'tsho, *Bod lugs sman rtsis kyi tshig mdzod bod dbyin shan sbyar*, 374; Mkhas grub, *Gso bya lus kyi tha snyad mdzod*, 135–37.

93 Casselman, *A Dictionary of Medical Derivations*, 350.

94 *Lgang bu'i kha*: Pad ma rab brtan and Sangs rgyas 'bum, *Gso ba rig pa'i ro bkra'i dpe ris kun gsal me long*, 94.

95 Nyi ma tshe ring and Mig dmar, *Rgya bod shan sbyar tshon khra can gyi ro bkra'i dpe ris*, 95, no. 13.

96 Pad ma rab brtan and Sangs rgyas 'bum, *Gso ba rig pa'i ro bkra'i dpe ris kun gsal me long*, 97; Nyi ma tshe ring and Mig dmar, *Rgya bod shan sbyar tshon khra can gyi ro bkra'i dpe ris*, 96, no. 6.

97 Jäschke, *A Tibetan-English Dictionary*, 159.

Various structures associated with the kidneys (*mkhal ma*), often called synonymously the "fruit of the kidney" (*mkhal ma'i 'bras bu*), are depicted on several thangkas. In thangka 49 and 50 we find the "kidney bed" (*mkhal ma'i yul*),[98] thangka 71 depicts perinephric fat (*mkhal tshil*), or terms of the vascular supply of the kidney (*mkhal rtsa nag*).[99] It is no surprise that modern anatomical atlases present more words with regard to smaller renal structures. However, none of the classical structures has received more attention than a urogenital organ, which is generally and unspecifically translated as the "reproductive vesicle" (*bsam se'u* or *bsam bse'u*), which is particularly difficult to identify.[100] It is not in the scope of this article to add other possibilities or to clarify its historical meaning, but I would like to demonstrate the variety of identifications in descriptions and depictions over time. Before I start with my evaluation of Tibetan illustrations, I would like to introduce the lexical situation on this term.

The first identification of the "reproductive vesicle" in a European language that I am aware of was made by Heinrich August Jäschke, who noted the structure as "seminal vesicle" and as possibly the ovaries.[101] The male gland (*glandula vesiculosa*) located below the urinary bladder was also taken by Das,[102] and later by Roerich, who also included the testicles.[103] Goldstein has it as gonads only,[104] and Tsering Takchö Drungtso (*tshe ring thag gcod drung 'tsho*) and Tsering Drölma Drungtso (*tshe ring sgrol ma drung 'tsho*) took Jäschke's suggestion as additional information, but they call it less specifically "vesicle of regenerative substances."[105] Jenny Bright, who examined contemporary Tibetan medical literature on menstruation, translates the term as "both the male and female reproductive sacs," leaving unclear what is actually meant.[106] The way "reproductive vesicle" is depicted in the *Illustrations to the Blue Beryl* indicates

98 Parfionovitch et al., *Tibetan Medical Paintings*, 269, no. 48; and 271, no. 69.

99 Parfionovitch et al., *Tibetan Medical Paintings*, 313, nos. 84 and 85.

100 See a full article on this issue: Isabella Würthner, "A Preliminary Study on the Function, Anatomy and Origin of the Term *bsam-se'u* in Tibetan Medical Literature," *Curare* 39, no. 1 (2016): 42–55.

101 Jäschke, *A Tibetan-English Dictionary*, 593.

102 Sarat Chandra Das, *A Tibetan-English Dictionary* (Delhi: Sri Satguru Publications, 1989 [repr. 1902]), 1317.

103 Roerich, *Tibetsko-russko-angliiskii slovar*, vol. 10, 175.

104 Goldstein, *The New Tibetan-English Dictionary of Modern Tibetan*, 1166.

105 Tshe ring thag gcod drung 'tsho and Tshe ring sgrol ma drung 'tsho, *Bod lugs sman rtsis kyi tshig mdzod bod dbyin shan sbyar*, 525.

106 Jennifer Bright, "'Female Nectar': A Study of Hybridity and Gender in Contemporary Tibetan Medical Literature on Menstruation," *Asian Medicine* 6, no. 2 (2010–11): 404; Jennifer Bright, *Women and Hormones in Tibetan Medical Literature* (Toronto, ON: Doctoral Dissertation at the University of Toronto, 2017).

that the structure is regarded to be located somewhere in the retroperitoneal space, although this is only one part in the debate. The *Illustrations to the Blue Beryl* contains at least five thangkas depicting the "reproductive vesicle" directly, and another five thangkas locating superficial gateways to the organ for the application of external therapies, such as moxibustion. Although there are varieties to the mode of counting bones, "reproductive vesicle" always corresponds to the thirteenth vertebra according to the Tibetan style, setting the location at the height around the eleventh thoracic vertebra. In the eighth thangka it is presented as a pair between the upper edge of the kidneys, a topography where an empirical anatomist would find the adrenal glands. Classic Tibetan literature describes and thangkas ten and fourteen depict an unpaired vascular supply, like it is the case of unpaired organs such as the heart, the liver, or the spleen, in contrast to paired vascular supply in the case with the kidneys or the lungs.

Although both the set stored in Lhasa as well as the set in Ulan-Ude are labelled accordingly in Tibetan right above the kidneys, the editors of the Ulan-Ude set attached the reference number falsely at the end of the spine.[107] This mistake is not a sheer coincidence, but a result of an observable descensus of the location at depictions in the course of time. A Buryat painting from Atsagat Monastery created in the 1920 questions the location of "reproductive vesicle": it is depicted well below the kidneys and labelled with an interrogative particle (*'am*), whereas other organs were not questioned.[108] Obviously under the influence of biomedical concepts, Tibetan-English dictionaries and images in Tibetan medical books published at the end of the twentieth century mainly identify the seminal vesicle and the gonads as the biomedical male equivalent of "reproductive vesicle," and determine consistently the ovaries as the female counterpart.[109] Although the seminal vesicle secretes a fluid which mixes with sperm—during ejaculation it is observable as semen—it is doubtfully whether that the concept of "reproductive vesicle" originally was

107 Parfionovitch et al., *Tibetan Medical Paintings*, 187, no. 17. Würthner already drew attention to the mistake ("A Preliminary Study on the Function, Anatomy and Origin of the Term *bsam-se'u*," 17).

108 The image can be found on the back side of the *Curare* issue 39 (2016), including Bolsokhoyeva, "Tibetan Medical Illustrations from Atsagat Medical College."

109 Dbang 'dus, *G.yu thog dgongs rgyan*, plates 21–22; Bsam gtan, *Gso rig snying bsdus skya rengs gsar pa*, plates 45–46; Tupten Püntsok 1999: 45–46, 146; Bod rang skyong ljongs sman rtsis khang, ed., *Bod lugs gso rig tshig mdzod chen mo*, 34, plates 30–31; Ting 'dzin, *Gso rig rgyud bzhi'i dka' gnad thor bu la dpyad pa*, 39 and 41; Nyi ma tshe ring and Mig dmar, *Rgya bod shan sbyar tshon khra can gyi ro bkra'i dpe ris*, 97, no. 21; 98, no. 3.; Mkhas grub, *Gso bya lus kyi tha snyad mdzod*, 136; Pad ma rab brtan and Sangs rgyas 'bum, *Gso ba rig pa'i ro bkra'i dpe ris kun gsal me long*, 98 and 99 (they only mention the ovaries as a biomedical pendant of *samseu*, with no male equivalent).

associated with this tiny structure located on the floor of the pelvis. This doubt was already pronounced by Fernand Meyer, who suggested to compare it, despite big differences, with the more subtle "triple burner" system in traditional Chinese medicine mentioned above.[110] Janet Gyatso referred to a consideration by Wangdü (*dbang 'dus*) "who maintained the term is a faulty rendering of a Chinese term phoneticized in Tibetan as *gsan rtsa'u*, but that the Tibetan understanding of the *bsam se'u* is unique to Yutok."[111] Isabella Würthner examined arguments that speak for or against this hypothesis in various Tibetan commentaries and concluded that the Chinese description does not fully correspond to the Tibetan.[112] Maybe Elisabeth Finckh was a bit hasty when she regarded the same relation of internal organs and certain vertebrae as conclusive evidence that "reproductive vesicle" would be identical with *san jiao*.[113] Nevertheless, in spite of the different systemic conceptions, a connection of ideas which may describe some observations from different perspectives should not be ignored. Some researchers assume that "reproductive vesicle" should be associated with the endocrine system.[114]

How do the authors of recent publications reconcile these historical developments? Tindzin tried to bring traditional terms and concepts in harmony with modern anatomical structures. He identified "reproductive vesicle" within the male reproductive system with both seminal vesicle and epididymis,[115] both of which develop together with the vas deference from the mesonephric duct during embryogenesis. They are all important for successful ejaculation and the epididymis are in fact "storage boxes" for the maturing sperm, but would this be proof enough to identify the historical "reproductive vesicle" primary as the male ejaculatory system? The identification and function of this structure is still debated intensely among Tibetan scholars and that is maybe the reason

110 Fernand Meyer, *Le système médical tibétain: Gso-ba Rig pa* (Paris: CNRS [Centre Nationale de la Recherche Scientifique], 2002 [repr. 1988]), 156; David L. Snellgrove, "Review of Fernand Meyer, *gSo-ba riq[sic]-pa, le système médical tibétain*," *Bulletin of the School of Oriental and African Studies* 46, no. 1 (1983): 173; Florian Ploberger, *Wurzeltantra und Tantra der Erklärungen der Tibetischen Medizin* (Schiedlberg: Bacopa, 2012), 85.

111 Gyatso, *Being Human in a Buddhist World*, 461, n. 96.

112 Würthner, "A Preliminary Study on the Function, Anatomy and Origin of the Term *bsam-se'u*," 47.

113 Elisabeth Finckh, *Der Tibetische Medizin-Baum: Texte und Illustrationen* (Uelzen: Medizin-Literar. Verl.-Ges, 1990), 76.

114 See, for example, Thub bstan phun tshogs, *Gso bya lus kyi rnam bshad* (Beijing: Mi rigs dpe skrun khang, 1999), 40–50, 146. For a broader discussion on different perspectives how traditional explanations may be compatible with biomedical hormonal regulation: see Bright, "Female Nectar."

115 Ting 'dzin, *Gso rig rgyud bzhi'i dka' gnad thor bu la dpyad pa*, 39–41.

why the Tibetan *Terminologia Anatomica* in publication by Pema Rapten and Sanggyé Bum does not associate the term with any male urogenital structure any more, whereas Nyima Tsering and Mikmar still hold on the identification with the "seminal vesicle" in the case of the male urogenital system.[116] In the former atlas, the seminal vesicle is called the "semen case" (*khu thum*), a portmanteau of semen (*khu ba*) and case (*thum bu*), and the epididymis is named rather metaphorical *sgong zur*, which means literally "egg edge."[117] Another name for epididymis is *rlig 'bras zur ma*,[118] or a portmanteau called *zur 'bras*,[119] as *zur ma* indicates something aside or at the edge and the testicles are called *rlig 'bras* in classical as well as modern Tibetan.[120]

As mentioned above, in the female body the "reproductive vesicle" is consistently equated with the ovaries, which are located in the lesser pelvis.[121] I could not find a single Tibetan synonym for ovary in any specialized medical textbook. Only general dictionaries compiled in the 1980s used other terms: Tashi Tsering suggested to name the ovaries "egg-container" (*sgong snod*),[122] and Goldstein has it as a "container of the (menstrual) blood of the womb" (*mngal khrag gi snod*).[123] In the atlas by Pema Rapten and Sanggyé Bum, the ovary and related tissues are the only anatomical structure being labeled as "reproductive vesicle," and the male anatomical equivalent is not connected to the term. Vascular supply by the *arteria ovarica* is named in Tibetan

116 Nyi ma tshe ring and Mig dmar, *Rgya bod shan sbyar tshon khra can gyi ro bkra'i dpe ris*, 95, no. 3.

117 Pad ma rab brtan and Sangs rgyas 'bum, *Gso ba rig pa'i ro bkra'i dpe ris kun gsal me long*, 89.

118 Nyi ma tshe ring and Mig dmar, *Rgya bod shan sbyar tshon khra can gyi ro bkra'i dpe ris*, 95, no. 13.

119 Mkhas grub, *Gso bya lus kyi tha snyad mdzod*, 134.

120 Taken strictly epididymis means "on" and "testicles," but it is resting on and beside each testis (see Casselman, *A Dictionary of Medical Derivations*, 129).

121 Dbang 'dus, *G.yu thog dgongs rgyan*, plate 22; Bod rang skyong ljongs sman rtsis khang, ed., *Bod lugs gso rig tshig mdzod chen mo*, plate 34; Bsam gtan, *Gso rig snying bsdus skya rengs gsar pa*, plate 21; Bod rang skyong ljongs sman rtsis khang, ed., *Bod lugs gso rig tshig mdzod chen mo*, plate 34; Tshe ring thag gcod drung 'tsho and Tshe ring sgrol ma drung 'tsho, *Bod lugs sman rtsis kyi tshig mdzod bod dbyin shan sbyar*, 374; Ting 'dzin, *Gso rig rgyud bzhi'i dka' gnad thor bu la dpyad pa*, 39 and 41; Pad ma rab brtan and Sangs rgyas 'bum, *Gso ba rig pa'i ro bkra'i dpe ris kun gsal me long*, 95, 98; Nyi ma tshe ring and Mig dmar, *Rgya bod shan sbyar tshon khra can gyi ro bkra'i dpe ris*, 89, no. 6; Mkhas grub, *Gso bya lus kyi tha snyad mdzod*, 135–37.

122 Tashi Tsering, *English-Tibetan-Chinese Dictionary* (Beijing: Nationalities Publishing House, 1991 [repr. 1988]), 686.

123 Melvin C. Goldstein and Ngawangthondup Narkyid, *English-Tibetan Dictionary of Modern Tibetan* (Dharamsala: Library of Tibetan Works and Archives, 1999), 217.

the "pulsating channel of the reproductive vesicle" (*bsam se'u'i 'phar rtsa*) and the *ligamentum suspensorium ovarii*, which are translated accurately as the "sustaining ligament of reproductive vesicle" (*bsam se'u'i 'degs chu*).[124] The male gonad artery is called the "pulsating channel of the testicle" (*rlig 'bras 'phar rtsa*).[125] Not even a tiny little structure can be found in images depicting the male body. Nothing in the "modern" male body resembles the important organ. That is surprising because Janet Gyatso stated that "both male and female sexual fluids ultimately have their source in the gonad-like *bsam se'u* in the body."[126] She also pointed out that the *Illustrations to the Blue Beryl* demonstrates a strong androcentric tendency,[127] and thangka number ten and fourteen certainly depict the "reproductive vesicle" in the height of the kidneys within a male body with visible outer genitalia. Thangka fourteen presents vascular supply for the organ in form of one of the eight major hidden channels just one vertebra above the kidneys.[128] It is obvious that the visual interpretation of the term has changed dramatically in the course of time. Its location descended from above the kidneys to the minor pelvis or even below, and it was reduced from an organ with male as well as female equivalents to the female ovaries only. The descensus of the location of this organ within depictions over the last 300 years should be critically evaluated. Nevertheless, it is worth to take a closer look at the vascular supply of the gonads. During embryonic development both the ovaries and testicles are located behind the kidneys before they descend to the pelvis or the scrotum. Due to this descensus, the paired arteries arise from the abdominal aorta just below the kidneys and travel down to supply the organs. Maybe it would be worthwhile to examine commentaries to Tibetan embryonic development to find more information on the "reproductive vesicle." So far, we have ended up with speculations and, as Fernand Meyer suggested already many years ago, for the sake of justice to the historical meaning of the organ and its physiology, it may be better not to determine its biomedical identification in modern anatomical atlases.[129]

An even more complicated development is observable in the scope of a less prominent question, a vascular triple originally associated with the urinary

124 *'Degs chu* is a portmanteau consisting of *'degs pa* (to sustain) and *chu ba* (tendon or ligament); Pad ma rab brtan and Sangs rgyas 'bum, *Gso ba rig pa'i ro bkra'i dpe ris kun gsal me long*, 100.

125 Mkhas grub, *Gso bya lus kyi tha snyad mdzod*, 224.

126 Gyatso, *Being Human in a Buddhist World*, 292.

127 Gyatso, "Looking for Gender in the Medical Paintings of Desi Sangye Gyatso"; Gyatso, *Being Human in a Buddhist World*.

128 Parfionovitch et al., *Tibetan Medical Paintings*, 200, nos. 110 and 115.

129 Meyer, *Le système médical tibétain*, 156.

bladder.[130] They are all part of 112 vulnerable blood vessels called "black life channels" (*srog rtsa nag po*) of the lower trunk mentioned just rudimentary in the *Four Tantras* and listed in detail in its commentaries. Called "water channel" (*chu rtsa*),[131] "life channel" (*srog rtsa*), and "existence channel" (*srid rtsa*), their names are a bit confusing as they break through the usual assignment in Tibetan classification of tissues. Maybe this is the reason why it is hard to define their location. On thangka nine of the *Illustrations to the Blue Beryl*, the vascular triple is shown in a picture depicting the male perineum,[132] and it is neither located inside the body nor associated with the urinary bladder. There is no female counterpart. In modern anatomical publications the vascular triple cannot be found at all, only the mentioned vascular triple depicted in Tindzin's atlas contains the term *chu rtsa* indicating the ureter. The red uterine artery is called "wind channel" (*rlung rtsa*) and the blue uterine vein is called "blood channel" (*khrag rtsa*).[133]

5 Conclusion

These are just a few examples of the transformation of Tibetan medical language and the depiction of internal organs over time. The process is characterized by the successive integration of "modern anatomical" knowledge. As Janet Gyatso has pointed out, in contrast to orthodox religious Tibetan paintings, the *Illustrations to the Blue Beryl* presents the ordinary material world with ordinary people in the unique painting style of the seventeenth century.[134] However, each tradition of anatomical depiction presents just an abstract image of the structure which should be illustrated. Classical Tibetan medical knowledge was often idealized with regard to Buddhist iconography, colorful and allowing a sense of humor. Although there is at least one thangka demonstrating the approach of illustrating "what is observed," it remains often unclear if the painter really knew what he actually painted.

---

130 *Sgang bu'i chu rtsa srog rtsa srid rtsa gsum* (Blo bzang chos grags, *Legs bshad gser gyi thur ma*, 20/24); If *sgang bu* is taken as a synonym for *lgang bu*, the urinary bladder (Roerich, *Tibetsko-russko-angliiskii slovar*, vol. 2, 276).

131 Usually *chu rtsa* belong to the group of white channels (*srog rtsa dkar po*), which are associated with neurovascular structures or tendons (Sabernig, "Anatomical Structures"; Sabernig, "Vulnerable Parts"), but in this case the name stands for a black life channel.

132 Parfionovitch et al., *Tibetan Medical Paintings*, 190, nos. 79–81.

133 Ting 'dzin, *Gso rig rgyud bzhi'i dka' gnad thor bu la dpyad pa*, 41.

134 Gyatso, *Being Human in a Buddhist World*, 27.

While preserving Tibetan style, the Atsagat-paintings created in the early twentieth century included some specific Buryat features and obviously integrated modern anatomical knowledge. The early publications after the cultural revolution demonstrate the ambition to adapt traditional knowledge within the frame of biomedical ideas. A highlight of this fruitful process is the book by Tindzin, with its challenging attempt to harmonize classical and modern knowledge and anatomical forms of depiction. In this respect, the result is certainly delighting, but in some cases, it is made clear that these diverging forms of knowledge are not always compatible. The example of difficulties in identifying the "reproductive vesicle" is just the tip of the iceberg.

On the other hand, it is obvious that in recent years many new medical words were coined carefully, mostly translated into Tibetan from Latin or English via preceding Chinese translations. At the moment the modern Chinese anatomical nomenclature appears more homogenous and standardized than its Tibetan counterpart. The atlas by Pema Rapten and Sanggyé Bum uses mainly topographical terminology, aims to be a clear translation of modern biomedical *Terminologia Anatomica*, and is indeed suitable as a reference book for clinical practitioners who want to study modern anatomy in the Tibetan language. The atlas by Nyima Tsering and Mikmar appears to be a bit less accurate with regard to scientific clearness, but it still includes an impressive amount of metaphorical vocabulary typical for Tibetan culture. These modern anatomical publications were not produced to clarify traditional vocabulary. The whole development marks a significant improvement for the professionalization and integration of traditional Tibetan medicine into the modern health care system, and the integration of biomedical knowledge into the Tibetan language. Some scholars have expressed fears that this development will degenerate traditional concepts, but if the cognitive levels of the concepts are clearly distinguished, traditional Tibetan medical and biomedical services may profit in the end.

References

Adams, Vincanne. "Complications in the Study of Efficacy of Tibetan Medicine within the Biomedical Context." In *Anthology of 2000 International Academic Conference on Tibetan Medicine*, edited by Apei Awang Jinmei [Ngag dbang 'jigs med], 928–34. Unpublished: 2000.

Balk, Michael. "A Bibliographical Survey of Medical Literature in Tibetan Language Based on the Post-war Holdings of the State Library in Berlin: A Strand of Pearls to Enlighten Researchers." *Curare* 39, no. 1 (2016): 88–94.

Blo bzang chos grags [Dar mo sman rams pa]. *Legs bshad gser gyi thur ma.* Bod kyi gso ba rig pa'i gna' dpe phyogs bsgrigs dpe tshogs, vol. 31. Beijing: Mi rigs dpe skrun khang, 2005.

Bod rang skyong ljongs sman rtsis khang, ed. *Bod lugs gso rig tshig mdzod chen mo.* Beijing: Mi rigs dpe skrun khang, 2006.

Bolsokhoyeva, Natalia, and Kseniya Gerasimova. "The Atlas of Tibetan Medicine: Treasures from The History Museum of Buryatia." In *The Buddha's Art of Healing: Tibetan Paintings Rediscovered*, edited by John Avedon, 33–60. New York, NY: Rizzoli, 1998.

Bolsokhoyeva, Natalia. "Tibetan Medical Illustrations from Atsagat Medical College and other Anatomical Achievements of the Buryat Lama and Physician D. Endonov." *Curare* 39, no. 1 (2016): 6–21.

Bolsokhoyeva, Natalia. "Tibetan Medical Illustrations from the History Museum of Buryatia, Ulan Ude." *Asian Medicine* 3 (2007): 347–67.

Bright, Jennifer. "'Female Nectar': A Study of Hybridity and Gender in Contemporary Tibetan Medical Literature on Menstruation." *Asian Medicine* 6, no. 2 (2010–11): 387–420.

Bright, Jennifer. *Women and Hormones in Tibetan Medical Literature*. Toronto, ON: Doctoral Dissertation at the University of Toronto, 2017.

Bsam gtan. *Gso rig snying bsdus skya rengs gsar pa*. Lhasa: Bod ljongs mi dmangs dpe skrun khang, 1997.

Bstan 'dzin don grub, ed. *Dpal ldan rgyud bzhi dpe bsdur ma*. Beijing: Krung go'i bod rig pa dpe skrun khang, 2005–2008.

Byams pa phrin las and Wang Lei. *Tibetan Medical Thangka of the Four Medical Tantras* [Bod lugs gso rig rgyud bzhi'i nang don bris cha ngo mtshar mthong ba don ldan]. Translated into English by Cai Jingfeng. Lhasa: Bod ljongs mi dmangs dpe skrun khang, 1994.

Casselman, William. *A Dictionary of Medical Derivations: The Real Meaning of Medical Terms.* New York, NY: The Pantheon Publishing Group, 1998.

Cha, Wung-Seok, and Hyuk-Sang Jung. "Body Perception in East Asian Culture." *Curare* 39, no.1 (2016): 75–87.

Das, Sarat Chandra. *A Tibetan-English Dictionary*. Delhi: Sri Satguru Publications, 1989 [repr. 1902].

Dbang 'dus. *Bod gangs can pa'i gso ba rig pa'i dpal ldan rgyud bzhi sogs kyi brda dang dka' gnad 'ga' zhig bkrol ba sngon byon mkhas pa'i gsung rgyun g.yu thog dgongs rgyan*. Beijing: Mi rigs dpe skrun khang, 1983.

Goldstein, Melvin C., T. N. Shelling, and J. T. Surkhang, eds. *The New Tibetan-English Dictionary of Modern Tibetan.* Berkeley: University of California Press, 2001.

Goldstein, Melvin C., and Ngawangthondup Narkyid. *English-Tibetan Dictionary of Modern Tibetan*. Dharamsala: Library of Tibetan Works and Archives, 1999.

Finckh, Elisabeth. *Der Tibetische Medizin-Baum: Texte und Illustrationen.* Uelzen: Medizin-Literar. Verl.-Ges, 1990.

Gyatso, Janet. *Being Human in a Buddhist World: An Intellectual History of Medicine in Early Modern Tibet.* New York, NY: Columbia University Press, 2015.

Gyatso, Janet. "Looking for Gender in the Medical Paintings of Desi Sangye Gyatso, Regent of the Tibetan Buddhist State." *Asian Medicine: Tradition and Modernity* 6, no. 2 (2010–2011): 217–92.

Gyatso, Janet. "Introduction." In *Body and Spirit: Tibetan Medical Paintings.* Edited by Laila Williamson and Serinity Young. Medical Tangkas painted by Romio Shrestha and Atelier, 3–13. American Museum of Natural History, New York; Seattle and London: University of Washington Press, 2009.

Hendriksen, Marieke M. A. *Elegant Anatomy: The Eighteenth-Century Leiden Anatomical Collections.* Leiden: Brill, 2015.

Jäschke, Heinrich August. *A Tibetan-English Dictionary.* Richmond: Curzon Press, 2003 [repr. 1881].

Kuriyama, Shigehisa. *The Expressiveness of the Body and the Divergence of Greek and Chinese Medicine.* New York: Zone Books, 1999.

Maciocia, Giovanni. 1994. *Die Grundlagen der Chinesischen Medizin: Ein Lehrbuch für Akupunkteure und Arzneimitteltherapeuten.* Geleitwort von Su Xin-Ming. Translated into German by Andreas Höll. Kötzting: Verlag für Traditionelle Chinesische Medizin.

McGrath, William A. "Vessel Examination in the *Medicine of the Moon King.*" In *Buddhism and Medicine: An Anthology of Premodern Sources*, edited by C. Pierce Salguero, 501–13. New York, NY: Columbia University Press, 2017.

Men-Tsee-Khang, trans. *The Basic Tantra and The Explanatory Tantra from the Secret Quintessential Instructions on the Eight Branches of the Ambrosia Essence Tantra.* Dharamsala, Himachal Pradesh: Dawa [Publisher], 2008.

Meyer, Fernand. "Introduction: The Medical Paintings of Tibet." In *Tibetan Medical Paintings: Illustrations to the 'Blue Beryl' Treatise of Sangs rgyas Rgya mtsho (1653–1705)*, edited by Yuri Parfionovitch, Gyurme Dorje, and Fernand Meyer, vol. 1, 2–13. London: Serindia Publications, 1992.

Meyer, Fernand. *Le système médical tibétain: Gso-ba Rig-pa.* Paris: CNRS (Centre Nationale de la Recherche Scientifique), 2002 [repr. 1988].

Michler, Michael, Jost Benedum, and Inge Michler. *Einführung in die Medizinische Fachsprache: Medizinische Terminologie für Mediziner und Zahnmediziner auf grundlage des Lateinischen und Griechischen, unter Mitarbeit von I Michler und M. Michler.* Berlin, Heidelberg, New York: Springer Verlag, 1981.

Mkhas grub. *Gso bya lus kyi tha snyad mdzod.* Chengdu: Si khron mi rigs dpe skrun khang, 2012.

Nutton, Vivian, ed. *The Unknown Galen.* London: Institute of Classical Studies, 2002.

Nyi ma tshe ring and Mig dmar. *Rgya bod shan sbyar tshon khra can gyi ro bkra'i dpe ris mthong ba don gsal*. Lhasa: Bod ljongs mi dmangs dpe skrun khang, 2012.

Pad ma dkar po [Blo gsal dbang po]. *Rgyud bzhi'i 'grel ba gzhan la phan pa'i gter*. Bod kyi gso ba rig pa'i gna' dpe phyogs bsgrigs dpe tshogs, vol. 52. Beijing: Mi rigs dpe skrun khang, 2007.

Pad ma rab brtan and Sangs rgyas 'bum. *Gso ba rig pa'i ro bkra'i dpe ris kun gsal me long*. Xining: Mtsho sngon mi rigs dpe skrun khang, 2011.

Parfionovitch, Yuri, Gyurme Dorje, and Fernand Meyer, eds. *Tibetan Medical Paintings: Illustrations to the 'Blue Beryl' Treatise of Sangs rgyas Rgya mtsho (1653–1705)*. London: Serindia Publications, 1992.

Persaud, T. V. N., Marios Loukas, and R. Shane Tubbs. *A History of Human Anatomy*. Springfield, IL: Charles C. Thomas, 2014.

Platzer, Werner, Kahle Werner, and Helmut Leonhardt. *Taschenatlas der Anatomie für Studium und Praxis*. Stuttgart: Thieme, 1991.

Ploberger, Florian. "Anatomical Terms of the 27 Chapters of the Subsequent Tantra (*Phyi ma'i rgyud*)." *Curare* 39, no. 1 (2016): 33–41.

Ploberger, Florian. *Wurzeltantra und Tantra der Erklärungen der Tibetischen Medizin*. Schiedlberg: Bacopa, 2012.

Rgya bod dbyin gsum shan sbyar deng rabs gso rig ming mdzod [Chinese-Tibetan-English Modern Medicine Dictionary]. Beijing: Mi rigs dpe skrun khang, 2011.

Roerich, Yuri Nikolayovitch. *Tibetsko-russko-angliiskii slovar* [Tibetan-Russian-English Dictionary]. Moskva: Izdat. Nauka, 1983–1993.

Sabernig, Katharina. "On a New Database of Tibetan Pharmacological and Anatomical Terms." In *The Proceedings of the Establishing Meeting for the Specialty Committee of Tibetan Medicine of the World Federation of Chinese Medicine Societies and First Annual Conference*, 675–81. Xining: 'Dzam gling krung mthun bod gso mthun tshogs gsar 'dzugs, 2015.

Sabernig, Katharina. "Anatomical Structures and the Structure of Anatomy in Tibetan Medicine: The Fourth Chapter of the Explanatory Tantra in its Commentaries." *Curare* 39, no. 1 (2016): 22–32.

Sabernig, Katharina. "Description and Depiction of Inner Organs in Classical and Modern Works." In *Lha ldan sman rtsis khang bgu brnyes nas lo ngo brgya 'khor ba'i rgyal spyi'i rig gzhung gros tshogs: 'Dzam gling krung gso mthun tshogs bod kyi gso rig ched las lhan tshogs kyi skabs gnyis pa'i lo tsogs: Dpyad rtsom phyogs bsgrigs*. Lhasa: 2016 [publisher not identified].

Sabernig, Katharina. "Vulnerable Parts: Locating and Defining Vital Areas of the Body in Tibetan Medicine." *Asian Medicine* 12, nos. 1–2 (2017): 86–118.

Sabernig, Katharina. "The Tree of Nosology." In *Cultural Systems of Classification: Sickness, Health and Local Epistemologies*, edited by Ulrike Steinert. Forthcoming.

Shaglakhaev, V. A. [Шаглахаев, В. А.], and N. D. Bolsokhoeva [Болсохоева, Н. Д.]. *Atlas tibetskoj mediciny v kul'turnom prostranstve Central'noj Azii* [Атлас тибетской медицины в культурном пространстве Центральной Азии; The Atlas of Tibetan Medicine in the Cultural Space of Central Asia]. Ulan-Ude: Izdatel'stvo RCMP MZ RB, 2010.

Snellgrove, David L. "Review of Fernand Meyer, *gSo-ba riq*[sic]*-pa, le système médical tibétain.*" *Bulletin of the School of Oriental and African Studies* 46, no. 1 (1983): 172–74.

Strandring, Susan [ed.-in-chief]. *Gray's Anatomy: The Anatomical Basis of Clinical Practice*. London: Elsevier, 2008

Tashi Tsering. *English-Tibetan-Chinese Dictionary*. Beijing: Nationalities Publishing House, 1991 [repr. 1988].

Taube, Manfred. *Beiträge zur Geschichte der medizinischen Literatur Tibets.* Sankt Augustin: VGH Wissenschaftsverlag, 1981.

Thiel, Walter. *Photographischer Atlas der Praktischen Anatomie.* Berlin: Springer, 1996–1999.

Thub bstan phun tshogs. *Gso bya lus kyi rnam bshad.* Beijing: Mi rigs dpe skrun khang, 1999.

Ting 'dzin. *Gso rig rgyud bzhi'i dka' gnad thor bu la dpyad pa'i gtam brgyad cu rtsa bzhi ba dang lus kyi gnas lugs grub cha'i dpe ris*. Chengdu: Si khron mi rigs dpe skrun khang, 2007.

Tshe ring thag gcod drung 'tsho and Tshe ring sgrol ma drung 'tsho. *Bod lugs sman rtsis kyi tshig mdzod bod dbyin shan sbyar* [Tibetan-English Dictionary of Tibetan Medicine and Astrology]. Dharamsala: Drungtso Publications, 2005.

Vesalius, Andreas. *De humani corporis fabrica*. Budapest, 1968 [repr. 1543].

Würthner, Isabella. "A Preliminary Study on the Function, Anatomy and Origin of the Term *bsam-se'u* in Tibetan Medical Literature." *Curare* 39, no. 1 (2016): 42–55.

Wujastyk, Dominik. "Interpreting the Image of the Human Body in Premodern India." *International Journal of Hindu Studies* 13, no. 2 (2009): 189–228.

Yang Ga. *The Sources for the Writing of the Rgyud bzhi, Tibetan Medical Classic.* Cambridge, MA: Doctoral Dissertation at Harvard University, 2010.

Ye shes bzang po [Gtsang sman]. *Bshad pa'i rgyud kyi gnas lugs le'u'i 'grel bshad rag tho dam pa snga ma'i zhal rgyud*. In *Gtsang sman pa'i sman yig phyogs bsgrigs*, 155–181. Bod kyi gso ba rig pa'i gna' dpe phyogs bsgrigs dpe tshogs, vol. 45. Beijing: Mi rigs dpe skrun khang, 2007.

Zur mkhar blo gros rgyal po. *Rgyud bzhi'i 'grel pa mes po'i zhal lung*. Bod kyi gso ba rig pa'i gna' dpe phyogs bsgrigs dpe tshogs, vol. 19. Beijing: Mi rigs dpe skrun khang, 2005.

CHAPTER 5

The Modern Biomedical Conception of Cancer and Its Many Potential Correlates in the Tibetan Medical Tradition

Tawni Tidwell

1 Introduction

As a rigorous comprehensive medical system and the primary health care system throughout Tibet and much of the Himalayan world, Tibetan medicine has a long history of addressing the full scope of human disease, including treating debilitating, life-threatening conditions. Over the last several decades, Tibetan medicine has had substantial clinical and research engagement with biomedical collaborations due to greater numbers of patients globally seeking Tibetan medical treatment for cases difficult to treat by biomedicine. Likewise, researchers have demonstrated increased interest in Tibetan medical interventions successfully treating challenging conditions,[1] such as specific types of cancers.[2]

1 Study examples include: W. J. Brzosko et al., "Influence of Padma 28 and the Thymus Extract on Clinical and Laboratory Parameters of Children with Juvenile Chronic Arthritis," *International Journal of Immunotherapy* 7, no. 3 (1991): 143–47; S. Jankowski et al., "Influence of Padma 28 on the Spontaneous Bactericidal Activity of Blood Serum in Children Suffering from Recurrent Infections of the Respiratory Tract," *Phytotherapy Research* 5, no. 3 (1991): 120–23; R. Korwin-Piotrowska et al., "Experience of Padma 28 in Multiple Sclerosis," *Phytotherapy Research* 6, no. 3 (1992): 133–36; Y. Matzner and S. Sallon, "The Effect of Padma-28, a Traditional Tibetan Herbal Preparation, on Human Neutrophil Function," *Journal of Clinical and Laboratory Immunology* 46, no. 1 (1995): 13–23; Mary Ryan, "Efficacy of the Tibetan Treatment for Arthritis," *Social Science and Medicine* 44, no. 4 (1997): 535–39; W. Split et al., "The Estimation of the Action of Padma-28 in the Treatment of Ischaemic Brain Stroke," *European Journal of Neurology* 5, no. 1 (1998): 9; Tenzin Namdul et al., "Efficacy of Tibetan Medicine as an Adjunct in the Treatment of Type 2 Diabetes," *Diabetes Care* 24, no. 1 (2001): 176–77; Markus Exner et al., "Anti-Inflammatory Mechanisms of the Tibetan Herbal Preparation Padma 28 in the Vessel Wall," *Forschende Komplementärmedizin* 13, no. 1 (2006): 13–17; Fritz Füllemann, "Padma 28 in the Treatment of Chronic Dental Pulpitis: An Observational Case Study in 49 Patients," *Forschende Komplementärmedizin* 13, no. 1 (2006): 28–30; Jörg Melzer et al., "Treating Intermittent Claudication with Tibetan Medicine

 | DOI:10.1163/9789004404441_006

Recent history indicates pressure on Tibetan medical practitioners and scholars to demonstrate science- and biomedical sensibilities in national and international contexts as an effort to establish a specific type of rationality and evidence-based approach for its survival and growth.[3] Tibetan medical physician-scholars have provided one-to-one categorical mapping between Euroamerican and Tibetan medical illness categories, influenced by these recent historical pressures, and aiming to garner recognition and legitimacy amidst the broader contemporary biomedical and scientific context in which Tibetan medicine is practiced and in dialogue. However, explanatory models which oversimplify nosologies and etiologies threaten to entangle Tibetan medical paradigms with those of biomedicine, ignoring historical, theoretical, etiological and practical distinctions of each system and how each tradition approaches disease and health. Although both medical systems engage a single body and human experience, each also assesses salient concerns of the body and experience differentially, and therefore applies a different set of diagnostic and treatment modalities to enact healing and wellness. As such, accurate, nuanced, and specific translations for disease categories, concepts and paradigms are becoming increasingly important. Comparisons of Tibetan

Padma 28: Does It Work?" *Atherosclerosis* 189, no. 1 (2006): 39–46; H. W. Zhang et al., "Fu xi ting lianhe zhong xiyao zhiliao gaoyuan diqu laonian yiyu zheng de linchuang yanjiu [Clinical Study on Effect of Fluoxetine Combined with Chinese Medicine or Tibetan Drugs in Treating Senile Depression in Plateau District]," *Zhongguo Zhongxiyi jiehe zazhi* [Chinese Journal of Integrated Traditional and Western Medicine] 26, no. 3 (2006): 202–204; Tenzin Choedon et al., "Anticancer and Cytotoxic Properties of the Latex of *Calotropis procera* in a Transgenic Mouse Model of Hepatocellular Carcinoma," *World Journal of Gastroenterology* 12, no. 16 (2006): 2517–22; Rigzin Sangmo et al., "Clinical Trial of Tibetan Medicine in the Treatment of Chronic Hepatitis B," *Journal of Men-Tsee-Khang* 4, no. 1 (2007): 32–49; Cynthia Husted and Lobsang Dhondup, "Tibetan Medical Interpretation of Myelin Lipids and Multiple Sclerosis," *Annals of the New York Academy of Sciences* 1172, no. 1 (2009): 278–96; Lobsang Dhondup and Cynthia Husted, "Tibetan Medicine and Regeneration," *Annals of the New York Academy of Sciences* 1172, no. 1 (2009): 115–22; Tenzin Choedon et al., "Pro-Apoptotic and Anticancer Properties of *Thapring*: A Tibetan Herbal Formulation," *Journal of Ethnopharmacology* 137, no. 1 (2011): 320–26; Cecile Vennos et al., "Clinical Studies on the Efficacy and Safety of Padma 28, a Complex Herbal Formulation from Tibetan Medicine: An Overview," *Complementary Medicine Research* 20, no. 2 (2013): 25–30.

2 Susan Bauer-Wu et al., "Tibetan Medicine for Cancer: An Overview and Review of Case Studies," *Integrative Cancer Therapies* 13, no. 6 (2014): 502–12.

3 Vincanne Adams, Renchen Dongzhu, and Phuoc V Le, "Translating Science: The Arura Medical Group at the Frontiers of Medical Research," in *Studies of Medical Pluralism in Tibetan History and Society*, ed. Sienna Craig et al. (Bonn: International Institute for Tibetan and Buddhist Studies, 2010), 111–36; Vincanne Adams, Mona Schrempf, and Sienna R. Craig, eds., *Medicine Between Science and Religion: Explorations on Tibetan Grounds* (New York, NY: Berghahn Books, 2011).

medical categories related to biomedical cancer and other neoplasms, such as *dréné* (*'bras nad*) and *drétren* (*'bras skran*) are instructive in that they provide fertile grounds to compare, relate, and distinguish biomedical and Tibetan medical understandings and approaches. Likewise, the severity of disease, the presence of concrete physical morphologies, and the importance of differential diagnostics for effective treatment each reflects an urgency for understanding such distinctions.

This paper provides an hermeneutical and praxis-based comparative analysis of the biomedical conception of cancer into the most proximate Tibetan medical etiological categories. Recent Tibetan medical clinical practice, scholarly work and public forums refer to cancer as *dréné* or *drétren* as a simple shorthand that appeals to the biomedical approach to disease classification. Elucidating a biomedical category like "cancer" indeed facilitates discussion and collaboration with biomedical modes of discourse but must be careful not to privilege a biomedical presentation and thereby diminish Tibetan medicine's own rigorously sophisticated indigenous nosology as well as occlude critical treatments that outcompete biomedical approaches. This paper analyzes the etiological and diagnostic bases for such a categorical collapse—using the *Four Tantras* (*rgyud bzhi*) as the analytical base with several modern commentarial contributions as clarifying additions, including *The New Dawn Compendium of Medicine* (*gso rig snying bsdus skya rengs gsar pa*) by Samten, one of the first publications to appeal to a biomedical sensibility in its presentation of Tibetan medical categories. I will propose a more complex mapping of biomedical cancer that draws upon the additional categories of *méwel* (*me dbal*), *surya* (*surya*), and other conditions related to "metabolic disruptions of nutritional essence" (*dwangs ma ma zhu ba*), as well as distinguishes noncancer *dréné* or *drétren*.

This work relies on the author's experience training in Tibetan medicine and working with contemporary Tibetan medical physicians in Xining and at the Dharamsala Men-Tsee-Khang, where an increasing number of Tibetan physicians are receiving biomedical and science training. The author integrates her own background in biocultural anthropology to develop epistemologic and ontological links between traditions to facilitate clinical research and treatment collaborations between the two traditions. This paper proposes that physicians of the Tibetan medical tradition try to maintain nosological distinctions between medical systems in referring to both general categories and specific conditions so as to retain the etiological paradigms that implicate diagnosis and treatment. The greater aim is to provide the most promising contributions to treatment of these illnesses, many of which are serious and life-limiting, from the Tibetan medical perspective and acknowledge the epistemological underpinnings that differentiate each tradition. This analysis engages the praxis level—clinical presentations and diagnostics—analyzing practical and therapeutic perspectives, as well as the theoretical level, drawing upon an hermeneutical analysis of the *Four Tantras* and several prominent commentaries relating to diagnostics of *dréné* (*'bras nad*), *tren* (*skran*), *méwel* (*me dbal*), *surya* (*surya*), and related conditions to engage their literal, etiological, and metaphorical significance.

In this paper, I begin with a starting point by describing recent discourse on cancer in Tibetan medicine. Then, I briefly outline the biomedical conception of cancers and neoplasms, followed by distinctions in units of analysis employed in biomedicine compared to those used in the *Four Tantras*. I then present the Tibetan medical understanding of *tren* and *dréné* as described classically in the *Four Tantras* and its commentaries, as a foundation for discussion. I subsequently present the integrative perspective of Menpa Samten, a preeminent Lhasa Men-Tsee-Khang physician of the mid-1980s and 90s. I will proceed to show that, likely due to the historical pressures of scientification constrictions, Samten's work is too narrow to encompass and map the broader scope of all the Euroamerican nosology of biomedical cancers and neoplasms into the Tibetan medical nosology.[4] I argue that the classical etiological presentations in the *Four Tantras* are sufficient to understand how biomedical cancers map into Tibetan nosology, with the clarifying contribution of Desi Sanggyé Gyatso's *Oral Instructions Supplement* (*man ngag lhan thabs*). I proceed to present the six defining characteristics of biomedical cancer followed by a map of the Tibetan medical conditions and links with an overarching etiological framework, highlighting three illuminating case studies from the biomedical context—skin cancer, leukemia and lymphoma—into the appropriate Tibetan medical context relating to subtypes within *méwel, surya*, and metabolic disruptions with abnormal blood proliferation.

---

4 Of important note, though *The New Dawn* carries his name as sole author, Samten's work is the product of the integrated insights and perspectives of many Tibetan senior physicians in Lhasa at the time (personal communication, Gönpo Kyab [*mgon po skyabs*], Gansu Provincial Tibetan Medical Research Institute [*kan su'u zhing chen bod kyi gso rig zhib 'jug gling*], June 2018).

2 An Historical Starting Point

In the early 1990s, Tibetan physicians formally addressed similar comparisons, such as those at the March 1996 conference at Dharamsala Men-Tsee-Khang,[5] and through conferences, publications and clinic reorganizations by those in Tibet.[6] Early discussions of such comparisons did not stem from rigorous analysis of the etiology of each disease and the attending medical epistemologies from which they arose.[7] Tibetan medical historian Olaf Czaja notes that the biomedical understanding of cancer among Tibetan physicians at the time was limited and thus neither theoretical nor clinical comparisons of diagnostics and treatment could be evaluated. The focal point of comparison was, simply, abnormal growth in the body without characterizing the origins, nature, context, or type of growth; and at times, primarily focusing on the life-threatening aspects of such growths.[8] As Czaja describes, efforts were focused on a one-to-one correlation between a biomedical disease category on one side and a Tibetan medical disease category on the other side, without recognizing their differential attendant epistemologies and etiologies that define the root of each tradition's fluorescence of conditions, and motivate only rare or even non-existent one-to-one correlations.[9] Today, we see a greater number of Tibetan physicians training in biomedicine and working alongside biomedical physicians such as at the Qinghai Provincial Tibetan Medical Hospital in Xining as well as various locales throughout Tibet and around the world. They are developing greater recognition of the etiological distinctions between cancer and *dréné*.

5 Olaf Czaja, "The *Four Tantras* and the Global Market: Changing Epistemologies of Drä (*'bras*) versus Cancer," in *Medicine Between Science and Religion: Explorations on Tibetan Grounds*, ed. Vincanne Adams et al. (New York, Oxford: Berghahn, 2011), 265–95.

6 Khro ru tshe rnam, *Gso rig rgyud bzhi'i 'grel chen drang srong zhal lung* [The Great Commentary on the *Four Tantras*: Oral Instructions of the Sages] (Chengdu: Si khron mi rigs dpe sgrun khang, 2000); Bsam gtan, *Gso rig snying bsdus skya rengs gsar pa* [The New Dawn Compendium of Medicine] (Lhasa: Bod ljongs mi dmangs dpe skrun khang, 2013); Lha mo skyabs, *Bod lugs 'bras nad gso rig* [Tibetan Medical Oncology] (Beijing: Mi rigs dpe skrun khang, 2009); 'Jam dbyangs bkra shis, *Bod kyi gso ba rig pa'i 'bras nad kyi nad thog rmang gzhi'i rig gzhung dpyad zhib* [Clinical, Basic Research, and Literature Analysis of Cancer (*Dréné*) in Tibetan Medicine] (Lhasa: Doctoral Dissertation at the Tibet University of Tibetan Medicine, 2015). Döntsé personal communications 2013, 2015.

7 As Czaja notes, "[I]n the case of cancer, Tibetan doctors hotly debated and thus were less self-assured about the identification of this 'modern' disease with their own traditional categories and aetiologies" (Czaja, "The *Four Tantras* and the Global Market," 272).

8 See, for instance, Lha mo skyabs, *Bod lugs 'bras nad gso rig*.

9 Czaja, "The *Four Tantras* and the Global Market," 273, 280.

In the general discourse in the Tibetan medical field, there is widespread acceptance that cancer and *dréné* are not identical forms of disease,[10] but the practical use of *drétren* and *dréné* as a short form for cancer is common.[11] After the attempt to clarify critical points from the 1996 Dharamsala Men-Tsee-Khang conference, many Tibetan medical scholars outside of Tibet have used the English transliteration *kensar* (*kan sar*) to differentiate biomedical conceptions of cancer from *drétren* and *dréné*.[12] Yet there still exists continued conflation of the terms in important works later on. For instance, despite expressing concern about using the term *dréné* synonymously for cancer in the conference, Menpa Dorje Rabten Neshar still uses the term *dréné* to refer to the cases in his cancer studies where patients were recruited after having a definitive biomedical diagnosis of cancer, and gives little description of the Tibetan medical diagnostics.[13] Understandably such records were developed to demonstrate effective treatment of biomedical cancer to a scientific and non-specialist audience and were not focused on demonstrating the Tibetan medical diagnostic categories or methods; however, such a convention set precedent for this slippage of a one-to-one correlation of cancer and *dréné*. Likewise, among Tibetan doctors in Tibet, there is the frequent synonymous use of *dréné* and the Chinese term for biomedical cancer (*aizheng* 癌症), as well as the use of *drétren* to describe malignant forms of tumors. This is demonstrated by the newly developed "Cancer-Tumor Department" (*'bras skran tshan khag*), established in 2014 at Qinghai Provincial Tibetan Medical Hospital in Xining, and the conferences organized along with its inception to generate greater scholarship, understanding, and standardized treatment approaches around these categories and related diagnostics and treatments.[14]

---

10 Dorjee Rabten Neshar, "Clinical Case Study of Cancer (*Dres-Ned*) Patients Treated at Men-Tsee-Khang's Bangalore Branch Clinic for the Period of 27 Months from November 2002 to February 2005," *sMan-rTsis Journal: Journal of Tibetan Medicine and Astrological Sciences* 4, no. 1 (2007): 50–68; Döntsé, personal communication, 2014; Namlhakhar, personal communication, 2014.

11 See, for instance, 'Jam dbyangs bkra shis, *Bod kyi gso ba rig pa'i 'bras nad kyi nad thog rmang gzhi'i rig gzhung dpyad zhib*; and Lde'u rong jo skyabs tshe ring, *Bod kyi gso rig las 'bras nad skor gyi dpyod gling*.

12 Even within Tibet, the English term has been inserted without attempt to translate. See, for instance, Dho lha, *Mchin pa'i Cancer la bod lugs gso rig gis brtag bcos zhib 'jug*.

13 Rabten Neshar, "Clinical Case Study of Cancer (*Dres-Ned*) Patients."

14 Through the course of developing my Tibetan medical graduating thesis (written and presented in Tibetan) and presenting its contents at Sorig Loling in June 2015 and the August 2017 conference in Lhasa commemorating the 100th Anniversary of the founding of Lhasa Men-Tsee-Khang, it generated much discussion among Tibetan physicians. Few disagreed with the content, but many remarked on its "new" approach of mapping one condition onto many in the Tibetan medical nosology and so forth. Perhaps the discussion

However, this synonymity is not apparent from, for example, recitations and studies of the *Four Tantras* and its various commentaries. Likewise, the distinctions between more aggressive and mild forms seem to form a gradient across both *dréné* and *tren* categories, as well as expand across other candidates of disease categories in the *Four Tantras*. These illness types seem to pose possible links to biomedical categories of cancer but are not identical due to many non-cancer diseases subsumed within these illness categories and etiologies, and many cancer subtypes mapping more effectively into other Tibetan medical illness categories with distinct etiologies.

In the next section, I briefly outline contemporary biomedical conceptions of tumors and cancers.

3 Biomedical Tumors and Cancer as Neoplasms

In biomedicine, the term "neoplasm" (literally, "new growth") refers to a group of cells that undergo abnormal, unregulated growth and form a mass or distribute diffusely in the body. When this abnormal growth of cells accumulates as a mass, it is referred to as a tumor.[15] All tumors are neoplasms.[16] Neoplasms can be either benign or malignant. Benign tumors remain confined to their original location enclosed in a fibrous capsule that neither invades surrounding tissues nor spreads to other body sites. A skin wart would even be considered a benign neoplasm. Malignant neoplasms have the capacity to both invade adjacent cells and tissues as well as spread to other tissues and organs. When a neoplasm is malignant, it is referred to as cancer. All cancers are malignant neoplasms. Both malignant and benign neoplasms are classified according to the type of cell and tissue from which they arise. Malignant tumors are

illuminated an inherent assumption among Tibetan physicians that in discussions with biomedical physicians and scientists they needed to demonstrate one-to-one categorical semblance with biomedical illness categories. In late fall 2014, the Cancer-Tumor Department invited specialists from all over Kham and Amdo to discuss *dréné* and *tren*, and how to understand cancer from the Tibetan medical perspective, including the various related conditions, diagnostics, and treatments. This was an invite-only private conference of about a dozen attendees. A close mentor and attendee of the conference, Gen Döntsé, recently appointed head doctor of the outpatient division of the Cancer-Tumor Department, said there was very little consensus among physicians or concrete directives of diagnostics or treatment developed (Döntsé, personal communication, 2014).

15 Geoffrey M. Cooper, *Elements of Human Cancer* (Boston, MA: Jones and Bartlett Publishers, 1992), 16.

16 Solid neoplasms are called tumors, masses, neoplastic cells, or neoplasia.

divided into four types: carcinomas, sarcomas, leukemias and lymphomas, and neuroectodermal tumors.

Carcinomas comprise 90 percent of all human cancers.[17] They arise from superficial cell layers called epithelial cells of the gastrointestinal tract, including the mouth, esophagus, and small and large intestines. They also include those of the skin, mammary glands, pancreas, lungs, liver, ovaries, gallbladder and urinary bladder.[18] There are two major biological functions of the epithelia that distinguish the two major categories of carcinomas that form from them: epithelial cells that form protective cell layers are called squamous cell carcinomas, and epithelial cells that secrete substances into the ducts or cavities they line are called adenocarcinomas.[19]

Malignant tumors that arise from nonepithelial tissues throughout the body derive from connective tissues, such as mesenchymal cells, and are called sarcomas. They comprise only about one percent of tumors. Mesenchymal cells differentiate into various functions such as those that support tendons and skin;[20] store fat;[21] form bone;[22] and comprise muscles.[23]

The second type of nonepithelial cancers stem from various blood-forming tissues and are thus called hematopoietic, literally meaning "to make blood."[24] These include cells of the immune system.[25] Leukemia (literally, "white blood") refers to disorders of white blood cells known as leukocytes, in which the hematopoietic cell lineages have become malignant. Unlike normal red blood cells, leukocytes are unpigmented and thus white in color. They do not coalesce into solid tumors, and instead move freely through circulation. This will be an important point in the comparison with both *dréné* and *tren* in the *Four Tantras* due to the latter's solid morphological characteristics as disease types. Lymphomas derive from two types of lymphocytes called B and T lymphocytes, collectively called lymphoid lineages, which are responsible for primary adaptive immune response in the body, recognizing indicators of potentially harm-

---

17 Cooper, *Elements of Human Cancer*, 17.

18 Robert A. Weinberg, *The Biology of Cancer* (New York, NY: Garland Science, 2006), 29.

19 Weinberg, *The Biology of Cancer*, 30.

20 Fibroblasts secrete collagen to support tendons and skin.

21 Adipocytes store fat in their cytoplast.

22 Osteoblasts assemble calcium phosphate in their collagen matrices.

23 Myocytes form muscles.

24 From "blood" (Grk. αἷμα) and "to make" (Grk. ποιεῖν). See Henry George Liddell and Robert Scott, *Liddell and Scott's Greek-English Lexicon* (London: Simon Wallenberg Press, 2007).

25 Like those destined to become erythrocytes (red blood cells), antibody-secreting (plasma) cells, and T and B lymphocytes (Weinberg, *The Biology of Cancer*, 32). See for instance Tristram G. Parslow et al., *Medical Immunology* (New York, NY: McGraw-Hill/Appleton and Lange, 2001).

ful foreign substances in the body called antigens. Disruptions to lymphocyte development and growth produce cells which aggregate to form solid tumor masses most often found in the lymph nodes, but also can be found dispersed as single-cell populations similar to leukemia.

The third and last major type of nonepithelial tumors derives from the central and peripheral nervous system and are called neuroectodermal tumors named after the cells from which they arise.[26] They comprise 1.3 percent of all diagnosed cancers but are responsible for double the number of deaths.[27]

Some unique types of cancers do not fit into the four categories (one epithelial, and three nonepithelial) described above, like those arising from specialized skin and eye retinal cells (melanomas), as well as specific cells in the lungs similar to those found in the adrenal glands of the kidneys.[28] These cells and related malignancies are unique in that they can switch their cell type and lineage demonstrating the cell plasticity that allows some carcinoma cells to invade adjacent normal tissues.[29] This will be relevant in the comparison with *dréné, méwel,* and *surya* etiology and the related Tibetan medical illnesses below.

4 Distinction in Units of Analysis: Cells and Tissues versus Bodily Constituents

Before discussing how the Tibetan medical perspective understands uncontrolled abnormal growths in the body that invade adjacent normal body regions and cause associated dysfunction, it is important to note a distinction on the primary unit of analysis in each tradition. When analyzing disease formation in Euroamerican medicine, the cell is a primary unit of analysis, along with a group of morphologically similar cells that interact to perform specific

26 For example, neuroectodermal tumors include gliomas, glioblastomas, neuroblastomas, schwannomas, and medulloblastomas.

27 Cooper, *Elements of Human Cancer*, 17.

28 These include melanomas and small-cell lung carcinomas (SCLCs). Melanomas derive from melanocytes, pigmented cells in the skin and retina. SCLCs have cells with attributes of neurosecretory cells like those in the neural crest of the adrenal glands above the kidneys.

29 These tumors likely originate in epithelial cells then switch their tissue lineage to those of a neuroectodermal lineage. This transition is called an epithelial-mesenchymal transition (EMT) and is the demonstrative characteristic of cell plasticity which enables some carcinoma cells to invade adjacent normal tissues (J. P. Thiery and J. P. Sleeman, "Complex Networks Orchestrate Epithelial-mesenchymal Transitions," *Nature Reviews Molecular Cell Biology* 7 [2006]: 131–42).

functions of the body.[30] Such a group of cells is called a tissue.[31] Biomedicine looks at how specific cells differentiate from the initial cells of life, further differentiate into specialized cells in utero, and, likewise, continually engage in such recapitulated morphological and functional processes throughout the life course. In Tibetan medicine, a primary unit of analysis in describing disease formation is the seven bodily constituents—that is, nutritional essence, blood, muscle, fat, bone, bone marrow, and regenerative fluid; the excrements, such as urine, feces, perspiration, as well as many others; and the vital, vessel, and sensory organs. In the *Four Tantras* and its commentaries, it is important to note that bodily constituents and the other units of analysis are defined by their function, and less by morphology. Likewise, for example, the bodily constituents are described according to how they develop in utero and how they differentiate from each other to form their specialized functions, similar to that of cells and tissues from the biomedical perspective. Thus, when comparing abnormal growth, in biomedicine, we refer to cells and tissues, and in Tibetan medicine we refer to bodily constituents, the vital, vessel, and sensory organs they comprise, and the effects on the excrements they exude.[32]

Furthermore, Euroamerican medicine delineates specific systems of body functions such as the nervous, circulatory, muscular, and reproductive systems with associated organs, pathways, fluids, metabolites, and so forth. Such systems are functional when in homeostasis or moving to new norms in heterostasis, yet can experience dysfunction and result in disease. Likewise, in Tibetan medicine, there are three main systems of body referred to as *nyépa* (*nyes pa*).[33]

30 As with histopathology, which analyzes microscopic changes in cells and tissues that indicate disease and abnormalities.

31 Sylvia Mader and Michael Windelspecht, *Human Biology* (New York, NY: McGraw-Hill Education, 2015), 44.

32 New initiatives in Tibetan medicine and across Buddhism have developed the terminology for cell, tissue and a vast number of scientific terms in biology, chemistry, physics, neuroscience, and the philosophy of science, in order to facilitate dialogue, generate greater understanding of science in the Tibetan fields of knowledge and across Tibetan society, and assist the traditions in mutual contributions of epistemologies, ontologies, and knowledge of body, mind, and the natural world (see, for instance, Emory-Tibet Science Initiative and its associated publications and projects). Thus, we are seeing increasing integrative perspectives of Tibetan medical understandings applied to contemporary delineations of body systems and units (e.g., cholesterol), and biomedical understandings contributing to Tibetan medical paradigms as well.

33 The three *nyépa* have experienced many approaches to their translation due to their multivalent meanings and applied use (Yonten Gyatso, "*Nyes pa*: A Brief Review of its English Translation," *The Tibet Journal* 4 (2005–2006): 109–18; Barbara Gerke, "Correlating Biomedical and Tibetan Medical Terms in *Amchi* Medical Practice," in *Medicine Between Science and Religion*, ed. V. Adams et al. [New York, NY: Berghahn Books, 2010], 127–52).

These are default functional energetic systems of pathways or activities that, in their default mode, link body constituent, organ, fluid, and energetic signaling dynamics to provide specific systemic functions in the body.

These three systems—known in Tibetan as *rlung* (*rlung*),[34] *tripa* (*mkhris pa*) and *béken* (*bad kan*)—have a vast number of functions, but, in short, relate to the functional dynamics and activities of motility, heat, and solidity/cohesion, respectively, in the body.[35] To retain the complexity of the original Tibetan terms, I will not translate them beyond these adjectival approximations, but will expand briefly on their functions for greater understanding of each system. The *rlung* system manages all motility in the body, similar to the neuroendocrine system in biomedicine.

Rlung controls respiration, swallowing, and articulation; physical, verbal and mental movement; exertion; sensory organ perceptual acuity; metabolic separation of nutrient and waste products and digestive waste elimination as well as similar downward-voiding activities of the uterus, urinary system, colorectal region, and so forth. *Rlung* also encompasses many other functions related to motility and signal-response in the body. The bodily constituents, organs, and sensory organs related to *rlung* pathways include bone, heart, colon, hearing and tactile sensory organs, colon, and the pathways supporting life (*srog*).

Tripa is related to the heat-producing functions in the body. It is responsible for thermoregulation, metabolic power and heat in digestion, cardiovascular functions, heart and blood constituents and activities, hunger and thirst, liver and gallbladder function, complexion and skin maintenance, and sharpness

---

See Gerke, "Correlating Biomedical and Tibetan Medical Terms," for an expanded discussion on the challenges of translating Tibetan medical terms into English; and see Czaja ("The Administration of Tibetan Precious Pills," *Asian Medicine* 10, nos. 1–2 [2015]: 36–89) for examples of some of the tensions. To retain a more literate translation of the term, since the Tibetan term refers to their activity as the primary instigators of disease and imbalance in the body, like a weakness that befalls the Achilles heel and results in systemic debilitation, Yonten Gyatso aptly translates them as "defaults" ("*Nyes pa*," 109–18). This article follows Gyatso's lead in partially using the translation terminology "default" for this term (*nyes pa*). Although the functional form is formally termed the three *duwa* (*'du ba*), the functional and pathological forms of *duwa* and *nyépa* are often both referred to as *nyépa* throughout the *Four Tantras* with context determining the version to which the term is referring. For related discussion, see Henk Blezer, "A New Sense of (Dark) Humor in Tibet: Brown Phlegm and Black Bile," this volume.

34 Although the standard phonetic conversion (Germano and Tournadre 2010) for rlung is "lung" (pronounced *lōōng*, meaning "winds;"), I retain the Wylie spelling "rlung" to distinguish the term and prevent confusion with the organ lung.

35 These are known as the elemental dynamics of wind, fire, and water and earth (*rlung/me/sa dang chu*), respectively. Here, I choose to use the adjective forms in translating the terms to facilitate a better recognition of how they are understood by the tradition and employed in a medical context.

of cognitive and intellectual processing. Its pathways relate to the blood, liver, gallbladder, small intestine, visual sensory organs, and perspiration.

Béken is related to solidity and cohesion in the body, namely, providing support for the body and mind; promoting physical and mental patience, tolerance, and imperturbability; facilitating sleep; producing connectivity in the joints; and smoothing and oiling functions of all organs, constituents, and fluids in the body. Its pathways relate to the nutritional essence, muscle, fat, bone marrow, regenerative fluid, feces, urine, olfactory and gustatory sensory organs, lungs, spleen, stomach, kidneys, and urinary bladder, as well as many of the other fluids and oils in the body.

In addition to their vast and diverse functions, these three systems can also incur innumerable imbalances and dysfunctions. I will refer to these three materio-energetic systems coordinating body constituent and organ functions as the "three default systems," or "defaults," for short. Imbalances and dysfunctions, such as disturbances, can refer to metabolic disruptions such as in *tripa* functions and pathways; disturbances in lymph and serum metabolites as with *béken*; neuroendocrine signaling dysfunction as in *rlung* pathways; and the associated improper bodily constituent development, activities, and pathways as well.

In the next section, I describe the understanding of *tren* and *dréné* as described classically in the *Four Tantras*, as well as several elaborations and additions in its commentaries.

5 *Tren* as Abnormal Growths and Accretions

Tren are defined as any abnormal mass formed in the body.[36] The definition for neoplasms in biomedicine demonstrates large similarity to many *tren* described in the *Four Tantras*. For example, of the various types of *tren* described in the *Four Tantras*, many are abnormal growths that arise from the bodily constituents. These kind of *tren* include: esophagogastric *tren* (*lhen skran*), masses in the uterus (*mngal skran*), *tren* developed in *rlung*-associated regions (*rlung skran*), channel *tren* in blood and lymph vessels and neural pathways (*rtsa skran*), *tren* related to blood formation processes and organs (*khrag skran*), and

36 Byams pa 'phrin las, ed., *Bod lugs gso rig tshig mdzod chen mo* [*Great Tibetan Medical Dictionary*] (Lhasa: Mi rigs dpe skrun khang, 2006), 44: "The name of a disorder in which hard, dense accreted masses form either by metabolic disruptions from waste products or nutritional essence of ingested materials" (*kha zas kyi snyigs ma ma zhu ba'am dwangs ma ma zhu ba las gyur pa'i lus kyi phyi nang gang rung du 'byung ba'i dbyibs gong bur 'dril la ngo bo sra mkhregs can gyi nad kyi ming ngo/*).

tren due to microorganisms (*srin skran*),[37] which can form in the liver, gallbladder, spleen, gut, colon, small intestine, and so forth, with differing prevalence and characteristics in each region. However, *tren* also include any abnormal mass formed from that which the body ingests that slowly accretes and hardens. Examples of these *tren* include: gallstones (*mkhris skran*), literally stone accumulations of the gallbladder (*mkhris pa'i rdo skran*); kidney stones (*mkhal ma'i rde'u skran*); and bezoars (*lhen skran, pho skran*) or gut boluses of indigestible material such as those that form from cellulose and other indigestible plant material, fruit pits, dense and sticking gum-like substances, or hair (*spu skran*). Clearly, those *tren* that arise primarily from abnormal growths and accumulations of the body constituents relate to the biomedical conception of neoplasm. Whereas those *tren* which form from that which the body ingests, relate to the biomedical conception of lithiasis—calculi, concretions, and calcifications.[38]

In the *Four Tantras*, abscesses also are part of the *tren* category,[39] as fluid-filled *tren*, also known as pus *tren* (*rnag skran*), fluid *tren* (*chu skran*), or *chuser*-filled *tren*.[40] *Chuser* (*chu ser*), which literally translates as "yellow fluid," is

---

37 Regarding *srin* (*srin*), see Byams pa 'phrin las, *Bod lugs gso rig tshig mdzod chen mo*, 955: "The 84,000 *sinbu* that reside as coemergent in the body and, in a balanced state, provide strength and radiance to the body and one's longevity as well as protect one's vitality and sensory organs. They accompany one's projection of dexterity. In imbalance, they produce diseases of various types" (*lus la lhan skyes su gnas pa'i srin bu brgyad khri bzhi stong la bya ste/ de dag rnam par ma gyur pa'i tshe lus kyi stobs mdangs bskyed cing/ tshe srog dbang po srung ba dang/ yang rtsal dod pa sogs kyi grogs byed pa dang/ rnam par gyur na nad rigs rnam pa sna tshogs skyed par byed pa'i las can no/*). On *Sinbü* (*srin bu, srin 'bu*), see Byams pa 'phrin las, *Bod lugs gso rig tshig mdzod chen mo*, 956: "A term for the coemergently existent and minutely small internal and external organisms that cause *srin* disease when disturbed. In terms of classification by type, there are those that collect in heaps, *rlung*-related that are elongated, *tripa*-related that are body hair- and needle point-like. Classified by location, there are those of lice and its eggs, eyes, teeth, skin, rectum, and genitalia, which are traditionally classified" (*lus la lhan skyes su mchis shing 'khrugs na srin nad du gyur ba'i phyi nang gi srin bu'am 'bu srin phra mo rnams kyi ming ste/ 'di la'ang rigs kyi sgo nas dbye na bad srin dru bu sdog pa 'dra ba dang/ rlung srin thur ma 'dra ba/ mkhris srin sha spu'am khab rtse 'dra ba/ gnas kyi sgo nas dbye na shig sro dang/ mig srin/ so srin/ pags srin/ gzhang srin/ mtshan ma'i srin bcas dbye srol mchis so/*).

38 Calculi are abnormal concretions, usually composed of mineral salts, which occur throughout the body most often in hollow organs and their passages. They are also called stones and suffixed by *-lith* (e.g., a broncholith is a pulmonary calculus; see J. M. Longmore, *Oxford Handbook of Clinical Medicine* [Oxford: Oxford University Press, 2010]).

39 G.yu thog yon tan mgon po, *Bdud rtsi snying po yan lag brgyad pa gsang ba man ngag gi rgyud* [The Secret Quintessential Instructions on the Eight Branches of the Ambrosia Essence Tantra] (New Delhi: Men-Tsee-Khang, 2008), 174–77.

40 At other times fluid-like pockets or eruptions known as *shuwa* (*shu ba*), a term also used to refer to blisters, scabs, abscesses, and some sores.

somewhat similar to the term "serous fluid" in biomedicine, except that *chuser* it encompasses a greater scope of the fluid types, processes, and metabolisms across bodily constituents and compartments throughout the body. *Chuser* is a composite term for the fluid that comprises intra- and extracellular fluid, interstitial fluid, pre-lymph fluid, blood serum, cerebrospinal fluid, and so forth. The metabolisms of these fluids across various body cavities, vessels, and spaces are seen to be one process that has its own metabolism, and which can undergo disturbances in how the fluids perfuse tissues, integrate nutrients, expel waste products, and so forth—all under the heading of *chuser* functions, pathways, and activities. In biomedicine, a fluid-filled neoplasm is often called a cyst, but an abscess is designated as a cavity caused by tissue damage that often fills with fluid or pus. Abscesses are technically not neoplasms unless the cells subsequently undergo abnormal growth.

Like the biomedical definition that abscesses are fluid-filled cavities that develop from tissue damage, fluid *tren* most often form from damage to the bodily constituents. *Chuser tren* often form secondary to primary *tren* due to damage incurred by *tren*-formation processes, and related *chuser* metabolism. The contrasting conceptions of neoplasms as abnormal cell growth in biomedicine compared to that of *tren* as abnormal mass formation in bodily constituents, excrements, and ingested material in the *Four Tantras* highlights the distinction between the two categories of neoplasm and *tren*.[41]

6 *Dréné* Etiology: a Subtype of Coemergent "Wounds"

In the *Four Tantras, dréné* is classified as a type of wound (*rma*), defined as damage to the skin or flesh level.[42] Such wounds can occur internally or externally, in or on specific organs or bodily constituents.[43] The *Four Tantras* broadly

41 Likewise, due to the pervasiveness of influences contributing to the development of *tren* in the body, and its relationship to long, slow temporal processes, the *Four Tantras* describe *tren* as one of the great chronic disorders (*gcong chen skran*). See G.yu thog yon tan mgon po, *Bdud rtsi snying po yan lag brgyad pa gsang ba man ngag gi rgyud*, 174. In biomedical diagnostics, the coarse appearance of some abscesses is often difficult to distinguish from neoplasms showing an ontological nuance in the categorical delineations (S. A. Klotz and R. L. Penn, "Clinical Differentiation of Abscess from Neoplasm in Newly Diagnosed Space-Occupying Lesions of the Liver," *Southern Medical Journal* 80, no. 12 [1987]: 1537–41).

42 G.yu thog yon tan mgon po, *Bdud rtsi snying po yan lag brgyad pa gsang ba man ngag gi rgyud*, 462: *'dzag pa dri nga tshor ba sdug bsngal bcas/ lus las 'phral du nyams shing rma ba la/ pags pa sha gdan ral phyir rma zhes bya/.*

43 G.yu thog yon tan mgon po, *Bdud rtsi snying po yan lag brgyad pa gsang ba man ngag gi rgyud*, 400.

subdivides "Wounds" into two major categories: "Coemergent Wounds" (*lhan skyes rma*) and "Incidental Wounds" (*glo bur rma*).[44] *Dréné* is a type of disease in the "Coemergent Wound" (*lhan skyes rma*) category.[45]

"Coemergent Wounds" are defined as "wounds that arise, not from an external source such as that of a knife, weapon, impaling object, or projectile, but spontaneously co-arise from an internal disturbance in the three default systems."[46] In the *Four Tantras*, "Coemergent Wounds" comprise eight diseases: *dréne*, hemorrhoids, burn-like irritations (*méwel*), sunburst-shaped irritations/ulcers (*surya*), lymph disorders, testicular swelling, leg-swelling disorders (*kangbam*) like varicose veins, perineal fistulas, and other internal ulcers, irritations, and tears. *Méwel, surya*, and lymph disorders will be further explained shortly as they become important when we look at all the candidate Tibetan medical conditions onto which biomedical neoplasms and, specifically, cancers map. "Incidental Wounds" (that is, external trauma-related wounds) include all acute types and locations of injuries—flays and lacerations (*bshus*), incisions (*bshags*), cuts (*bcad*), avulsions and cleavages (*rnam par bcad*), partial avulsions and dismemberments (*rab tu 'phyang ba*), fall injuries (*lhung*), breaks and fractures (*grums*), punctures and penetrations (*phug pa*)—and three location classes of the injury—head and neck, chest and abdomen, and limbs.[47]

Etiologically in the *Four Tantras*, *dréné* initially arises from damage to a bodily constituent in the form of a wound due to "trauma, disturbance, or metabolic un-ripening" of nutrient essences propagated to each of the bodily constituents.[48] Consequently, poor blood quality develops, and the winding coalescing processes of eddies in the flow of aggravated *rlung*[49] forms a growth in the region qualifying it as a *dré*, literally meaning "fruiting mass." As with other illnesses in the *Four Tantras*, the causes of a disease provide the "initial conditions" from which a disease gains the potential to arise. However, it is the compounding conditions that provide the driving influences for the

---

44 G.yu thog yon tan mgon po, *Bdud rtsi snying po yan lag brgyad pa gsang ba man ngag gi rgyud*, 462.

45 G.yu thog yon tan mgon po, *Bdud rtsi snying po yan lag brgyad pa gsang ba man ngag gi rgyud*, 400–13.

46 Byams pa 'phrin las, *Bod lugs gso rig tshig mdzod chen mo*, 1007: *phyi'i mda' rdo dang gri mtshon sogs phog pa las byung ba ma yin par nang gi 'du ba 'khrugs pa'i nad dang lhan cig tu skyes pa'i rang bzhin du byung ba'i rma'i ming /.*

47 G.yu thog yon tan mgon po, *Bdud rtsi snying po yan lag brgyad pa gsang ba man ngag gi rgyud*, 462.

48 G.yu thog yon tan mgon po, *Bdud rtsi snying po yan lag brgyad pa gsang ba man ngag gi rgyud*, 400: *rgyu ni 'grams 'khrugs kha zas ma smin pa/.*

49 G.yu thog yon tan mgon po, *Bdud rtsi snying po yan lag brgyad pa gsang ba man ngag gi rgyud*, 400: *ngan khrag rgyas te rlung gis bsgril nas 'byung/.*

manifestation of actual disease. The four compounding conditions (*rkyen bzhi*) the *Four Tantras* identifies that precipitate imbalance and disease comprise: seasonality and place, non-human external factors,[50] diet, and lifestyle (*dus gdon zas spyod*). I will provide a brief introduction to the "causes" (*rgyu*) of *dréné* below, which provide the foundation for disease development. However, it is important to keep in mind these compounding conditions, or "conditions" in short, that apply to each cause, provide the inciting influences that drive disease initiation and progression.

6.1 *"Trauma" as a Cause*

"Trauma" (*'grams pa*) refers to pervasion, impact, injury, or harm. It indicates trauma or injury to a bodily constituent or organ.[51] Since *dréné* is considered a type of wound in the *Four Tantras*, this cause is further understood by the overarching understanding of wounds as trauma to the skin (*pags pa*) and muscle layers (*sha*) in the *Four Tantras*. For example, Jampa Trinlé's (1928–2011) edited work, the *Great Tibetan Medical Dictionary* (*bod lugs gso rig tshig mdzod chen mo*), describes this impact on the skin constituent (*pags la gram pa*) as "the spreading or dispersion across the skin,"[52] which has a clinical presentation on the superficial and sub-dermal regions as irritations and local damage such as rash, pustules, pox, wounds, bruising, and so forth.

6.2 *"Disturbance" as a Cause*

"Disturbance" (*'khrugs pa*) refers to a disturbance in the function, pathways, and related constituents of the three default systems. The *Four Tantras* describes a disturbance as an influence that stems from the four conditions in which one of these conditions adversely affects one or more of the respective defaults causing proliferation, deficiency, or disturbance in the flow and function of the defaults.[53] For example, the natural light (*yang ba*) and rough (*rtsub*

50 This condition known as *dön* (*gdon*) has wide and diverse connotations: on one side they are described as evil spirits and on the other side they are harmful environmental influences that cause a range of mental, skin, and serous fluid (*chu ser*) disorders. Many of the other disorders in the Tibetan medical nosology can be caused or influenced by *dön* as well, though presenting with the same symptomology as other causes.

51 Byams pa 'phrin las, *Bod lugs gso rig tshig mdzod chen mo*, 135.

52 Byams pa 'phrin las, *Bod lugs gso rig tshig mdzod chen mo*, 446: *pags la gram pa / pags pa'i steng du khyab pa'am 'thor ba'i don/.*

53 G.yu thog yon tan mgon po, *Bdud rtsi snying po yan lag brgyad pa gsang ba man ngag gi rgyud las rtsa ba'i rgyud bshad pa'i rgyud phyi ma'i rgyud kha skong dang bcas pa* [Root Tantra, Explanatory Tantra, and Subsequent Tantra from the Secret Quintessential Instructions on the Eight Branches of the Ambrosia Essence Tantra] (New Delhi: Men-Tsee-Khang, 1999), 73–77.

pa) qualities of early summer (*so ga*) that relate to similar qualities in the environment, one's body, and dietary and lifestyle behaviors cause *rlung* to accumulate in the body.[54] Because there is an accompanying warmth of the season, *rlung* does not proliferate. However, due to the moist cold qualities produced by the summer monsoon season, *rlung* proliferates in the midsummer and an increase in *rlung* disorders is common. According to the *Four Tantras*, the fall season has more oily and warm qualities which cause such *rlung* imbalances to naturally subside.[55] However, an excessively dry, rough and cool fall will cause the *rlung* to continue to proliferate and thus, fully manifested *rlung* conditions will result.

In the same way, dietary and lifestyle conditions can cause underlying imbalances to manifest. When a default system moves from its own default region to that of another system's default region, it is referred to as a "disturbance," and symptoms will manifest in that region characteristic of both the region and the penetrating default system.

6.3 *"Unriped Constituents" as Cause*

Improper metabolic ripening of the bodily constituents refers to the inability of the digestive system to properly identify nutrient (*dwangs ma*) from waste (*snyigs ma*). According to the *Four Tantras*, fire-accompanying *rlung* (*me mnyam rlung*) is responsible for this differentiation of nutrient and waste. When fire-accompanying *rlung* does not function properly, there is separation error in the identification and differentiation of nutrient and waste. Improper differentiation leads to waste product falling into the nutrient pathways that normally carry nutritional essence from ingested dietary content to properly build, develop, and maintain all the bodily constituents. When waste product enters the nutrient stream, radiance-transforming *tripa* (*mdwangs sgyur mkhris pa*) cannot properly produce normal healthy blood; that is, this subtype of *tripa* cannot properly "ripen" the blood (*zungs khrag ma smin pa*), and consequently that blood cannot develop the other bodily constituents as needed. When this improper blood resides for long durations in the liver, the patient develops a "metabolic disruption of the nutritional essence" (*dwangs ma ma zhu ba*) condition.

---

54 This is due to exacerbating the natural qualities (i.e., defining characteristics) of *rlung*. See G.yu thog yon tan mgon po, *Rtsa ba'i rgyud bshad pa'i rgyud phyi ma'i rgyud kha skong dang bcas pa*, 60: *rlung gi mtshan nyid rtsub cing yang ba dang/ grang zhing phra la sra zhing g.yo ba yin/.*

55 G.yu thog yon tan mgon po, *Rtsa ba'i rgyud bshad pa'i rgyud phyi ma'i rgyud kha skong dang bcas pa*, 75.

6.4 *Inciting Causal Factors: Impure Blood Proliferation and* rlung *Aggravation*

In the *Four Tantras*, what makes *dréné* distinct from *tren* is the coincident causal factor[56] that ultimately forms a *dré*. This is the excess production of poor quality (or impure) blood and the intensity of a coalescing force of aggravated *rlung*.[57] The *Four Tantras* describes the full etiology of *dréné* as: "Due to trauma, disturbance, or metabolic un-ripening, bad blood proliferates and *rlung* condenses [the constituents] to form [*dréné*]."[58] Thus from the generation of diseased blood and the compounding factor of *rlung* condensing the involved constituents, masses coalesce in the body like a gnarl on a tree, hence the name *dréné*, where *dré* is a growth, like a whorled growth on an oak or an edible fruit.

Dréné are further classified according to type in terms of etiological distinctions of the primary default system imbalance driving their formation—*rlung, tripa*, blood, and *béken*, where blood here, similar as for other illnesses described in the *Four Tantras*, is technically a bodily constituent but treated similar to an additional default system etiologically.[59] Type classifications in the text also include an etiology linked to damage caused by a weapon (*mtshon*) and that which has morphological characteristics like a bird egg (*bye 'dras*). *Dréné* are also classified in the *Four Tantras* according to "external" and "internal" location, where, "external" refers to more anatomically superficial layers of the constituent from which the *dré* grows, namely, muscle, bone, and blood, as well as lymph and neural channels.[60] "Internal" locations refer to more anatomically deep regions and aspects of organs described where the

56 Subsequent to the three causes setting the initial causal conditions.

57 G.yu thog yon tan mgon po, *Bdud rtsi snying po yan lag brgyad pa gsang ba man ngag gi rgyud*, 400.

58 G.yu thog yon tan mgon po, *Bdud rtsi snying po yan lag brgyad pa gsang ba man ngag gi rgyud*, 400: *rgyu ni 'grams 'khrugs kha zas ma smin pa/ ngan khrag rgyas te rlung gis bsgril nas 'byung/*.

59 Blood (*khrag*), as well as *chuser* (*chu ser*) and microorganisms (*srin*), as intermittently treated similar to additional default systems, require more space than the scope of this paper to address and so will be left unexplained for now. For now, note that the gloss of type classifications provided for *dréné* in the *Four Tantras* explicitly contextualizes them like default system types (G.yu thog yon tan mgon po, *Bdud rtsi snying po yan lag brgyad pa gsang ba man ngag gi rgyud*, 400: *nyes pa'i rigs kyi dbye/*).

60 G.yu thog yon tan mgon po, *Bdud rtsi snying po yan lag brgyad pa gsang ba man ngag gi rgyud*, 400.

dré grows, namely, lung, heart, liver, spleen, kidney, stomach, large and small intestines, rectum, and urinary bladder.[61]

Interestingly, in the *Four Tantras* lymph gland *dré* (*'bras rme*)[62] are not placed as one of the locations (*gnas*) in the *dréné* chapter, but are delineated in the separate lymph disorders chapter along with goiters, thyroid disorders, and other conditions categorized in the *Four Tantras* with lymph gland conditions (*rmen bu'i nad*).[63] However, the *Four Tantras* does recognize a similar blood-*rlung* etiology for lymph gland *dré* as the other *dréné*.[64]

6.5 *Important Commentarial Addition to Understanding of* Dréné *in the* Four Tantras

As many contemporary physician-scholars of Tibetan medicine have reviewed the commentarial scholarship written on *dréné* in their writings,[65] they acknowledge that most commentaries retain the classical sub-categories within *dréné* in the *Four Tantras*, with the exception of Desi Sanggyé Gyatso's (1653–1705) *Oral Instructions Supplement.*

As Czaja describes in his 2011 article mentioned above, Desi Sanggyé Gyatso delineates the additional category of "infection-derived *dré*" (*gnyan 'bras*),[66]

61 G.yu thog yon tan mgon po, *Bdud rtsi snying po yan lag brgyad pa gsang ba man ngag gi rgyud*, 401.

62 G.yu thog yon tan mgon po, *Bdud rtsi snying po yan lag brgyad pa gsang ba man ngag gi rgyud*, 410.

63 G.yu thog yon tan mgon po, *Bdud rtsi snying po yan lag brgyad pa gsang ba man ngag gi rgyud*, 409–11.

64 G.yu thog yon tan mgon po, *Bdud rtsi snying po yan lag brgyad pa gsang ba man ngag gi rgyud*, 409: *rgyu rkyen drag shul rkyen gyis 'grams pa'am/ rlung khrag 'khrugs pa rmen bu la brten skrangs/ phal cher ske mjing mig zur sne sa mang/.*

65 See for instance, Lha mo skyabs, *Bod lugs 'bras nad gso rig*; 'Jam dbyangs bkra shis, *Bod kyi gso ba rig pa'i 'bras nad*; Lde'u rong jo skyabs tshe ring, *Bod kyi gso rig las 'bras nad skor gyi dpyod gling*; and Dho lha, *Mchin pa'i Cancer la bod lugs gso rig gis brtag bcos zhib 'jug*, among others.

66 I choose to translate *nyendré* (*gnyan 'bras*) here as infection-derived due to its clinical use and understanding. *Nyen* illnesses (*gnyan nad*) are described as a class of illnesses with particularly intense suffering that come from those microorganisms, toxin-containing entities, and *barbata* from the external environment, as well as those which reside in the body primarily as blood microorganisms, with a round, appendage-less, and red appearance. The term itself confers the severity of the class of illnesses. See Byams pa 'phrin las, *Bod lugs gso rig tshig mdzod chen mo*, 281: *ngo bo phyi rol yul gyi dug can srin bu par pa ta dang nang lus la gnas pa'i khrag srin rkang med zlum la dmar ba gnyis lhan cig tu bsdungs pa las gyur pa'i nad rigs gdug pa can zhig gi ming ste/ nges tshig nad kyi nyen che bas na gnyan nad ces bya'o/.* One of the noteworthy additions that Desi Sanggyé Gyatso makes throughout the *Supplement*, is the addition of *nyen* to various illnesses which are considered more serious. For example, he classifies the treatments for brain infection (*gnyan*

describing a condition that forms a *dré* from infection. This additional category of *dré* provides a nice addition to the *dréné* portfolio as a strong candidate for linking the Tibetan medical framework for abnormal growths to biomedical conceptions of both malignant and benign neoplasms, particularly forms that are related to the proliferation of pathogenic microorganisms, toxins, and carcinogens in the environment. From the biomedical perspective, many neoplasms begin from initial infections of viruses and pathogens, such as liver cancer developing from a chronic infection of the hepatitis B virus. Desi Sanggyé Gyatso also notes a strong connection to a degenerate era with numerous environmental and food toxins, similar to the innumerable familiar and yet-to-be-recognized carcinogens described today. Czaja describes that infection-derived *dré* was one of the only categories considered at the 1996 Dharamsala Men-Tsee-Khang conference convened on the topic of cancer.[67] Although "infection-derived *dré*" provides one part of the mapping project, it is certainly not sufficient by itself.

Considering the above presentation of *dréné*'s categorization and etiology, I would like to highlight several commonalities with biomedical cancer. First, the categorization of *dré* as a wound is similar to the biomedical term "ulcer," which, in biomedicine, refers to an open sore on an external or internal surface of the body breaking the skin and mucous membranes, and in Tibetan medicine, refers to damage to the internal or external skin and/or muscle constituents.[68] Second, defining wound as damage to the bodily constituents has specific resonance to cellular and tissue damage and consequent growth in the

---

nad mgor babs klad gzer), infection-derived pains (*gnyan nad gzer thung ngam stod gzer/*), infection-derived abdominal cramps (*gnyan rims pho glang/*), infection-derived *méwel* (*gnyan rims me dbal/*), which are burn-like infections and ulcers, infection-derived lymph disorders (*gnyan rims rmen bu/*), among several others (Sangs rgyas rgya mtsho, *Man ngag yon tan rgyud kyi lhan thabs zugs rngu'i tsha gdung sel ba'i katpua* [Oral Instructions Supplement] [Dharamsala: Tibetan Medical and Astro Institute, 2005], *xi–xii*). Desi Sanggyé Gyatso introduces *nyendré* (*gnyan 'bras*) in both his chapter on treating *nyen* illnesses, as well as in the *dréné* treatment chapter (Sangs rgyas rgya mtsho, *Man ngag yon tan rgyud kyi lhan thabs*, 195, 366). In contemporary use among Tibetan physicians in Xining, Lhasa, and Dharamsala, *nyenné* is a category of contagious disease that often delineates those classes of disease that are most infectious and transmittable to instigate epidemics. For example, the plague, Ebola, and SARS would be classified as *nyenrim* illnesses (*gnyan rims*), a particularly contagious form of *nyen*. *Nyen* conditions are often identified as those derived from a virus, bacteria, amoeba, or other pathogenic-vector. *Rim* conditions are those that spread and infect others.

67 Czaja, "The *Four Tantras* and the Global Market," 275.

68 In the biomedical context, an ulcer is an open wound that fails to heal, whereas in the Tibetan medical context the wound term refers simply to damage of the skin and/or muscle layers.

biomedical context. In the *dréné* case, damage occurs through trauma, disturbance or unripened bodily constituents similar to the conception of internal cellular damage, pathway signal disregulation and unripened cell proliferation in the biomedical context, which we will see in more detail as we look at the particulars of the six characteristics defining cancer later. Thirdly, the specific body constituent region in which a *dréné* wound appears correlates well with the respective tissue layers in which cancer occurs. In the *Four Tantras*, the terms "skin" (*lpags*, or *skyi lpags*) and "muscle," in addition to integumentary skin and muscle, respectively, are also used to describe layers of an organ, which relate similarly to the biomedical distinction of epithelial and connective tissue cells of organs. Epithelia are sheets of cells that line the walls of cavities, channels, organs, and the integumentary system or external covering of the body—the skin. Beneath the epithelial cell layer is a basement membrane often referred to as basal lamina, which separates epithelial cells from the underlying layer of supporting connective tissue cells called the stroma.[69] In contemporary anatomical depictions in Tibetan medicine, the epithelial layer is called *pak* (*pags, lpags*; skin or outer layer), *kyimo* (*skyi mo*; outer skin or layer), or *tum* (*thum*; sheath).[70] The basal lamina (*rmang leb*) and stroma (*mang rdzas phra phung*) are considered to be connected to the epithelial layer as distinguished from the muscle (*sha, sha grim*) as bodily constituents.[71] Although using these terms to link to biomedical terms make them appear as neologisms, the concepts outlined above and related disease etiologies and treatments, precede their use in the *Four Tantras* and correlation to the biomedical terms.[72] These terms also illuminate the conceptions of skin and muscle[73] unique to the Tibetan medical

69 Jean Kanitakis, "Anatomy, Histology and Immunohistochemistry of Normal Human Skin," *European Journal of Dermatology* 12, no. 4 (2002): 390.

70 'O rtsogs chen, *Rgya bod dbyin gsum shan sbyar deng rabs gso rig ming mdzod* [Chinese-Tibetan-English Modern Medicine Dictionary] (Beijing: Mi rigs dpe skrun khang, 2011), 470; Pad ma rab brtan and Sangs rgyas 'bum, *Gso ba rig pa'i ro bkra'i dpe ris kun gsal me long* [All-Clarifying Mirror of Vivid Medical Dissectional Diagrams] (Xining: Mtsho sngon mi rigs dpe skrun khang, 2011), 92, 116.

71 'O rtsogs chen, *Rgya bod dbyin gsum shan sbyar deng rabs gso rig ming mdzod*, 239, 241.

72 For example, the various conceptions of *chuser* accumulation around specific organs and internal fascia rely on understandings of an outer layer for each organ and bodily constituent that is specified as the "skin layer" (*skyi pags*) of the heart, liver, and lungs, for example. Treatments such as paracentesis specifically address such accumulated *chuser* conditions adjacent and between these layers.

73 The term "muscle" provides the most appropriate translation for the Tibetan term *sha* because of its function and compositional distinction from "fat" (*tshil*) as described in the *Four Tantras*. G.yu thog yon tan mgon po, *Rtsa ba'i rgyud bshad pa'i rgyud phyi ma'i rgyud kha skong dang bcas pa*, 54: "Muscle covers; fat lubricates" (*sha yis g.yogs/ tshil gyis snum/*). The term "flesh" in English is defined as describing "soft substance consisting

tradition. Skin and muscle are defined by the function of "covering the bones."[74] Thus, on one hand, skin (*pags pa*) is subsumed under the same functionality as muscle (*sha*)—to cover the body. However, muscle is seen to closely relate to and be permeated by blood since it is formed from the blood constituent,[75] so vascularized connective tissue would provide a better corollary for the Tibetan term "muscle" (*sha*), and epithelia would provide a better corollary for the Tibetan term "skin" (*pags pa*). Fat, distinguished from both muscle and skin in the *Four Tantras*, is defined by its oiling and lubricating qualities with the associated characteristics,[76] and would relate to adipose tissue as well as interstitial fat constituents, such as those found in blood, around organs, and in joint spaces. Since epithelia spawn the most common human cancers—the carcinomas that are responsible for more than 80 percent of cancer-related deaths in the Euroamerican world[77]—this distinction is important for our depiction of cancer from the perspective of the *Four Tantras*. The fourth commonality

---

of muscle and fat that is found between the skin and bones of an animal or a human" (Oxford Dictionary Online). This hybrid fat-muscle soft substance is not the understanding with the term *sha*. In the *Four Tantras*, fat is also described to arise from muscle in the development of the bodily constituents. G.yu thog yon tan mgon po, *Rtsa ba'i rgyud bshad pa'i rgyud phyi ma'i rgyud kha skong dang bcas pa*, 56: "From blood, muscle develops; from muscle, fat develops; from fat, bone develops; from bone, bone marrow develops" (*khrag las sha/ sha las tshil 'gyur tshil las rus par 'gyur/ rus las rkang 'gyur*). As a corollary, in biomedicine, fat cells (i.e., adipocytes) arise from the precursor cells for muscle cells (i.e., myocytes) called mesenchymal cells (Terence Ryan and Sergio Curri, "Genesis of Adipocytes," *Clinics in Dermatology* 7, no. 4 [1989]: 9–24). Likewise, bone cells (osteoblasts) and cartilage cells (chondrocytes) also derive from mesenchymal cells (Donald Phinney and Darwin Prockop, "Concise Review: Mesenchymal Stem/Multipotent Stromal Cells: The State of Transdifferentiation and Modes of Tissue Repair—Current Views," *Stem Cells* 25, no. 11 [2007]: 2896–902).

74 For muscle, see G.yu thog yon tan mgon po, *Rtsa ba'i rgyud bshad pa'i rgyud phyi ma'i rgyud kha skong dang bcas pa*, 54: "Blood moistens and sustains life, muscle covers" (*khrag gis brlun shing srog 'tsho sha yis g.yogs*). For skin, the embryology chapter of the *Explanatory Tantra* describes, "At the twenty-first week, skin encases the fetal body" (G.yu thog yon tan mgon po, *Rtsa ba'i rgyud bshad pa'i rgyud phyi ma'i rgyud kha skong dang bcas pa*, 43: *rtsa gcig pa la phyi yi pags pa g.yogs/*). Whereas in the eighteenth week muscle has already formed: "In the fifth month, that is the eighteenth week, muscle and fat form" (G.yu thog yon tan mgon po, *Rtsa ba'i rgyud bshad pa'i rgyud phyi ma'i rgyud kha skong dang bcas pa*, 43: *zla lnga bdun phrag bco brgyad sha tshil chags/*), distinguishing muscle from skin, where fat arises from muscle according to the developmental sequence of bodily constituents.

75 G.yu thog yon tan mgon po, *Rtsa ba'i rgyud bshad pa'i rgyud phyi ma'i rgyud kha skong dang bcas pa*, 56.

76 G.yu thog yon tan mgon po, *Rtsa ba'i rgyud bshad pa'i rgyud phyi ma'i rgyud kha skong dang bcas pa*, 54.

77 Weinberg, *The Biology of Cancer*, 29.

between *dréné* and cancer is the compounding, or inciting, conditions from which *dréné* forms, which are similar to the current understanding of the various causes of neoplasms and their transformation into malignant neoplasms types,[78] which we will discuss further later.

Dréné and *tren* as abnormal masses form obvious candidates in linking both *dréné* and *tren* to biomedical conceptions of neoplasms: both benign tumors as well as malignant cancers. However, like *tren, dréné* is a more complex disease category where not all *dréné* would be considered neoplasms from the biomedical perspective, especially those that comprise the initial stages of tissue damage only. And furthermore, those *dré* which would be considered neoplasms would not all be considered malignant. As *dréné* and *tren* are classically described in the *Four Tantras*, linking them as a single category to benign and malignant neoplasms seems a reasonable beginning in the correlation to the biomedical category of cancer. As such, we can understand the motivation to do so by one of the first Tibetan medical physicians Menpa Samten to author a text integrating perspectives from both Euroamerican and Tibetan traditions of medicine.

7 *Dré-Tren*: Collapsing Categories, Sidelining the Three Default Systems

In the *New Dawn Compendium of Medicine*, Menpa Samten re-maps Tibetan etiologies according to the physiological systems described in biomedicine with sections on the respiratory system (*'byin rngub kyi ma lag*), circulatory system (*'khor rgyugs kyi ma lag*), digestive system (*'ju byed kyi ma lag*), nervous system (*chu rtsa'am dbang rtsa'i ma lag*), and so forth. The great medical scholar-lama Troru Tsenam Rinpoché (1928–2004) praised the text as the first major work integrating perspectives from Tibetan and Euroamerican biomedicine. Educated during the 1970s and 80s with strong foundations in classical Chinese, Samten was one of the first Tibetan medical physicians to be able to read biomedical literature published in Chinese and assimilate such perspectives into Tibetan medical understandings and sensibilities.[79] He wrote the

78 See for instance O. H. Warburg, *The Metabolism of Tumours: Investigations from the Kaiser Wilhelm Institute for Biology, Berlin-Dahlem* (London: Arnold Constable, 1930); O. H. Warburg, "On the Origin of Cancer Cells," *Science* 123 (1956): 309–14; O. H. Warburg, "On Respiratory Impairment in Cancer Cells," *Science* 124 (1956): 269–70; M. G. Vander Heiden et al., "Understanding the Warburg Effect: The Metabolic Requirements of Cell Proliferation," *Science* 324 (2009): 1029–33.

79 Jamyang Gyatso, personal communication, 2018.

New Dawn Compendium of Medicine to appeal to a biomedical sensibility at a time when presenting Tibetan medicine in such a way that it could dialogue with biomedical physicians and scholars was important. At this time, reforms orchestrated by Chinese socialism included "direct revision of Tibetan medicine through Chinese biomedicalization" focused on eliminating important parts of Tibetan medical theory claiming that it contained "religious or superstitious elements."[80] Thus, at the time of the publication of Samten's text in 1985, the scientification of Tibetan medicine was well underway.[81] Anthropologist and medical historian Theresia Hofer shows how central institutions like Men-tsee-Khang made a practice of leading such initiatives to survive, avoiding the marginalization that Medical House (*sman grong*) and monastery physicians incurred on the periphery.[82] The anatomical charts in the front matter of Samten's text use biomedical drawings with Tibetan terms designating anatomy, in contrast to the classical depiction of anatomy in the stylistic drawings of the medical thangkas commissioned by Desi Sanggyé Gyatso.[83] Drawing upon the biomedical drawings, and a distinctly biomedical sensibility of seeing the body,[84] might have afforded Samten and his colleagues an additional strategy to help Tibetan medicine survive, recover, and/or find its place during these challenging political times. Fortunately, Samten's efforts to present Tibetan medical nosology in such a way that could be understood by the biomedical community allowed for an appreciation of and dialogue with Tibetan medical approaches to disease diagnostics and treatment that is still drawn upon by contemporary Tibetan doctors in collaborative contexts.[85] In Samten's choices of disease categorization and presentation, he deemphasized classifications according to the *nyépa*, presumably so as to make them more

80 Vincanne Adams et al., eds., *Medicine Between Science and Religion*, 18.

81 Vincanne Adams and Fei-Fei Li, "Integration or Erasure? Modernizing Medicine at Lhasa's Mentsikhang," in *Tibetan Medicine in the Contemporary World: Global Politics of Medical Knowledge and Practice*, ed. Laurent Pordié (London and New York: Routledge, 2008), 105–31; Adams et al., "Translating Science: The Arura Medical Group at the Frontiers of Medical Research," 111–36.

82 Theresia Hofer, *Medicine and Memory in Tibet: Amchi Physicians in an Age of Reform* (Seattle: University of Washington Press, 2018).

83 For a description, see for instance Katharina Sabernig, "On the History of the Murals in the Medical College at Labrang Monastery," *Asian Medicine* 7 (2012): 358–83.

84 See Shigehisa Kuriyama, *The Expressiveness of the Body and the Divergence of Greek and Chinese Medicine* (New York, NY: Zone Books, 2002) for a related account on disparate cultural views of the body depicted vis-à-vis anatomical drawings in classical Greek medicine and classical Chinese medicine.

85 Jamyang Gyatso, personal communication, 2018.

accessible to a biomedical audience. In this modern nosology, Samten defines *dré-tren* categorically as follows:

> *Drétren* primarily arise from the causative condition of a nutritional essence metabolic disturbance [in] the stomach, liver and so forth from which abnormal excess products grow in uncertain locations in the vital and vessel organs and bodily constituents. Turning into a mass, it absorbs the body's essential nutrients. [The growths] obstruct the pathways of the bodily constituents and due to harming the critical sensory organ faculties and so forth, it is an illness which incites great fear and concern for [one's] life.[86]

Samten's description of his newly classified, combined category of *drétren* retains an etiology consistent with both the classical descriptions of *dré* and *tren* in the *Four Tantras* and in Desi Sanggyé Gyatso's later contribution of the *Oral Instructions Supplement.* However, Samten integrates a biomedical lens in his account by describing products (*grub cha*) and nutrient compounds (*dwangs ma'i bcud rdzas*), for instance, and is the first to overtly place *dré* and *tren* in a single category beyond the group of nutritional essence metabolic disturbance illnesses from two of the four subtypes of the chronic metabolic disturbances: namely, twisting (*'tril ba*) and spreading (*byer ba*) natures of the disturbance.[87] Categorically placing *dré* and *tren* together, he makes an overt link to biomedical descriptions of cancer, integrating perspectives from both Euroamerican and Tibetan medical traditions. He does not describe the "types" (*rigs*) of *dréné* as described in the *Four Tantras* that employ the etiological distinctions from imbalances in the default systems driving the formation of *dré.* In doing so, he omits the subtypes within both *dré* and *tren* that do not threaten one's life and are considered easy to treat. For example, in the *Four Tantras,* old blood *tren* are considered one of the easiest illnesses to treat.[88]

---

86 Bsam gtan, *Gso rig snying bsdus skya rengs gsar pa*, 276: *'bras skran zer ba de ni phal cher dwangs ma ma zhu ba'i rkyen gyis pho mchin sogs lus zungs don snod kyi gnas nges med du rgyun ldan min pa'i grub cha 'thol pa 'tshar skyes byung ba dang/ gong bur bsgril nas lus khams kyi dwangs ma'i bcud rdzas 'jib 'then byed pa dang/ lus zungs kyi bu ga'i rgyu lam bkag pa/ gal che'i dbang rten la gnod 'tshe gtong ba sogs byas nas mi'i tshe srog la 'jigs snang tshabs chen bskul ba'i nad cig red/.*

87 G.yu thog yon tan mgon po, *Bdud rtsi snying po yan lag brgyad pa gsang ba man ngag gi rgyud*, 169: *'dril bas skran rnams skyed par byed pa ste/* [...] *byer bas dug mdze me dbal 'or du lhung/ 'bras dang sur ya dreg dang grum bu dang/ mig ser rtsa skran rkang 'bam du mar 'gyur/* [...] *nad rnams phal cher dwangs ma ma zhus skyed/.*

88 G.yu thog yon tan mgon po, *Rtsa ba'i rgyud bshad pa'i rgyud phyi ma'i rgyud kha skong dang bcas pa*, 170: *'on kyang rims la yul dus mtshungs pa dang/ chu 'gags nad la gnod bya mnyams pa dang/ khrag skran rnying pa gso ba sla zhes bya/.*

Instead, he lists the other classic categories from the *Four Tantras* of external and internal forms of *dréné*, as well as those categorized by location (*gnas*) of growth formation, and identifies which types of *tren* should be suitably linked within the *dré-tren* category.

The *tren* that Samten puts in the *drétren* category comprise: gastroesophageal *tren* (*lhen skran*),[89] which is subsumed in the larger category of gastric *tren* (*pho skran*), *tren* of fat constituent (*tshil skran*), *tren* of the ovaries and related reproductive pathways (*bsam se'u'i skran*), uterine and cervical *tren* (*mngal skran*), and skin *tren* (*pags skran*). He describes that *tren* is named because it is a mass (*gong bu*) that aggregates (*bsgril ba*) into a distinct, isolated entity (*kher rkyang du*) anywhere in the body.[90] Samten makes the distinction that *tren* do not have the characteristic of propagating to other areas of the body.[91] Thus, one can infer that for Samten, *tren* are benign tumors, and *dré* are malignant.

However, as we have seen from the above analysis, Samten's characterization exaggerates a simplification of the *tren* and *dréné* etiologies in order to collapse them into a single category, providing a one-to-one correlation with benign tumors and malignant cancers. The nosological complexity and its attendant epistemological and ontological perspectives get jettisoned in the process. As shown above from the classical depiction in the *Four Tantras*, several *tren* types are not neoplasms or tumors, and some *tren* types that are neoplasms can become malignant. Likewise, some *dré* are benign and do not spread in the body. Furthermore other diseases in Tibetan medicine, such as *méwel* and *surya* have subtypes which are malignant growths and spread like malignant cancers, which we will discuss further below. Likewise, in Samten's characterization of *tren*, skin *tren* is not skin cancer as one might assume. Instead, he describes it as a clogged hair follicle that forms a mass, which is also not a neoplasm.[92] Samten calls metabolic disruptions due to waste products in the stomach "bezoars," glossing them as "adhesive products in gastric juices."[93] Samten does

89 The Tibetan term *lhen* refers to the juncture between the esophagus (*mid pa*) and stomach (*pho ba*). It describes an anatomical position between the two organs as well as an external location proximal to that juncture upon which an important moxibustion point resides called the *lhen sang* (*lhen gyi me gsang*). A mass growing at the esophageal-gastric juncture is called a *lhen tren* and is classified in the *Four Tantras* (G.yu thog yon tan mgon po, *Bdud rtsi snying po yan lag brgyad pa gsang ba man ngag gi rgyud*, 175) as well as in Samten's *New Dawn Compendium of Medicine* (Bsam gtan, *Gso rig snying bsdus skya rengs gsar pa*, 276).

90 Bsam gtan, *Gso rig snying bsdus skya rengs gsar pa*, 277.

91 Bsam gtan, *Gso rig snying bsdus skya rengs gsar pa*, 277: *gnas bzhan du mched mi 'gro ba/.*

92 Bsam gtan, *Gso rig snying bsdus skya rengs gsar pa*, 282: *pags skran zer ba de ni phal che ba ba spu'i bu ga 'gags pa'i rkyen gyis lus zungs kyi snyigs ma phyir don mi thub par skran du 'dril nas 'bur rdog don pa'i nad cig red/.*

93 Bsam gtan, *Gso rig snying bsdus skya rengs gsar pa*, 280: *pho chur 'byar tshi skye ba/.*

not mention any blood *dré* and keeps lymph *dré* in the lymph gland category as is classically found for lymph *dré* in the *Four Tantras*, as described earlier.

8 Retaining Epistemologies and Etiologies: Providing a Map

In sidelining the *nyépa* as important etiological distinctions for each illness, simplifying the categories of *dréné* and *tren* to force a single category, and disregarding the etiological cousins of other nutritional essence metabolic disturbances as candidate links, I argue that Samten's fairly recent modern symphysis is insufficient in providing a comprehensive mapping of biomedical neoplasms into the suitable Tibetan medical categories, despite its important historical contribution to this project. In the following, I present the six characteristics predominantly recognized by cancer biologists currently as the defining criteria for cancer, then I attempt to provide a mapping for the characteristics that still retains the classical categories and etiological understandings found primarily in the *Four Tantras* with the addition of infection-derived *dré* provided by Desi Sanggyé Gyatso's *Oral Instructions Supplement.*

8.1 *Six Defining Characteristics of Cancer*

Cancer biologists have shown that, under a microscope, a malignant cell has a dilated nucleus, thin rim of cytoplasm, and an autonomous engine to continue dividing, driven by mutations to the genetic code.[94] Such cells are immortal, inhibiting the cellular instructions for apoptosis (normal cell death) as well as senescence (the delay of normal cellular cycles).[95] As early as 1858, physician and biologist Rudolf Virchow, known for his advancement of public health, argued that cancer is the result of inflammation due to injury or response to an external agent such as bacteria or pathogen,[96] which causes swelling and immune system activation, and consequently causes cells to proliferate. This cell proliferation would lead to an outgrowth of malignant cancer.[97] Virchow's early insights on cancer development in cells remain highly relevant today for current understandings. Chronic inflammation over a long period of time,

94 Douglas Hanahan and Robert A. Weinberg, "The Hallmarks of Cancer," *Cell* 100, no. 1 (2000): 57.

95 J. M. Adams and S. Cory, "The Bcl-2 Apoptotic Switch in Cancer Development and Therapy," *Oncogene* 26 (2007): 1324–37.

96 M. Schäfer and S. Werner, "Cancer as an Overhealing Wound: An Old Hypothesis Revisited," *Nature Reviews Molecular Cell Biology* 9 (2008): 628–38.

97 Siddhartha Mukherjee, *The Emperor of All Maladies: A Biography of Cancer* (New York, NY: Scribner, 2010), 340.

such as decades, is still recognized as contributing to the transformation of a benign neoplasm into malignancy and is currently gaining greater research attention for its integral role.[98]Although there are one hundred distinct types of cancer and many subtypes of tumors specific to an organ and tissue, there are commonalities in the disruption of the distinct regulatory circuits that manage normal cell proliferation and homeostasis, such as that resultant from chronic inflammation and pathogenic agents.[99] Cancer biologists Robert Weinberg and Douglas Hanahan have dedicated their research careers to understanding the genetic basis for cancer and are considered two of the foremost authorities. Weinberg discovered the first human oncogene and the first tumor suppressor genes, and his work led to the discovery of over one hundred cancer cell types. Douglas Hanahan developed the first transgenic mouse models for cancer. Their seminal papers published in January 2000 and updated 2011 review have provided the foundation for contemporary studies and further cancer research development by providing the six functional capabilities that cells acquire to transform normal cells into malignancy:

1. Self-sufficiency in growth signals,
2. Insensitivity to growth-inhibitory (antigrowth) signals,
3. Evasion of programmed cell death (apoptosis),
4. Limitless replicative potential,
5. Sustained angiogenesis (or the development of blood supply), and
6. Tissue invasion and metastasis.[100]

In the following section, I will provide a brief description of each functional capacity recognized.

---

98 Carlos Cordon-Cardo and Carol Prives, "At the Crossroads of Inflammation and Tumorigenesis," *The Journal of Experimental Medicine* 190, no. 10 (1999): 1367–70; A. Zumsteg and G. Christofori, "Corrupt Policemen: Inflammatory Cells Promote Tumor Angiogenesis," *Current Opinion in Oncology* 21 (2009): 60–70.

99 Cooper, *Elements of Human Cancer*.

100 D. Bonnet and J. E. Dick, "Human Acute Myeloid Leukemia is Organized as a Hierarchy That Originates from a Primitive Hematopoietic Cell," *Nature Medicine* 3 (1997): 730–37; Hanahan and Weinberg, "The Hallmarks of Cancer," 57; G. Bergers and L. E. Benjamin, "Tumorigenesis and the Angiogenic Switch," *Nature Reviews Cancer* 3 (2003): 401–10; Adams and Cory, "The Bcl-2 Apoptotic Switch," 1324; I. Amit et al., "A Module of Negative Feedback Regulators Defines Growth Factor Signaling," *Nature Genetics* 39 (2007): 503–12; Z. Ahmed and R. Bicknell, "Angiogenic Signaling Pathways," *Methods in Molecular Biology* 467 (2009): 3; V. Baeriswyl and G. Christofori, "The Angiogenic Switch in Carcinogenesis," *Seminars in Cancer Biology* 19 (2009): 329–37; S. E. Artandi and R. A. DePinho, "Telomeres and Telomerase in Cancer," *Carcinogenesis* 31 (2010): 9–18; K. Pietras and A. Ostman, "Hallmarks of Cancer: Interactions with the Tumor Stroma," *Experimental Cell Research* 316 (2010): 1324–31. Their 2011 update (Hanahan and Weinberg, "Hallmarks of Cancer: The Next Generation," *Cell* 144, no. 5 [2011]: 646–74) expands on their initial 2000 article.

Self-sufficiency in growth signals. For self-sufficiency in growth signals, signals must originate internally. Normal cells require mitogenic growth signals before they move from a quiescent state into an active proliferative state, growing their mass and dividing to produce new cells. Such signals originate elsewhere in the body and enter the cell through transmembrane receptors. Cancer cells have their own set of oncogenes that mimic normal growth signals. Hanahan and Weinberg describe that normal cells require growth factors (GFs) from different cell types to stimulate proliferation; however, cancer cells acquire the ability to synthesize GFs themselves, to which they themselves are also responsive—creating a positive feedback loop. They also have an overexpression of cell surface receptors, making them hyper-responsive to ambient levels of growth factors that would not normally trigger proliferation.

Insensitivity to antigrowth signals. Similar to their positively acting counterparts, growth-inhibitory signals must be received by transmembrane cell surface receptors to induce intracellular signaling circuits. Such signals function in two ways: a cell may be forced from its proliferative cycle into a quiescent state until another extracellular signal permits; or cells may be induced into a post-mitotic state that permanently relinquishes their proliferative potential. Cancer cells neither produce nor respond to growth-inhibitory signals.

Apoptosis evasion. All normal cells have a latent form of programmed cell death (apoptosis) that is triggered by physiological signals and unfolds in a choreographed series of steps—the cell membrane is disrupted, the cytoplasmic and nuclear skeletons break down, the cytosol is extruded, chromosomes degraded, and nucleus fragmented. This occurs in a matter of 30–120 minutes, and the resultant shriveled cell corpse is engulfed by nearby cells in a tissue and disappears, usually within twenty-four hours.[101] Sensors and effectors are two components that determine whether the apoptotic program is put into play. Sensors determine the normality of the intracellular environment and effectors receive that signal to enact the apoptotic program. Detected abnormalities include DNA damage, survival factor insufficiency, and hypoxia. Malignant cancer cells are able to evade the apoptotic program.[102] The most common way cancer cells lose proapoptotic regulation is through a mutation involving a tumor suppressor gene (the p53 tumor suppressor gene) and the resulting functional inactivation of its product (the p53 protein). The survival signaling circuit can be activated by extracellular factors.[103]

---

101 Hanahan and Weinberg, "The Hallmarks of Cancer," 61.

102 Adams and Cory, "The Bcl-2 Apoptotic Switch."

103 Such as such as IGF-1/2 or IL-3 (G. Evan and T. Littlewood, "A Matter of Life and Cell Death," *Science* 281, no. 5381 [1998]: 1317–22). For an example of related immune-mediated

Limitless replication. So far we have seen that three acquired abilities—growth signal autonomy, insensitivity to antigrowth signals, and resistance to apoptosis—lead to an uncoupling of a cell's growth program from signals in its environment.[104] This could be enough to create vast cell populations, but studies have identified another independent program that limits cell multiplication. Once normal cell populations progress to a certain number of doublings, they enter what is called "senescence," where they stop growing. If certain elements are disabled, cells can continue multiplying for additional generations until a crisis state occurs of massive cell death. However, a variant sometimes arises that has the trait of immortality, which allows cancer cells to gain limitless replicative potential.[105]

Sustained angiogenesis. All normal cells in a tissue must reside within 100 millimeters of a capillary blood vessel in order to retrieve oxygen and nutrients required for cell function and survival.[106] Most new aberrant proliferating cells or lesions lack angiogenic ability, which curtails their expansion capacity. Thus, malignant neoplasms are unique in that they develop angiogenic ability, or the capacity to develop their own blood supply.[107]

Tissue invasion and metastasis. The ability for primary tumor masses to spawn pioneer cells that move out to invade adjacent tissues and distant sites where they set up new colonies—that is, metastases—are the cause of the great majority of human cancer deaths.[108] Although Euroamerican medical science does not understand invasion and metastasis well, which it locates as genetic and biochemical determinants, it does recognize that several proteins are implicated in tethering cells to their surrounding tissue, which,

equilibrium with cancer, see M. W. L. Teng et al., "Immune-mediated Dormancy: An Equilibrium with Cancer," *Journal of Leukocyte Biology* 84 (2008): 988–93.

104 Adams and Cory, "The Bcl-2 Apoptotic Switch," 1324.

105 Studies have shown the primary counting device for cell generations is telomeres—that is, the ends of chromosomes. Various treatments that allow for telomere repair help to lengthen lifespan and vitality, but would also increase the incidence of malignant tumor cells since 85–90% of such cells upregulate expression of the telomerase enzyme, allowing them to maintain telomere length above a critical threshold, and thus permitting unlimited replication (Wright et al., "Expression of c-erb B-2 Oncoprotein: A Prognostic Indicator in Human Breast Cancer," *Cancer Research* 49 [1989]: 2087–90; Hanahan and Weinberg, "The Hallmarks of Cancer," 63).

106 Hanahan and Weinberg, "The Hallmarks of Cancer," 63.

107 Ahmed and Bicknell, "Angiogenic Signaling Pathways," 3. Loss of p53 tumor suppressor protein occurs in most human tumors. This can simultaneously cause thrombospondin-1 levels to fall, which allows endothelial cells to be liberated from angiogenic suppression effects (A. Patenaude et al., "Involvement of Endothelial Progenitor Cells in Tumor Vascularization," *Microvascular Research* 79 [2010]: 217–23).

108 M. B. Sporn, "The War on Cancer," *Lancet* 347, no. 9012 (1996): 1377–81.

when altered, provide cells with invasive and metastatic capabilities.[109] This is the final capacity for cancer cells to achieve in order to gain all six of its defining characteristics.

8.2 *Tibetan Medical Etiological Links to the Six Characteristics*

Reflecting on these six defining characteristics as outlined above by Hanahan and Weinberg, I propose specific etiological links drawing from the *Four Tantras* that identify the Tibetan medical disease categories related to biomedical cancer and neoplasms. I recognize a correlating association between chronic inflammation and the Tibetan medical conception of aggravated *rlung* and the development of poor quality blood (*ngan khrag rgyas pa*). Contemporary biomedical researchers understand inflammation as a normal protective physiologic response that coordinates immune cells, blood vessels, and molecular mediators to eliminate the initial cause of tissue and cellular injury. However, in its chronic form, a perceived threat by the body persists aggressive cells systemically over time and causes chronic damage. Since *rlung* regulates cellular signaling, neuroendocrine functions, immune activation, and the mobility of proper constituents in the blood, chronic inflammation relates to *rlung* activities coordinated with related blood constituents. Illnesses that relate to biomedical conceptions of cancer would draw upon these two characteristics of disease ecology.

Growth/anti-growth signals and rlung-tripa activity. Contemporary Tibetan physicians link abnormal cell proliferation from the biomedical perspective to a combination of aggravated *rlung* and *tripa* activity due to their role in growth of the bodily constituents, and particularly abnormal blood qualities.[110] Likewise, they link *rlung* activity to cellular responsiveness since *rlung* manages signal transmission in the body.[111] Thus, in order to interpret Hanahan and Weinberg's six functional capacities of malignant cells in terms of a Tibetan medical sensibility, I highlight the role of a combined influence of *rlung* and blood-related *tripa* (that is, unrestrained cell proliferation and particular

109 These proteins called cell-cell adhesion molecules (CAMS) are classes of immunoglobulins and calcium-dependent cadherins. Integrins and proteases also play a key role in invasive and metastatic potential (Hanahan and Weinberg, "The Hallmarks of Cancer," 65).

110 Jamyang Gyatso, personal communication, 2018; referring to G.yu thog yon tan mgon po, *Rtsa ba'i rgyud bshad pa'i rgyud phyi ma'i rgyud kha skong dang bcas pa*, 39: *sa med mi 'grub chu med sdud mi nus/ me med mi smin rlung med 'phel mi 'gyur/*.

111 Jamyang Gyatso, personal communication, 2018; referring to G.yu thog yon tan mgon po, *Rtsa ba'i rgyud bshad pa'i rgyud phyi ma'i rgyud kha skong dang bcas pa*, 58: *nyes pa'i las ni rlung gis dbugs 'byin rngub/ bskyod dang las spyod shugs 'byin gnod bya rgyu/ dbang po gsal dang lus rjes 'dzin par byed/*.

supply access in blood and lymph vessels) and excess aggravated *rlung* alone (that is, cellular signaling in growth, mobility, and perpetuity).

Limitless replication and abnormal proliferation of the body constituents. To generate an aggregation in the body of limitless proliferation from the perspective of the *Four Tantras* requires the synchronization of resources in order to provide the mass, growth, and ripening of those bodily constituents. The capacity to dominate control of the first two constituents—nutritional essence and blood—are required for excess development and proliferation of any of the other constituents. Thus, I argue that the disorders in the *Four Tantras* related to cancer would direct nutritional essence advantageously, and result from excess blood, as is the case with nutritional essence metabolic disorders. To provide greater growth, such disorders must also excessively mobilize *rlung* and *tripa* activities while dominating mass accumulation functions of *béken.*

Apoptosis evasion and rlung. As discussed above, contemporary Tibetan physicians describe cell signaling as a *rlung* activity. The ability to maintain function would require continual mobilization of resources from that ingested into the body. The *Four Tantras* characterizes all mobilization as *rlung* activity. Thus, apoptotic evasion would likely be linked to the hyperactivity of *rlung.*

Sustained angiogenesis and abnormal proliferation of blood. Angiogenesis around abnormal cell masses relates well to the condition of abnormal blood excess in the *Four Tantras.* A quality common with the general nutrient essence metabolic disturbance, as well as the specific conditions like *dréné,* channel *tren,*[112] *méwel,* and *surya.*

Metastatic capacities as a result of diminished béken and aggravated rlung. Due to the adhesive qualities required to tether a cellular mass to its original site, metastatic occurrences would relate to the down-regulating of the adherence-promoting activity of *béken* and the upregulation of etiological variants of the conditions discussed above.

The etiological links to the six defining characteristics of biomedical cancer outlined above relate to a subset of nutritional essence metabolic disturbances in the *Four Tantras,* namely *dréné,* channel *tren, méwel, surya,* and blood proliferation compounded by aggravated *rlung.* As such they provide an etiological context upon which biomedical cancer mapped. Furthermore, there are a few conditions for biomedical cancer to form that assists our analysis.

112 G.yu thog yon tan mgon po, *Bdud rtsi snying po yan lag brgyad pa gsang ba man ngag gi rgyud,* 176: *dwangs ma ma zhu ngan khrag rgyas pa de/ mchin dri glo mkhal rgyu grog pho ba'i rtsar/ 'grims pa sa gcig 'dril pa rtsa yi skran/.*

An enabling characteristic for cancer formation in biomedicine is genome instability, which allows for the six characteristics mentioned above to develop. Karyotypic order, or the number and appearance of the chromosomes within a cell, is fastidiously maintained by innumerable DNA monitoring and repair enzymes. Likewise, mitosis, or regulated cell division, provides an important checkpoint in the cell's life to ensure that mutations are rare. Increased mutability has been posited to account for the significant frequency with which cancers appear in human populations.[113] Because of the number of steps and alterations required, cancers tend to be rare early in the human lifetime and take hold later in life, similar to the condition required for "metabolic disruptions of the nutritional essence" to progress into these advanced and chronic conditions. Causes of genome instability and cellular damage still relate back to Virchow's initial two causal trajectories of cellular and tissue damage due to inflammatory response and pathogenic agents, as well as the related genetic susceptibilities. I point out that the two-fold driving forces in transforming benign neoplasms to malignant cancer bear a striking resemblance to the dual categories in Desi Sanggyé Gyatso's *Oral Instructions Supplement.* The latter's two major subcategories of *dré* formation comprise: (1) "wound-derived *dré*" (*rma 'bras*), which resembles Virchow's inflammation response due to injury; and (2) "infection-derived *dré*," which resembles the response to an external pathogenic agent, as in the case of general *nyenné* described above. In some, these forms of damage to the development and maintenance of bodily constituents results from a metabolic disruption as described in the *Four Tantras*. In the next section, I will describe how this conceptual perspective shapes the correlation between biomedical cancers and related illnesses in the *Four Tantras*.

9 "Metabolic Disruptions" as Broader Context: More Candidate Illnesses

Many conditions, including both *dréné* and *tren* result from "metabolic disruption" (*ma zhu ba*) conditions. In fact, the *Four Tantras* identifies metabolic disruptions as the root of all chronic illness.[114] It describes that proper

113 Lawrence A. Loeb, "Mutator Phenotype May Be Required for Multistage Carcinogenesis," *Cancer Research* 51 (1991): 3075–79.

114 G.yu thog yon tan mgon po, *Bdud rtsi snying po yan lag brgyad pa gsang ba man ngag gi rgyud*, 168: "The cause of chronic illness, 'metabolic disruptions,' has six general points" (*ma zhu gcong gi rgyu la spyi don drug/*).

development of life-sustaining blood (*zungs khrag*) is not only important for developing the various bodily constituents, organs, fluids, vessels, channels, and so forth, but its malfunction is the primary mechanism for developing chronic conditions propagated from the liver and the downstream developing body constituents and processes. According to the *Four Tantras*, there are two main types of metabolic disruptions: waste product disruptions[115] and nutritional essence disruptions.[116] Waste product disruptions occur when ingested contents remain in the stomach or colon and coalesce from excess *béken* mucosal and viscous digestive constituents, such that the waste products of the ingested materials are overly coated, stagnate, and adhere to tract walls, where they remain for long time periods, eventually forming hardened masses and accretions. Nutritional essence metabolic disruptions, where waste product infiltrates the nutrient stream pathways and causes disruption in liver function and proper blood production as described further in the above section, have four subtypes: (1) wrapping or condensing (*'dril ba*), (2) leaking or dropping (*zags pa*), as with fluid, (3) dispersing or spreading (*byer ba*), and (4) posturing (*'gyings pa*).[117] These four types characterize processes that lead to an underlying metabolic disruption condition to develop into various illnesses. For example, *tren* arise from the wrapping (*'dril ba*) condition, and *dréné* and channel-type *tren* arise from the spreading (*byer ba*) condition. Both *dréné* and *tren* arise from abnormalities in the processes driving proper formation of the bodily constituents, which comprise all bodily components, organs, fluids, and their respective products.[118] Disturbance in proper constituent development produces abnormalities at subsequent levels, creating adhesions, aggregations, and masses.

In reviewing these etiologically-similar classes of illnesses outlined in the *Four Tantras*, several other candidate Tibetan medical illnesses upon which biomedical neoplasms, both benign and malignant, map become apparent. Particularly in the spreading condition of metabolic disruptions of nutritional essence, the *Four Tantras* lists: toxin disorders, leprosy (*mdze*), *méwel* (burn-like irritations), secondary edema, *dré, surya* (irritations and ulcers that spread

115 G.yu thog yon tan mgon po, *Bdud rtsi snying po yan lag brgyad pa gsang ba man ngag gi rgyud*, 189: *snyigs ma ma zhu ba/.*

116 G.yu thog yon tan mgon po, *Bdud rtsi snying po yan lag brgyad pa gsang ba man ngag gi rgyud*, 189: *dwangs ma ma zhu ba/.*

117 G.yu thog yon tan mgon po, *Bdud rtsi snying po yan lag brgyad pa gsang ba man ngag gi rgyud*, 169.

118 G.yu thog yon tan mgon po, *Rtsa ba'i rgyud bshad pa'i rgyud phyi ma'i rgyud kha skong dang bcas pa*, 23, 54: "nutritional essence, blood, muscle, fat, bone, bone marrow and regenerative fluid" (*dwangs ma khrag sha tshil rus rkang khu ba*).

like sun-rays), gout, arthritis, jaundice, channel *tren* in blood and lymph vessels and nerves, and *kangbam* (which includes various leg disorders like varicose veins).[119] From this list, I integrate *méwel* and *surya* into my analysis of the prospective Tibetan medical disorders upon which biomedical malignant and benign neoplasms map, as well as note why *tren* of specific channels (*rtsa*) in the body, which include blood vessels, nerves, and lymph vessels,[120] is uniquely distinguished from the other *tren* types within this group. Now the expanded collection of illnesses in the *Four Tantras* onto which I propose biomedical cancer maps include: *dréné* and *tren*, but also include "*béken* throat obstructions" (*bad kan mgul 'gags*),[121] which are growths in the esophagus known as esophageal *dré* (*mid 'bras*);[122] *méwel; surya*; proliferation of diseased blood (*nad khrag 'phel ba*); proliferation of bone marrow (*rkang mar*); and lymph gland *dré* (*'bras rmen*) from the chapter on lymph disorders (*rmen bu'i nad*) as well as the subcategory spreading condition (*byer ba*), dispersing or spreading, in proliferating "metabolic disruptions."

In the next section, I will briefly analyze how biomedical categories of cancer map onto these Tibetan medical categories by looking at three instructive conditions—skin cancer, leukemia, and lymphoma describing how they are etiologically and diagnostically distinguished.

9.1 *Skin Cancer and* Méwel

Skin cancer provides an illustrative case when considering its place in the Tibetan medical nosological system because there is no skin *dré* beyond what I have described above in the *Four Tantras*, Desi Sanggyé Gyatso's *Oral Instructions Supplement*, and Samten's modern synthesis regarding

---

119 G.yu thog yon tan mgon po, *Bdud rtsi snying po yan lag brgyad pa gsang ba man ngag gi rgyud*, 169: *byer bas dug mdze me dbal 'or du lhung/ 'bras dang sur ya dreg dang grum bu dang/ mig ser rts skran rkang 'bam du mar 'gyur/.*

120 "Channels" (*rtsa*) also include ligaments (*chu ba*) and tendons (*rgyus pa*), as seen in the white channel category that includes *chu rtsa, rlung rtsa, dbang rtsa, rgyus rtsa*, and *srog rtsa dkar po*. See Zur mkhar pa blo gros rgyal po, *Rgyud bzhi'i 'grel pa mes po'i zhal lung* (Beijing: Krung go'i pod kyi shes rig dpe skrun khang, 2005), 205, 216–7; Sangs rgyas rgya mtsho, *Gso ba rig pa'i bstan bcos sman bla'i dgongs rgyan rgyud bzhi'i gsal byed bai durya sngon po'i malli ka* [Blue Beryl] (Dharamsala: Tibetan Medical & Astro Institute, 1994); 'Jam dbyangs bkra shis, *Bod kyi gso ba rig pa'i 'bras nad*, 39.

121 *Béken* throat obstructions (*bad kan mgul 'gags*) are a specific disease category within the *béken* default system that have a similar etiology to *dré* of the stomach and esophagus, in which esophageal *dré* are one of the most predominant forms and thus often described as synonymous conditions.

122 Sangs rgyas rgya mtsho, *Man ngag yon tan rgyud kyi lhan thabs*; Lha mo skyabs, *Bod lugs 'bras nad gso rig*, 110.

obstructed hair follicles. Although skin (*pags pa*) is not enumerated among the seven bodily constituents (*lus zungs*),[123] it is recognized as a region specific to *tripa* pathways and activities. In short, the skin is one of the regions where *tripa* resides.[124]

Since the skin (*pags pa*) in the *Four Tantras* is subsumed under the same functionality as muscle (*sha*)—to cover the body—as described above, one might initially consider skin cancer as a type of "flesh *dré*" (*sha 'bras*), where "flesh" is being used here as a hybrid skin/muscle term instead of its common use as a muscle/fat substance: "Specifically, flesh *dré* resembles a frozen moist turnip."[125] One would also assume that it shares the general diagnostics of "a subtle trembling pulse"[126] for all *dré* that manifest externally, as well as their characterization: "swollen, hard, and stiff, and manifesting little pain."[127] It would also have all the subtypes of *dréné: rlung, tripa*, blood, *béken*, wound-induced (*mtshon 'bras*), and small bird egg-sized (*bye 'bras*).[128]

However, I propose that the category of *méwel* in its aggressive form has a more instructive and convincing link to biomedical conceptions of skin cancer, and as many contemporary Tibetan physicians frequently note, more mild forms of *méwel* link to the biomedical clinical presentation of *Herpes simplex* as well as other inflammatory dermal conditions and infections.[129] *Méwel* is described as a disorder of burn-like irritations on superficial parts of the external and

---

123 The *Bod lugs gso rig tshig mdzod chen mo* does not define "skin" or "bodily constituent" well. The *Yutok Gonggyen* (Dbang 'dus, *Gso ba rig pa'i tshig mdzod g.yu thog dgongs rgyan* [Beijing: Mi rigs dpe skrun khang, 1973], 602) does not define skin well, but it does refer to several accounts of the bodily constituents: *lus zungs/ byang pa rnam rgyal grags bzang gis mdzad pa'i bshad rgyud kyi 'grel ba bdud rtsi'i chu rgyun las/ lus 'dzin par byed pa'i phyir lus zungs zhes so/ zhes dang/ zla zer las/ zungs kyi sgra ni 'dzin pa'i don no/ zhes gsungs so/.* Thus, the bodily constituents are those which uphold the body, a repository for the body.

124 As described in the *Explanatory Tantra*, G.yu thog yon tan mgon po, *Rtsa ba'i rgyud bshad pa'i rgyud phyi ma'i rgyud kha skong dang bcas pa*, 79: "The regions in which *tripa* resides include the navel, stomach, blood, sweat, nutritional essence, chuser, eyes, and skin" (*mkhris gnas lte ba pho ba khrag dang rngul/ dwangs ma chu ser mig dang pags pa ste/*).

125 G.yu thog yon tan mgon po, *Bdud rtsi snying po yan lag brgyad pa gsang ba man ngag gi rgyud*, 400: *khyad par sha 'bras nyung gsher 'khyags pa 'dra/.*

126 G.yu thog yon tan mgon po, *Bdud rtsi snying po yan lag brgyad pa gsang ba man ngag gi rgyud*, 400: *rtsa rgyud phra la 'dar/.*

127 G.yu thog yon tan mgon po, *Bdud rtsi snying po yan lag brgyad pa gsang ba man ngag gi rgyud*, 400: *skrangs pa sra brtan na zug chung la/.*

128 A "small bird egg-sized" type of *dréné* (*bye 'bras*) is glossed as the size and shape of a small bird's egg (*bye 'bras kyi rtags ni/ 'bras nad gang yang sgrangs pa'i dbyibs dang che chung bye'u'i sgo nga tsam*).

129 Personal communications, Menpa Gyamtso (*rgya mtsho*), Taktsang Lhamo Kirti Monastery (*stag tshang lha mo kirti dgon*); Menpa Sangee Bohm (*sangs rgyas 'bum*), Qinghai Provincial Tibetan Medical Hospital Skin Department, July 2018.

internal body that have a proclivity to spread.[130] Earlier, we have discussed how the term "skin" in the *Four Tantras* refers to external skin as well as the superficial layers on organs: "Sites where *méwel* manifest include the skin and vital organs, specifically the heart."[131] The *Four Tantras* describes the *méwel* etiology as follows: "By means of diet, behavior, and non-human external influences (*gdon*), blood and *tripa* proliferate and *chuser* and heat are aggravated by *rlung* [to produce *méwel*]."[132] Here, we see links to the six characteristics outlined above with aggravated *rlung*, blood, and *tripa* proliferation from the wound-derived etiology. Since skin conditions (*lpags nad*) in the *Four Tantras* are considered to arise from disturbances by microorganisms (*srin*); serous, interstitial and pre-lymphatic fluid metabolic imbalances (*chu ser*); harmful non-human external influences (*gdon*); and disruptions in the three default systems;[133] *méwel* has a particular association with the skin and superficial layers of organs.

From the biomedical understanding, skin cancer develops from abnormal cells in the skin and has the capacity to spread to other areas of the body. The three major types develop from the epithelia (squamous cell skin cancer [SCSC]), basal lamina (basal cell skin cancer [BCSC]), and melanocytes (melanoma). BSCS grows slowly and can damage surrounding tissue but is unlikely to spread to distant regions or result in death. It is often painless and may be shiny with blood vessels running over it or raised like an ulcer. SCSC is more likely to spread and has a hard lump with scaly top, but can also manifest as an ulcer. Melanomas are the most aggressive, starting as a mole that changes size, shape and color, has irregular edges and variegated coloring and can be itchy or bleed.[134] Each of these types can have a wound-like (ulcer) or burn-like appearance on the skin similar in description to *méwel*. Compared to *dréné*, even

130 G.yu thog yon tan mgon po, *Bdud rtsi snying po yan lag brgyad pa gsang ba man ngag gi rgyud*, 407: "Producing external burn-like wounds that spread" (*phyir byung mes tshig rma dang 'dra zhing mched/*).

131 G.yu thog yon tan mgon po, *Bdud rtsi snying po yan lag brgyad pa gsang ba man ngag gi rgyud*, 407: *gnas ni pags pa don snying rnams la gnas/*.

132 G.yu thog yon tan mgon po, *Bdud rtsi snying po yan lag brgyad pa gsang ba man ngag gi rgyud*, 407: *rgyu rkyen zas spyod gdon gyis khrag mkhris 'phel/ chu ser tsha ba rlung gis bus pa'o/*.

133 G.yu thog yon tan mgon po, *Bdud rtsi snying po yan lag brgyad pa gsang ba man ngag gi rgyud*, 396: "Skin conditions are produced by the accumulation of *sin* and *chuser* in the body, along with a disturbance in *dön* and *duwa*" (*rgyu ni srin dang chu ser 'phel ba la/ gdon dang 'du ba 'khrugs pas lpags nad skyed/*), where *duwa* are the balanced forms the functional default systems, properly termed "*nyépa*" when experiencing dysfunction.

134 Sajjad Rajpar and Jerry Marsden, *ABC of Skin Cancer* (Malden, MA: Blackwell Publishing, 2008).

if "skin *dré*" were subsumed within "flesh *dré*," *méwel* provides a more consistent skin-specific etiology in the *Four Tantras* and a skin cancer presentation of morphology and symptoms.

In *The New Dawn Compendium of Medicine*, Samten creates a new seemingly redundant category called "wound *dré*" (*rma 'bras*) in which he locates skin wounds of the limbs, trunk, face, neck, and so forth, to presumably provide a categorical link in *dréné* to skin cancer.[135] Additionally, he places *méwel* under skin illnesses (*pags pa'i nad*). This is an instructive modern move in shifting the nosology of *méwel* and delineating a separate category under *drétren* called wound *dré*. Samten omits internal *méwel*, such as that which affects the internal organs, from his depiction to present it as an exclusively skin-specific disorder, and minimizes its intensity to focus on its rash-like spreading forms. Thus, one can say that wound *dré* provides the territory onto which Samten maps biomedical conceptions of skin cancer, without distinctions for how to map different types based on the Tibetan diagnostic paradigm. However, the redundancy of adding "wound" to *dré* seems unnecessary to create a new category for skin cancer; and the re-characterization of *méwel* as a mild external skin condition facilitates his focus of a categorical collapse in linking cancer to *drétren* and recasts *méwel* accordingly. It is interesting to note that Samten's reframing of *méwel* informs prevalent clinical diagnostics of *méwel* today, as mentioned above, for various biomedical *Herpes* virus clinical presentations.

9.2 Surya *as a* Dréné *Cousin and Better Candidate for Many Carcinomas*

In the *Four Tantras*, *surya*, a Tibetan transliteration for the Sanskrit term "sun," indicates a disorder in which irregularly-shaped external or internal sores form with streaks or heterogeneous edges like the rays of the sun and tend to spread along channels and re-erupt in other regions of the body.[136] Such internal and external sores tend to ulcerate and leak pus, blood, and abnormal (literally, "putrid") flesh.[137] Its etiology arises from excess proliferation of blood due to dietary and lifestyle conditions; blood quality disturbances due to injury, trauma, or improper venesection; contagious disease (*rims nad*); toxins; and excess

135 Bsam gtan, *Gso rig snying bsdus skya rengs gsar pa*, 280: *nad rtags ni thog mar pags pa mthug po chags pa nas rim bzhin skrangs 'bur chen po don dang/ skrang po mkhregs shing 'bar 'bur yin par dkyil ngos nas rma khung rdol te dri ngan can gyi khrag ngan chu ser 'dzad med 'dzags te/ nyung ma 'khyags/.*

136 G.yu thog yon tan mgon po, *Bdud rtsi snying po yan lag brgyad pa gsang ba man ngag gi rgyud*, 408; Shes rab chos 'phel, ed., *Lhan skyes rma gso ba* [Coemergent Wounds Treatment] (Beijing: Mi rigs dpe skrun khang, 2011), 46.

137 G.yu thog yon tan mgon po, *Bdud rtsi snying po yan lag brgyad pa gsang ba man ngag gi rgyud*, 408.

heat in the channels that has not been properly therapeutically released. Such causal conditions lead to the development of poor blood quality and serous fluid imbalances that collect in the vital and vessel organs as well as the blood vessels, lymph vessels, and nerve channels. *Rlung* aggravation[138] compounds these processes, and the consequent swelling and pus lead to the formation of a *dré*-like growths.[139] *Surya* relates to the six characteristics of cancer in its *rlung* aggravation, proliferating *tripa*-derived blood abnormalities, and trauma- or pathogen-inflicted wound etiology.

Furthermore, as described above, *surya* arises from the spreading (*byer ba*) condition of nutritional essence metabolic disruptions like *dréné, méwel,* and *tren* of the blood vessels, lymph, and neural channels. Along with *méwel,* it specifically indicates the ability to spread throughout the body along these channels, which is not explicitly described for *dréné* or *tren*. *Surya* primarily affects the lungs, liver, stomach, colon, and kidneys, and specifically affects the skin (*pags pa*) and muscle (*sha*) constituents of the body, such as with skin cancer, and cancers of the superficial cell layers. Likewise, distinctly compared to *dréné, surya* explicitly enters and affects the vessels of the body, which provide an etiological relationship to cancers of the blood vessels, neural tissues, and lymph glands, such as lymphomas.

Here, we return to the concept of skin and muscle in the *Four Tantras* as also applying to layers of the vital and vessel organs, as well as external protective layer of skin, such as with epithelial and endothelial cells in the biomedical designation. As described above, epithelial cells are the outermost layer of skin, but also line cavities and surfaces of organs and blood vessels throughout the body.[140] Endothelium is a specialized form of epithelium which lines

---

138 G.yu thog yon tan mgon po, *Rgyud chung bdud rtsi snying po* [The Ambrosia Essence Smaller Tantra], in *Cha lag bco brgyad* [Eighteen Supplements] (Beijing: Mi rigs dpe sgrun khang, 2005), 534.

139 G.yu thog yon tan mgon po, *Bdud rtsi snying po yan lag brgyad pa gsang ba man ngag gi rgyud*, 408: *gyur tshul zas spyod gyis khrag 'phel dang/ mtshon khrag lus dang 'grams khrag gtar ma 'chun/ rims dug tsha ba rtsar babs ma gtar bas/ khrag ngan chu ser don snod rtsa mig 'dus/.*

140 Various types of epithelial cells occur. For example, simple squamous epithelium comprise the air sacs in the lungs, the lining of the heart, blood vessels and lymphatic vessels; simple cuboidal epithelium reside in the secretory glands and kidney tubules; simple columnar epithelium are ciliated tissues in bronchi, uterine tubes and uterus and smooth types along the digestive tract; pseudostratified columnar epithelium line the trachea and upper respiratory tract; stratified squamous epithelium line the esophagus, mouth and vagina; and stratified cuboidal epithelium comprise the sweat glands, salivary glands and mammary glands; among others (Sylvia Mader and Michael Windelspecht, *Human Biology* [New York, NY: McGraw-Hill Education, 2015]).

various blood and lymphatic vessels. Epithelial layers contain no blood vessels, so they must receive nourishment from the underlying connective tissue and the various substances diffused from the basement membrane.

From the physiological development of constituents in the *Four Tantras*, muscle arises from blood. Since skin is seen to cover muscle, a reasonable corollary would be muscle as the endothelial and underlying connective tissues (again, recall the "wrapping" function of muscle in the *Four Tantras*). Due to the abnormal growth of skin and muscle constituents of the external surfaces of the body, as well as vital and vessel organs, and blood, lymph and neural vessels, *surya* must be added to the set of diseases in the Tibetan medical canon onto which biomedical malignant and benign neoplasms are mapped, and may be the primary candidate onto which most carcinomas and adenocarcinomas map.[141]

9.3 *Leukemia and Nutritional Essence Metabolic Disturbances*

Leukemia has provided a stumbling block for many Tibetan physicians discussing how cancer maps into the Tibetan medical nosology and how we, as Tibetan physicians, understand and approach conditions of leukemia clinically. On one hand, many physicians assert that leukemia is merely blood *dré* (*khrag 'bras*), one of the classic types described in the *Four Tantras* mentioned earlier. However, the *Four Tantras* describes *dré* derived from blood (*khrag las gyur pa'i 'bras nad*) as primarily forming *dréné* of the breast (*nu ma*) and uterus (*mngal*). In describing the medicine compounding for treating *dré* derived from blood and *tripa*, the *Four Tantras* states: "[*Dré* derived from] blood and *tripa* [is treated with the orchid] *pushel-tsé*,[142] *Rubia manjith*,[143] the three [sacred]

141 This is because, as described above, ninety percent of cancers arise from epithelial cells as squamous cell carcinomas and adenocarcinomas (Cooper, *Elements of Human Cancer*, 17). Interestingly, Samten does not include *surya* in any of the categories in the *The New Dawn* (Bsam gtan, *Gso rig snying bsdus skya rengs gsar pa*, 1–16). This disease has eluded many Tibetan physicians with whom I spoke in India as well as in central and eastern Tibet, perhaps due to the unfamiliarity with organ morphologies affected by cancer that might present more as a *surya* condition. I speculate that Samten's motivation to leave out *surya* stems from an effort to streamline Tibetan nosology to provide one-to-one correlations with that of biomedicine, which is the method this article challenges.

142 *Coelogyne corymbosa* (*pu shel rtse*), *Dendrobium densiflorum* (*smyug pu shel rtse*). See Tshe ring nor bu, *Bod lugs gso ba rig pa'i skye dngos sman rdzas sngo 'bum kun btus* [Comprehensive Collection of Tibetan Medical Biological Specimens] (Dharamsala: Men-Tsee-Khang, 2013), 391.

143 On *Rubia manjith* (*btsod*), see Tshe ring nor bu, *Bod lugs gso ba rig pa'i skye dngos sman rdzas sngo 'bum kun btus*, 187. Species identification based on specimens used at Dharamsala Men-Tsee-Khang.

fruits,[144] pine resin,[145] licorice,[146] turmeric,[147] a *Berberis* species,[148] black juniper berries,[149] and common juniper berries."[150] Likewise, in the skin illnesses chapter of the *Oral Instructions Tantra*, it says: "The two yellows, *Saussurea lappa*,[151] *dukmo-nyung*,[152] and smoky mineral exudate treat blister conditions, vitiligo, rashes, and all skin conditions without exception."[153] Here, "the two yellows" are the familiar turmeric (*yung ba*) and *Berberis* species (*skyer pa*), as found in the treatment for the blood-derived *dréné*. Thus, it might appear that from the treatment perspective, one would link *dré* derived from blood more to skin cancer than cancers of biomedical blood or bone marrow.[154]

---

144 On *Terminalia chebula, Terminalia bellerica, Emblica officinalis* (*a ru ra, ba ru ra, skyu ru ra*), see Tshe ring nor bu, *Bod lugs gso ba rig pa'i skye dngos sman rdzas sngo 'bum kun btus*. Species identification based on specimens used at Dharamsala Men-Tsee-Khang.

145 On pine resin (*shel ta* = Chi. *songxiang* 松香), see Dga' ba rdo rje, *'Khrungs dpe dri med shel gyi me long* [Mirror of Crystal Pure Living Specimens] (Beijing: Mi rigs dpe skrun khang, 2011), 126.

146 On *Glycyrhiza glabra* (*shing mngar*), see Tshe ring nor bu, *Bod lugs gso ba rig pa'i skye dngos sman rdzas sngo 'bum kun btus*, 345. Species identification based on specimens used at Dharamsala Men-Tsee-Khang.

147 On *Curcuma longa* (*yung ba*), see Tshe ring nor bu, *Bod lugs gso ba rig pa'i skye dngos sman rdzas sngo 'bum kun btus*, 283. Species identification based on specimens used at Dharamsala Men-Tsee-Khang.

148 On *Berberis* spp (*skyer pa*), see Tshe ring nor bu, *Bod lugs gso ba rig pa'i skye dngos sman rdzas sngo 'bum kun btus*, 82, 84. Species identification based on specimens used at Dharamsala Men-Tsee-Khang.

149 On *Juniperus indica* (*spa 'brum*), see Tshe ring nor bu, *Bod lugs gso ba rig pa'i skye dngos sman rdzas sngo 'bum kun btus*, 402. Species identification based on specimens used at Dharamsala Men-Tsee-Khang.

150 On *Juniperus communis* (*shug 'bru*), see Tshe ring nor bu, *Bod lugs gso ba rig pa'i skye dngos sman rdzas sngo 'bum kun btus*, 355. Species identification based on specimens used at Dharamsala Men-Tsee-Khang. G.yu thog yon tan mgon po, *Bdud rtsi snying po yan lag brgyad pa gsang ba man ngag gi rgyud*, 404: *khrag mkhris pu shel rtse btsod 'bras bu gsum/ shel ta shing mngar yung skyer spa shug 'bru/*.

151 On *Saussurea lappa* (*ru rta*), see Tshe ring nor bu, *Bod lugs gso ba rig pa'i skye dngos sman rdzas sngo 'bum kun btus*, 310. Species identification based on specimens used at Dharamsala Men-Tsee-Khang.

152 On *Holarrhena floribunda, Wrightia tinctoria*, and *W. tomentosa* (*dug mo nyung*), see Tshe ring nor bu, *Bod lugs gso ba rig pa'i skye dngos sman rdzas sngo 'bum kun btus*, 340–41. Species identification based on specimens used at Dharamsala Men-Tsee-Khang.

153 G.yu thog yon tan mgon po, *Bdud rtsi snying po yan lag brgyad pa gsang ba man ngag gi rgyud*, 397: *ser po gnyis dang ru rta dug mo nyung/ dud pa'i lde gus shu ba bkra dang/ g.yan pa lpags nad ma lus sel bar 'gyur/*.

154 The way the Tibetan medical tradition understands blood (*khrag*) compared to biomedical understandings of blood is a topic that warrants a separate discussion beyond the scope of the present chapter.

Menpa Khyenrab Gyamtso,[155] former Vice Principal and one of the senior lecturers of Dharamsala Men-Tsee-Khang, with experience seeing patients in Europe, north America and throughout India, explained leukemia through the lens of "metabolic disruptions of the nutritional essence" and its spreading condition (*byer ba*), or *dréné*-producing variant. He said that although the *Four Tantras* may not specifically describe an illness with a one-to-one correlation with biomedical leukemia, one must think about how Tibetan medicine understands the formation of abnormal constituents in the body, and Tibetan medicine's unique perspective on blood (*khrag*). He is a strong proponent of adhering to the Tibetan medical paradigm as presented in the *Four Tantras* and its commentaries—its distinct epistemology—and not dismissing it to privilege explanations more akin to biomedicine; although he also identifies mapping biomedical conditions into Tibetan medicine as important for collaborative discussions with science and biomedicine. He says that leukemia would be a classic manifestation of the spreading (*byer ba*) condition of "metabolic disruptions" because the genesis of healthy, life-sustaining blood (*zungs khrag*) is not properly developed in the body. Thus, from a treatment perspective, we would need to treat the "metabolic disruptions" and the inability of the body to produce proper blood, which Tibetan medical physicians see as stemming from the liver (*mchin pa*).

An initial analysis might interpret leukemia in Tibetan medical terms as proliferation of the white constituents in blood (*khrag dkar 'phel ba*).[156] Since blood is developed from nutritional essence, and the fluid that becomes blood is not termed so until it transits through the liver and gains the proper constituents and qualities, the condition of deficiency of blood (*khrag zad pa*) in the *Four Tantras*[157] could be understood as an imbalance in the body, which impairs the capacity to produce proper healthy blood. The symptoms associated with a deficiency of blood are described as "slackening of the channels, rough skin, and a yearning for cold and sour foods."[158] For both acute and chronic leukemia, common symptoms include excessive bleeding, easy bruising, frequent

155 Khenrab Gyamtso, personal communication, 2015.

156 See, for example, discussion in Tawni Tidwell [Rangjung Lhamo], "Phi lugs gso rig gi kan sar (Cancer) zhes pa'i nad rigs de bod lugs gso rig gi 'bras nad dang surya skran rigs gang la sbyar rung bar dpyad pa" [A Comparative Analysis: Mapping Biomedical Cancer into Tibetan Medical Etiological Categories], *Bod man slob gso dang zhib 'jug* [Tibetan Medical Education and Research Journal] 4 (2016): 98–113.

157 As described in the chapter on "Defining Characteristics of Illnesses" in the second part of the *Four Tantras* (G.yu thog yon tan mgon po, *Rtsa ba'i rgyud bshad pa'i rgyud phyi ma'i rgyud kha skong dang bcas pa*, 79–85).

158 G.yu thog yon tan mgon po, *Rtsa ba'i rgyud bshad pa'i rgyud phyi ma'i rgyud kha skong dang bcas pa*, 82: *khrag zad rtsa lhod lpags rtsub bsil skyur dang /*.

infections, joint/bone pain and tenderness, night sweats and fevers, enlarged spleen and lymph nodes, fatigue, loss of appetite, muscle weakness, shortness of breath, and weight loss. Thus, the symptoms for blood deficiency do not match those for leukemia.

Proliferation of bone marrow (*rkang 'phel*), as described in the *Four Tantras*, might also provide a likely strong candidate. Its symptoms are described as "a feeling of heaviness in one's body from proliferation of vitality essence (*bcud*) throughout the whole body causing difficulty moving, sitting, flexing or extending; poor eyesight, and thickening and enlargement of bone heads and thicker regions at joint sections."[159] Although "bone marrow proliferation" is a more likely candidate onto which to map leukemia from the biomedical etiological perspective, the associated symptoms do not encompass the breadth of the biomedical symptoms for leukemia nor the severity that, say, *dréné* would. These distinctions highlight the etiologic differences in each system.

A final category of blood proliferation (*khrag 'phel ba*) provides a likely association. The *Four Tantras* describes this condition: "Blood proliferation manifests as *méwel*, internal *dré*, spleen disorders, leprosy (*mdze*), *tren*, blood and *tripa* disorders, jaundice, gum illnesses, difficulty moving, and reddening of the eyes, urine, and skin."[160] Here we see a theoretical framework for an underlying condition that drives the formation of both *dréné*, *méwel*, and *tren* and can provide a useful understanding for commonalities among these conditions, including leukemia, skin cancer, and lymphoma. Since leukemia rarely forms aggregations or masses, except secondary to accumulations at lymph nodes, it would not be considered a *tren* or a *dréné* from the Tibetan medical perspective. However, as Khyenrab Gyamtso identifies, here is the etiological link to "metabolic disruptions of the nutritional essence" and its spreading condition (*byer ba*), as a collection of related illnesses that includes *dréné* in the Tibetan medical epistemology and ontology.

---

159 G.yu thog yon tan mgon po, *Rtsa ba'i rgyud bshad pa'i rgyud phyi ma'i rgyud kha skong dang bcas pa*, 81: *rkang 'phel lus lci mig g.yung tshigs kha sbom/*. Further explained in Khro ru tshe rnam, *Gso rig rgyud bzhi'i 'grel chen drang srong zhal lung* [The Great Commentary on the *Four Tantras*: Oral Instructions of the Sages] (Chengdu: Si khron mi rigs dpe sgrun khang, 2000), 257: *rkang 'phel ba'i rtags su lus yongs la bcud kyis khyab pa'i stobs kyis lus lci ba ste 'gro 'dug dang 'gul skyod la sogs pa dka' zhing/ mig g.yung ba ste gsal por mi mthong ba dang/ tshigs kha ste tshigs mdud kyi mgo bo rnams sbom zhing che bar 'gyur ba/*.

160 G.yu thog yon tan mgon po, *Rtsa ba'i rgyud bshad pa'i rgyud phyi ma'i rgyud kha skong dang bcas pa*, 80–81: *khrag 'phel me dbal khong 'bras mcher pa'i nad/ mdze skran khrag mkhris nad dang mig ser dang/ rnyil nad skyod dka' mig dang gcin lpags dmar/*.

9.4 *Lymphoma and Lymph* Dré

In the *New Dawn Compendium of Medicine*, Samten keeps the category of lymph illnesses (*rmen bu'i nad*) within the "Coemergent Wounds" (*lhan skyes rma*) section of illnesses to which *dréné, méwel,* and *surya* belong classically. However, he focuses on a new addition called "rapid-spreading infectious disease" (*gnyan nad 'khyam po*), taken from the description Desi Sanggyé Gyatso provides in the *Oral Instructions Supplement.* Samten focuses on the association with infection (*gnyan nad*), but also recognizes its potential for gaining a nature of chronic illness or mass accumulation, as with *dréné*. Here the classic signs of lymphoma are even described: swelling at lymph nodes and at joints; fevers, significant sweats, and ease of infection; lethargy, malaise, and weight loss; and itching. Samten even distinguishes *rlung, tripa,* and *béken* variants in this case.[161] This etiologic link relates to the condition of abnormal blood proliferation in the case of leukemia, where an internal *dré* manifests in the lymph glands that at times forms actual *tren* or *dré*-like masses, and at other times remains in the antecedent condition.

However, the *Four Tantras* outlines an appropriate category within the lymph gland disorders chapter of lymph *dré*,[162] as described earlier, which retains the same etiologic underpinnings of blood and *rlung* compounding metabolic disruptions, such as with *dréné, tren, méwel,* and *surya*. I argue that the classic category of lymph *dré* in the *Four Tantras*, with the broader context of nutritional essence metabolic disturbance, is a sufficient correlate for biomedical lymphoma. Though this lymphoma-lymph *dré* link appears to be a one-to-one relationship between the biomedical category and Tibetan medical category, it retains the contemporary epistemological and ontological distinctions of each respective tradition's units of analysis, pathways, and systems, such as the *nyépa* in the *Four Tantras*, and the larger etiological contexts. The infection addition of Desi Sanggyé Gyatso situates a subclass of lymph gland disorders related to infection but is unnecessary in the depiction of lymphoma.

10 Shared Commonalities with Biomedical Cancer and Neoplasms

The pathology of *dré*, channel *tren, méwel, surya,* and blood proliferation disorders engage several common processes central to the Tibetan medical understanding of similar disease origins and trajectories, specifically digestive

---

161 Bsam gtan, *Gso rig snying bsdus skya rengs gsar pa*, 321.

162 G.yu thog yon tan mgon po, *Bdud rtsi snying po yan lag brgyad pa gsang ba man ngag gi rgyud*, 409–11.

and metabolic processing and blockages; the relationship between digestion and the differential managing of "nutrients" (*dwangs ma*) and "waste products" (*snyigs ma*) specific to blood production-metabolism; and pathogenic relationships to these processes. Additionally, they all draw upon disturbances to nutritional essence metabolism, with compounding conditions of coarse and subtle levels of specific physiologic pathways disruptions, due to their connection to blood impurities and *rlung* aggravation.

Their etiology also provides convincing resemblance to the six defining characteristics for biomedical cancer. As cellular hyperplasia, which is recognized as the disturbed, pathological growth of cells,[163] which the term neoplasm denotes, biomedical cancer is understood to result from a set of mutations that produce oncogenes allowing a dominant gain in function and tumor suppressor genes inducing a recessive loss of function. Its origins are understood to be a complex array of layers deriving from genetic, environmental, social, psychological, dietary, and related factors. Oncogenesis and tumor formation are seen to be a multi-step and co-emergent process that generates these genetic alterations with multiple rate-limiting steps producing these incremental growth advantages, as we see in the compounding conditions that incite or diffuse each of the conditions in the *Four Tantras* presented.[164]

Furthermore, it is interesting to note that the language of co-emergent wounds in the biomedical literature around cancer is prolific[165]—even to the extent of a "genetic lesion." A lesion is seen as circuit injury in which the cell must follow reprogrammed circuitry from the incurred damage and repair.[166] This might sound similar to the overarching category of "coemergent wounds" (*lhan skyes rma*) in which *dréné, méwel*, and *surya* are subcategories. The idea of multiple conditions coming together to form biomedical cancer might also sound familiar from the Tibetan medical perspective, since the use of the term "coemergent" (*lhan skyes*), again as in the name of this larger category, to describe the lesion and development of *dréné, méwel*, and *surya* is also common.

As Hanahan and Weinberg describe the six characteristics a cell must procure in order to become malignant, not all cancer cells acquire each characteristic

163 Mukherjee, *The Emperor of All Maladies*, 340.

164 Hanahan and Weinberg, "The Hallmarks of Cancer," 57.

165 See for instance H. F. Dvorak, "Tumors: Wounds That Do Not Heal," *New England Journal of Medicine* 315 (1986): 1650–59; J. W. Harper and S. J. Elledge, "The DNA Damage Response: Ten Years After," *Molecular Cell* 28 (2007): 739–45; A. F. Hezel and N. Bardeesy, "LKB1; Linking Cell Structure and Tumor Suppression," *Oncogene* 27 (2008): 6908–19; M. Schäfer and S. Werner, "Cancer as an Overhealing Wound: An Old Hypothesis Revisited," *Nature Reviews Molecular Cell Biology* 9 (2008): 628–38.

166 Hanahan and Weinberg, "The Hallmarks of Cancer," 66.

by the same chronology or mechanism.[167] Similarly, Tibetan medicine describes that the conditions that must assemble in order to produce *tren, dréné, méwel,* or *surya* can come in variable combinations and sequences. Much of the research on cancer has focused on cancer cells propagated in culture and dissected into molecular components; however, the biological reality of tumor formation shows that it is not just an isolated event driven by cell-autonomous processes. Instead, most tumors removed from a living person, including their metastatic outgrowths, are complex mixtures of several cell types within a tissue mass,[168] similar to the complex mass described as *dré* in the *Four Tantras* and its commentaries that are likened to a gnarled mass growing on a tree with a distorted aggregation of combined bodily constituent types (i.e., varied cells types). Although one type of constituent predominates the genesis of the *dréné* mass, the mass itself is a "whorl" of various bodily constituents that get aggregated. Thus, the characteristics needed to form masses would necessarily require different bodily constituent types to co-constitute the aggregation. For instance, "nutrients" develop "the objects that incur injury" (*gnod bya*), that is, the seven bodily constituents and three excrements.[169] Blood moistens, fat lubricates, bone supports and stabilizes, bone marrow transforms regenerative essence (*bcud*), the distilled vital essence required by the body for sustenance and growth, and the regenerative constituents that hold the reproductive seed in the womb.[170] Contributions from several of the bodily constituents are needed to generate an aggregation in the body for *tren, dréné, méwel, surya,* and the other mapped conditions because of the compounded etiology derived from the proliferation of improper blood and aggravated condition of *rlung*, which can theoretically affect all bodily constituents.[171] The diagram below provides the correlated conditions from the *Four Tantras* and its commentaries in which I propose relate most closely to biomedical conceptions of cancer.

Such a mapping highlights the etiological and categorical similarities and distinctions between the two systems. As such, practitioners and researchers

167 Hanahan and Weinberg, "The Hallmarks of Cancer," 66.

168 Hanahan and Weinberg, "The Hallmarks of Cancer," 67.

169 G.yu thog yon tan mgon po, *Bdud rtsi snying po yan lag brgyad pa gsang ba man ngag gi rgyud*, 54: *de la dwangs mas gnod bya 'phel bar byed.* The "agents producing the harm" (*gnod byed*) are the three default systems.

170 G.yu thog yon tan mgon po, *Rtsa ba'i rgyud bshad pa'i rgyud phyi ma'i rgyud kha skong dang bcas pa*, 54: *khrag gis brlan srog 'tsho sha yis g.yogs/ tshil gyis snum dang rus pas brten pa dang/ rkang gis bcud 'gyur khu bas mngal 'dzin byed/.*

171 G.yu thog yon tan mgon po, *Bdud rtsi snying po yan lag brgyad pa gsang ba man ngag gi rgyud*, 400.

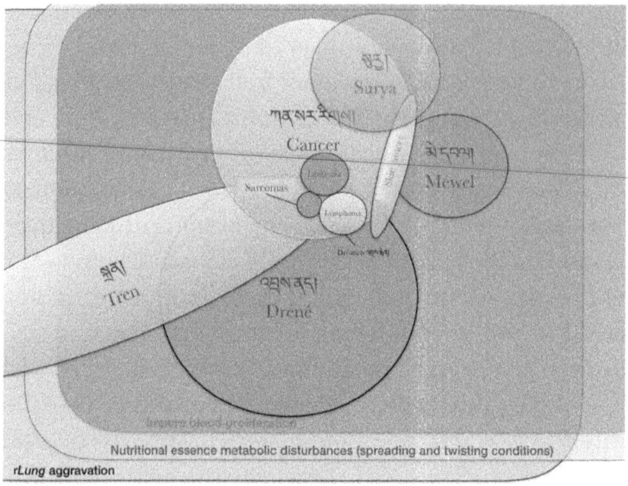

FIGURE 5.1 Biomedical cancer and correlating Tibetan medical conditions

from both systems can more explicitly dialogue on contributions in diagnostics and treatment from each approach.

10.1 *Potential Contributions to Biomedical Conceptions of Cancer*

From the biomedical understanding, it is not completely certain whether cancer cells have true autonomy—ancillary cells, such as fibroblasts and endothelial cells, have received little attention and may play an important role in the cell-to-cell (paracrine) and systemic (endocrine) signals.[172] As highlighted above, cellular signaling is understood by contemporary Tibetan physicians to be controlled by *rlung* functions. Thus, excess, deficiency, and abnormalities in such signaling would likely have *rlung* imbalance origins as described in the *Four Tantras*. The mapping between Tibetan medical and biomedical disease etiologies allows for contributions from the Tibetan medical paradigm to inform biomedical analyses of cancer development. From the Tibetan medical perspective, these overlooked cells in the biomedical paradigm could potentially play a critical role in cancer modulation vis-à-vis the etiological links I have outlined above between cancer and *dréné, tren, méwel, surya,* and the various related metabolic disturbances, as well as the high association of *rlung* activity with that of the different subtle signaling pathways, which would correlate to these aspects of the neuroendocrine system. Thus, I argue that biomedical physicians could potentially benefit from considering the Tibetan

172 Hanahan and Weinberg, "The Hallmarks of Cancer," 59.

medical insights of these disorders highlighted here by placing greater attention on these overlooked cells and the role they may place in cancer genesis. From a treatment perspective, calming the *rlung* would have an intimate relationship with the continued incitation of growth among the cancer cells, which has been seen in the Tibetan medical treatments of cancer reviewed by Bauer-Wu and colleagues.[173] Furthermore, inflammatory cells may be assisting cancer cells rather than suppressing them.[174] This has yet to be studied well.

Likewise, the Tibetan medical approach of supporting proper blood generation and maintenance of normal bodily constituents may contribute to modes of managing angiogenesis in the early stages of cancer development. From what I have outlined above, Tibetan physicians' treatment of poor blood (*ngan khrag*) could be a critical target therapy in tumor treatment and suppression. The relentless quality of dominating the body's resources gives cancer the characteristic of insatiability in nutrient acquisition. Supporting proper nutritional essence metabolism from the Tibetan medical perspective is a target intervention to prevent the development of this defining characteristic that mobilizes cancer. Furthermore, since apoptotic pathways are still operative in cancer cells, Tibetan treatments used for cancer might restore such pathways through *rlung* treatments, as described above, and contribute to how etiological processes driving biomedical cancer might be viewed through the lens of the *Four Tantras*.

11 Conclusion

In this paper I have argued that *dréné* is not cancer, and *tren* are not synonymous to biomedical neoplasms. To conflate either of the two poses a serious threat to the etiological lenses with which each medical system sees the body. Many cancers can be *dréné* and vice versa; many neoplasms are *tren*, and vice versa. However, *méwel, surya*, and abnormal blood proliferation, and the related nutritional essence metabolic disturbances in the *Four Tantras* and its prominent commentaries provide a wider landscape onto which biomedical benign and malignant neoplasms map.

---

173 Bauer-Wu et al., "Tibetan Medicine for Cancer," 502–12.

174 Cordon-Cardo and Prives, "At the Crossroads of Inflammation and Tumorigenesis"; L. M. Coussens et al., "Inflammatory Mast Cells up-Regulate Angiogenesis during Squamous Epithelial Carcinogenesis," *Genes and Development* 13, no. 11 (1999): 1382–97; J. D. Hudson et al., "A Proinflammatory Cytokine Inhibits p53 Tumor Suppressor Activity," *The Journal of Experimental Medicine* 190, no. 10 (1999): 1375–82.

In conclusion, in order to facilitate discussions of various conditions between practitioners of Tibetan medicine and Euroamerican medicine, it is imperative to retain the nosologies of each medical tradition with their attendant epistemologies, such that the collapse of categories does not jettison the very paradigmatic and unique tools that Tibetan medicine can offer to the diagnostics and treatment of some of the most devastating illnesses of our time. By translating cancer as *drétren*, I argue that the epistemology based in the *Four Tantras* that Tibetan medical practitioners engage is lost, namely the view of how the mind and body integrally interrelate, the development of disease from the mental affliction roots that drive the three default systems, the role of digestive and metabolic function in the formation of all of the bodily constituents, and the relationship of the three default systems with each organ, bodily constituent, and excrement—as well as how each of these factors relate to diagnostics and treatment. Collapsing cancer into *dréné* would be like collapsing the immune system and the neuroendocrine system into understandings of *rlung*.

Differences in evidence according to those implementing contemporary epistemologies rooted in each tradition's intellectual history must be recognized. For example, Menpa Sönam Wangdü cautions Tibetan doctors against claiming to "cure" cancer since the measure for curing cancer would be not a single metastatic cell left.[175] However, this might not be the case for Tibetan medicine—if the condition is under control (in balance, so to speak) for the rest of the person's life, there still may be abnormal cells and tissues present without dysfunction or life threat.[176] The same holds for pathogens (*srin, srin 'bu*),[177] like viruses and bacteria. Tibetan medical practitioners might treat a condition but not eradicate populations of the pathogen. Euroamerican medicine practitioners are beginning to appreciate this approach. For example, a cutting-edge treatment for melanoma is done through bolstering the immune system exclusively, which also does not focus on eradication of metastatic cells, but boosting the body's own physiologic controls of proper cell production and elimination of abnormal cells.[178] Likewise, our understanding of the microbiome shows that eradicating populations of bacteria are not ideal in treating disease. Like the 84,000 *sin* (*srin*) that reside in our body,[179] which help digestion, increase bodily strength, and facilitate a healthy complexion, I am encouraged to see this Euroamerican medicine-Tibetan medicine link vis-à-vis

175 Czaja, "The *Four Tantras* and the Global Market," 276.

176 Actually, this approach is seen increasingly with some new biomedical perspectives on treating cancer. For example, see M. W. L. Teng et al., "Immune-mediated Dormancy."

177 See fn 37 for an explanation of this term.

178 See MD Anderson Cancer Center, "Immunotherapy: Research Platform for the Moon Shots Program"; for more on this approach.

179 See for instance, Czaja, "The *Four Tantras* and the Global Market," 289, n. 25.

recent microbiome research. Treating the body like a micro-ecosystem and returning balance provides a more optimum solution to health across the life course. Allowing for mapping approaches that encourage practitioners of each system to retain their distinct current epistemologies, etiologies, and nosologies is important in order to facilitate fruitful conversation between Euroamerican and Tibetan medicine, and for developing cogent comparisons of beneficial treatments and approaches for serious illness.

Bibliography

Tibetan-language Sources

Blo bzang 'phrin las. *Mkhas dbang dung dkar blo bzang 'phrin las mchog gis mdzad pa'i bod rig pa'i tshig mdzod chen mo shes bya rab gsal* [White Conch Dictionary]. Beijing: Krung go'i bod rig pa dpe skrun khang, 2002.

Bsam gtan. *Gso rig snying bsdus skya rengs gsar pa* [The New Dawn Compendium of Medicine]. Lhasa: Bod ljongs mi dmangs dpe skrun khang, 2013 [repr. 1985].

Bsod nams tse ring. *Dag yig gsar bsgrigs* [Orthographic Tibetan Dictionary]. Xining: Mtsho sngon mi rigs dpe sgrun khang, 1979.

Byams pa 'phrin las, ed. *Bod lugs gso rig tshig mdzod chen mo* [Great Tibetan Medical Dictionary]. Lhasa: Mi rigs dpe skrun khang, 2006.

Dga ba'i rab rje. *'Khrungs dpe dri med shel gyi me long* [Mirror of Crystal Pure Living Specimens]. Ed. by Chab mdos Khul sman rtsis Khang. Beijing: Mi rigs dpe skrun khang, 2011.

Dge 'dun 'jam dbyangs rgya mtsho. *Bod kyi gso ba rig pa'i rnam bshad*. Unpublished manuscript, 2018.

Dbang 'dus. *Gso ba rig pa'i tshig mdzod g.yu thog dgongs rgyan*. Beijing: Mi rigs dpe skrun khang, 1973.

G.yu thog yon tan mgon po. *Bdud rtsi snying po yan lag brgyad pa gsang ba man ngag gi rgyud* [The Secret Quintessential Instructions on the Eight Branches of the Ambrosia Essence Tantra]. New Delhi: Men-Tsee-Khang, 2008.

G.yu thog yon tan mgon po. *Bdud rtsi snying po yan lag brgyad pa gsang ba man ngag gi rgyud*. Lhasa: Bod ljongs mi dmangs dpe skrun khang, 1982.

G.yu thog yon tan mgon po. *Bdud rtsi snying po yan lag brgyad pa gsang ba man ngag gi rgyud las rtsa ba'i rgyud bshad pa'i rgyud phyi ma'i rgyud kha skong dang bcas pa* [Root Tantra, Explanatory Tantra, and Subsequent Tantra from the Secret Quintessential Instructions on the Eight Branches of the Ambrosia Essence Tantra]. New Delhi: Men-Tsee-Khang, 1999.

G.yu thog yon tan mgon po. *Rgyud chung bdud rtsi snying po* [The Ambrosia Essence Smaller Tantra]. In *Cha lag bco brgyad* [Eighteen Supplements]. Beijing: Mi rigs dpe sgrun khang, 2005.

'Jam dbyangs bkra shis. *Bod kyi gso ba rig pa'i 'bras nad kyi nad thog rmang gzhi'i rig gzhung dpyad zhib* [Clinical, Basic Research, and Literature Analysis of Cancer (*Dréné*) in Tibetan Medicine]. Lhasa: Doctoral Dissertation at Tibet University of Tibetan Medicine, 2015.

Khro ru tshe rnam. *Gso rig rgyud bzhi'i 'grel chen drang srong zhal lung* [The Great Commentary on the *Four Tantras*: Oral Instructions of the Sages]. Chengdu: Si khron mi rigs dpe sgrun khang, 2000.

Lde'u rong jo skyabs tshe ring. *Bod kyi gso rig las 'bras nad skor gyi dpyod gling* [Discussion on Dréné in Tibetan Medicine]. Beijing: Krung go'i bod rig pa dpe skrun khang, 2017.

Lha mo skyabs. *Bod lugs 'bras nad gso rig* [Tibetan Medical Oncology]. Beijing: Mi rigs dpe skrun khang, 2009.

'O rtsogs chen. *Rgya bod dbyin gsum shan sbyar deng rabs gso rig ming mdzod* [Chinese-Tibetan-English Modern Medicine Dictionary]. Beijing: Mi rigs dpe skrun khang, 2011.

Pad ma rab brtan and Sangs rgyas 'bum. *Gso ba rig pa'i ro bkra'i dpe ris kun gsal me long* [All-Clarifying Mirror of Vivid Medical Dissection Diagrams]. Xining: Mtsho sngon mi rigs dpe skrun khang, 2011.

Rdo lha. *Mchin pa'i Cancer la bod lugs gso rig gis brtag bcos zhib 'jug* [Tibetan Medical Diagnostics and Treatment of Liver Cancer]. Xining: Master's Thesis at Tibetan Medical College of Qinghai University, 2018.

Sangs rgyas rgya mtsho. *Gso ba rig pa'i bstan bcos sman bla'i dgongs rgyan rgyud bzhi'i gsal byed bai durya sngon po'i malli ka* [Blue Beryl]. Dharamsala: Tibetan Medical & Astro Institute, 1994.

Sangs rgyas rgya mtsho. *Man ngag yon tan rgyud kyi lhan thabs zugs rngu'i tsha gdung sel ba'i katpua, ra dus min 'chi zhags bcod pa'i ral gri* [Oral Instructions Supplement]. Dharamsala: Tibetan Medical & Astro Institute, 2005.

Shes rab chos 'phel, ed. *Lhan skyes rma gso ba* [Coemergent Wounds Treatment]. Dus rab 21 pa'i bod lugs gso rig dngos tshan slob gso'i 'char 'god slob deb [21st Century Tibetan Medicine Standard Textbook Series: Foundations], vol. 7. Beijing: Mi rigs dpe skrun khang, 2011.

Skyem pa tshe dbang. *Rgyud bzhi'i rnam bshad*. Xining: Mtsho sngon rigs dpe skrun khang, 2000.

Tidwell, Tawni [Rangjung Lhamo]. "Phi lugs gso rig gi kan sar (Cancer) zhes pa'i nad rigs de bod lugs gso rig gi 'bras nad dang surya skran rigs gang la sbyar rung bar dpyad pa" [A Comparative Analysis: Mapping Biomedical Cancer into Tibetan Medical Etiological Categories]. *Bod man slob gso dang zhib 'jug* [Tibetan Medical Education and Research Journal] 4 (2016): 98–113.

Tshe ring nor bu. *Bod lugs gso ba rig pa'i skye dngos sman rdzas sngo 'bum kun btus* [Comprehensive Collection of Tibetan Medical Biological Specimens]. Dharamsala: Men-Tsee-Khang, 2013.

Zur mkhar pa blo gros rgyal po. *Rgyud bzhi'i 'grel pa mes po'i zhal lung*. Beijing: Krung go'i pod kyi shes rig dpe skrun khang, 2005.

European-language Sources

Adams, J. M., and Cory, S. "The Bcl-2 Apoptotic Switch in Cancer Development and Therapy." *Oncogene* 26 (2007): 1324–37.

Adams, Vincanne, and Fei-Fei Li. "Integration or Erasure? Modernizing Medicine at Lhasa's Mentsikhang." In *Tibetan Medicine in the Contemporary World: Global Politics of Medical Knowledge and Practice*, edited by Laurent Pordié, 105–31. London and New York: Routledge, 2008.

Adams, Vincanne, Renchen Dongzhu, and Phuoc V Le. "Translating Science: The Arura Medical Group at the Frontiers of Medical Research." In *Studies of Medical Pluralism in Tibetan History and Society*, edited by Sienna Craig, Mingji Cuomo, Frances Garrett, and Mona Schrempf, 111–36. Bonn: International Institute for Tibetan and Buddhist Studies, 2010.

Adams, Vincanne, Mona Schrempf, and Sienna R. Craig, eds. *Medicine Between Science and Religion: Explorations on Tibetan Grounds*. New York, NY: Berghahn Books, 2011.

Ahmed, Z., and R. Bicknell. "Angiogenic Signaling Pathways." *Methods in Molecular Biology* 467 (2009): 3–24.

Amit, I., A. Citri, T. Shay, Y. Lu, M. Katz, F. Zhang, G. Tarcic, D. Siwak, J. Lahad, J. Jacob-Hirsch, et al. "A Module of Negative Feedback Regulators Defines Growth Factor Signaling." *Nature Genetics* 39 (2007): 503–12.

Artandi, S. E., and R. A. DePinho. "Telomeres and Telomerase in Cancer." *Carcinogenesis* 31 (2010): 9–18.

Baeriswyl, V., and G. Christofori. "The Angiogenic Switch in Carcinogenesis." *Seminars in Cancer Biology* 19 (2009): 329–37.

Bauer-Wu, Susan, Tenzin Lhundup, Tawni Tidwell, et al. "Tibetan Medicine for Cancer: An Overview and Review of Case Studies." *Integrative Cancer Therapies* 13, no. 6 (2014): 502–12.

Bergers, G., and L. E. Benjamin. "Tumorigenesis and the Angiogenic Switch." *Nature Reviews Cancer* 3 (2003): 401–10.

Bonnet, D., and J. E. Dick. "Human Acute Myeloid Leukemia is Organized as a Hierarchy That Originates from a Primitive Hematopoietic Cell." *Nature Medicine* 3 (1997): 730–37.

Brzosko, W. J., A. Jankowski, W. Prusek, and H. Ollendiek. "Influence of Padma 28 and the Thymus Extract on Clinical and Laboratory Parameters of Children with

Juvenile Chronic Arthritis." *International Journal of Immunotherapy* 7, no. 3 (1991): 143–47.

Choedon, Tenzin, Ganeshan Mathan, Soneera Arya, Vijay L Kumar, and Vijay Kumar. "Anticancer and Cytotoxic Properties of the Latex of *Calotropis Procera* in a Transgenic Mouse Model of Hepatocellular Carcinoma." *World Journal of Gastroenterology* 12, no. 16 (2006): 2517–22.

Choedon, Tenzin, Dawa Dolma, and Vijay Kumar. "Pro-Apoptotic and Anticancer Properties of *Thapring*: A Tibetan Herbal Formulation." *Journal of Ethnopharmacology* 137, no. 1 (2011): 320–26.

Cooper, Geoffrey M. *Elements of Human Cancer*. Boston, MA: Jones and Bartlett Publishers, 1992.

Cordon-Cardo, Carlos, and Carol Prives. "At the Crossroads of Inflammation and Tumorigenesis." *The Journal of Experimental Medicine* 190, no. 10 (1999): 1367–70.

Coussens, L. M., W. W. Raymond, G. Bergers, et al. "Inflammatory Mast Cells up-Regulate Angiogenesis during Squamous Epithelial Carcinogenesis." *Genes and Development* 13, no. 11 (1999): 1382–97.

Czaja, Olaf. "The Administration of Tibetan Precious Pills." *Asian Medicine* 10, nos. 1–2 (2015): 36–89.

Czaja, Olaf. "The *Four Tantras* and the Global Market: Changing Epistemologies of Drä (*'bras*) versus Cancer." In *Medicine Between Science and Religion: Explorations on Tibetan Grounds*, edited by Vincanne Adams, Mona Schrempf, and Sienna R. Craig, 265–95. New York, Oxford: Berghahn, 2011.

Dorjee Rabten Neshar, "Clinical Case Study of Cancer (*Dres-Ned*) Patients Treated at Men-Tsee-Khang's Bangalore Branch Clinic for the Period of 27 Months from November 2002 to February 2005." *sMan-rTsis Journal: Journal of Tibetan Medicine and Astrological Sciences* 4, no. 1 (2007): 50–68.

Dhondup, Lobsang, and Cynthia Husted. "Tibetan Medicine and Regeneration." *Annals of the New York Academy of Sciences* 1172, no. 1 (2009): 115–22.

Dvorak, H. F. "Tumors: Wounds That Do Not Heal. Similarities Between Tumor Stroma Generation and Wound Healing." *New England Journal of Medicine* 315 (1986): 1650–59.

Evan, G., and T. Littlewood. "A Matter of Life and Cell Death." *Science* 281, no. 5381 (1998): 1317–22.

Exner, Markus, Marianne Raith, Gregor Holzer, Bernhard Gmeiner, Oswald Wagner, and Stylianos Kapiotis. "Anti-Inflammatory Mechanisms of the Tibetan Herbal Preparation Padma 28 in the Vessel Wall." *Forschende Komplementärmedizin* 13, no. 1 (2006): 13–17.

Fedi, P., S. R. Tronick, S. A. and Aaronson. "Growth Factors." In *Cancer Medicine*, edited by J. F. Holland, R. C. Bast, D. L. Morton, E. Frei, D. W. Kufe, and R. R. Weichselbaum, 41–64. Baltimore, MD: Williams and Wilkins, 1997.

Füllemann, Fritz. "Padma 28 in the Treatment of Chronic Dental Pulpitis: An Observational Case Study in 49 Patients." *Forschende Komplementärmedizin* 13, no. 1 (2006): 28–30.

Gendun Gyamtso (Dge 'dun 'jam dbyangs rgya mtsho). Translated by Tawni Tidwell. *Principles of Tibetan Medicine: A Textbook of the Explanatory Treatise* [*Bod kyi gso ba rig pa'i rnam bshad*]. Unpublished manuscript, forthcoming.

Gerke, Barbara. "Correlating Biomedical and Tibetan Medical Terms in *Amchi* Medical Practice." In *Medicine Between Science and Religion: Explorations on Tibetan Grounds*, edited by V. Adams, M. Schrempf, and S. Craig, 127–52. New York, NY: Berghahn Books, 2010.

Gerke, Barbara. *Taming the Poisonous: Mercury, Toxicity and Safety in Tibetan Medical Practice*. Heidelberg Studies on Transculturality. Heidelberg: Heidelberg University Publishing, forthcoming.

Germano, David and Nicolas Tournadre. "THL Simplified Phonetic Transcription of Standard Tibetan." *The Tibetan and Himalayan Library*, 2010. Accessed online 10 January 2018. <http://www.thlib.org/reference/transliteration/#!essay=/thl/phonetics/s/bl>.

Gyatso, Yonten. "*Nyes pa*: A Brief Review of its English Translation." *The Tibet Journal* 4 (2005–2006): 109–18.

Hanahan, Douglas, and Robert A. Weinberg. "The Hallmarks of Cancer." *Cell* 100, no. 1 (2000): 57–70.

Hanahan, Douglas, and Robert A. Weinberg. "Hallmarks of Cancer: The Next Generation." *Cell* 144, no. 5 (2011): 646–74.

Harper, J. W., and S. J. Elledge. "The DNA Damage Response: Ten Years After." *Molecular Cell* 28 (2007): 739–45.

Hezel, A. F., and N. Bardeesy. "LKB1; Linking Cell Structure and Tumor Suppression." *Oncogene* 27 (2008): 6908–19.

Hofer, Theresia. *Medicine and Memory in Tibet: Amchi Physicians in an Age of Reform*. Seattle, WA: University of Washington Press, 2018.

Hudson, J. D., M. A. Shoaibi, R. Maestro, et al. "A Proinflammatory Cytokine Inhibits p53 Tumor Suppressor Activity." *The Journal of Experimental Medicine* 190, no. 10 (1999): 1375–82.

Husted, Cynthia, and Lobsang Dhondup. "Tibetan Medical Interpretation of Myelin Lipids and Multiple Sclerosis." *Annals of the New York Academy of Sciences* 1172, no. 1 (2009): 278–96.

Jankowski, S., A. Jankowski, S. Zielinska, M. Walczuk, and W. J. Brzosko. "Influence of Padma 28 on the Spontaneous Bactericidal Activity of Blood Serum in Children Suffering from Recurrent Infections of the Respiratory Tract." *Phytotherapy Research* 5, no. 3 (1991): 120–23.

Kanitakis, Jean. "Anatomy, Histology and Immunohistochemistry of Normal Human Skin." *European Journal of Dermatology* 12, no. 4 (2002): 390–99.

Klotz, S. A., and R. L. Penn. "Clinical Differentiation of Abscess from Neoplasm in Newly Diagnosed Space-Occupying Lesions of the Liver." *Southern Medical Journal* 80, no. 12 (1987): 1537–41.

Korwin-Piotrowska, R., D. Nocon, A. Stankowska-Chomicz, A. Starkiewicz, J. Wojcicki, and L. Samochowiec. "Experience of Padma 28 in Multiple Sclerosis." *Phytotherapy Research* 6, no. 3 (1992): 133–36.

Kuriyama, Shigehisa. *The Expressiveness of the Body and the Divergence of Greek and Chinese Medicine*. New York, NY: Zone Books, 2002.

Liddell, Henry George, and Robert Scott. *Liddell and Scott's Greek-English Lexicon*. London: Simon Wallenberg Press, 2007.

Loeb, Lawrence A. "Mutator Phenotype May Be Required for Multistage Carcinogenesis." *Cancer Research* 51 (1991): 3075–79.

Longmore, J. M. *Oxford Handbook of Clinical Medicine*. Oxford: Oxford University Press, 2010.

Mader, Sylvia, and Michael Windelspecht. *Human Biology*. New York, NY: McGraw-Hill Education, 2015.

Matzner, Y., and S. Sallon. "The Effect of Padma-28, a Traditional Tibetan Herbal Preparation, on Human Neutrophil Function." *Journal of Clinical and Laboratory Immunology* 46, no. 1 (1995): 13–23.

MD Anderson Cancer Center. "Immunotherapy: Research Platform for the Moon Shots Program." Accessed online at: https://www.mdanderson.org/cancermoonshots/research_platforms/immunotherapy.html on 3 February 2018.

Melzer, Jörg, Reto Brignoli, Curt Diehm, Jürgen Reichling, Dai-Do Do, and Reinhard Saller. "Treating Intermittent Claudication with Tibetan Medicine Padma 28: Does It Work?" *Atherosclerosis* 189, no. 1 (2006): 39–46.

Mukherjee, Siddhartha. *The Emperor of All Maladies: A Biography of Cancer*. New York, NY: Scribner, 2010.

Namdul, Tenzin, Ajay Sood, Lakshmy Ramakrishnan, Ravindra M. Pandey, and Denish Moorthy. "Efficacy of Tibetan Medicine as an Adjunct in the Treatment of Type 2 Diabetes." *Diabetes Care* 24, no. 1 (2001): 176–77.

Oxford Dictionary Online. "Flesh." Oxford: Oxford University Press, 2018. Accessed online 30 January 2018. <https://en.oxforddictionaries.com/definition/flesh>.

Parslow, Tristram G., Daniel P. Stites, Abba I. Terr, and John B. Imboden. *Medical Immunology*. New York, NY: McGraw-Hill/Appleton and Lange, 2001.

Patenaude, A., J. Parker, and A. Karsan. "Involvement of Endothelial Progenitor Cells in Tumor Vascularization." *Microvascular Research* 79 (2010): 217–23.

Phinney, Donald, and Darwin Prockop. “Concise Review: Mesenchymal Stem/Multipotent Stromal Cells: The State of Transdifferentiation and Modes of Tissue Repair—Current Views.” *Stem Cells* 25, no. 11 (2007): 2896–902.

Pietras, K., and A. Ostman. “Hallmarks of Cancer: Interactions with the Tumor Stroma.” *Experimental Cell Research* 316 (2010): 1324–31.

Rajpar, Sajjad, and Jerry Marsden. *ABC of Skin Cancer*. Malden, MA: Blackwell Publishing, 2008.

Ryan, Mary. “Efficacy of the Tibetan Treatment for Arthritis.” *Social Science and Medicine* 44, no. 4 (1997): 535–39.

Ryan, Terence, and Sergio Curri. “Genesis of Adipocytes.” *Clinics in Dermatology* 7, no. 4 (1989): 9–24.

Sabernig, Katharina. “On the History of the Murals in the Medical College at Labrang Monastery.” *Asian Medicine* 7 (2012): 358–83.

Sangmo, Rigzin, Dawa Dolma, Tenzin Namdul, T. Tsepel, and Ravindra M. Pandey. “Clinical Trial of Tibetan Medicine in the Treatment of Chronic Hepatitis B.” *Journal of Men-Tsee-Khang* 4, no. 1 (2007): 32–49.

Schäfer, M., and S. Werner. “Cancer as an Overhealing Wound: An Old Hypothesis Revisited.” *Nature Reviews Molecular Cell Biology* 9 (2008): 628–38.

Split, W., M. Szydlowska, and W. Brzosko. “The Estimation of the Action of Padma-28 in the Treatment of Ischaemic Brain Stroke.” *European Journal of Neurology* 5, no. 1 (1998): 9.

Sporn, M. B. “The War on Cancer.” *Lancet* 347, no. 9012 (1996): 1377–81.

Teng, M. W. L., J. B. Swann, C. M. Koebel, R. D. Schreiber, and M. J. Smyth. “Immune-mediated Dormancy: An Equilibrium with Cancer.” *Journal of Leukocyte Biology* 84 (2008): 988–93.

Thiery, J. P., and J. P. Sleeman. “Complex Networks Orchestrate Epithelial-mesenchymal Transitions.” *Nature Reviews Molecular Cell Biology* 7 (2006): 131–42.

Vander Heiden, M. G., L. C. Cantley, and C. B. Thompson. “Understanding the Warburg Effect: The Metabolic Requirements of Cell Proliferation.” *Science* 324 (2009): 1029–33.

Vennos, Cecile, Jörg Melzer, and Reinhard Saller. “Clinical Studies on the Efficacy and Safety of Padma 28, a Complex Herbal Formulation from Tibetan Medicine: An Overview.” *Complementary Medicine Research* 20, no. 2 (2013): 25–30.

Warburg, O. H. *The Metabolism of Tumours: Investigations from the Kaiser Wilhelm Institute for Biology, Berlin-Dahlem*. London: Arnold Constable, 1930.

Warburg, O. H. “On the Origin of Cancer Cells.” *Science* 123 (1956): 309–14.

Warburg, O. H. “On Respiratory Impairment in Cancer Cells.” *Science* 124 (1956): 269–70.

Weinberg, Robert A. *One Renegade Cell: The Quest For The Origin Of Cancer*. New York, NY: Basic Books, 1999.

Weinberg, Robert A. *The Biology of Cancer*. New York, NY: Garland Science, 2006.

Wright, C., B. Angus, S. Nicholson, J. R. C. Sainsbury, J. Cairns, W. J. Gullick, P. Kelly, A. L. Harris, and C. H. W. Horne. "Expression of c-erb B-2 Oncoprotein: A Prognostic Indicator in Human Breast Cancer." *Cancer Research* 49 (1989): 2087–90.

Zhang, H. W., C. Y. Wang, H. N. Xu, X. Zhao, Q. Dai, J. Li, X. Du, et al. "Fu xi ting lianhe zhong xiyao zhiliao gaoyuan diqu laonian yiyu zheng de linchuang yanjiu [Clinical Study on Effect of Fluoxetine Combined with Chinese Medicine or Tibetan Drugs in Treating Senile Depression in Plateau District]." *Zhongguo Zhongxiyi jiehe zazhi* [Chinese Journal of Integrated Traditional and Western Medicine] 26, no. 3 (2006): 202–204.

Zumsteg, A., and G. Christofori. "Corrupt Policemen: Inflammatory Cells Promote Tumor Angiogenesis." *Current Opinion in Oncology* 21 (2009): 60–70.

PART 2

Medicine and Religion in Context

CHAPTER 6

The Nine-Fold Magical Cord Cycle: Investigating *'Phrul gyi the gu brgu skor*, a Wartime Medical Manual

Tsering Samdrup

1 Introduction

This paper investigates a recently discovered digital copy of a rare manuscript on traumatology or wound-healing practice (*rma dpyad*) entitled the *Nine-fold Magical Cord Cycle* (*'phrul gyi the gu brgu skor*). Tibetan medical histories list a handful of titles from the Tibetan imperial period, most of which are no longer extant. In his medical history, for instance, Belo Tsewang Künkhyap ('Be lo tshe dbang kun khyab) mentions an anatomy text that has a title very similar to our text: The *Nine-fold Cord of Anatomy* (*ro bkra thag gu dgu sbyor*). He reports that it was written by an imperial court doctor named Biji Zhen Pashilaha (bi ji zhen pa shi la ha),[1] but it is probably not related to our text since it seems anatomy is the central focus, while our text is primarily concerned with healing wounds.[2] Not many medical texts from the Tibetan imperial period (*btsan po'i rgyal rabs*) have survived and, with the exception of the handful of manuscripts that were found at Dunhuang and are now preserved in various collections scattered around the world, the few that have survived are not without revisions made by later authors, editors, and commentators. Thus, a critical question for scholars working on Tibetan medical history arises, as expressed by Dan Martin: "Just how much, and in what precise ways, was Tibetan medicine blessed with an eclectic spirit, which forged a number of local and international influences into something quite new and thoroughly Tibetan?"[3] This

1 Bi ji zhen pa shi la is also written as Bi ji tsan pa shi la ha in other instances; see Dan Martin, "Greek and Islamic Medicines' Historical Contact with Tibet: A Reassessment in View of Recently Available but Relatively Early Sources on Tibetan Medical Eclecticism," in *Islam and Tibet Interactions along the Musk Routes*, ed. A. Akasoy et al. (Farham, VT: Ashgate Press, 2011), 117–43.

2 'Be lo tshe dbang kun khyab, *Gso ba rig pa'i khog dbub kun gyi bu yig sgo brgya 'byed pa'i lde mig* (Undated manuscript), 30a.

3 Dan Martin, "An Early Tibetan History of Indian Medicine," in *Soundings in Tibetan Medicine: Anthropological and Historical Perspectives*, ed. M. Schrempf (Leiden: Brill, 2007), 320.

 | DOI:10.1163/9789004404441_007

paper attempts to follow this strand of thought by examining a rare medical text from the past on healing wounds entitled the *Nine-fold Magical Cord Cycle*.

After Christopher Beckwith published his pioneering article on how Tibetan medicine is influenced by Chinese, Indian, and especially Persian-Greek medical traditions during the Imperial Tibet Era,[4] much research has been done, by both Tibetan and non-Tibetan scholars on the origin of Tibetan medicine or the historical interactions it had with foreign cultures in the past.[5] In particular, Yang Ga's ground-breaking study on the origins of the *Four Tantras* (*rgyud bzhi*) meticulously details a few of the central questions that have previously been discussed regarding the historiography of Tibetan medicine: the crucial one being the centuries-old debate among Tibetan medical practitioners and scholars over the origin of *Four Tantras*.[6] As Ronit Yoeli-Tlalim correctly pointed out, the "multi-cultural character of Tibetan medicine" has not been neglected in many of the Tibetan medical historiographies from the past.[7] However, there are still nativists that argue for an essentialist stand on Tibetan medicine being uniquely Tibetan, namely *Four Tantras* have been adapted from the *Four Collections* (*'bum bzhi*) of Bön,[8] which they argue, is purely Tibetan.

Since there are no commentaries and traditional readings of the *Nine-fold Magical Cord Cycle* available to us, it is impossible to present a traditionalist reading, or the second plane of philology that Sheldon Pollock suggests in his advice for making sense of texts on three planes.[9] The *Nine-fold Magical*

---

4 Christopher I. Beckwith, "The Introduction of Greek Medicine into Tibet in the Seventh and Eighth Centuries," *Journal of the American Oriental Society* 99, no. 2 (1979): 297–313.

5 Christopher I. Beckwith, "Tibetan Treacle: A Note on Theriac in Tibet," *The Tibetan Society Bulletin* 15 (1980): 49–51; Samten G. Karmay, "Vairocana and the *rGyud-bzhi*," *Tibetan Medicine* 12 (1989): 19–31; Martin, "Greek and Islamic Medicines' Historical Contact with Tibet"; Ronit Yoeli-Tlalim, "On Urine Analysis and Tibetan Medicine's Connections with the West," in *Studies of Medical Pluralism in Tibetan History and Society*, ed. S. Craig et al. (GmbH: IITBS, 2010), 195–211; Ronit Yoeli-Tlalim, "Central Asian Melange: Early Tibetan Medicine from Dunhuang," in *Scribes, Texts, and Rituals in Early Tibet and Dunhuang*, ed. B. Dotson et al. (Wiesbaden: Ludwig Reichert Verlag, 2013), 53–60.

6 Yang Ga, *Sources for the Writing of the Rgyud bzhi: Tibetan Medical Classic* (Cambridge, MA: Doctoral Dissertation at Harvard University, 2010).

7 Yoeli-Tlalim, "Central Asian Melange," 53.

8 Phun tshogs, "G.yung drung bon gyi sman gzhung lo rgyus" [A History of Bön Medicine], in *Krung go'i mtho rim bod sman zhib 'jug bgro gleng 'dzin grwa'i rtsom yig gces bsdus* (Lhasa: Bod rang skyong ljongs sman rtsis khang, 1998), 53–56; A rgya, "Gso dpyad 'bum bzhi las gso rig dpal ldan rgyud bzhi'i 'byung khungs dang bsgyur tshul gleng ba rgya tsho'i chu thigs," [Discussing How the Four Tantras Originated from the Four Collections of Bön] *Gangs ljongs bod lugs gso rig* 2 (2005): 9–17.

9 The three planes of philology suggested by Pollock, in his own words, are: "its moment of genesis; its reception over time; and its presence to my own subjectivity" (S. Pollock, "Philology

Cord Cycle presents the Buddha's words or instruction (*sangs rgyas bcom ldan 'das kyi bka'*) as the origin of the text, however, it is very hard to find a Buddhist theme throughout the entire content except the narrative at the beginning. Instead, it features archaic characteristics, including terms such as "ritualist physician" (*sman bon*) for the physician who also participates in the scattering rituals.[10] I propose that the *Magical Cord Cycle* is a quintessential manual on wound healing of military origin, primarily concerned with wounds caused by weaponry, that was probably recorded around the eleventh century at the latest. The core instructions of the text may have also been composed during the Tibetan imperial period, for it appears to be a compilation deriving from multiple sources and origins. Without a physical copy of the text, it is nearly impossible to date it with any accuracy, but a probable dating could be done with palaeographic methods and other forms of textual analysis. All in all, this text does not have the "unedited" authority of Dunhuang manuscripts, but it still sheds light on how medicine was practiced by Tibetans in the past, and even the *editedness* of the text is intriguing for understanding how Tibetan medicine evolved since its inception in Imperial Tibet. Below I shall discuss the extant manuscript of the *Nine-fold Magical Cord Cycle* by considering the manuscript, title, authorship, dates, and content. With a discussion of the manuscript in details, it is very likely that while some questions will be resolved, many more will be raised.

2 The Manuscript and Dates

The *Nine-fold Magical Cord Cycle* was written in a readable, headless (*dbu med*) cursive style on a double-sided loose-leaf rectangular paper with six lines of writings on each side of the leaf. The text consists of ten folios numbered with the first ten Tibetan letters (*ka–tha*), and unfortunately one page of the scan is missing (8b, *nya*) from our copy of the file. The leaves look rather short and relatively small, indicating that it may have been used as a handbook or manual. It is also observable that this manuscript does not bear the characteristics of later Tibetan texts, with a title page and drawings on the title page; in fact,

in Three Dimensions," *Postmedieval: A Journal of Medieval Cultural Studies* 5, no. 4 [2014]: 399).

10 In terms of its etymology, this term is a combination of *sman*, or medicine and *bon*, which means the ritualist of the native religion of Tibet, Bön, and it is not a common compound noun for physicians in many of the extant Tibetan medical texts. However, this very term appears in Dunhuang manuscripts at least for twice (PT 1042: line 77; PT 1043: line 72) and it probably denotes a physician who also performs rituals. Thus, I use "ritualist physician" as translation for the term *sman bon*.

there is no title page for this text at all. The colophon (*mdzad byang*) is brief, providing merely the title of the text.[11] Unlike the usual practice in traditional formality of Tibetan writings, the name of the writer and sources are not mentioned in the colophon, but rather near the beginning of the text, and the name of the scribe and the date of writing are not mentioned anywhere in the text.

According to Sam van Schaik's palaeographic method for dating Tibetan scripts, this text probably falls into his category of tenth-century post-imperial Buddhist headless style of IOL Tib J 321, IOL Tib J 341, etc.[12] In addition, this text preserves many archaic forms of Tibetan writing, such as added *ya* subfixes (*mya* instead of *ma*), archaic diction (*bro 'tshal pa* instead of *na ba* for "being sick"), and the interchange of letters within quadruples (*glad* instead of *klad, gyi* instead of *kyi*, and *ched* instead of *chen*).[13] The *Magical Cord Cycle* manuscript includes the post-postscript (*yang 'jug*) *da* as well. Despite these archaic features, the text is written in a straightforward prose style, resembling many Dunhuang manuscripts and older medical texts, such as the ones unearthed in the stupa of Gatang Bumpaché (*dga' thang 'bum pa che*), all of which predate the eleventh century.[14] Finally, the work shows no influence from South Asian literature—it lacks the complex and playful use of language from the *Mirror of Poetry* (*kāvyādarśa* = *snyan ngag me long*) and there is no observable influence from the *Essence of the Eight Branches* (*aṣṭāṅgahṛdayasaṃhitā* = *yan lag brgyad pa'i snying po bsdus pa*). Based on palaeographical investigations, primarily the use of archaic language, and content, it is likely that this manuscript was composed in the tenth or eleventh century, however, it is still just an educated speculation, which may be verified by a carbon-dating technique if we were to acquire the physical copy.

---

11 The whole colophon states: "this is end of what is known as the nine-fold magical cord cycle" (*'phrul gyi the gu brgu skor bya ba// rdzogs s.ho//*).

12 For the features of Tibetan script styles throughout history, see S. van Schaik, "Dating Early Tibetan Manuscripts: A Paleographical Method," in *Scribes, Texts and Rituals in Early Tibet and Dunhuang*, ed. B. Dotson et al. (Weisbaden: Reichert Verlag, 2013), 126–27.

13 "Quadruple" refers to the seven and a half sets of four consonants that make up the thirty letters of the Tibetan alphabet.

14 For studies on the manuscripts from *dga' thang 'bum pa che*, see Samten Karmay, "Queen of the World and Her Twenty-seven Daughters," *Journal of the International Association for Bon Research* 1 (2013): 19–35; and Lcags mo mtsho, *Gtam shul dga' thang 'bum pa che nas rnyed pa'i bon gyi gna' dpe'i zhib 'jug* [Study of Manuscripts Found in Dga' thang 'Bum pa che] (Beijing: Krung go'i bod rig pa dpe skrun khang, 2016). Karmay believes that these manuscripts from at least prior to the eleventh century (p. 21) while Lcags mo mtsho argues they are from the mid-eighth to the ninth century (p. 221).

3 Title

Titles of traditional Tibetan texts are often poetic and flowery, without much indication of the content. Glorifying the subject matter in an exaggerated way, titles often serve as ornamental elements.[15] As stated above, the *Nine-fold Magical Cord Cycle* (*'phrul gyi the gu brgu skor*) is the title of the manuscript given in the colophon, unfortunately, without any further information. The term "magical" (*'phrul gyi*) often appears in Dunhuang manuscripts for describing the king or emperor (*btsan po*). *'Phrul gyi lha bstan po*, for example, can be translated as the "magically-powered god king,"[16] and therefore *'phrul gyi* should be translated as "magical" or "magically-powered" in this context as well. The next word, "cord" (*the gu*), seems to be a variant spelling for *tha gu, thi gu*, and *the ku*. The text itself suggests the meaning of "cord" where a *the ku* is used to measure a patient's head to locate moxibustion spots (6a [*cha*]). Although "nine" or "nine-fold" (*brgu*) is a problematic syllable, it appears to be a variant spelling of *rgu* or *dgu*. Because nine is the largest single-digit number, it is also can be interpreted as many, all, and everything (*yod rgu*/*yod dgu*) in Tibetan. "Cycle" (*bskor* or *skor*) can refer to a topic, group, or type, but here it means a cycle of practices. Similar titles can be found in Tibetan medical histories, for instance, as mentioned earlier, Belo Tsewang Künkhyap mentions a text titled *Nine-fold Cord of Anatomy* (*ro bkra thag gu dgu sbyor*) in his medical history, where *sbyor* functions as a synonym of *bskor*.[17] Thus, it seems common for texts on anatomy (*ro bkra*) and wound-healing to include expressions such as "cord" (*thag gu* or *the gu*) and "nine-fold cycle" (*dgu sbor* or *brgu skor*). Another wild, but probably unlikely interpretation of the title is that it could be entirely an ornamental one, referencing the nine-fold braided cord of *zaok* (*za 'og*), or the brocade of Tri Songdetsen (*khri srong lde btsan*) employed

---

15 More on the characteristics of traditional Tibetan texts, see G. Smith, *Among the Tibetan Texts: History and Literature of the Himalayan Plateau* (Somerville, MA: Wisdom Publications, 2001); and U. Roesler, "Classifying Literature or Organizing Knowledge? Some Considerations on Genre Classifications in Tibetan Literature," in *Tibetan Literary Genres, Texts, and Text Types: From Genre Classification to Transformation*, ed. J. Dheingans et al. (Leiden: Brill, 2015), 29–53.

16 See translations and discussions of the term *'Phrul gyi lha bstan po* in Dawa Norbu, *China's Tibet Policy* (Richmond: Curzon Press, 2001), 130–31. Richardson translates *'phrul* as "supernaturally wise" for his translation of the *skar chung* inscription (E. H. Richardson, *A Corpus of Early Tibetan Inscriptions* [London: Royal Asiatic Society, 1985]).

17 'Be lo tshe dbang kun khyab, *Gso ba rig pa'i khog dbub*.

while testing pulse palpation skills of the physicians from nine different foreign countries before they become dynasty physicians.[18]

4 Authorship

The *Magical Cord Cycle* is a text with multiple origins, and the text acknowledges them in certain ways. Though the text does not identify an individual author who composed it, it rather attributes its authorship to the Buddha via a Vedic-themed origin story at the exact beginning of the text. The story begins with the following scene: the gods and demigods were once fighting over the wish-fulfilling tree (*shing yongs su sa brtsol* or *shing yongs kyi sa brtol*). The deadly battle between the two parties came to an end with the humans siding with the gods and cannibal demons (*srin po*),[19] aiding the demigods. In response to this battle, the Buddha ordered someone to write these instructions for wound-healing practice (*rma dpyad*).[20] Importantly, in the origin story at the beginning of the text the syllable for "person" or "people" is written as *mi* (no *ya* subfix), whereas it is written in the archaic form of *myi* everywhere else in the body text. This detail has led me to speculate that the origin story is a later addition written by a different person, probably a subsequent scribe.

The Buddha is referred to as a source later in the text, again, by providing an origin story along with other alternative sources:

> This is a practical manual that belongs to the wife from the Chokro clan, Karmo Nyen. It is also known as the practice from Zahor and [the

18 For a narrative in which a cord is used for such testing, see Zur mkhar blo gros rgyal po, *Shes bya spyi'i khog dbugs* (Chengdu: Si khron mi rigs dpe skrun khang, 2001); on the nine physicians, see Martin, "Greek and Islamic Medicines' Historical Contact with Tibet"; and on the origin of this narrative, see W. A. McGrath, *Buddhism and Medicine in Tibet: Origins, Ethics, and Tradition* (Charlottesville, VA: Doctoral Dissertation at the University of Virginia, 2017), 186.

19 Here I am following van der Kuijp's translation of the term ("Zahor and its Contribution to Tibetan Medicine, Part One: Some Names, Places, and Texts," *Journal of Tibetology* 6 [2010]: 21–50).

20 *'Phrul gyi the gu brgu skor bya ba* (Undated manuscript), 1a (*ka*): *lha dang lha ma yin gnyis 'thab nas// shing yongs su sa brtol la ma mtsal// rtsa ba dang 'bras la// 'brum bu dang rtsa ba phyed lhas thob// rtsa ba phyed lha me yin gyis thob// shing yongs kying sa brtsol la ma bjal nas// lha dang lha ma yin gnyis 'thabs// mtshon gi char skal pa chen po bsab so// lha'i rogs ni mis bgyis// la ma yin gyi rogs srin rin pos bgyis// gcig sha la gcig za// gcig khrag la gcig 'thung// de nas sangs rgyas bcom ldan 'das kyis bka' stsal nas rma dpyad sdod cig byung//.*

practice] with practical applications. This practice is what the Buddha instructed. It should be appreciated.[21]

In this recognition of several distinct sources, Zahor (*za hor*) is mentioned. Though neighbouring countries have been posited as sources of medical knowledge in many Tibetan medical histories, Zahor is comparatively less common to see as a source in these writings. As Leonard van der Kuijp discusses in depth in his sequential essays on Zahor, there are a few medical works attributed to Zahor in Urgyen Lingpa's (*u rgyan gling pa*) *Chronicle of the Ministers* (*blon po bka'i thang yig*), but the *Magical Cord Cycle* is not among them.[22] Where is Zahor? van der Kuijp states that sources suggest "Za hor was roughly found in the area is now occupied by Dacca."[23] Therefore, it is possible that practices from Zahor are included in this text, though it is beyond scope of this paper to detect them at the moment.

Another source attribution of the text is to the "wife from Chokro clan, Kharmo Nyen." From this information we can only tell that she is a woman from the famous Chokro clan,[24] probably a consort queen of the Tsenpo since the name bears the identification of "wife" (*bza'*). Historians of Tibet have identified a few Chokro consorts to the Tibetan kings from the eighth century to post-imperial times.[25] The most well-known "wife from Chokro clan" was Tri Tsukdetsen, a.k.a. Relpachen's (r. 815–838) consort who had to kill herself in a probable setup.[26] However, there *is* a woman from Chokro who was famous

21 *'Phrul gyi the gu brgu skor bya ba*, 2b (*kha*): *dpyad ni cog ro gza'*[=*bza'*] *dkar mo gnyan gyi dpyad ces bya' 'o // za hor gyi dpyad zhes kyang bya 'o // 'di ni dpyad kyi lag len zhes kyang bya 'o // sangs rgyas bcom ldan 'das kyis bka' stsal pa'i dpyad lags so // thugs rje che bar bya'o //.*

22 The tittles mentioned are the *Thirteen Arcane Treasures* (*Gsan mdzod bcu gsum*), *Eight Destructions of* [*or: Eight Distinctions between*] *the Life and Death of the Cannibal Demons* (*Srin po'i shi gsos byer brgyad*), and the *Great Medical Tantra of the Demi-gods* (*Lha ma yin gyi gso rgyud chen*). van der Kuijp believes that none of these texts are extant ("Zahor and its Contribution to Tibetan Medicine, Part One," 21–22).

23 van der Kuijp, "Zahor and its Contribution to Tibetan Medicine, Part One," 21.

24 For more on the Chokro (Cog ro) clan, see B. Dotson, "At the Behest of the Mountain: Gods, Clans and Political Topography in Post-imperial Tibet," in *Old Tibetan Studies: Dedicated to the Memory of R. E. Emmerick*, ed. C. Scherrer-Schaub (Leiden: Brill, 2003), 159–205.

25 For several instances of royal wives from the Chokro clan in Tibetan history, see Bsod nams rgyal mtshan, *The Mirror Illuminating the Royal Genealogies: An Annotated Translation of the XIVth Century Tibetan Chronicle: rGyal-rabs gsal-ba'i me-long*, trans. P. K. Sorensen (Wiesbaden: Harrassowitz Verlag, 1994), 411, 426, 438, and 467.

26 For the probable setup and death of this wife from Chokro clan, see Dung dkar blo bzang 'phrin las, *Dung dkar blo bzang 'prhin las kyi gsung rtsom phyogs bsgrigs* (Beijing: Krung go'i bod rig pa dpe skrun khang, 1997), 44.

for medicine, the "Deity of Horses, Girl from Chokro" (*cog ro bu mo rta yi lha*) from the reign of Tri Songdetsen (r. 755/56–797). She is mostly well-known for hippology and hippiatry, as her name suggests,[27] but it is entirely possible that her expertise extends beyond veterinary medicine, perhaps even including the *Magical Cord Cycle*. Though she is known as Tayi Lha, or the "Deity of Horses," it is very likely that she received her name through her profession as a veterinarian rather than having it as her proper name. Therefore, it is possible that she is known as Karmo Nyen as well due to her specialization in the general field of medicine.

A recently published facsimile collection of medical manuscripts from Potala and the Fifth Dalai Lama's private library at Drepung Monastery (*'bras spungs dgon*) in Lhasa includes a text entitled the *Great Treatise: Twenty Branches* (*stan cos* [*bstan bcos*] *chen po yan lag nyi shu pa*). This text narrates a story that during the reign of Tri Detsuktsen (*khri lde gtsug btsan*, r. 712–755), the *Lamp That Illuminates the Red Register of the Upper Torso* (*byang khog dmar byang gsal ba'i sgron me*)[28] was made available as a treasure text (*gter ma*) and presented by the king to Drangti Gyelnyé Kharpuk (*brang ti rgyal mnyes mkhar phug*) as a reward for his three years of service as a minister in Domé (*mdo smad*). There were other texts presented with it, and a certain *Nine-fold Cord Cycle* (*thig gu dgu skor*) was among them.[29] Other than displaying the presence of this text in Tibetan medical histories, this narrative probably suggests the *Magical Cord Cycle* was used by the followers of the Drangti to project the relevance of the Drangti clan during the Yarlung dynasty (*yar klung rgyal rabs*). Finally, two versions of a commentary for a medical text entitled the *Black-blood Drip: A Commentary of the Four-fold Magical Cycle* (*'phrul gyi bzhi skor gyi 'grel ba khrag 'dzag nag po*) in the same facsimile collection published in Lhasa covers a similar topic of wound-healing with our manuscript,[30] however, there are very few instances where this work resembles our manuscript in terms of content and style.

27 Ye shes stobs rgyal, *Bod kyi rta'i gso dpyad gzhung lugs bdams bsgrigs* (Lhasa: Bod ljongs bod yig dpe rnying dpe skrun khang, 1990).

28 For a discussion of this text in relation to the *Four Tantras* (*Rgyud bzhi*), see Yang Ga, *Sources for the Writing of the Rgyud bzhi*, 44–54.

29 Xizang Zangyi xueyuan, *Zhongguo Zangyiyao yingyin guji zhenben* (Lhasa: Bod ljongs mi dmangs dpe skrun khang, 2013), vol. 14; and a similar narrative is provided by Yang Ga, *Sources for the Writing of the Rgyud bzhi*, 44–45.

30 Xizang Zangyi xueyuan, *Zhongguo Zangyiyao yingyin guji zhenben*, vol. 9.

5 Medical Healing

Diagnostics and therapeutics are the two general topics discussed extensively in the *Magical Cord Cycle*, although some typological frameworks are presented as well. In terms of the structure of the text, it can be divided into the following five sections:

1. The origin of the text.
2. Types of head-wounds, healing head-wounds, wounds of the upper torso, wounds of the joints, and wounds of the "the spine/muscles of the brain/head" (*glad pa'i then thag*).
3. Six types of diagnosis, including the diagnosis of tumors and pox (*'bras*), suppuration (*chu ser*), and healing "fractures [?]" (*rus kho tse*).
4. Addition methods for healing head-wounds, healing wounds of four major joints and limbs, head/brain typologies, and healing wounds at the top head channel.
5. Colophon (with title in it).

Topically, this text treats head wounds as the primary focus (from pages 1b [*ka*] to 6b [*cha*] and in the latter part of the text), while including other types of wounds and categories of the head/brain (*glad rigs*). Though other early medical texts discuss wounds and traumatology,[31] they usually cover other topics as well, and our manuscript is primarily concerned with healing wounds caused most often by various kinds of weapons such as arrows. It is not hard to imagine why these texts would focus on traumatology, given the injuries caused by the violence and warfare in Tibet for centuries, and the practicality of such manuals. The preponderance of traumatological texts also suggests a military origin for these works, as Matthew Kapstein indicates while introducing Anne-Marie Blondeau's study of the Tibetan medical manuscripts found at Dunhuang.[32]

In terms of diagnosis, this text discusses inspection of the eyes, tongue, urine, diet, as well as a method called "investigating omens" (*rten 'brel brtag pa*).[33] In terms of diagnostics, examination of patient's eye is done through judging the colour of his/her sclera (*dmyig* [*mig*] *sprin*); according to our text,

31 Dunhuang manuscripts, *The Moon King: A Medical Practice* (*So ma ra dza*), *Lamp That Illuminates the Red Register of the Upper Torso* (*Byang khog dmar byang gsal ba'i sgron me*), and *The Yellow-edged Volume of Biji* (*Bi ji po ti kha ser*) are some examples among many.

32 Anne-Marie Blondeau, "Medical Traditions," in *Sources of Tibetan Tradition*, ed. K. R. Schaeffer et al. (New York, NY: Columbia University Press, 2013), 114–15.

33 For a discussion on present-day use of the term *rten 'brel* in Amdo, see T. Thurston, "An Introduction to Tibetan *Sa bstod* Speeches in A mdo," *Asian Ethnology* 71, no. 1 (2012): 49–73.

it is a sign of illness if the sclera appears red or yellow and it foreshadows that the patient's bone has a problem if his/her sclera is turned upwards.[34] For examining the tongue, an extremely grey and red tongue is unfavorable and means suppuration is active; it is a sign for illness if the edge of the tongue is grey.[35] For therapies or treatment methods, moxibustion (*me btsa'*), bloodletting (*gtar ka*), bathing (*lums*),[36] compress therapy (*dugs*), ritual scattering (*byol*),[37] and minor surgeries are implemented for different purposes in this text. Sometimes multiple therapies are performed for one situation according to the degree of seriousness of the wound. After looking for a systemic way of organizing the medical knowledge through the pages, I was able locate some categories listed in the content. The text sometimes states the categories without further information on subcategories.

1. Eight types of head/brain (*glad [klad] rigs rnam pa brgyad*)[38]
2. Thirteen types of head (*'go [mgo] rigs rnam pa bcu gsum*)[39]
3. Three types of salt (*tsha [tshwa] sna gsum*)[40]
4. Four aggregators (*'du ba rnam bzhi*)[41]
5. Five solid organs (or viscera) and six hollow organs (or bowels; *don snying rnam pa lnga dang nang glol rnam pa drug*)[42]

34 *'Phrul gyi the gu brgu skor bya ba*, 3b (*ga*): *dmyig sprin pa dmar na nad yod do// dmyig sprin pa ser nan ad yod// dmyig sprin pa gyen la zlog rus pa skyon yod//.*

35 *'Phrul gyi the gu brgu skor bya ba*, 3b (*ga*): *lce skya tshabs che yang na lce dmar na yang nang[=ngan] // chu ser gyi nad 'phyo te ngan// lce kha skya bkra ru 'dug na yang ngan bas nad yod do//.*

36 At least three types of *lums* or bathing are mentioned in the *'Phrul gyi the gu brgu skor bya ba*, namely "five-grain bathing" (*'bru sna lnga'i lums*; 7b [*ja*]), "excrement bathing" (*brun lums*; 7a [*ja*]), and the "grand bath" (*lums po che*; 2b [*kha*]).

37 *Byol* denotes "to escape" and "to avoid" and since it connotates there is a practitioner who is doing the avoiding, thus I use scattering here.

38 The text lists eight types of head/brain with their characteristics, they are: "flesh head/brain" (*sha glad*), "beehive" (*bung tshang*), "dog head/brain" (*kyi [=khyi] glad*), "butter head/brain" (*mar glad*), "yoghurt head/brain" (*zho glad*), "sparrow head/brain" (*by'u glad*), "water head/brain" (*chu glad*), and "curd head/brain" (*phrum glad*). *'Phrul gyi the gu brgu skor bya ba*, 9a (*ta*)–9b (*tha*).

39 The text does not provide a list of these thirteen types of head.

40 Three types of salt are: black salt (*kha ru ru thsa*, it is very likely *potassium permanganate*, see the description in De'u dmar bstan 'dzin phun tshogs, *Shel gong shel phreng* [Beijing: Minzu chubanshe, 2005], 370–71), "bear salt" (*dom bu thsa*), and "glass-piece salt" (*shel drum tsha*, which probably refers to *sal ammoniac*).

41 For a discussion of *'du ba*, see Martin, "Greek and Islamic Medicines' Historical Contact with Tibet," 132; and Henk Blezer, "A New Sense of (Dark) Humor in Tibet: Brown Phlegm and Black Bile," in the present volume.

42 This is a variant wording for *don lnga snod drug*, a Tibetan medical concept that shares similarities with the Chinese medical concept of the *wuzang liufu* 五脏六腑. For a

6. Four major joints (*tshigs chen bzhi*)[43]
7. Six grand channels (*rtsa chen po drug*)[44]
8. 360 channels (*rtsa sum brgya drug bcu*)[45]
9. Four spines/muscles of the brain/head [?] (*glad pa'i then thag bzhi*)[46]

Plants and animal parts are the primary *materia medica* mentioned in this section of the text. For instance, three different types of bile (*khris* [*mkhris*] *pa*)[47]—bear bile (*dom khris* [*mkhris*]), vulture/fish[?] bile (*rgya khris* [*mkhris*]),[48] and the great bile or human bile (*khris* [*mkhris*] *chen*)—are mentioned here for curing the splitting of bone and flesh (*sha rus bye ba sdom mo*).[49] Previous scholarship has discussed some *materia medica* in Tibetan medicine, especially in their search for foreign origins. Among them, "theriac" (*dar ya kan*) is relatively well researched,[50] and it appears in the *Magical Cord Cycle* as a valuable medicine. It states that a lice-sized prescription of theriac should be used to treat an arrow wound in the head by applying it externally.[51] "Bamboo concretion"

---

discussion of this topic, see W. A. McGrath, "Vessel Examination in the *Medicine of the Moon King*," in *Buddhism and Medicine: An Anthology of Premodern Sources*, ed. C. P. Salguero (New York, NY: Columbia University Press, 2017), 502–503.

43 The text does not provide any further details except methods of curing wounds in those joints once an arrow has hit them, which are probably references to the two elbow joints and two knee joints. *'Phrul gyi the gu brgu skor bya ba*, 6b (*cha*)–7b (*ja*).

44 According to the text, the six grand channels are: two channels on the right and left side of neck-joint, another two on the thighs [?], and two on the heels. *'Phrul gyi the gu brgu skor bya ba*, 3b (*ga*): *rtsa chen drug mchis na// 'jing 'khor g.yas g.yon gnyis na gnyis mchis// sha yi rgya mtsan martsa* [*na rtsa*] *gnyis gnas so// sha'i sre mjug na rtsa ched na po gnyis gnas so//.*

45 The text does not provide any further information except that they stem from the six grand channels (*rtsa chen po drug*).

46 For the locations of four muscles/spines of the head/brain, the text mentions, one is at the back of neck, one is on the forehead, and two are at the back of both ears. *'Phrul gyi the gu brgu skor bya ba*, 3a (*ga*): *glad pa'i then thag cig ni// ltag khung na mchis// then thag cig ni dpral 'dzi 'u na mchis// glad pa'i then thag cig ni// rna ltag g.yas g.yon gnyis na mchis//.*

47 Traditionally the three biles in Tibetan medicine are bear bile (*dom mkhris*), human bile (*mi mkhris*), and fish bile (*nya mkhris*) (Dbang 'dus, *Bod gangs can pa'i gso ba rig pa'i dpal ldan rgyud bzhi sogs kyi brda dang dka' gnad 'ga' zhig bkrol ba sngon byon mkhas pa'i gsung rgyun g.yu thog dgongs rgyan zhes bya ba bzhugs so* [Beijing: Minzu chubanshe, 1983], 62). Sometimes the bile of a human, bear, vulture, and fish are listed together as the four biles (*mkhris chen bzhi*). See De'u dmar bstan 'dzin phun tshogs, *Shel gong shel phreng*, 468.

48 Though it is not clear what *rgya* means here, it is probably a variant form for writing either vulture or fish since usually these two appears with human and bear when it comes to biles.

49 *'Phrul gyi the gu brgu skor bya ba*, 1a (*ka*).

50 Beckwith, "Tibetan Treacle"; Yoeli-Tlalim, "On Urine Analysis and Tibetan Medicine's Connections with the West."

51 *'Phrul gyi the gu brgu skor bya ba*, 6a (*cha*).

(*cu gang* < Chi. *zhuhuang* 竹黃) is another substance contained in the text, which is a loanword and very likely from Chinese. Saffron (*gur gum*), cane sugar (*bu ram*), and camphor (*ga bur*) are also common medicinal ingredients with foreign names that are prescribed in this text for different kinds of traumatological practices.[52]

In addition to the cosmopolitan substances, there is also one distinctively Tibetan substance mentioned in this text, or at least a material that can only be found in places where there are yaks. According to the *Magical Cord Cycle*, the hide and blood of a four-year-old male dzo (*mdzo po sum drus kyi pags pa dang khrag*) can be used for different purposes,[53] such as cleaning bone fractures (*rus kho tse bkru ba*) and compressing method (*dugs*).[54] There also is a combination of uncommon substances—such as human sperm, dog, sperm,[55] goat sperm,[56] sheep sperm, pig sperm, and women's cervical mucus (*mngal snabs*)—that is to be consumed after boiling them in two ladles of wine (*chang*).[57] This concoction is to be used for curing withering, pustulating wounds that were caused by improper behaviour (*rma spyod pas dred pa*). A few types of steaming therapy are also mentioned in the text, but most interesting of all is the performance of the "Grand Bathing" (*lums po che*). It should be prescribed to a patient who has been hit on the lower part of the "neck [?]" (*snyu sha*) and collar bone (*sgrog rus*) by a weapon. The procedure is described as following: one load (*khal*) of salt,[58] one load of leaves (it does not specify what kind of leaves), one load of melde leaves (*sne'u*),[59] and one load of bird droppings boiled in one load of water. When the water has dried out, one should make the patient lie down in the supine position and press (*gnan pa*)

52 R. Yoeli-Tlalim, "Re-visiting 'Galen in Tibet,'" *Medical History* 56, no. 3 (2012): 355–65.

53 Dzo (*mdzo*) are the cross-breed of a yak and cow. For terms and ways to determine the age of yaks in Amdo, see Chos bstan rgyal, *Following the Herds: Rhythms of Tibetan Pastoral Life in A Mdo*, ed. G. Roche (Xining: Asian Highlands Perspectives, 2014). They use *Nyos bcos* for the three-year-old male yaks, but it seems *nyis drus* or *nyis grus* should be the correct rendering. Though *sum drus* or *sum grus* is not a common term used for four-year-old male yaks nowadays, it is deducible from *nyis drus* that *sum drus* is a four-year-old male yak, or dzo in our case.

54 *'Phrul gyi the gu brgu skor bya ba*, 5a (ca) and 6b (*cha*).

55 The text specifically describes that it is the sperm of *khyi rgya bo*, or a black dog with brown facial stripes and socks.

56 The text also mentions that the goat is *rgya bo*, or black with brown facial stipes and socks.

57 *'Phrul gyi the gu brgu skor bya ba*, 8a (*nya*): *de la bcos pa'i thabs ni // myi'i sa bon / ra rgya bo'i sa bon / lug khra'i sa bon / bud myed kyi mngal snabs la phag gi sa bon // de rnams chang skyogs do dang skol la lto ru gtang ngo // des ni thub par 'ong //.*

58 One *khal* probably equals to 25–30 lbs.

59 Melde leaves (*sne'u*) derive from a fast-growing weedy annual plant in the genus *chenopodium* known as *chenopodium album*.

as if one were pressing barley to make wine.[60] The quill of a vulture's feather is also supposed to be used as the tube for a dropper made specifically for applying medicinal compounds into the patient's wounds. Almost all the therapeutic practices ensure that there is an alternative cure if one practice does not do the job, thus different forms of the phrase "this will cure the problem, if not ..." (*des thub par mchi'o ... ma thub na*) is a common occurrence throughout the text.

6 Ritual Healing

When it comes to studying the *Magical Cord Cycle*, as well as other works of ancient medical traditions, one often must confront the constructed dichotomy of "medical" and "ritualistic" practices. These categories, of course, were never an oppositional division for the practitioners and authors of these texts, nor did they exist in the clear-cut way that they are often presented in secondary scholarship.

Rituals illustrated in the *Magical Cord Cycle* are exemplary of what Geoffrey Samuel has described as "operating simultaneously on both mind and body, individual and social context."[61] Ronit Yoeli-Tlalim has also contributed to our understanding of such rituals with her brief but very informative study of Duhuang Tibetan medical texts. There she describes instructions for "ransom" (*glud*) ritual practices found at Dunhuang, especially using IOL Tib J 756 as the primary source.[62] Although she identifies three occasions where a ransom ritual is performed in the Dunhuang manuscript in question, she misidentifies one such instance because she mistakes a variant spelling for the verb *glud* ("to give to drink") as a ransom ritual for the treatment of poisoning.[63]

Though rituals are integrated with other types of medical therapies in this text, it seems that major rituals are performed as a last resort for patients. Two actors involved in ritual performance for the sick or injured are the "ritualist

60 *'Phrul gyi the gu brgu skor bya ba*, 2b (*kha*): *de la lums po che bgyi 'tshal te tsha khal cig // shing lo khal cig // skye sne'u khal cig // bya brun khal cig // chu khal cig gi nang du btsos te // chu skams tsam na nad pa gan rgyal du bsnyal la // chang gnan pa ltar byas la lums de ltar bgyi 'o //*.

61 G. Samuel, "The Effectiveness of Goodness, or, How Ritual Works," *Anthropological Forum: A Journal of Social Anthropology and Comparative Sociology* 11 (2001): 76.

62 R. Yoeli-Tlalim, "Between Medicine and Ritual: Tibetan 'Medical Rituals' from Dunhuang," in *Tibetan and Himalayan Healing: An Anthology for Anthony Aris*, ed. C. Ramble and U. Roesler (Kathmandu: Vajra Books, 2015).

63 Yoeli-Tlalim, "Between Medicine and Ritual," 751. To help understand *glud* as a verbal equivalent to *blud* or *ldud*, meaning "give to drink" in Old Tibetan, it is helpful to consider the verbs *lud* and *glud* in IOL Tib J 733: lines 27–29.

physician" (*sman bon*) and the "wound healer" (*rma mkhan*).[64] This particular ritual, known as "scattering" (*byol thabs*), is performed in the text when the patient is possessed by a ghost spirit (*'dre*). The ritual is performed as a continuation of a compress therapy (*dugs*). It is described in the text as follows:

> For compressing the ghost spirit, one measure (*bre*) of barley should be offered to the gods (*lha*) and one measure of the five grains [barley, rice, wheat, beans, and sesame] should be offered to the spirits (*lha srin*). When practicing the compressing therapy, the ritualist physician (*sman bon*) should generate anger, and the "wound healer" (*rma mkhan*) should contemplate on his essential deity while also performing the compress therapy. One should throw one measure of the five grains and prostrate to the four directions while performing the healing ritual. If the patient is in possession of a severe ghost spirit, this [compress therapy] can be performed three or four times. This should be enough to cure it. One can also perform it on a patient possessed by an even more severe ghost spirit. Also, for the patient with an even more severe ghost spirit, one should perform the scattering (*byol thabs*) ritual. One should remove the patient from the bed, put a dead dog in the patient's bed and cover it with patient's clothing while several ritualists act as if they are protecting it. This will cure [the patient].[65]

Regardless of their precise relationship, one thing can be stated for certainty here: ritualist physicians and wound healers had different roles to play in the process of healing the wounded in collaboration. Healers deal mostly with the physical bodies of patients whilst ritualists treat the illnesses healers diagnosed as having something to do with spirits.

Of all the subjects covered in the passage cited above, the scattering ritual (*byol thabs*) begs for closer examination. Scattering rituals are one alternative

64 The sheer existence the term, "wound-healer/surgeon" (*rma mkhan*), clearly differentiates the doctor in charge of healing wounds from other types of physicians.

65 *'Phrul gyi the gu brgu skor bya ba*, 2a (*kha*)–2b (*kha*): *de ni 'dre la dug byin ba ni te 'dre yul 'byin ba yin te // gnyan te nas dkar mo bre gang ni lha la yon du sngos // 'bru sna lnga la mngon gyi tshugs su bra gang du byas te // lha srin la yon du bsngo // dugs de byed pa'i dus su sman bon kyis zhe sdang bskyed // rma mkhan gis rang gi snying po lha bsgoms // da ci'i dugs de byed pa'i dus su 'bru sna lnga la bre gang la // phyogs bzhir gtor ro // phyogs bzhir lha phyag bgyi 'o // nad pa 'dre che ba la dugs de 'dra ba phogs gsum bzhi bgyi 'o // des nit hub par chi te // nad pa 'dre che bat hams cad la // de ltar bgyi 'o // nad pa 'dre che ba la // nad pa'i mal nas phyung ste // byol thabs gtang ngo // nad pa'i mal du kyi ro cig bcug la // nad pa'i gos kyis kyang g.yog go // sman bon 'gas kyang bsrung ba ltar bya 'o // des ni thub par mchi 'o//.*

for curing serious illnesses, wounds in our case, in the Tibetan medical tradition. Scattering rituals repeatedly appear in the *Tale of Retaliation* (*gnag rabs*) manuscript, which maintains "bad omens of evils will appear, which cannot be defeated by anything other than scattering rituals,"[66] and "evils and ill-omens cannot be defeated without scattering rituals; scattering rituals defeat all the evil spirits."[67] Though the *Tale of Retaliation* is not a medical, but a ritual text, it deals mostly with subduing evil spirits harmful to the people.

The *Magical Cord Cycle* is not exceptional in this sense that it employs both medical therapeutics and ritualistic healing to balance out the healing of wounds. It is also evident from the participation of two specialists in the scattering ritual, namely the ritualist physician and the wound-healer, that the curing of the severe conditions was done in a collaboration of the ritualists and surgeons. As Yoeli-Talalim observed from studying Dunhuang Tibetan manuscripts,[68] ritual aspect of the healing is prevalent in Tibetan traditional medicine. Dogs are frequently used for therapeutic purposes in this text, which is probably due to their association with ghosts (*'dre*) in Tibetan culture.[69] Later the text specifically mentions covering the wound with the skin of a four-eyed dog (*gyi* [*khyi*] *rgya bo dang dmig bzhi*) to cure the wounds in the four major joints.[70] As is the case in most ransom rituals (*glud*), the role of the dog in the scattering ritual can also be interpreted as sending an animal (or effigy) in the place of the patient, so that the patient might avoid the unfortunate consequences brought on by the spirit possession.

In the *Magical Cord Cycle*, omens and the behaviour of patients are also considered for the diagnosis and classification of the patient's wounds. For instance, the text maintains that it is inauspicious if the patient looks up in the sky and clouds, if the patient's hands are restless, if the patient is afraid of the condition, if the patient walks toward animals and water, if the patient's dog barks at the wound-healer (*rma mkhan*), or if the patient and his or her family members are unfriendly to the wound-healer.[71] In addition, the patient's

66 Lcags mo mtsho, *Gtam shul dga' thang 'bum pa che nas rnyed pa'i bon gyi gna' dpe'i zhib 'jug*, 280: *'d-i dud kyi ltas ngan byung/ c-is kyang mi thub byol gyis thub/*.

67 Lcags mo mtsho, *Gtam shul dga' thang 'bum pa che nas rnyed pa'i bon gyi gna' dpe'i zhib 'jug*, 283: *bḍud dang ltas ngan cis yang myi thub byol gyis thub/ 'dre gang byol gyis ldog*.

68 Yoeli-Tlalim, "Between Medicine and Ritual."

69 People of Amdo in eastern Tibet where I grew up have said that putting the tears of a four-eyed black and tan dog (*rgya bo mig bzhi*, see the next footnote for why it is known as "four-eyed") over one's eyes will make that person able to see ghosts (*'dre*).

70 *'Phrul gyi the gu brgu skor bya ba*, 7b (*ja*). In Tibetan, *rgya bo mig bzhi*, or a four-eyed dog is usually a black and tan dog with two brown dots over its eyes.

71 *'Phrul gyi the gu brgu skor bya ba*, 3b (*ga*): *dmyig rtsa gnam srin gnyis kyi 'tshams su lta na ngan no// lag pa gnas sa ru nyug na ngan no// nad 'jigs na ngan no// ska pa sems can snyag*

diet, especially the ways in which he or she consumes food, is also taken as a primary sign for the seriousness of his or her illness; it is inauspicious if the patient eats like a musk deer eating grass,[72] if the patient sips water in a sucking fashion, or if the patient eats like a sparrow [?] (*tshod ma phye'u*), chewing only three times, or not swallowing and only chewing.[73]

7 Conclusion

Though it is not a manuscript of great length, the *Nine-fold Magical Cord Cycle* presents a vast amount of medical knowledge, from diagnosis to external therapies and the prescription of *materia medica*, as well as anatomical typologies. Though attributing its origins to the Buddha is typical of post-*Four Tantras* medical texts, thereby legitimizing medical knowledge,[74] the *Magical Cord Cycle* is best understood as a pre-twelfth-century work for the palaeographical reasons outlined above and other features, such as the absence of later post-*Four Tantras* systematized Tibetan medical knowledge in the text. As a result, the *Magical Cord Cycle* demonstrates that it is not impossible to have texts claiming Buddha origins prior to the twelfth century, even if the date of this text remains speculative due to the limited information available. Even without fully knowing the historical background, the content of the *Magical Cord Cycle* is valuable enough to provide us with nuances not only about early medical practices but also about social relations in Tibet. The text depicts the social relationship between wound-healers and patients, as well as the collaboration medical and ritual specialists in the case of severe conditions. Moreover, the manuscript also presents instructions for doctors to diagnose patients using divination, stating that it is a bad omen when a patient's dog barks at the doctor, which possibly suggests that dogs should be kept away when doctors come to visit. Future studies of this text can focus on further detailing the *materia medica* and external therapies that appear in this and other early extant manuscripts on Tibetan medicine. The probable early date and wide array of information found in the *Magical Cord Cycle* makes it an exceptionally valuable manuscript that merits further exploration.

---

na ngan no nad pa chu snyag na ngan no// rma mkhan la nad pa yi khyi za na ngan no nad pa dang khyim bdag rma mkhan la ngom zung gnag na yang ngan no//.

72 It probably denotes acting in a vigilant fashion while one is eating.

73 *'Phrul gyi the gu brgu skor bya ba*, 4a (*nga*): *gla ba rtswa za ba ltar byed na ngan no// chu 'jib chu ru 'thung na ngan no// tshod ma phye'u zas za ba ltar phogs gsum lcag lcag zer na ngan no// khong par myi za bar blcag blcag zer na ngan no//.*

74 Yang Ga, *Sources for the Writing of the Rgyud bzhi*, 4–21.

Acknowledgements

I am grateful for William McGrath's careful edits and numerous helpful comments on this chapter. I also want to express my gratitude to Palgon Thar of Gansu Provincial Tibetan Medical Research Centre (Kan su'u zhing chen bod kyi gso rig zhib 'jug khang) for providing constructive suggestions and pointing to numerous relevant references; all remaining errors are, of course, my own.

Primary Sources

'Phrul gyi the gu brgu skor bya ba [Nine-fold Magical Cord Cycle]. Undated manuscript. Dunhuang Tibetan Manuscripts IOL Tib J 733; PT 1042; and PT 1043.

Bibliography

A rgya. "Gso dpyad 'bum bzhi las gso rig dpal ldan rgyud bzhi'i 'byung khungs dang bsgyur tshul gleng ba rgya tsho'i chu thigs" [Discussing How the Four Tantras Originated from the Four Collections of Bön]. *Gangs ljongs bod lugs gso rig* 2 (2005): 9–17.

Blondeau, A. "Medical Traditions." In *Sources of Tibetan Tradition*, edited by K. R. Schaeffer, M. T. Kapstein, and G. Tuttle, 114–18. New York, NY: Columbia University Press, 2013.

Beckwith, C. I. "The Introduction of Greek Medicine into Tibet in the Seventh and Eighth Centuries." *Journal of the American Oriental Society* 99, no. 2 (1979): 297–313.

Beckwith, C. I. "Tibetan Treacle: A Note on Theriac in Tibet." *The Tibetan Society Bulletin* 15 (1980): 49–51.

'Be lo tshe dbang kun khyab. *Gso ba rig pa'i khog dbub kun gyi bu yig sgo brgya 'byed pa'i lde mig/ 'be lo tshe dbang kun kyab kyi gsung thor bu'i skor bzhugs so*. Undated manuscript.

Bsod nams rgyal mtshan. *The Mirror Illuminating the Royal Genealogies: An Annotated Translation of the XIVth Century Tibetan Chronicle: rGyal-rabs gsal-ba'i me-long*, translated by P. K. Sorensen. Wiesbaden: Harrassowitz Verlag, 1994.

Chos bstan rgyal. *Following the Herds: Rhythms of Tibetan Pastoral Life in A Mdo*, edited by G. Roche. Xining: Asian Highlands Perspectives, 2014.

Dawa Norbu. *China's Tibet Policy*. Richmond: Curzon Press, 2001.

Dbang 'dus. *Bod gangs can pa'i gso ba rig pa'i dpal ldan rgyud bzhi sogs kyi brda dang dka' gnad 'ga' zhig bkrol ba sngon byon mkhas pa'i gsung rgyun g.yu thog dgongs rgyan zhes bya ba bzhugs so*. Beijing: Minzu chubanshe, 1983.

De'u dmar bstan 'dzin phun tshogs. *Shel gong shel phreng*. Beijing: Minzu chubanshe, 2005.

Dotson, B. "At the Behest of the Mountain: Gods, Clans and Political Topography in Post-imperial Tibet." In *Old Tibetan Studies: Dedicated to the Memory of R. E. Emmerick, Proceedings of the Tenth Seminar of the IATS, 2003*, edited by C. Scherrer-Schaub, 159–205. Leiden: Brill, 2003.

Dung dkar blo bzang 'phrin las. *Dung dkar blo bzang 'prhin las kyi gsung rtsom phyogs bsgrigs*. Beijing: Krung go'i bod rig pa dpe skrun khang, 1997.

Fenner, T. "*rGyud bzhi*: A Tibetan Medical Tantra." In *Tibetan Literature: Studies in Genre*, edited by J. I. Cabezon and R. R. Jackson, 458–69. Ithaca, NY: Snow Lion, 1996.

Karmay, S. G. "Queen of the World and Her Twenty-seven Daughters." *Journal of the International Association for Bon Research* 1 (2013): 19–35.

Karmay, S. G. "Vairocana and the *rGyud-bzhi*." *Tibetan Medicine* 12 (1989): 19–31.

Lcags mo mtsho. *Gtam shul dga' thang 'bum pa che nas rnyed pa'i bon gyi gna' dpe'i zhib 'jug* [Study of Manuscripts Found in Dga' thang 'Bum pa che]. Beijing: Krung go'i bod rig pa dpe skrun khang, 2016.

Martin, D. "An Early Tibetan History of Indian Medicine." In *Soundings in Tibetan Medicine: Anthropological and Historical Perspectives. PIATS 2013: Tibetan Studies: Proceedings of the Tenth Seminar of International Association for Tibetan Studies, Oxford, 2003*, edited by M. Schrempf, 307–26. Leiden: Brill, 2007.

Martin, D. "Greek and Islamic Medicines' Historical Contact with Tibet: A Reassessment in View of Recently Available but Relatively Early Sources on Tibetan Medical Eclecticism." In *Islam and Tibet Interactions along the Musk Routes*, edited by A. Akasoy, C. Burnett, and R. Yoeli-Talalim, 117–43. Farham, VT: Ashgate Press, 2011.

McGrath, W. A. *Buddhism and Medicine in Tibet: Origins, Ethics, and Tradition*. Charlottesville, VA: Doctoral Dissertation at the University of Virginia, 2017.

McGrath, W. A. "Vessel Examination in the *Medicine of the Moon King*." In *Buddhism and Medicine: An Anthology of Premodern Sources*, edited by C. P. Salguero, 501–13. New York, NY: Columbia University Press, 2017.

Phun tshogs. "G.yung drung bon gyi sman gzhung lo rgyus" [A History of Bön Medicine]. In *Krung go'i mtho rim bod sman zhib 'jug bgro gleng 'dzin grwa'i rtsom yig gces bsdus*. Lhasa: Bod rang skyong ljongs sman rtsis khang, 1998.

Pollock, S. "Philology in Three Dimensions." *Postmedieval: A Journal of Medieval Cultural Studies* 5, no. 4 (2014): 398–413.

Richardson, E. H. *A Corpus of Early Tibetan Inscriptions*. London: Royal Asiatic Society, 1985.

Roesler, U. "Classifying Literature or Organizing Knowledge? Some Considerations on Genre Classifications in Tibetan Literature." In *Tibetan Literary Genres, Texts, and Text Types: From Genre Classification to Transformation*, edited by J. Dheingans et al., 29–53. Leiden: Brill, 2015.

Samuel, G. "The Effectiveness of Goodness, or, How Ritual Works." *Anthropological Forum: A Journal of Social Anthropology and Comparative Sociology* 11 (2001): 73–91.

Smith, G. *Among the Tibetan Texts: History and Literature of the Himalayan Plateau.* Somerville, MA: Wisdom Publications, 2001.

Thurston, T. "An Introduction to Tibetan *Sa bstod* Speeches in A mdo." *Asian Ethnology* 71, no. 1 (2012): 49–73.

Tsering Thakchoe and Tsering Dolma. *Tibetan-English Dictionary of Tibetan Medicine and Astrology*. Archana: Drungtso Publications, 2005.

van der Kuijp, L. "Zahor and its Contribution to Tibetan Medicine, Part One: Some Names, Places, and Texts." *Journal of Tibetology* 6 (2010): 21–50.

van Schaik, S. "Dating Early Tibetan Manuscripts: A Paleographical Method." In *Scribes, Texts and Rituals in Early Tibet and Dunhuang*, edited by B. Dotson, K. Iwao, and T. Takeuchi, 119–35. Weisbaden: Reichert Verlag, 2013.

Xizang zangyi xueyuan. *Zhongguo Zangyiyao yingyin guji zhenben*, vols. 9 and 14. Lhasa: Bod ljongs mi dmangs dpe skrun khang, 2013.

Yang Ga. *Sources for the Writing of the Rgyud bzhi: Tibetan Medical Classic*. Cambridge, MA: Doctoral Dissertation at Harvard University, 2010.

Ye shes stobs rgyal. *Bod kyi rta'i gso dpyad gzhung lugs bdams bsgrigs*. Gangs can rig mdzod, vol. 13. Lhasa: Bod ljongs bod yig dpe rnying dpe skrun khang, 1990.

Yoeli-Tlalim, R. "Between Medicine and Ritual: Tibetan 'Medical Rituals' from Dunhuang." In *Tibetan and Himalayan Healing: An Anthology for Anthony Aris*, edited by C. Ramble and U. Roesler. Kathmandu: Vajra Books, 2015.

Yoeli-Tlalim, R. "Central Asian Melange: Early Tibetan Medicine from Dunhuang." In *Scribes, Texts, and Rituals in Early Tibet and Dunhuang*, edited by B. Dotson, K. Iwao, and T. Takeuchi, 53–60. Wiesbaden: Ludwig Reichert Verlag, 2013.

Yoeli-Tlalim, R. "On Urine Analysis and Tibetan Medicine's Connections with the West." In *Studies of Medical Pluralism in Tibetan History and Society. PIATS 2006: Tibetan Studies: Proceedings of the Eleventh Seminar of the International Association for Tibetan Studies, Konigswinter 2006*, edited by S. Craig, Mingji Cuomu, F. Garrett, and M. Schrempf, 195–211. GmbH: IITBS, 2010.

Yoeli-Tlalim, R. "Re-visiting 'Galen in Tibet.'" *Medical History* 56, no. 3 (2012): 355–65.

Zur mkhar blo gros rgyal po. *Shes bya spyi'i khog dbugs.* Chengdu: Si khron mi rigs dpe skrun khang, 2001.

CHAPTER 7

Knowledge, Imagery, and the Treatment of Communicable Disease in the *Vase of the Amṛta of Immortality*: A Preliminary Analysis of a Nyingma Medical Corpus

Carmen Simioli

1 Introduction: The *Vase of the Amṛta of Immortality* and Its Status in the History of Tibetan Medicine

Throughout the centuries, societies have formulated varieties of philosophical, medical, alchemical, and religious responses to outbreaks of pestilence and communicable diseases.[1] Tibetan medical sources from the tenth to the late seventeenth century describe complex but uniform epistemological postures concerning the causalities of *rimtsé* (*rims tshad*) or "epidemic fevers" and *nyenné* (*gnyan nad*) or "infectious diseases," which subsumes eighteen harsh infective and malignant diseases. In Tibetan medical collections from the tenth century onwards, we find references to these ailments, which were explained as physical disorders, but, as in many other cultural contexts,[2] demonology played a significant role in understandings of their pathogenesis. Accordingly, it can be observed that in these sources the empirical approach to the diagnosis of diseases is often interrelated with divination and religious curative methods.

When addressing the issue of epidemics and infective diseases, we shall consider to what extent the theories and the practices of Buddhist Tantric medicine came to exert influence on Tibetan medical tradition, and in particular which textual traditions played a prominent role in codifying Tibetan

1 For alchemical responses, see Chiara Crisciani and Michela Pereira, "Black Death and Golden Remedies: Some Remarks on Alchemy and the Plague," in *The Regulation of Evil: Social and Cultural Attitudes to Epidemics in Late Middles Ages*, ed. Agostino Paravicini Bagliani and Francesco Santi (Firenze: Sismel-Edizioni del Galluzzo, 1998), 7–40. For religious responses, see Andrew Cunningham, "Epidemics, Pandemics and the Doomsday Scenario," *Historically Speaking* 7 (2008): 29–31.

2 Siam Bhayro and Catherine Rider, eds., *Demons and Illness from Antiquity to the Early-Modern Period* (Brill: Leiden, 2017).

 | DOI:10.1163/9789004404441_008

epidemiology.[3] The medical literature on *nyenné* and *rimné* reflects, in a wider sense, the comprehensive nature of Tibetan medical system, which encompasses other complementary disciplines, such as alchemy, iatrochemistry, and magic (*las la sbyor ba*, lit. the "application of [ritual] activities"). Although, in the course of time, the differentiation between the respective literary genres has generally become clear cut, medical texts on epidemics were closely connected to the alchemical literature of "extracting essences" (*bcud len* = Skt. *rasāyana*), treatises of iatrochemistry (*dngul chu'i grub pa'i bstan bcos* = Skt. *rasasiddhiśāstra*), and "grimoires" (*sngags be'u bum*, lit. "collections of mantras and spells"; *las sna tshogs be'u bum*, lit. "collections of ritual acts").[4] The expectation of finding a valid remedy for mortal disorders, which, as anticipated, were conceived as liminal entities in the midst of corporeal and spiritual reality, prompted pharmacological research on the one hand, and the redaction of ancient ritual literature on the other. Thus, the historical connection between medical and ritual literature can be found in the search for a universal medicine prepared by means of alchemical techniques.

What today is known as the *Four Tantras* (*rgyud bzhi*), the seminal treatise of the Tibetan medical tradition attributed to Yutok Yönten Gönpo (*g.yu thog yon tan mgon po*, twelfth century), is the result of a long process of reception, systematization, and canonization of diverse medical theories and practices, which reached its climax during the fourteenth century.[5] In this source, among

3 On Tantric medicine see for example Vesna Wallace's consummate essay on the *Kālacakratantra*: Vesna A. Wallace, "Medicine and Astrology in the Healing Arts of the *Kālacakratantra*," in *As Long as Space Endures: Essays on the Kālacakra Tantra in Honor of H. H. The Dalai Lama*, ed. Edward A. Arnold (Ithaca, NY: Snow Lion Publications, 2009), 179–91.

4 On the definition of *rasāyana* in Sanskrit medical and alchemical literature see Dagmar Wujastyk, "Acts of Improvement: On the Use of Tonics and Elixirs in Sanskrit Medical and Alchemical Literature," *History of Science in South Asia* 5, no. 2 (2017): 1–36. On Tibetan *rasāyana* see Barbara Gerke, "Treating Essence with Essence: Re-inventing *bcud len* as Vitalising Dietary Supplements in Contemporary Tibetan Medicine," *Asian Medicine: Tradition and Modernity* 7, no. 1 (2012): 196–224; and Barbara Gerke, "Treating the Aged and Maintaining the Health: Locating *bcud len* Practices in the *Four Medical Tantras*," *Journal of International Buddhist Studies* 35, nos. 1–2 (2012): 329–62. On *rasaśāstra* in Tibetan literature, see Carmen Simioli, "Alchemical Gold and the Pursuit of the Alchemical Elixir," *Asian Medicine: Tradition and Modernity* 8, no. 1 (2013): 43–77. For a detailed definition of magic as category of knowledge and expertise in the Tibetan context see Bryan J. Cuevas, "'The Calf's Nipple' (*Be'u bum*) of Ju Mipham (*'Ju mi pham*): A Handbook of Tibetan Ritual Magic," in *Tibetan Ritual*, ed. José Ignacio Cabezón (Oxford: Oxford University Press, 2010), 165–86.

5 Since the cosmopolitan imperial epoch (seventh-eighth centuries CE), the Tibetan medical system started to assimilate and integrate elements from other medical traditions. See Christopher I. Beckwith, "The Introduction of Greek Medicine into Tibet in the Seventh and Eighth Centuries," *Journal of the American Oriental Society* 99, no. 2 (1979): 297–313; Dan Martin, "An Early Tibetan History of Indian Medicine," in *Soundings in Tibetan Medicine*, ed.

the diverse *rasāyana* formulations, mercurial compounds clearly epitomize the ideal of the universal panacea. Not unlike the Āyurvedic concept of the *rasāyana* that "pacifies all disorders" (*sarvopaghāta śamanīya*), the countermeasure called the "precious reversal suppressant, universal pacifier of all the diseases" (*zhi bye kun log gnon rin po che*) can dispel any kind of harsh disease, including epidemics, and can even protect from demonic attacks and poisoning.[6] Since alchemy and magic represent two categories of operative knowledge that share the same philosophical substratum of "dependent arising" (*rten 'brel* = Skt. *pratītyasamutpāda*), they permeate each other. Therefore, along with the alchemical idea of the manipulation of substances to create a perfect medicine, we find the secret potencies of *materia medica* that pertain to natural magic (the sympathies and the antipathies existing in the whole of nature), as well as ritual practices (invocations, the use of incantations to summon and also exorcisms), and also the conjunct preparation of magic diagram or circles (*'khor lo*) and sacred images (*gzugs brnyen*), which typify image magic.[7]

Mona Schrempf (Leiden: Brill, 2007), 307–25; Dan Martin, "Greek and Islamic Medicines' Historical Contact with Tibet," in *Islam and Tibet: Interactions along the Musk Routes*, ed. Anna Akasoy et al. (Burlington, VT: Ashgate Publishing Company, 2011), 117–44; William A. McGrath, "Vessel Examination in the *Medicine of the Moon King*," in *Buddhism and Medicine: An Anthology of Premodern Sources*, ed. C. Pierce Salguero (New York, NY: Columbia University Press, 2017), 501–13; Anna Akosay and Ronit Yoeli-Ylalim, "Along the Musk Routes: Exchanges between Tibet and the Islam World" in *Asian Medicine, Tradition and Modernity* 3 (2007): 217–40 ; Ronit Yoeli-Tlalim, "On Urine Analysis and Tibetan Medicine's Connections with the West," in *Studies of Medical Pluralism in Tibetan History and Society*, ed. Sienna Craig et al. (Halle: International Institute for Tibetan and Buddhist Studies GmbH, 2010), 195–211; Ronit Yoeli-Tlalim, "Re-visiting 'Galen in Tibet,'" *Medical History* 56, no. 3 (2012): 355–65; Ronit Yoeli-Tlalim, "Central Asian Mélange: Early Tibetan Medicine from Dunhunag," in *Scribes, Texts, and Rituals in Early Tibet and Dunhuang*, ed. Brandon Dotson, Kazushi Iwao, and Tsuguhito Takeuchi (Wiesbaden: Reichert-Verlag, 2013), 53–60; and Ronit Yoeli-Tlalim, "Between Medicine and Ritual: Tibetan 'Medical Ritual from Dunhuang,'" in *Tibetan and Himalayan Healing: An Antology for Anthony Aris*, ed. Charles Ramble and Ulrike Roesler (Kathmandu: Vajra Publications, 2015), 739–46. For further analysis of this process of unification, standardization, and modes of knowledge transmission in the Tibetan medical system, see William A. McGrath, *Buddhism and Medicine in Tibet: Origins, Ethics, and Tradition* (Charlottesville, VA: Doctoral Dissertation at the University of Virginia, 2017).

6 This formulation appears in the *Ultimate Tantra* (*phyi'i rgyud*) of the *Four Tantras*. See *Bdud rtsi snying po yan lag brgyad pa gsang ba man ngag gi rgyud* (Lhasa: Bod ljongs mi rigs dpe skrun khang, 1982), 601/9–12.

7 Image magic with its astrological and philosophical implications, as well as its divinatory, medical and apotropaic uses, have been largely investigated in western studies. For a detailed study on textual amulets see Don C. Skemer, *Binding Words: Textual Amulets in the Middle Ages* (Philadelphia, PA: University of Pennsylvania Press, 2006). For a theoretical approach to the concept of *simulacra* in Tibetan Buddhism see Stephan Beyer, *The Cult of Tara: Magic*

These disciplines are part of the instructional corpus of the Tibetan medical tradition, which is an immense body of practical occult lore, grounded in Tantric Buddhist knowledge. These narratives and ritual practices were gathered up over the centuries and condensed in the literature of "accomplishing medicine" (*sman sgrub*), a genre structured according to the model of *Mahāyogatantra* that flourished in Tibet between the twelfth and the thirteenth centuries.[8] In these scriptures, alchemy and various forms of magic merged with evocation rituals (*sgrub thabs*) aimed at producing a ritually empowered "*amṛta* of immortality" (*'chi med bdud rtsi*).

The *Great Vase of the Amṛta of Immortality* (*'chi med bdud rtsi bum chen*; hereafter *Vase of Amṛta*), whose contents will be examined in this study, belongs to this literary genre. I will be using two redactions of the *Great Vase*: the first is included in the nineteenth century *Precious Treasury* (*rin chen gter mdzod*) redacted by Jamgön Kongtrül Lodrö Thayé (*'jam mgon kong sprul blo gros mtha' yas*, 1813–1899) and Jamyang Khyentse Wangpo (*'jam dbyangs mkhyen brtse'i dbang po*, 1820–1892); the second belongs to the *Collection of Prominent Medical Works Ascribed to Padmasambhava* (*slob dpon pad 'byung gi sman yig gces bsdus*), which is a volume included in the publication series of ancient medical works redacted by the Arura Medical Institute and Tibetan Medical Research Association in Tsongön (Kokonor, Qinghai).[9] The *Vase of Amṛta* formally conforms to the category of treasure texts (*gter ma*), the revealed-scripture tradition ascribed to Padmasambhava, and is a medical oriented textual cycle completely devoted to the cure of *nyenné* and *rimtsé*. Other titles are, indeed, contained within the corpus of the *Vase of Amṛta*, each alluding to its contents and structure, such as the *Medical Corpus in Eight Branches* (*gzhung yan lag brgyad pa*), the *Trilogy of Tantras of the Medical Methods* (*gso dpyad rgyud don skor gsum pa*), or the *Three Precious Heaps of Medical Methods*

and Ritual in Tibet (Dehli: Motilal Banarsiddass, [1973] 2001); for an analysis of an iatromantic image see Ronit Yoeli-Tlalim, "A Tibetan Image of Divination: Some Contextual Remarks," in *Imagining Chinese Medicine*, ed. Vivienne Lo and Penelope Barrett (Leiden: Brill 2018), 429, fig. 9.

8 On "accomplishing medicine" see for example: Francis Garrett, "The Alchemy of Accomplishing Medicine (*sman sgrub*): Situating the *Yuthok Heart Essence* Ritual Tradition," *Journal of Indian Philosophy* 37, no. 3 (2009): 207–30; and Cathy Cantwell, "The Medicinal Accomplishment (*sman sgrub*) Practice in the Dudjom Meteoric Iron Razor (*gnam lcags spu gri*) Tradition: Reflections on the Ritual and Meditative Practice at a Monastery in Southern Bhutan," *Journal of the Oxford Centre for Buddhist Studies* 8 (2015): 49–95.

9 (1) *'Chi med bdud rtsi bum pa*, in *Rin chen gter mdzod* (Paro: Stod lung mtsur phu'i par khang, 1980), vol. 46 (*ngo, ha*), 1.1–124.1 (hereafter *'Chi med bdud rtsi bum pa* [1]); and (2) *'Chi med bdud rtsi bum pa*, in *Slob dpon pad 'byung gi sman yig gces btus* (Beijing: Mi rigs dpe skrung khang, 2006), 1–193 (hereafter *'Chi med bdud rtsi bum pa* [2]).

(*gso dpyad rin chen spungs bag gsum pa*).[10] Another significative appellation is the *Scroll of Quintessential* [*Teachings*] (*yang thig gces shog dril*), which alludes to the Nyingma doxographical category of pith instructions.

Despite being redacted in these rather late collections, the rediscovery of the *Vase of Amṛta* is specifically attributed to Dorbum Chökyi Drakpa (*rdor 'bum chos kyi grags pa*), a mysterious yogin from Ngari (*mnga' ris*). We find scattered references to Dorbum within the *Vase of Amṛta*, regarding his physical appearance and his tantric implements: he was a yogin of small stature (*bong thung*) and had a particular spot on his forehead, which caused him to be also known as the "one endowed with the peacock brilliant mark" (*'od kor rma bya'i mdongs can*); and he owned a fanged skull (*ga li* [=*ka li*] *rkan so can*).[11] The *Vase of Amṛta* provides us with the approximate date of its rediscovery that took place "in the year of the sharp-minded hare" (*blo gsal yos bu lo la 'don*). A detailed description of this event is to be found in Dorbum's hagiography: according to this work, the yellow scroll of the *Vase of Amṛta* emerged directly from the hearth of Hayagrīva, the "resplendent subjugator of arrogant beings" (*zil dregs zil gnon*) at the temple of Jang Tradüntsé (*byang pra dun rtse*).[12]

The chapter on the calcite (*cong zhi*) theriac in the modern redaction of the *Vase of Amṛta*, which should correspond to the final section and the colophon of nineteenth-century version of the *Vase of Amṛta*, reveals that this manuscript is a scribal work. The copyist (*yi ge pa*), who calls himself as Sönam Rinchen (*bsod nams rin chen*), provides us with a few temporal and geographical data. After restating the role of Dorbum as treasure-finder (*gter ston*), the copyist starts narrating the account of a so-called "sky-holder" (*gnam 'chang*), who connected the transmission of the manuscript to the "noble clan of those [wearing] shining thunderbolt-proof [armor?] in the lineage of Minyak" (*mi nyag rigs la thog thub mdongs kyi rus*). The copy was written "during the waxing period of the moon in the fourth Mongolian month of the [male] earth-dog year (*sa khyi hor zla bzhi pa'i yar ngo la*), when 2496 years had passed after the Nirvāṇa of the Buddha, in the sacred land with the horned Khyung mountain

10 *'Chi med bdud rtsi bum pa* (1), 6v/5–7r/6; and *'Chi med bdud rtsi bum pa* (2), 9/6–24. The first title refers to the exposition of the issue of epidemics in eight points (primary and secondary causative factors; time and place of the outbreak; diagnosis; ritual protections and therapeutic countermeasures); the other refer to its major subdivisions in the three main tantras devoted to the general exposition of the contents, diagnosis, therapeutics, and apotropaic rituals.

11 *'Chi med bdud rtsi bum pa* (1), 115v/6; *'Chi med bdud rtsi bum pa* (2), 55/6–8.

12 'Jam mgon kong sprul blo sgros mtha' yas, *Gter ston brgya rtsa'i rnam thar* (Lhasa: Bod ljongs mi dmangs dpe skrun khang, 2007), vol. 1, 137/ 9–17.

as its center."[13] Although I have not been able to date this copy of the manuscript based on the provided chronological data, these elements allow us to state that this copy was first redacted no earlier than the thirteenth century.[14]

Despite the paucity of historical data provided by these manuscripts, however, the *Vase of Amṛta* has an intriguing lineage history that connects it both to the Nyingma treasure tradition and to the Tibetan medical tradition. In the *Current of the River Ganges: Enumeration of the Received Teachings on the Vast and Profound Sacred Dharma* (*Gang ga'i chu rgyun*; hereafter *Current of the River Ganges*), the Fifth Dalai Lama Ngawang Lozang Gyatso (*ngag dbang blo bzang rgya mtsho*, 1617–1682) clearly identified the *Vase of Amṛta* as a "northern treasure" (*byang gter*) and connected it to important religious and medical figures, such as the "treasure finder" (*gter ston*) Trashi Topgyel (*bkra shis stobs rgyal*, 1550–1603) and the physicians of the famous Drangti (*brang ti*) and Zur families, even connecting the *Vase of Amṛta* back as far as the twelfth-century Yutok. Although a definitive historical study of the medical lineage of the *Vase of Amṛta* is beyond the scope of the present chapter, we will consider the inter-textual lineage of the *Vase of Amṛta* in the thirteenth and fourteenth centuries, as well as its transmission in the influential medical collections of the seventeenth century.

The intertextual lineage links the *Vase of Amṛta* to the iatrochemistry of mercury procedures (*dngul chu btso bkru*) that originated in Orgyenpa Rinchen Pel's (*o rgyan pa rin chen dpal*, 1229/30–1309) alchemical system and that were transmitted through important collections, such as the Drangti's *Great Measure of Gold* (*gser bre chen mo*) and Lhatsün Rinchen Gyatso's (*lha btsun rin chen rgya mtsho*, fourteenth century) *Collection of Drongtsé* (*'brong rtse be'u bum*). Moreover, the *Vase of Amṛta* probably served as source for the fourteenth-century redaction of the chapter on precious stones remedies of the *Ultimate Tantra* of the *Four Tantras*.[15] Fragments of the *Vase of Amṛta* are

---

13 Compare *'Chi med bdud rtsi bum pa* (2), 101/1–112/9; with the final section and the colophon of *'Chi med bdud rtsi bum pa* (1), 118r/–123r/6.

14 The manuscript of the *'Chi med bdud rtsi bum pa* (2) might have been written after the Mongolian final conquest of Tangut reign in 1226 and the consequent settlement of Tanguts in the eastern territorial areas of Tibetan plateau. Certainly, it was composed later than the introduction of the "Mongolian month" (*hor zla*) to the Tibetan calendar in the thirteenth century by the Drogön Chögyel Pakpa Lodrö Gyeltsen (*'gro mgon chos rgyal 'phags pa blo gros rgyal mtshan*, 1235–1280), who was the preceptor of Kublai Khan.

15 See Dpal ldan rgyal mtshan, *Brang ti lha rje'i rim brgyud kyi man ngag gser bre chen mo* (Lhasa: Bod ljongs mi dmangs dpe skrun khang, 2005),144–78; Lha btsun Rin chen rgya mtsho, *'Brong rtse be'u bum dkar po* (Beijing: Mi rigs dpe skrun khang, 2005), 278/20–283/24. See also Carmen Simioli, "The 'Brilliant Moon Theriac' (*Zla zil dar ya kan*): A Preliminary Study of Mercury Processing according to the *Vase of Amrita of Immortality*

included in other sections of the *Great Measure of Gold* and consist of short recipes and spells for curing specific *rim* and *nyen* diseases, such as the *rim* disease of the gall bladder and the bile duct (*mkhris rims*), or the *rim* disease affecting the gastrointestinal tract (*rgyu gzer*). The treasure text is referred to as the *Innermost Essence of the Vase of Amṛta* (*bdud rtsi bum pa yang snying*) and Guru Padmasambhava's "oral pith instruction source" (*man ngag* = Skt. *upadeśa*) transmitted through the Drangti medical system.[16] With this information in mind, it might be possible to assume that at least sections of the *Vase of Amṛta* circulated widely and were preserved in the indirect medical textual tradition from the thirteenth century onward.

At the turn of the seventeenth century, the speculative models, which guided the interpretation and classification of epidemic fevers and infective diseases in Tibet, were well-established conceptions rooted in the study of the *Four Tantras*, as well as in the study of formative magical and alchemical scriptures. Sanggyé Gyatso (*sangs rgyas rgya mtsho*, 1653–1705), regent (*sde srid*) of the Fifth Dalai Lama and leading academic theorist of medicine, composed several commentarial works on the *Four Tantras*, including a subsidiary collection entitled the *Camphor That Dispels the Torments of Fevers, the Sword That Cuts off the Lasso of Untimely Death: Supplements to the Excellent Tantra of Oral Instructions* (*man ngag yon tan rgyud gyi lhan thabs zug rngu'i tsha gdung sel ba'i kat pu ra dus min 'chi zhags gcod pa'i ral gri*; hereafter *Supplements to the Instructional Tantra*). The contents and structure of its chapters devoted to *nyenrim* reflect the clear authorial intent of systematizing all of the notions on these diseases distilled from authoritative medical and religious sources in a coherent and legitimate body of knowledge. Sanggyé Gyatso also supplemented the instructions of the *Four Tantras* with a plethora of recipes, spells to consecrate medicines, and protective rituals derived from tantric sources, presenting them as an expansion of something inherent in the medical classic.[17]

In the twenty-sixth chapter on "contagious fever" and "Nepalese disease" (*bal nad*), and in thirtieth chapter on the "*nyen* disease afflicting the brain" (*klad gzer*), Sanggyé Gyatso states his indebtedness to several tantras of the "early translation" (*snga 'gyur*) and of the "late translation" (*phyi 'gyur*) schools. He tried to produce a perfect "synthesis of the pith instructions drawn from

('*Chi med bdud rtsi bum pa*) and Its Influence on Tibetan Pharmacological Literature," *Revenue d'Etudes Tibétaines* 37 (2016): 391–419.

16 *Brang ti lha rje'i brgyud kyi man ngag gser bre chen mo*, 203/3–204/13; 236/13–237/8; 252/17–253/6.

17 On the secret recipes of the *Supplements*, see Tony Chui, "'Secret Medicine' in the Writings of Sanggyé Gyatso: The Encoded Esoteric Material of Therapeutics," in the present volume.

the 'treasure texts' ascribed to Padmasambhava."[18] The contents of the *Supplements to the Instructional Tantra* reflect not only the place of magic in Sanggyé Gyatso's medical thought, but it can also offer a perspective on the status of specific ritual magic texts in the history of Tibetan medicine. Plumbing the intricate web of literary references in the *Supplements to the Instructional Tantra*, we find that Sanggyé Gyatso quoted passages from a treasure text entitled the *Great Guru's Vase of Amṛta* (*gu ru chen po'i bdud rtsi bum pa*),[19] which can be identified as the *Vase of Amṛta* on the basis of intertextual analysis. As we can infer from the *Current of the River Ganges*, upon which Sanggyé Gyatso relied to describe the contents of the *Vase of Amṛta* in his medical historiography, the *Vase of Amṛta* in question seems to coincide with the *textus receptus* preserved in the nineteenth-century *Precious Treasury* collection.[20] The influential role of this scripture in the *Supplements to the Instructional Tantra* was certainly due to the Fifth Dalai Lama's lineage of transmission.

In the seventeenth century, the *Vase of Amṛta* became one of the most authoritative sources concerning the treatment of epidemics and poisoning. Deumar Tendzin Püntsok (*de'u dmar bstan' dzin phun thsogs*, b. 1672), important theorist and physician, frequently cites the *Vase of Amṛta* in his chapter devoted to the treatment of the "black disease, union of the three" (*nag po gsum sgril*). Like the Drangti physicians, Deumar calls it the *Innermost Essence of the Vase of Amṛta* and classifies it as an oral instruction.[21]

The lineage of transmission of the *Vase of Amṛta* can be traced up to nineteenth century. The *Precious Treasury* collection not only preserves the *textus receptus* of the *Vase of Amṛta* but includes a series of related instructional texts, such as the *Essential Daily Practices of the Vase of Amṛta* (*bdud rtsi bum pa'i rgyun khyer snying dril*), the transmission and guiding explanations of the *Vase of Amṛta* authored by the luminary Jamgön Kongtrül, who worked alongside with the treasure finder Jamyang Khyentsé Wangpo for the preservation of the

18 Sangs rgyas rgya mtsho, *Man ngag gi yon tan rgyud gi lhan thabs* (Xining: Mtsho mi rigs dpe skrung khang, 1991), 175/11–176/3.

19 Sangs rgyas rgya mtsho, *Man ngag gi yon tan rgyud gi lhan thabs*, 184/8.

20 I have compared the catalogue of contents provided in the *Gang ga'i chu rgyun* and the contents of *'Chi med bdud rtsi bum pa* (1) and *'Chi med bdud rtsi bum pa* (2). For references see the previous note and Ngag dbang blo bzang rgya mtsho, *Zab pa dang rgya che ba'i dam chos kyi yig gang ga'i chu rgyun*, in *Gsung 'bum* (Gangthok: Sikkim Research Institute of Tibetology, 1991–95), vol. 1 (*gsan yig ka*), 340/1–345/9. See also Gavin Kilty, trans., *Mirror of Beryl: A Historical Introduction to Tibetan Medicine* (Boston, MA: Wisdom Publications, 2009), 177–85.

21 De'u dmar btan'dzin phun tshogs, *Gso rig gces btus rin chen phreng ba* (Xining: Mtsho sgnon mi rigs dpe skrun khang, 1993), 205/14–218/3.

treasure text tradition.[22] This work has been included in a modern extended edition of the *Yutok Heart Essence* (*g.yu thog snying thig*), an anthology of ritual practices related to different medical lineages.[23] This brief conspectus provides us with some noteworthy elements. The medical lineage of the *Vase of Amṛta* can be traced back to the fourteenth century, when it was considered an authoritative recipe book and spell book whose excerpts circulated through important medical collections and were part of the secret oral transmissions connected to medical lineages. Its influential role was mainly related to the codification of mercurial procedures. Its importance increased in the seventeenth century due to Nyingma lineage of the Fifth Dalai Lama. Its history is intertwined with the renaissance of the treasure-tradition within the non-sectarian (*rigs med*) movement of the nineteenth century. The presence of Jamgön Kongtrül's text in the modern redaction of the *Yutok Heart Essence* shows that the ritual practice based on the *Vase of Amṛta* is effectively part of a set of accomplishing medicine rituals connected to the medical tradition still being practiced today.

Drawing on the contents of the *Vase of Amṛta*, it is possible to determine other relevant elements that can allow us to better situate the *Vase of Amṛta* in the broader contexts of medical and alchemical literatures. Specific passages will illustrate how in the *Vase of Amṛta*, the alchemical quest for the long-life elixir and the search for the ultimate remedy against pestilences and poisons came to be conflated. The core part of this paper will be devoted to the analysis of the whole spectrum of diagnostic methods and rituals described in the *Vase of Amṛta*: its contents stretch from medical rubrics to divinatory prognosis (*kha dmar*). The work also deals with the preparation and consecration of "medical compounds" (*sbyor ba*) known as theriac (*dar ya kan*), the preparation of magical "unguents" (*phyug sman*), and "protective amulets" (*srung 'khor*), or ritualized therapies. Before discussing the contents of the *Vase of Amṛta*, it is necessary to first briefly introduce the concept of *nyenné* and *rimné*

22 Jamgön Kongtrül, *Bdud rtsi bum pa'i rgyun khyer snying dril*, in *Rin chen gter mdzod* (Paro: Stod lung mtsur phu'i par khang, 1980), vol. 47 (*ci, ha–a*), 1r/1–3r/1. The *Index of Treasure Texts Dealing with the Protection* [*From Epidemics*] (*Srung ba'i kha byang*) by Jamyang Khyentsé Wangpo, includes the *Vase of Amṛta*, among other important magic-medical sources. See *Slob dpon pad 'byung gi sman yig gces btus*, 367–89.

23 *G.yu thog snying thig* (Beijing: Mi rigs dpe skrun khang, 2007), 11–13. This has been edited by the Arura Institute and Medical Research Association in Tsongön. Based on the Lhasa Chakpori (*lcags po ri*) redaction of the collection authored by Karma Jigmé Sengé (*karma 'jigs med seng ge*, nineteenth century), this anthology has been expanded with the addition of writings composed by authors from different historical periods.

as expressed in ancient authoritative and canonical sources from the tenth to the seventeenth century.

2 The Etiology of *Nyenné* and *Rimné* According to Canonical Medical Sources: Physical Causation, Morbific Airs, and Demonic Poisons

This preliminary investigation intends to probe the coexistence of different explanatory models and the considerable uniformity of the medical discourse on *nyenné* and *rimné* from the twelfth to seventeenth century. Its core focuses on the analysis of sections from the *Instructional Tantra* (*man ngag rgyud*) of the *Four Tantras*, which has been compared with the *Sons' Benefit* (*bu don ma*), an ancillary treatise ascribed to Yutok Yönten Gönpo. We will also briefly refer to a medical source predating the *Four Tantras*, known as the *Moon King* (*zla ba'i rgyal po*). This analysis of the *Instructional Tantra*, will be complemented, when considered necessary, with references to exegetical writings such the *Blue Beryl* (*baidurya sngon po*) and the *Supplements to the Instructional Tantra* authored by Sanggyé Gyatso.

The Tibetan etiology of *nyenné* and *rimné* ultimately developed in the context of ancient Āyurvedic concepts. The selected sources provide a three-folded epidemic causality: diseases are determined by natural factors, supernatural factors, and are related to a moral causality. The taxonomy of *nyenné* and *rimné* proposed by both the *Sons' Benefit* and the *Instructional Tantra* notably corresponds with the etiological models provided by the Tibetan translation of the *Compendium of the Essence of the Eight Branches* (*yan lag brgyad pa'i snying po bsdus pa* = Skt. *aṣṭāṅgahṛdayasaṃhitā*; hereafter, *Essence of the Eight Branches*),[24] the well-known classic of Āyurveda authored by Vāgbhaṭa (*pha khol*).

According to these scriptures, the "three disturbing elements" (*nyes pa gsum*) and blood (*khrag*) are the dominant physiological models for interpreting *nyenrim*. *Rimné* are classified in four categories corresponding to each of the cited "disturbing elements" as well as their "combination" (*'dus pa*).[25] These

24 *Yan lag brgyad pa'i snying po bsdus pa*, in *Sbyor ba brgya ba dang yan lag brgyad pa'i snying po bsdus pa sogs* (Beijing: Mi rigs dpe skrun khang, 2005), 309/12–316/11.

25 There are six classes of *rim* diseases forming three couples of diseases, each associated with one of the "three disturbing factors": a) Epidemics fevers associated with "wind" (*rlung rims*), i.e. febrile states associated with insomnia called *yerbu* (*yer bu*), are characterized by intensive shivering, called *darbu* (*'dar bu*), which manifests in the prodromal phase of the disease; b) epidemic fever associated with "bile" (*mkhris rims*), i.e. *lepgen* (*leb rgan*), are characterized by yellow watery eyes and mucus, the disease of atrocious pain

three elements are potential pathogenic factors influenced by wrong behaviors, in particular excessive exhausting actions (*drag shul*), an imbalanced dietetic regimen (*kha zas ma snyoms*), and unusual changes in the climate that happen when the "seasons display inappropriate features" (*dus bzhi'i 'byung ba dman lhag log*; lit. the "elements of the four seasons are less or more than appropriate, or the opposite").[26] The fourth class of *rim* diseases is conceived as a clear manifestation of demonic assaults. The term used to identify the disease-carrier demon is *dön* (*gdon*), which refers to an evil uncanny force sent by non-human beings and therefore referred to as negative influence of malevolent "elemental beings" (*'byung po*).

In order to gain a clear picture of how *nyenné* and *rimné* are interpreted in the *Instructional Tantra*, we will now turn to the concept of contagion. In the *Instructional Tantra*, the term *rim*, which literally means "gradual," is glossed as follows: (a) it refers to a disease that enters the body thorough the nose and subsequently affects the other "entrances" (*'jug sgo*), i.e. it manifests by penetrating the skin, then gradually affects the flesh, the channels, the bones, and the organs; (b) it describes the contagious nature of the disease, which can spread through impure solid substances (*dri dngos*) or "air" (*rlung*) and "smoke" (*du ba*) emanating from the "disease breeding ground" (*nad yod sa*), and by infecting one after another, finally reaching "epidemic proportions" (*yams su rims kyis 'gos pa*).[27]

Among the causes for such contagions, "impurity" (*dri ma*) is primary. The term refers to physical defilements, deriving from the contact with impure substances (human and animal), the pungent odors of infected bodies (*nad dri*), and the effluvia that infest insalubrious places. This concept is further developed within the context of the subgroup of *nyen* diseases. According to the *Instructional Tantra*, unpleasant smells descend from the sky as pestilential vapors that are disseminated by irate goddesses, become morbific stains that enter the body, and affect the organism. The *Sons' Benefit* refers to the celestial miasmas of diverse colors exhaled by mother goddesses (*ma mo*)

of the brain (*glad zer*); c) epidemics associated with "phlegm" (*bad kan rims*), i.e. diseases characterised by aphasia and mental torpor (*rmongs bu*), are diseases characterized by a state of dullness and muteness (*lkugs pa*). *Bu don ma* (Beijing: Mi rigs dpe skrung khang, 2009), 84/1–86/10. For a further analysis of the *Bu don ma*, see Henk Blezer, "A New Sense of (Dark) Humor in Tibet: Brown Phlegm and Black Bile," in the present volume.

26 *Bdud rtsi snying po yan lag brgyad pa gsang ba man ngag gi rgyud*, 641/13–14.

27 *Bdud rtsi snying po yan lag brgyad pa gsang ba man ngag gi rgyud*, 243/11–12. See also Sangs rgyas rgya mtsho, *Gso ba rig pa'i bstan bcos sman bla'i dgongs rgyan rgyud bzhi'i gsal byed baidur sngon po'i mallika* (Lhasa: Bod ljongs mi dmangs dpe skrun khang, 1982), 642/1–4.

as disturbances that provoke specific *rim* diseases.[28] The morbific stains are invisible entities called *parpata*, categorized as *sinbu* (*srin bu*), which are described at length in Sanggyé Gyatso's *Blue Beryl* and *Supplements to the Instructional Tantra*.

Nevertheless, "impurity" also refers to moral faults that occur due to social and religious transgressions, as well as the desecration of nature and the dwellings of supernatural beings, which determine demonic influences.[29] The *Moon King* identifies "impurity" (*mi gtsang*), "malice" (*'khon*), and the "bad smell of burning impure animal substances" (*gzhog pa*) as the "immediate causes" for the onset of *gaklhok* (*gag lhog*), a specific class of contagious disease characterized by swelling throat and ulcers. According to this text, the "disturbances" (*'khrugs*) of "planetary gods" (*gza'*), "lunar mansions" (*rgyu skar*), "ferocious goddesses" (*ma mo*), and "local deities" (*sa bdag*) are causative factors of poxes (*'brum bu*).[30] This idea is reiterated in the eighty-first chapter of the *Blue Beryl*: the demonic assaults of *nyen* spirits (*gnyan gdon*) are provoked by (1) the destruction or (2) the profanation of deities' dwellings. Here "impurity" refers to polluting substances (*grib can*)—human odor, garbage, leftovers, and so forth—thrown into spirits' abodes. Fireplaces are also considered impure when the burning stoves (*thab*) leak various substances such as water (water extinguishes fire and leaves wet ash), blood, butter, or milk. Other impure substances include "burning animal parts," such as skin, fur, and bones, which produce "foul smoke" (*dud ba ngan*). Impurity can also be more abstract, referring to the "performance of wanton actions" (*'jol nyog spyod pa*), such as slaughtering animals, Buddhist monks or Bönpos who have no time to properly perform the "preliminary practices, *sādhana* meditation, and ritual activities" (*snyen sgrub las gsum*), or contaminating spirit dwellings with impure substances used for "black curses" (*mthu gtad*).

28 The female spirits called *ma mo* are ichnographically represented as wrathful sorceresses with emaciated and pendant breasts, bringing sacks full of diseases. In some cases, the *ma mo* are hybrid figures with animal heads. See René de Nebesky-Wojkowitz, *Oracles and Demons of Tibet: The Cult and Iconography of the Tibetan Protective Deities* (Delhi: Book Faith India, 1993), 269–72. *Bu don ma*, 84/3–4.

29 See Giuseppe Tucci, *Le Religioni del Tibet* (Roma: Edizioni Mediterranee, 1996), 217.

30 *Sman dpad zla ba'i rgyal po* (Leh: Tashigang, 1989), 69r/3–6. This disease is a classified as a hybrid *nyenrim* disease; its onset is characterized by the eruption of pustules and bulla caused by excessive impure blood and "yellow fluids" (*chu ser*, lit. "yellow water") beneath the skin; the process of suppuration starts from the feet and spreads overall the body. There are two categories of poxes: 1) "white poxes" (*'brum dkar*) caused by the combination of phlegm, wind, and cold disorder (*bad rlung grang ba shas che*); and 2) "black poxes" determined by bile and blood (*mkhris khrag shas che*). See Byams pa 'phrin las et al., *Bod lugs gso rig tshig mdzod chen mo* (Beijing: Mi rigs dpe skrun khang, 2006), 599.

The idea of contagion is related to a multidimensional perception of "impurity," which involves magical-religious conceptions and also has moral connotations. This aspect reflects, again, a correspondence with ideas developed in Vāgbhaṭa's work, and it is also comparable to the similar category of "errors of judgment" found in the *Compendium of Caraka* (*carakasaṃhitā*):[31] the individual predisposition to be affected by contagious fevers is rooted in negative mental attitudes and emotions, such as harboring hate, ager, fear, longing, and suffering, which are conceived as immediate causes of *rim* fevers.[32] When moral degeneration and decadence penetrate every social level, contagious fevers reach epidemic proportion. This point is particularly stressed in the *Instructional Tantra* and even more radically, as we will see, in the prophetic *Vase of Amṛta*, which starts with the narration of the fall of human society as the cause of pestilence and demonic forces.

Another fundamentally remarkable correspondence between the *Instructional Tantra* and the *Vase of Amṛta* concerns the idea of poison in relation to demonic influences. While Vāgbhata's *Essence of the Eight Branches* clearly distinguishes the scents of plants (*sman dri*), poisons (*dug*), and demonic attacks (*gdon gzhugs*) as three different causes of *rim* diseases, the *Instructional Tantra* describes "poisonous influences of malevolent spirits" (*'byung bo'i gdug*) as a possible cause of contagion. This interpretation is restated in later exegetical sources, such as the *Blue Beryl* and the *Supplements to the Instructional Tantra*.[33]

3 Etiology and Taxonomy of *Nyen* and *Rim* according to the *Vase of Amṛta*

The etiological models described in the *Vase of Amṛta* are consistent with those already examined. Both the natural and the demonic aspects of *nyenrim* are considered concomitant, but in the context of this prophetic literature, the moral and the supernatural causes of the disease are emphasized. According to the *Vase of Amṛta*, human arrogance and misbehaviors outrage

31 See Dominik Wujastyk, *The Roots of Āyurveda: Selections from Sanskrit Medical Writings* (London: Penguin Books, 2001), 79–91.

32 *Yan lag brgyad pa'i snying po bsdus pa* 312/23–313/4; *Bdud rtsi snying po yan lag brgyad pa gsang ba man ngag gi rgyud*, 243/9–10; and *Gso ba rig pa'i bstan bcos sman bla'i dgongs rgyan rgyud bzhi'i gsal byed baidurya sngon po'i mallika*, 641/14–19. See also Sangs rgyas rgya mtsho, *Man ngag gi yon tan rgyud gi lhan thabs*, 97/6–7.

33 See the previous note. See also Olaf Czaja, "*The Four Tantras* and the Global Market: Changing Epistemologies of *Drä* (*'bras*) versus Cancer," in *Medicine Between Science and Religion*, ed. V. Adams et al. (New York, NY: Berghahn Books, 2011), 286.

the demons and gods of the eight classes (*sde brgyad*), and in turn the ferocious *mamo* exhale noxious (*dug can*) breath (*kha rlangs*), which forms clouds in order to disseminate deadly diseases. The final five hundred years of our cosmic eon are called a "dark age" (*snyigs dus*) of moral and spiritual degeneration, characterized by the dissolution of the social order and by the downfall of religious vows, wars, famine, and the diffusion of pestilence. The nature of the disease is vividly described using an imaginative and codified language, as can be inferred from this passage of the *Vase of Amṛta*, entitled *Treatment for the All-Encompassing Oblivion: The Amṛta of Riving the Dead* (*cog 'gyel bcos thabs bdud rtsi shi sos*):

> [...] During the five hundred eons of degeneration, atrocious and horrific diseases [will appear]. They will be called the "poisonous all-encompassing oblivion," or the untimely death that befalls unexpectedly, baring its teeth with a sardonic grin. Trying to dispel them will be like facing a raging fire. They will be the death that comes under the conditions conducive to epidemic infections, and they will be difficult to cure. The mere sound of them will strike terror [...].[34]

The *nyen* disease described in the *Vase of Amṛta* comes under the category of the "black poisonous all-encompassing oblivion" (*ha la cog 'gyel nag po*),[35] a complex concept that simultaneously defines both the virulent and the deadly aspects of the pathology. Its symptoms are compared to those of a potent "poison" (*ha la*). Its fatal nature is expressed by the term *chokgyel* (*cog 'gyel*), which portrays the image of a multitude of falling corpses claimed by the disease, which "steals their life-supporting breath" (*lus srog dbugs 'jags par byed pa*).[36]

The dramatic description is ultimately accomplished with the demonic embodiment of the disease, which is represented by a ferocious sardonic mask. *Nyen* refers to a particular class of liminal beings dwelling in natural abodes, but at the same time it also identifies a particular class of diseases, heralds of divine ire, pathologies that are characterized by the presence of a noxious

34 *'Chi med bdud rtsi bum pa* (1), 71v/1–3.

35 *'Chi med bdud rtsi bum pa* (1), 73/7.

36 The *Great Dictionary of Tibetan Medicine* describes this *nyen* disease, which mainly affects the brain and the heart, as follows: *dug can srin bus bskyes pa'i gnyan nad stobs chen snying dang klad pa la phog nad yod do kun 'gyel te srog 'dor byas pa'i don* (Byams pa 'phrin las et al., *Bod lugs gso rig tshig mdzod chen mo*, 998).

parasite in the organism (*dug can srin*), which is related to the increasing impure yellow serum (*chu ser*) and blood.[37]

The term *nyen*, which already connotes the malignant nature of the diseases, is often correlated to specific adjectives, such as "wild" (*rgod pa*), thereby revealing the interpretation of the disease as an aggressive force, similar to a wild animal that can feed on human flesh. This is the initial phase of the disease, which corresponds to the demon's bite (*gdon gyi so bas bzung ba*).[38] The description of the disease called *lhokpa* (*lhog pa*), which subsumes different kinds of ulcers and swelling sores, is a paradigmatic representation of the fiery essence of *nyenné*. *Lhokpa* is described as follows:

> [Among] the signs of the disease [by which one can diagnose *lhokpa*] there is the [taxonomic] category of the four elements. The *lhokpa* disease associated with the wind element [is characterized by] pale and soft [pustules], the swelling is temporary and pulsating, and it is similar to a belly full of yogurt. The *lhokpa* associated with the fire element is bloody and painful, it manifests as a strong fever that flares up quickly and is permeated with a heat, which possess the quality of a flaming immeasurable mansion. The *lhokpa* disease associated with the water element is a swelling disease, soft and wet, and characterized by cool vesicles, which, to using a metaphor, [are cold] as a blue glacial turquoise lake. The *lhokpa* disease associated with the earth element is firm and solid; the swelling is firm and black in color and spreads over the head. It is similar to an iron pan turned upside down with the opening [on the ground]. Besides, there are the two categories of *wild* and *wildest*. The wild one spreads as quickly as a running elephant, the pain is strong, and it rides on the channels. The *wildest* is characterized by a large swelling [similar to] a volcano and it spreads radiating towards the edge [of the wounds]. It is also called the thorny plant with nine heads.[39]

Here *wild* (*rgod*) and *wildest* (*yang rgod*) represent two distinct categories of this disease, or two different degrees of the same disease. This taxonomy and the related terminology are also kept in later works on *nyenné*, such as *Supplements to the Instructional Tantra*.[40] The preservation of this metaphorical

37 *'Chi med bdud rtsi bum pa* (2) 40/ 17–18. See also the *Guru's Lesser Vase* (*gu ru bdud rtsi bum chung*), which also was rediscovered by Dorbum. *Slob dpon gso rig gces btus*, 193/10–11: […] *ming ni srin bu par pa ta zhes bya ba yin//*.

38 *'Chi med bdud rtsi bum pa* (2), 10/15.

39 *'Chi med bdud rtsi bum pa* (2), 123/19–124/11.

40 Sangs rgyas rgya mtsho, *Man ngag gi yon tan rgyud gi lhan thabs*, 208/13–209/8.

language is indicative of a certain level of coherence of the intellectual representation of these ulcers in pre-modern Tibetan medicine.[41] Interestingly, this same description is found in the *Son's Benefit*, where this description is said to drawn upon an oral pith instruction text (*man ngag*).[42]

According to the *Vase of Amṛta*, the natures of all the diseases are identical, but what differs is the specific organ or part of the body that is affected. The five macro-categories of *nyenné* are distinguished as follows: when the disease manifests externally (*phyi ru byung ba*), it becomes the aforementioned *lhokpa* (*lhog pa*), which has also three subcategories of "doe disease" (*yu mo*),[43] the "*lhok* disease affecting internal [organs]" (*khong lhog*), and the "*lhok* disease affecting the calf" (*byin lhog*). When *lhokpa* affects the throat (*gre bar byung ba*), it is *gakpa* (*gag pa*); when it affects the viscera (*don la babs pa*), it is *zertung*; when it affects the hollow organs (*snod par babs ba*), it is "the pain afflicting the gastrointestinal tract" (*rgyu zer*) and "pain afflicting the upper part of the body" (*stod zer*).[44] Along with these five, the texts enumerate the following *rimné* and *nyenrim* diseases: "epidemic influenza" (*chams rims*); "white and black poxes" (*'brum dkar dang nag*), and other similar diseases called *bekgé* (*beg ge*), "yellow-eye disease" (*mig zer*), or even the "disease affecting the brain" (*klad zer*); "plague" (*byis rims*, lit. "an epidemic [spread] by rats"); "dysentery" (*dmar bshal*); "twisted esphagus" (*mid 'chus*); and "sardonic grin" (*'dzum ltag dgye*), which aligns with the category of tetanus.[45]

41 In the history of ancient Eurasian medical systems, there are analogous cases. For example, the Hippocratic Corpus describes the nature of ulcers as "wild" or even "ferocious," using a vocabulary inherited from Greek tragedies. Indeed, as the Hippocratic doctors transformed the metaphorical language of tragedy into technical language, medical scholars drew upon the imaginative and religious representation of disease provided in visionary works such as the *'Chi med bdud rtsi bum pa*. For a further reading on the Hippocratic concept of epidemics see Jacques Jouanna and Neil Allias, trans., "Disease as Aggression in Hippocratic Corpus and Greek Tragedy: Wild and Devouring Diseases," in *Greek Medicine from Hippocrates to Galen*, ed. Philips van der Eijk (Leiden: Brill, 2012), 81–96.

42 *Bu don ma*, 121/1–122/2.

43 "Doe disease" (*yu mo*) is a swelling disease characterized by spotted pustules similar to small pox. *'Chi med bdud rtsi bum pa* (1), 111v/4–112v/1.

44 *'Chi med bdud rtsi bum pa* (1), 63v7/1–69v/4.

45 The disease causes spasms that affect the facial muscles resulting in the appearance of a sardonic grin; it causes spasms of the back muscles and the consequent arching of the neck bones and spine. See *'Chi med bdud rtsi bum pa* (1), 93r/5–93v/4.

3.1 *Diagnosis and Divinatory Prognosis of* Nyenrim *According to the* Vase of Amṛta

The following section will be devoted to the examination of the diagnostic techniques described in the *Vase of Amṛta*: we will observe how the hermeneutics of pathology are based on a detailed differential description of the diseases, which starts from the general symptomatology and proceeds to the specific symptoms, and lead to the localization and the identification of the noxious demons. The passages reveal a methodical accuracy that is a distinctive feature of a medical mentality: the spectrum of the symptoms, which *in itinere* becomes more and more specific, serves as frame of reference to isolate the significative morbific features, reconstruct the taxonomy of the pathology (see the above description of ulcers), and consequently apply the right cure.[46] The description provides us with a sophisticated depiction of the internal body, which is the result of overlapping models of physiology that originated in tantric and medical matrices. The analyzed sections unfold an internal landscape of intricate paths (*lam*) connecting functional organs to hollow organs and sense organs (section 3.2), and hint to the visionary system of subtle light channels called "lamps" (*sgron ma*) of the Nyingma Great Perfection (*rdzog chen*) tradition (sections 3.2 and 3.3). The discussion will illustrate the inextricable twofold nature of the diagnostic process described in the *Vase of Amṛta*, at the same time divinatory and based on empirical observation.

The main diagnostic sections of the *Vase of Amṛta* are: (a) the root diagnostic tantra, entitled *Union of the Sun and Moon* (*rtags pa nyi zla kha sbyor*), otherwise called the *Mañjuśrī Heart Essence: Union of the Sun and Moon* (*'jam pa'i dbyangs kyi thugs kyi bcud nyi zla kha sbyor*);[47] (b) its commentary entitled the *Exegetical Tantra Mañjuśrī Heart Essence: Union of the Sun and Moon*, otherwise called the *Exegetical Tantra: The Sun Illuminating the Diagnostic Signs* (*brtags pa nyi ma'i snang gsal bshad rgyud*);[48] (c) the *Innermost Pillar of the Vital Force* (*yang gsang srog gyi ka chen*);[49] and (d) the *Great Treasure of Vital Strength* (*srog gter chen gyi gyad*).[50] Both the *Mañjuśrī Heart Essence* texts begin with the invocation of Mañjuśrī, the primordial Buddha Vagiśvara, and

46 On empiricism in Tibetan medicine see Janet Gyatso's groundbreaking work: Janet Gyatso, *Being Human in a Buddhist World: An Intellectual History of Medicine in Early Modern Tibet* (New York, NY: Columbia University Press, 2015).

47 *'Chi med bdud rtsi bum pa* (1), 7v/1–9v/1; *'Chi med bdud rtsi bum pa* (2), 10–12.

48 *'Chi med bdud rtsi bum pa* (1), 9v/1–12v/5; *'Chi med bdud rtsi bum pa* (2), 10–19.

49 *'Chi med bdud rtsi bum pa* (1), 44v/4–45v/6; *'Chi med bdud rtsi bum pa* (2), 47–52.

50 *'Chi med bdud rtsi bum pa* (1), 35v/4–38r/1. In the *'Chi med bdud rtsi bum pa* (2), 40–44; the title is the *Medical Compounds of the Great Treasure of the Vital Strength* (*srog gter chen gyi sbyor ba*).

his Bodhisattva youthful form, Kumāra. Being the embodiment of transcendent wisdom, he discerns the different aspects of these fatal diseases and can guide the practitioner during the diagnosis, thus the signs will appear clear to him as the "vision of the rising sun light" (*rtags nyin shar dang 'dra*). The diagnostic procedure is conceived as a process of divine inspiration (*rtogs pa dang ldan pa dang zhing lha'i nga rgyal dang ldan*).[51] As we can infer from an analysis of the corpus, however, the diagnostic instructions in the root and exegetical tantras are also based on the detailed empirical observation of general and specific symptoms (*spyi dang byed brag gi brtags*) that manifest in connection with the three aspects of the diseases, which are "wind" (*rlung*), fever (*tshad*), and *nyen*. This is the reason why the disease is called the "black one, union of the three" (*nag po sum sgril*). Although, as we shall see, the progression of the disease is associated with the three humors, the connection of the demoniac disease with deviant winds is particularly stressed and points to an ancient medical conception, developed in different medical contexts. The *Carakasaṃhitā* describes the normal and abnormal function of wind with its divine creative and destructive powers, in nature and humanity.[52] The perverted wind-demonic force (*guiqi* 鬼气) also characterizes epidemics and the class of *xie* 邪 diseases in traditional Chinese medicine.[53]

In order to diagnose the disease, the physician observes changes in the patient's physical appearance and the physiopathology of pain through "channel examination" (*rtsa brtags*) and "uroscopy" (*chu brtags*). According to this system, every disease is associated with the "three disturbing factors," as well as with "cold" (*grang*) or "heat" (*tsha*) manifestations of the febrile states and with the "categories of the five elements" (*'byung ba lnga'i rigs*). The prodromal phase of the disease, which is called the "gray unripened state of the disease" (*skya rims ma smin*), is related to "wind" and fever. In this phase, the demonic attack is detectable through the interpretation of "turbid dreams" (*rmi lam nyag nyog*). The following excerpt describes the "wind" aspect of the disease:

> In the case of "wind," the pain is acute at dawn and in the evening (*tho rangs dang dgong shin tu rlang*); ocular bulbs are painful and the person may faint (*mig ril na 'gyel snyoms byed*); buzzing in the ears (*rna 'ur*) and despair (*snying mi dga'*) arise, as well as febrile states characterized by

51 *'Chi med bdud rtsi bum pa* (2), 18/4–5.

52 Priyavrat Sharma, *Carakasaṃhitā: Text with English Translation* (Varanasi: Chaukhambha Orientalia, 2014), 81–84.

53 Vivienne Lo and Sylvia Schroer, "Deviant Airs in Traditional Chinese Medicine," in *Asia Medicine in Globalisation* (Philadelphia, PA: University of Pennsylvania Press, 2005), 45–66.

> intensive shivering (*'dar bu*). The symptoms are similar to those of "cold diseases that belong to the category of the element water" (*grang ba'i nad ltar g.yo 'byung chu'i rigs*); the pain is so strong that the bones of the lower part of the body seem to boil (*ro smad kyi rus pa khol*). The "pulse is empty and submerged" (*rtsa stong bying*) or "scarcely perceptible" (*nyams chung*); feces and urine are retained and fever moves through the circulatory system (*rtsa chu dal ba rtsa kha tsha ba 'ong*).[54]

The state of fever places these diseases under the "category of the fire element" (*'byung me'i rigs*), which are characterized by intense "shivering and straight body hair" (*phrum ser khyer*), "dry nose and mouth" (*kha sna skams*), and a "quick pulse" (*rtsa mkhyogs*). The intermediate and increasing state of the disease (*'bar rgyas rtags*) is the visible sign of *nyen.* During this phase the disease manifests the symptoms of "phlegm" (*bad kan*), "bile" (*mkhris pa*), or combined disorders (*'dus pa*). The first category is characterized by a "black tongue" (*lce nag*), "deterioration of the sense faculties" (*dbang po nyams*), a submerged and "profound pulse" (*gting rtsa*), or a "subtle pulse" (*phra rtsa*) and an "accelerated pulse" (*myur rtsa*). The latter category is associated with the "element space" (*'byung nam mkha'i rigs*) and shows all the symptoms together (*kun 'dus pa*). The disease process culminates in irreversible injuries of functional organs (*don la 'babs*). It should also be said that this diagnostic section finds correspondences in the general description of symptoms provided in the *Sons' Benefit* and the *Four Tantras.*[55]

3.2 *Pathogenic Demonic Pulses in the* Vase of Amṛta

The "pulses of obstructive beings" (*bgegs rtsa*) are the abnormal pulses of functional organs and reveal the class and the nature of demonic forces. Every functional organ is associated with a sense organ and one of the five elements, which are considered "mounts of the obstructive forces" (*bgegs 'byung ba bzhi nam kha' dang lnga rta la zhon*). These pulses show clear similarities with descriptions provided in the *Ultimate Tantra* (*phyi'i rgyud*) of the *Four Tantras* and with the medical literature predating it, such as the *Lamp of Sunrays* (*nyi zer sgron ma*) attributed to Nāgārjuna. Every organ corresponds to a specific class of elemental beings. According to the *Vase of Amṛta,* "king spirits" (*rgyal po*) are related to the heart; "demons of madness" (*smyo 'dres*) are related to the lungs; "serpent spirits" (*klu*), "earth lord spirits" (*sa bdag*), and "haunting

54 *'Chi med bdud rtsi bum pa* (2), 14/1–8.

55 *Bu don ma*, 84–99; *Bdud rtsi snying po yan lag brgyad pa gsang ba man ngag gi rgyud*, 243 et passim.

ghosts" (*bstan*) are related to the liver; "mother goddesses" (*ma mo*) and serpent spirits are related to the kidneys; and "cannibal demons" (*sa srin*) are related to the intestines.[56]

These obstructive forces are localized through: (a) their entrances (*'jug sgo*); (b) their "wandering pathways" (*'grims pa'i srang*); (c) "regions and residences" (*yul gnas*); and (d) "fortresses" (*rdzong*).[57] A geographic imaginary is involved in the construction of the environment for the description of the pulses. (a) The demon of the regal caste (*rgyal rigs*) mounts the fire element and enters the body from the life-force *cakra* (*srog 'khor*) aperture of Brahmā at the top of the head. The demon of the servile class (*dmangs rigs*) mounts the water element and enters the body from the door of the "karmic wind of formative actions" (*'du byed las kyi rlung*) or from "nerves and tendons of the heel of the foot" (*rkang mthil chu rgyus sgo*). The demon of the aristocratic class (*rje rigs*) mounts the wind element and enters the body from "right subtle channel" (*ro ma'i sgo*). The Brahmin demon (*bram ze*) mounts the earth element and enters the body from the "door of the left subtle channel" (*rkyang ma sgo nas 'jug*). The outcaste demon (*gdol ba can*) is a "friend of the space element" (*nam mkhar 'grog*) and enters the body from the central "all-vibrating channel" (*kun 'dar ma*).

(b) The king demon wanders from the triangular path of the heart to the tongue. The aristocratic demon wanders from the "snowy mountain path of the lungs" (*gangs ri glo ba'i lam*) to the nose (*dri 'dzin lam*); the Brahmin wanders from the "quartz-mountain path of liver" (*mchong ri mchin lam*) to the eyes (*gzugs' dzin lam*); the servant wanders from the "kidney path of *nyen*" (*mkhal ma gnyan lam*) to the ears (*sgra 'dzin lam*); and the outcaste wanders from the "spleen path" (*mtsher lam*) to the lips.

(c) The king demon's domain is the "triangular region of the heart" (*zur gsum snying gi yul*), and its residence is the intestines (*rgyu ma nag du gnas*); the aristocratic demon's domain is the snowy mountain of the lungs while its "residence is the colon" (*long gi nang gnas*); the Brahmin's region is the quartz mount of the liver; its residence is the gallbladder (*mkhris pa'i nang gnas*); the servant's region is the cold region of the kidneys, while its residence is the

56 *'Chi med bdud rtsi bum pa* (1), 43v/2. See also *Bdud rtsi snying po yan lag brgyad pa gsang ba man ngag gi rgyud*, 565/15–566/4; *Rtsa yig cha nyi zer sgron ma* (Beijing: Mi rigs dpe skrun khang, 2008), 368/8–21. For a further inquiry into the concept of demonic diseases in Tibetan medicine see Susannah Deane, "Madness and the Spirits: Examining the Role of Spirits in Mental Illness in the Tibetan Communities of Darjeeling," in the present volume.

57 *'Chi med bdud rtsi bum pa* (1), 42r74–43r/5; *'Chi med bdud rtsi bum pa* (2), 48/7–49/17.

urinary bladder (*lgang pa*). The outcaste's region is the secret spleen and its residence is the stomach (*pho ba'i nang du gnas*).

(d) The king demon lives in the heart-fortress, the "mind-lake of memory" (*tsi ta dran pa'i mtsho*); the aristocratic demon lives the kidney-fortress, the "tent-like-lake of the breath" (*gur khyim dbugs gi mtsho*); the Brahmin lives in the liver-fortress, the "quartz-mountain and lake of blood" (*mchong ri khrag gi mtsho*); the servant lives in the kidneys-fortress, the "lake of urine and cold disease" (*grang ba chu'i mtsho*); and the outcaste lives in the spleen-fortress, the "lake of fever and composite disorders" (*tsha ba 'dus pa'i mtsho*).

3.3 *The Signs and Pulses of Death*

The "final signs of death" (*tha ma 'chi rtags*) are detected through the observation of "dissolving sense-faculties" (*dbang thim*) and can be predicted by examining the channels (*'phar rtsa sgo nas brtags*) and by interpreting premonitory secret signs. In this section, we will analyze the first two methodologies, while the third will be considered in the next section. In particular, we will observe that, according to the text, each external sign of a limited or absent sense faculty corresponds to an internal sign concerning an injured or collapsed functional organ, which ultimately reveals the dissolution of the related elemental constituent (*don lnga'i khams nyams*).

The dying process is essentially the "dissolution of the five elements" (*'byung ba thim*) and takes place when the elements fade one into another, in reverse order to that of the birth process.[58] The *Vase of Amṛta* does not refer to the visions experienced during this dissolution, which are usually found in other tantric texts. The breathing process indicates radical changes of the directions of subtle winds, which start from the nostrils (*sna rlung g.yas g.yon 'gyu chad log*). When the earth element dissolves into the water element, the spleen is injured and the sensation of intense heaviness prevails. The process continues with the water fading into fire, which corresponds to dysfunctions of the kidneys, indicated by the dissolution of the sense-faculty of hearing. Subsequently, the element fire fades into the wind causing deficiency of body heat. This is a sign that the disease has reached the liver and therefore leads to the dissolution of the faculty of sight. Then consciousness dissolves into the wind elements and "breath is reversed" (*dbugs ldog*); it connotes injury to the lungs and the dissolution of the faculties of smell. When the heart is injured, the faculty of taste is hindered.

58 The second chapter of the *Explanatory Tantra* (*bshad rgyud*) of the *Four Tantras* is devoted to the description of the birth process or "formation of the body." See *Bdud rtsi snying po yang lag brgyad pa'i gsang ba man ngag gi rgyud*, 16/7–20/7.

Death pulses also show clear similarities with the description provided in the *Ultimate Tantra* and the *Lamp of Sunrays*. Among these pulses there are: (a) those regarding the signs that a "disease of the water class that manifests in the case of a disease belonging to the class of the fire element" (*chu rtags me la byung*), which means that the fevers and the pulses typical of a febrile state show characteristics that are usually associated with cold diseases; and (b) the process opposite to the previous one that occurs when the "signs of the diseases usually associated with the class of the fire element manifest in case of a disease characterized by the element water" (*me rtgas chu la byung*).[59] This irregular manifestation is considered to be a result of the deceiving action of these demonic diseases. In another section of the text is said that, when hot and cold diseases present anomalous signs (*tsha grang ma snyoms*), the physician should be able to discern the real cause of the diseases through his or her penetrative knowledge, similar to an arrow of awareness (*rig pa'i mda'*), or like the blacksmith's instrument, which can "dismember the illusory body" (*sgyu lus dum bur btub*) created by the demons.[60] In this passage it is affirmed that, to cure the *nyen* disease, it is indispensable to rely on the scriptures, to know the nature of the disease (*ngo 'dzin*) and then accordingly apply the right cure (knowing the potencies of the medical substances; apply moxibustion or bloodletting; dietary and behavioral prescriptions). When these criteria and measures are insufficient, however, the physician will not fail due to the inspiration of the invoked divinity.

What follows is a description of the death pulses expressed through similes of the exegetical tantra, the *Union of the Sun and Moon*, which again includes some correspondences with the above mentioned *Four Tantras* and *Lamp of Sunrays*.

> When the pulse resembles a frog jumping in the water, one is about to die.[61]
>
> When the pulse resembles a falling drop or a bird that pecks grain from the ground, one is about to die.[62]

59 *'Chi med bdud rtsi bum pa* (2), 17/10.

60 *'Chi med bdud rtsi bum pa* (2), 8/1–4 and 21/1–4. See similar definition of the demonic pulse in the *Gso ba rig pa'i bstan bcos sman bla'i dgongs rgyan rgyud bzhi'i gsal byed baidur ya sngon po'i mallika*, 1537/10: [...] *rtsa mi snyoms pa*.

61 This corresponds to the death pulse of a combination of phlegm and bile.

62 This corresponds respectively to the death pulse of phlegm and the union of phlegm and wind.

> When the pulse resembles a great banner blowing in the wind, one is about to die.[63]
> When the pulse resembles to dropping saliva of a bull, one is about to die.[64]

As we can see here in the *Vase of Amṛta* we find only seven of the eleven pulses of death described in the *Ultimate Tantra*, excluding those regarding the weak pulse of a strong person, the pulse of long debilitated person, and the deviations in the bile pulse.[65]

3.4 *Premonitory Signs of Death*

Two groups of extraordinary premonitory signs are provided by the *Pillar of the Vital Force* (*srog gyi ka chen*) and by the *Treasure of the Vital Force* (*srog gter chen gyi gyad*). All the signs are obscure metaphors correlated to exact interpretative keys. The *Treasure of the Vital Force* compares these signs to the hermetic images appearing in a mirror (*brtags pa 'phrul kyi me long*), therefore creating a parallel between this divinatory prognosis and *prasenā* divination.[66] What follows is the translation of the signs described in the *Pillar of Vital Force*:

> If on the top of the mountain of the magical wheel the turquoise mist disappears, one is about to die.
> If the vapor emanated from the head dissolves, one is about to die.
> If the signs of pristine cognition disappear in the lamp-radiance of the ocean, one is about to die.
> If the iris, queen of the eye, appears soulless, one is about to die.[67]
> If the pillar of the Sky and Earth is destroyed in the space, one is about to die.
> If the two forearms in the space appear like being cut off in the middle, one is about to die.

---

63 This corresponds to the death pulse of wind.

64 This corresponds to the death pulse of combined humors.

65 *'Chi med bdud rtsi bum pa* (2), 17/15–20. See also *Rtsa yig cha nyi zer sgron ma*, 371/8–372/1. *Rgyud bzhi*, 565/4–6.

66 *'Chi med bdud rtsi bum pa* (2), 43/11–12. On *prasenā* divination see William A. McGrath, "Tantric Divination and Empirical Diagnosis: A Genealogy of Channel *Prasenā* Rituals in the Tibetan Medical Tradition," in the present volume.

67 *'Chi med bdud rtsi bum pa* (2), 51/9–10: [...] *rgya mtsho mdangs kyi sgron ma la ye shes rang rtags yal na 'chi.* The iris (*mig gi rgyal mo*) is the residence of the subtle channel where inner wisdom manifests on the outside through vivid eye light.

If the sound of the *ḍākinī* ceases within the inner recess of the forest, one is about to die.
If there are no sounds in the ears, one is about to die.[68]
If one of the five guards that stay together, stands up one is about to die.
If the artery of the ring finger pulsates, one is about to die.[69]
If the sun rises on the wheel of magical manifestations, one is about to die.
If the body heat of the legs vanishes, one is about to die.[70]
If from the *maṇḍala* of water and great bliss, the moon goes down, one is about to die.
If semen is emitted, one is about to die.[71]

The sign of the pulsating ring finger similarly occurs in the *Ultimate Tantra* as a sign of the demonic forces, or *nyen*: the "life-force channel" (*bla rtsa*), which is connected to the concept of life essence (*srog*) and life span (*tshe*), can be detected thought the pulse of the ring finger.[72] The *Exegetical Tantra* (*bshad rgyud*), the second treatise of the *Four Tantras*, includes the premonitory signs of death regarding optical illusions appearing in the space, the examination of unusual shapes of the body shadow, as well as the analysis of iris luminosity.[73] These series of metaphors remind one of the cryptic images described in the *Union of the Sun and Moon* (*nyi zla kha sbyor*) of the *Seminal Essence* (*snying thig*) scriptures of the Great Perfection (*rdzogs chen*), part of the *Collected Instructions* (*man ngag sde*).[74] The following quotations are two examples of

68 *'Chi med bdud rtsi bum pa* (2), 51/12–13: *nag 'dabs gsang ba'i brag phug tu/ mkha' 'gro'i rang sgra chag na 'chi/ rna ba'i sgra chag na 'chi//.*

69 *'Chi med bdud rtsi bum pa* (2), 51/13–14: *sdud byed so ba mi lnga nad so ba mi gcig lang na 'chi/ srin lag gi rtsa ba 'phar na//.*

70 *'Chi med bdud rtsi bum pa* (2), 51/14–15: *sprul ba 'khor lo'i grong khyer nas nyi ma gyen la 'dzeg na 'chi / rkang pa'i drod yal na 'chi//.*

71 *'Chi med bdud rtsi bum pa* (2), 51/15–16: *bde chen chu'i dkyil 'khor nas zla ba thur du babs na 'chi/ sa bon 'dzag na 'chi//.*

72 *Baidurya sngon po*, 1559/1–4.

73 *Bdud rtsi snying po yan lag brgyad pa'i gsang ba man ngag gi rgyud*, 32/11; 33/1–5;37/7–16.

74 According to Ronald Davidson (*Tibetan Renaissance: Tantric Buddhism in the Rebirth of Tibetan Culture* [New York, NY: Columbia University Press, 2005], 228–29), the *Collected Instructions* (*man ngag sde*) most probably were compiled around the eleventh and the twelfth centuries. See also the *Instructions on the Six Lamps from the Aural Transmission from Zhang zhung of the Great Perfection* (*rdzogs pa chen po zhang zhung snyan rgyud las sgron ma drug gig dams pa*): its sixth and last chapter is very similar to the *Nyi zla kha sbyor* section on the signs of death but contains further explanations. *Zhang zhung snyan rgyud zhang zhung snyan rgyud las sgron me drug gi gdams pa*. In *Zhang zhung snyang rgyud kyi gsung pod* (Lun grub steng: Sde dge par khang, [n.d.]), 10a/5–11a/6.

the paradigmatic correspondence: "When the pillar of the Sky and Earth is destroyed, one is about to die" (*gnam sa gnyis kyi ka gdun de/ bar snang chag na 'chi*); "If the sound of the *ḍākinī* ceases within the inner recess of the forest, one is about to die" (*nag 'dabs gsang ba'i brag phug tu/ mkha' 'gro'i rang sgra chag na 'chi*).[75] Therefore, we might assume that some diagnostic methods and divinatory techniques exposed in the *Vase of Amṛta* have connections with, and could derive from, the notions developed in the context of the early *Seminal Essence* literature.

At this stage of the research, the exact history of transmission of these diagnostic techniques cannot be established with certainty. However, the congruences among the various texts point to different literary traditions and narrative nuclei as possible sources for the development of demonic pulses on one hand, and for the prediction of signs of death on the other. The first represents a syncretistic literary tradition based on development of pulse taking, which shows clear similarities with Chinese sphygmology, and had integrated elements of the ancient Indian Buddhist demonology, magical healing, and exorcistic methods emblematically represented by specific categories of tantras, such as the *Garuḍatantras* (see section 4). In this tantric literature the ailments of the human body are attributed to divine factors, and magico-religious means are utilized in the cure. In the Tibetan medical context, the syncretic elaboration of pulse-taking and demonology (*bhūtavidyā*) is well represented by the scriptures ascribed to Nāgārjuna, such as the *Moon King* and the *Lamp of Sunrays*. This second literary tradition has developed from a hermeneutic sensibility that originated in the tantric investigation of ontological and soteriological themes. In this literature the examination of the nature of the mind and death and dying processes are associated with yogic and contemplative techniques for experiencing them. The cited *Seminal Literature* sources are paradigmatic examples of these concepts.

75 *'Chi med bdud rtsi bum pa* (1), 44v/3–49v/1. The first verse is explained as an optical illusion that arises when staring at the forearms fixed in a particular position. For an analysis on the corresponding verses in the *Union of the Sun and Moon*, see Giacomella Orofino, *Sacred Tibetan Teachings on Death and Liberation* (Bridport, Dorset: Prims-Unity Press, 1990), 33, 93. See also *Nyi zla kha sbyor chen mo gsang ba'i rgyud*, in *Rnying ma rgyud bcu bdun* (Dpal yul rdzong: A 'dzom chos sgar par khang, 2000), 28r/1–6; and *Zhang Zhung snyan rgyud las sgron ma drug gi gdams pa* (Lun grub steng: Sde dge par khang, [n.d.]), 10a/5–11a/6.

3.5 *Knowing the Body and Defining the Nature of the Diagnostic Process: Overlapping Models of Physiology*

The *Vase of Amṛta* provides us with a complex image of the body that integrates elements of different medical systems with demonology and tantric physiology. In the following, this imagery will be used as a guiding thread for reexamining the previous sections. In light of these therapeutic systems, we will also consider the diagnostic processes as a joining of divination and observation.

As seen, the architecture of the body is organized according to spatial and temporal patterns. The perspectives are pushed inwards, moving from material embodiment (skin, muscle, bones, organs, and arteries) to the luminescent innermost essence of being (subtle channels, winds, and awareness). Accordingly, it can be observed that the first step of the diagnostic process is the perception of the body through visual observation (patient's physical appearance and mental status), pulse taking, and urine analysis. Therefore, the signs (*rtags*) are interpreted in order to formulate a series of inferences and establish a prognosis. This process is complemented by speculative models: the medical approach to the diseases is underpinned by the theoretical apparatus of Buddhist cosmology, physiology, and knowledge of the nature of mind and its structures. The disease process is not only outlined according to Āyurvedic humoral physiopathology, but it also mirrors the dissolution of the elements (earth, fire, water, wind, and space), which regulates the state of constant metamorphosis of the entire universe.

The internal body is depicted as a microcosm, a reflection of the tantric knowledge of subtle channels. It evolves around an axial construction, the vital pilaster (*srog gi ka chen*) formed by three right, left, and central channels (*ro ma, skyang ma,* and *kun 'dar ma*). The first two are connected on a more physical level to breath and blood, while the third is connected to emptiness, thus its materiality is considered very subtle. The channel of "karmic wind of formative actions" (*'du byed las kyi rlung*) is associated to the triad: this corresponds to the channel of "karmic wind" (*las kyi rlung*), related to the arising of discursive thoughts and karmic propensity, which is in several Great Perfection sources and is described as abiding in the lungs or located between lungs and heart.[76] This channel might correspond to the "life channels" (*tshe'i rtsa*) of vital breath, also described in Tibetan medical literature, such as the *Exegetical Tantra*.[77] According to *Vase of Amṛta*, consciousness and conceptual thoughts

---

76 Daniel Scheidegger, "The First Four Themes of Klong chen pa's *Tshig don bcu cig pa*," *Revue d'Etudes Tibétaines* 16, no. 2 (2009): 67–68.

77 Janet Gyatso, *Being Human in a Buddhist World: An Intellectual History of Medicine in Early Modern Tibet* (New York: New York University Press, 2015), 202.

arise due to the karmic wind, whereas the mind itself is located at the center of the heart: the word *citta* (*tsit ta*) defines both the mind and the heart, which is considered its palace, and is connected to memory (*dran pa*).

The text is consistent with the conception of mind luminosity developed in the *Seminal Literature* of the Great Perfection. It shows similarities with the conception of luminous channels or "lamps" (*sgron ma*), and in particular the *Vase of Amṛta* refers to the capacity of "pristine awareness" (*ye shes*) to show its luminosity (*mdangs*) through the eyes, elements that also indicate the presence of a channel connecting heart to the eyes.[78] Cognition (*shes pa*) is associated to another channel called the "vital channel" (*srog rtsa*). Its affliction causes alteration of the mental status (*shes 'khrul*), as well as bloody eyes and pain radiating all over the torso. This channel seems to be connected both to the nervous system and the cardio-vascular system, as well as to the life-force (*bla rtsa*) channel since it can be detected at the ring finger channel (*srin lag*).[79] Indeed, according to the *Vase of Amṛta*, cognition is also related to different organs: it relates to the heart, whose role seems to be associated with the clarity of thoughts, therefore, when the heart is affected by *nyen*, thought loses its clarity (*dran pa mi gsal shes pa 'tshub*, lit. "unclear memory and turbid/confused cognition"). Cognition is also related to the liver and spleen, which, when damaged, determine different levels of "heavy cognition" (*shes lci; shes pa shin tu lci*).[80] In the first case, the problem occurs because liver cannot purify the blood, causing a disease that aligns to jaundice (*mkhris nad*, lit. "disease of the gallbladder"; *mig ser*, lit. "yellowish eyes"); consequently this disorder affects the brain (*klad gzer*), causing a loss of brain functions and bloody eyes.[81] An injured spleen affects the formation of concepts and mental focus (*dmigs thams cad g.yo bar byed*).[82] We can assume that, even though the text does not refer to the "vital channel" as "black or white vital channels" (*srog dkar nag*), a distinction applied in the medical literature, it describes the vital channel in terms of the functions associated to these two categories of channels. The text provides us with the description of the location of the "vital channel" in the physical body. Its upper extremity coincides with the *cakra* on the top of the head (*srog 'khor spyi gtugs*). There also are scattered references within the chapters explaining the secret points of moxibustion (*me btsa' gsang dmigs*): the secret point of the vital channel is located at the sixth vertebral digit, which

78 For further inquiry on "lamps" and their categories see Daniel Scheidegger, "Lamps in the Leaping Over," *Revue d'Etudes Tibétaines* 8, no. 10 (2005): 40 et passim.

79 *'Chi med bdud rtsi bum pa* (2), 63/13–18.

80 *'Chi med bdud rtsi bum pa* (2), 15/14–16/1.

81 *'Chi med bdud rtsi bum pa* (2), 15/21–24; 177/4–5.

82 *'Chi med bdud rtsi bum pa* (2), 12/ 17–18.

is not far from the "equidistant point between the black and white" (*dkar nag mtshams*), and the so-called "secret point of the heart" located at the intersection of the horizontal line between the nipples and the vertical distance between the throat cavity and the breast bones.[83] Therefore, we can assume that the "vital channel" extends from the head crown downward, passing through the throat and heart, and connecting to the brain and the eyes.

This microcosm conforms to precise heuristic schemata of correspondences and contrapositions: geographical elements, citadels and paths establish a web of connections among functional organs (heart, liver, kidneys, spleen, and lungs) and hollow organs (intestine, colon, gallbladder, urinary bladder, and stomach). This system of correspondences between the two groups of organs derives from Chinese influence.[84] The contraposition of mountains and lakes denotes the nature of organs in terms of solidity and softness, and in particular the watery aspect indicates the function, or the faculty associated to each vital organ. The description involves anatomical details, such as those regarding the intrathoracic triangular region with the heart at its center covered by the tent-shaped lungs, an image that recalls the medical representation of the body reproduced in the famous seventeenth-century medical paintings.

The landscape of the body is inhabited by wandering spirits that move through the channel-paths, which connect the functional organs to the sense organs. Therefore, by observing the sense faculties and detecting the deviating pulses, it is possible to understand which demonic classes have afflicted the patient. The notion of five demonic fortresses is similar to the description of spirit castles (*mkhar*) inhabited by pathogenic demons in the *Diagnostic Signs and Cures of the Eighteen Kuṣṭha Diseases Based on the Tantra of Peaceful and Irate Manifestations* (*mdze rigs bco brgyad kyi rtags rdo rje bde khros kyi dgongs pa las byung ba*), ascribed to Nāgārjuna.[85] According to this work, a certain group of symptoms reveal the demonic fortress, and consequently the right cure is administered. In the *Vase of Amṛta* the internal landscape might be considered to be a demonological chart, envisioned in order to individuate the hiding spirits. It illustrates specific body areas or points that are to be manipulated through different categories of moxibustion, such as "burning

83 *'Chi med bdud rtsi bum pa* (2), 125/16.

84 The *Vase of Amṛta* does not include a clear formulation of the "triple burner" (*sam se'u*), the sixth hollow organ of Chinese medicine, which was assimilated in Tibetan medicine through works like the *Moon King*. See William A. McGrath, "Vessel Examination in the Medicine of the Moon King," in *Buddhism and Medicine: An Anthology of Premodern Sources*, ed. C. Pierce Salguero (New York, NY: Columbia University Press, 2017), 501–13.

85 Klu sgrub, *Mdze rigs bco brgyad kyi rtags rdo rje bde khros kyi dgongs pa las byung ba*, in *Slob dpon klu sgrub kyi sman yig* (Beijing: Mi rigs dpe skrun khang, 2008), 140–42.

moxibustion" (*me bsreg*) or "warming moxibustion" (*sdigs me*), and bloodletting (*gtar*), which are prescribed as external therapies in the case of ulcers, swelling diseases, poxes, and diseases afflicting the internal organs of the upper and lower parts of the body (*stod gzer* and *rgyu gzer*). In this context, the therapies are ritualized and reconfigured as methods to tear away the demonic *nyen* from the body.

The healer is also instructed to observe the body in search of the wandering *nyen* spirits. This should take place within the "vital channel" from the crown of the head to the "red eye-channel" (*mig dmar*) below the navel at the groin area, at the armpit point (*dpung dzum*), at the "*ratna* point of the wind channel" (*rtsa rlung rat na*), and at the heart secret point. Then, applying the "moxa to close the channel" (*rtsa'i 'bros 'phrang bsdoms*), the practitioner should block the demonic flow by burning a circumscribed area at the its perimeter and then in the middle, where the *nyen* abides.[86] Other two emblematic descriptions regard the "warming interdependent moxibustion" (*sdigs rten 'brel gyi me*) and the "mirror moxibustion" (*me long btugs me*). The first consists of burning the secret points of the first vertebral digit at the nape of the neck, the sixth vertebral digit and at the secret point of heart, while reciting mantras to tear away the serpent spirits from the body. The latter starts with an examination of the pulse and an analysis of a patient's feces (*'khru mdog*) to individuate the injured hollow organ. Afterwards the mirror-moxibustion should be performed using a mirror as an implement: it has to be applied directly on the skin and where it reflects a specific form or, we might say when the practitioner scries a significant vision, that point or area should be burned or pierced, since this would be considered the demonic residence.[87]

A lengthy description of these two kinds of moxibustions is also provided by Deumar: when performing the first kind of moxibustion, the practitioner should visualize himself/herself as red fiery goddess and recite the mantra of interdependence. In the second case, the evoked divinity dissolves in a consecrated mirror (*pra thim*), which is then used for moxibustion.[88]

In the *Vase of Amṛta*, the body is a system intelligible on multiple levels. The evidence and visions of its nature and alterations change according to the methodology of diagnosis. The signs are structured according to physician's experiential understanding of the body and its functions; moreover, the

86 *'Chi med bdud rtsi bum pa* (2), 125/13–18.

87 *'Chi med bdud rtsi bum pa* (2), 140/21–24: [...] *mdun rgyab du me long btsugs pa de la gzugs kyi rtags me long la snang ba de la btsod kyi me btsas bsreg.*

88 De'u dmar bstan 'dzin phun tshogs, *Lag len gces rigs sdus pa sman kun bcud du sgrub pa'i las gyi cho ga kun gsal snang mdzod ces bya ba bzhugs* in *Dri med shel gong dang dri med shel phreng dang lag len gces bsdus* (S. W. Tashigang: Leh, 1970), 565/6–566/9.

interpretation is substantiated by acquired knowledge based on the textual tradition (*zhung bzhin*, lit. "according to the scriptures") and divine inspiration. In respect to the latter aspect, it should be said that in different passages the text affirms that the interpretation of signs and the medical practice is guided by Mañjuśrī or by a wrathful divine manifestation (see the next section). In this sense the terminology "arrow of awareness" used to penetrate the illusion created by demons and understanding the nature of the disease, assumes the value of contemplative "state of awareness" (*rig pa*), which allows the physician to discern the three causes of the disease (*nyen*, fever, and wind) and individuate the injured/afflicted organ. This divine arrow represents the trace of the ancient divination and exorcistic ritual of sucking away (*'jib rgyab*) the disease, which is alleged to be of Bön origin. This practice is carried out by setting up a special divination-arrow (*mda 'dar*) to pierce the demon residence found by a mirror and a bowl to collect the puss from the infected blood and serum.[89] In the *Vase of Amṛta*, the *Reversal Suppressant [Ritual] of Sucking [the Infection] with the Adamantine Sow's Tongue* (*log gnon phag mo'i ljags 'jibs*) clearly refers to this practice: the healer is the manifestation of the Black Sow Goddess who devours the *nyen* with her meteoric lips, a lancet (*gtsag bu*) is used to cut the pustules of ulcers is envisioned as the "fangs of a wild boar" (*phag rgog mche bar bsgom*), and the purulent serum sucked away from the scars becomes nectar.[90] The use of mirror as a scrying implement associated with the practice of moxibustion and the ritualized therapies to exorcise pathogenic demons not only substantiates the divinatory aspect of the diagnosis, but also shows how different methodologies have been adapted and assimilated in the Tibetan medical tradition.

4 Magical Protection and Invulnerability: How to Realize the Vajra Armor and Manipulate the Secret Potencies of *Materia Magica*

In the *Vase of Amṛta*, ritual magic (evocation rituals), image magic (preparation of textual amulets), natural magic (uses and consecration of *materia magica*), and alchemy merge into complex apotropaic rituals for averting disease-carrier demons. The *Long [Ritual] Vajra Armor of Meteoric Metal* (*nam lcags rdo rje'i khrab ring*) and the *Armor that Protects the Vital Force* (*srog gi srung gi*

89 de Nebesky-Wojkowitz, *Oracles and Demons of Tibet*, 365–66.
90 *'Chi med bdud rtsi bum pa* (1), 110r/1; *'Chi med bdud rtsi bum pa* (2), 152/11.

go cha)[91] describe the powerful practice of "vajra armor" (*rdo rje'i khrab*, otherwise called *go cha* or *go khrab*), which allows for the achievement of magical invulnerability, of an unspoiled divine and immortal body. Not different from the *kavaca* rituals found in diverse Hindu traditions,[92] "vajra armor" includes a certain set of practices: the recitation of magical formulas, the summoning of a divinity to enter the practitioner's body, and the transformation into a divine being. It also involves the preparation of protective textual amulets (*srung 'khor*, lit. "protective wheel"), magical unguents (*phyug sman*), pills (*ril bu*), and powders (*phur ma*). The preliminary purification process consists of lengthy recitations of *sūtras* (*mdo sde*), "dietary prescriptions" (*mi 'phrod za*, lit. "unwholesome food"), and sexual abstinence. The central practice includes two phases: (1) "internal protection" (*nang gi srung*), which involves incantations, amulets and empowerments of medical substances; and (2) "secret protection" (*gsang srung*), or the meditative practice centered on the wrathful blue Khyung (*garuḍa*).

Given the venomous nature attributed to *nyenné* and *rimné* diseases, the *Vase of Amṛta* represents the conflation of a long-life nectar and an alexipharmic antidote. Different sets of substances called the "nine heroes" (*dpa' bo rnam dgu*),[93] which belong to different categories of *materia medica*, are the fulcrum of arcane alchemical procedures aimed at transforming substances into an antidote for poisons and other diseases. The definition of the "nine heroes" indicates their intrinsic therapeutic potencies and occult virtues (*nus mthu*),[94]

91 *'Chi med bdud rtsi bum pa* (1), 12v/1–16v3; *'Chi med bdud rtsi bum pa* (2), 24–29; and *'Chi med bdud rtsi bum pa* (1), 104r/1–117v/6; respectively.

92 For a further inquiry see Karel R. Van Kooij, "Protective Covering (*Kavaca*)," in *Selected Studies on Ritual in the Indian Religions*, ed. Ria Kloppenborg (Leiden: Brill, 1983), 118–29; and Bühnemann, "Maṇḍala, Yantras and Cakra."

93 The lists of substances provided in the *'Chi med bdud rtsi bum pa* present some variations. According to *'Chi med bdud rtsi bum pa* (2), 24/16–18; the nine substances are *gla ba, gu gul, gi wang, shin kun, shu dag, sman chen, a ru ra, ldong ros*, and *sgog skya*. According to *'Chi med bdud rtsi bum pa* (2), 65/8–10; there are ten substances, i.e. *gul nag, bong nga nag po, spru nag, gla ba, shing kun, shu dag, mu zi, stag sha, ldong ros*, and *sa tshur*. According to *'Chi med bdud rtsi bum pa* (2), 70/12–1; (a) the substances used for preparing the protective unguent are: *gla ba, gu gul, shing kun, shu dag, rma chen, ldong ros, gi wang, tharnu*, and *sgog skya*; and (b) the substances used for the medicinal powders are: *sha chen, spru nag, stag sha, gla ba, mu zi, bong nga, yung ba*, and *ru rta*.

94 *Mthu* means power and in general is used to indicate black curse. In this context, it refers to the magical protective and reversal or exorcistic power (*bzlog pa*) of substances and amulets. *'Chi med bdud rtsi bum pa* (1), 14v/6–15r/1; *'Chi med bdud rtsi bum pa* (2), 27/2–9: [...] *thams chad 'tshogs pa'i zu gu la sogs pa nus mthu yis// nad kyi bkal ba byung gyur rang la 'gos pa mi srid do//*[...] *'chi bdag bdud las bzlog par 'gyur* [...].

which are mainly apotropaic virtues. In this group there are substances of animal origin such, as musk[95] and bezoar stones,[96] which are considered excellent antidotes for poisoning. There are also plant exudate such as the guggul gum resin,[97] whose medical and ritual uses are well documented since ancient Vedic times. There are substances of mineral origin such as sulfur and realgar, two important ingredients of mercurial medicine.[98] The text enumerates the myrobalan fruit,[99] famous for its rejuvenating potencies, along with plants used for curing different kinds of communicable and malignant diseases,

95 *Gla ba*. It is categorized as "essence medicines" (*rtsi sman*). Most probably it corresponds to the male musk deer, responsible for the production of musk (*gla rtsi can*), which is used in Tibetan medicine. It can be identified with the Siberian *Moschus moschiferus Linnaleus*, see for example Dga' ba rdo rje, *'Khrungs dpe dri med shel gyi me long* (Beijing: Mi rigs dpe skrun khang, 1995), 102; however, there are other possible identifications. See Olaf Czaja, "The Substitution of *Materia Medica* in Tibetan Medicine: An Inquiry into Traditional Tibetan Treatises," *East Asian Science, Technology and Medicine* 46 (2017): 174–75. According to Jampa Trinlé et al. (Byams pa 'phrin las et al., *Bod lugs gso rig tshig mdzod chen mo*, 116–17) *gla rtsi* can cure "poisoning" (*dug nad*), "kidney diseases" (*mkhal nad*), *nyen* fevers, and infective "*sin* diseases" (*srin nad*). For detailed references on ancient medical uses of musk in Tibetan and Arabic medicine see Akosay and Yoeli-Tlalim, "Along the Musk Routes," 217–40.

96 *Gi wang*. See for example Dga' ba rdo rje, *'Khrungs dpe dri med shel gyi me long*, 99; and Byams pa 'phrin las et al., *Bod lugs gso rig tshig mdzod chen mo*, 127–28. Both sources describe *giwang* as a powerful remedy to cure poisoning, *rim* diseases, different kinds of fever such as the fevers in infants (*byis pa'i tshad*), febrile states connected to several organs and in particular those affecting the liver and the bile duct (*mchin mkhris gtsor rgyur don snod kyi tshad sel*), and episodes of hysteria followed by collapse and shivering (*smyo 'bog brgyal dang 'dar ba*).

97 *Gu gul* also belongs to the category of "essence medicines"; according to Gawa Dorjé (Dga' ba rdo rje, *'Khrungs dpe dri med shel gyi me long*, 120) it is identifiable as *Commiphora mukul* and is particularly efficacious in annihilating different kinds of obstructive spirits and planetary hindrances (*bgegs skrod, 'dre klu, bdud dug gsod; gza' gsod*); according to Jampa Trinlé (Byams pa 'phrin las et al., *Bod lugs gso rig tshig mdzod chen mo*, 98–99) this substance is particularly efficacious in curing "leprosy" (*mdze nad*) and other categories of *nyenrim* diseases.

98 *Mu zi* and *ldong ros*. See for example Dga' ba rdo rje, *'Khrungs dpe dri med shel gyi me long*, 72–73; 67–68.

99 *A ru ra* is commonly identified with the chebulic myrobalan fruit. See for example Dga' ba rdo rje, *'Khrungs dpe dri med shel gyi me long*, 167–69. It is considered a very potent *rasāyana* substance. It cures different kinds of fever and eye diseases, and "dispels evil forces" (*gdon sel ba*).

epidemics, and poison-induced fevers, such as *ferula*,[100] costus,[101] turmeric,[102] locoweed,[103] the purgative root of *tharnu* (*thar nu*),[104] *Notopterygium*,[105] and the poisonous black aconite.[106]

---

100 There are several identifications of *shing kun* plant, the majority belong to the *Ferula* species. For a detailed discussion see Czaja, "The Substitution of *Materia Medica* in Tibetan Medicine," 195–96. According to Gawa Dorjé (Dga' ba rdo rje, *'Khrungs dpe dri med shel gyi me long*, 299–300) and Jampa Trinlé et al. (Byams pa 'phrin las et al., *Bod lugs gso rig tshig mdzod chen mo*, 912–13) there are two variants of the *shu dag* plant both from the aquatic *Araceae* species: the white one (*shu dag dkar po*) is identifiable with *Acorus gramineus Soland*; the black one (*shu dag nag po*) is identifiable with *Acorus calamus*. Most probably, the author of the *'Chi med bdud rtsi bum pa*, refers to the latter because this variant, according to the mentioned sources, "can overcome diseases characterized by 'impure serum' (*chu ser*), bad wounds and 'putrefactions' such as the *gaklhok* disease" (*gag lhog rma ngan rul ba rnams gcod la chu ser skam*) and can also "bring out *nyen* fever" (*gnyan tshad gyen du 'dren par byed pa*).

101 *Ru rta* is commonly identified with plants of the *Asteraceae* family commonly known as *Costus*. For a detailed discussion see Czaja, "The Substitution of *Materia Medica* in Tibetan Medicine," 194–95. For further references on the therapeutic potential of *Saussurrea Lappa*, see Kulsoom Zahara et al., "A Review of Therapeutic Potential of *Saussurea lappa*: An Endangered Plant from Himalaya," *Asian Pacific Journal of Tropical Medicine* 7, no. 1 (2014): 60–69.

102 *Yung ba*, according to Gawa Dorjé, is identifiable with *Curcuma longa*, a perennial plant of the *Zingiberaceae* family, particularly effective against envenomation and *nyen* diseases. See Dga' ba rdo rje, *'Khrungs dpe dri med shel gyi me long*, 192.

103 *Stag sha* is usually identified as a locoweed species. See Czaja, "The Substitution of *Materia Medica* in Tibetan Medicine," 197–98. According to Jampa Trinlé (Byams pa 'phrin las et al., *Bod lugs gso rig tshig mdzod chen mo*, 321–22) there are two variants of *stag sha*, both can cure *nyen* fevers, poison-induced fevers (*dug tshad*), different *nyen* diseases and "swelling diseases" (*skrangs po'i rigs*), such as *lhog pa*, and chronic diseases (*'bras nad*) that most closely aligns with the biomedical category of cancer. On this topic see Twani Tidwell, "The Modern Biomedical Conception of Cancer and Its Many Potential Correlates in the Tibetan Medical Tradition," in the present volume.

104 *Thar nu* is a purgative root, which can cure *lhog pa* and *nyen* fevers. See Byams pa 'phrin las et al., *Bod lugs gso rig tshig mdzod chen mo*, 336.

105 *Spru nag*. Gawa Dorjé (Dga' ba rdo rje, *'Khrungs dpe dri med shel gyi me long*, 240) identifies it with the *Notopterygium forbesii Boiss*. This plant can cure *nyen* and *rim* diseases, "toothache" (*so na ba*), can stop "hemorrhages" (*khrag shor ba*), leprosy, urological, and gastrointestinal disorders, can cure diseases connected to the *yama* type of *sinbu* (*ya srin*), a kind of animalcule or parasite, which according to Tibetan medical texts can affect eyes and ears, thus the *yama* disease most closely aligns to sinusitis.

106 *Bong nga nag po* is usually identified as a "black variant of aconite" belonging to the *Aconitum* species of *Ranunculaceae* family. See for example Dga' ba rdo rje, *'Khrungs dpe dri med shel gyi me long*, 244–45. In the *rasaśāstra* literature, this poisonous plant is enumerated among the "five major poisons" (*dug chen lnga*) used to process mercurial compounds. See Simioli, "Alchemical Gold and the Pursuit of the Alchemical Elixir," 62. Both Gawa Dorjé (Dga' ba rdo rje, *'Khrungs dpe dri med shel gyi me long*, 245) and Jampa Trinlé (Byams pa 'phrin las et al., *Bod lugs gso rig tshig mdzod chen mo*, 661) agree in identifying

The nine heroes should also be understood in term of their other appellation, "reversal suppressants" (*log gnon*). In the *Scroll of Reversal Suppressant Antidotes* (*log gnon gnyen po'i shog dril*), all the substances are defined as the "heroes that defeat Yama, the Lord of Death" (*'chi bdag 'joms pa'i dpa bo*).[107] According to the *Vase of Amṛta* these virtues can be exploited to empower a series of medical compounds, such as the five types of theriac (*dar yak an*).[108] Theriac combines a plethora of ingredients, many even potentially venomous, such as aconite, toxic animal substances, such as frog meats, or different kinds of minerals, including mercury, which are substantially detoxified (*'dul ba*, lit. "subjugated") through complex alchemical processes.

These compounds are otherwise known as the "five nectars" (*bdud rtsi lnga*) and are hence associated with a category of consecrated substances that play a key role in the tantric context of "accomplishing medicine" literature and rituals.[109] To be effective, the group of hero-substances undergoes a consecration ceremony of accomplishing medicine (*rab gnas sman grub*), which starts with an evocation ritual (*spyang dren pa*) aiming at transforming the substances in ambrosia. Both the celebrant and the medicine become recipients of divine

---

sman chen with a variant of *bong nga nag po*: according to Gawa Dorjé, it corresponds to the *Aconitum kongboense Lauener*, which is otherwise called *btsan dug sman chen*. *Rma chen* is not identified, most probably it is a corrupted transcription of *sman chen*.

107 *'Chi med bdud rtsi bum pa* (1), 96v/6–97v/1. See Simioli, "Brilliant Moon Theriac." Their formulations are not unique to the *Vase of Amṛta*. See for example the *Medical Compound of the Nine Black Substances to Overcome Every Disease and Evil Force* (*nag po dgu sbyor ba nad gdon kun 'joms*) preserved in the *Bye bya ring srel*. See Zur mkhar ba mnyams nyid rdo rje, *Man ngag bye ba ring bsrel pod chung rab 'byams gsal ba'i sgron me* (Lanzhou: Kan su'u mi rigs dpe skrun khang, 1993), 727/6–728/16.

108 The five key substances of the theriac compounds in the *'Chi med bdud rtsi bum pa* are: mercury (*dngul chu*), as the key element of the "brilliant moon-theriac" (*zla zil dar ya kan*) [*'Chi med bdud rtsi bum pa* (1), 88r/2–93r/5; *'Chi med bdud rtsi bum pa* (2), 87–92]; calcite (*cong zhi*), which is the key substance of the "fat-theriac" (*tshil bu dar ka yan*) [*'Chi med bdud rtsi bum pa* (1), 118r/5–123r/6; *'Chi med bdud rtsi bum pa* (2), 101/2–112/9]; locoweed (*stag sha*) that acts as the key substance of the "meat-theriac" (*sha dar ya kan*) [*'Chi med bdud rtsi bum pa* (1), 86r/46–88r/2; *'Chi med bdud rtsi bum pa* (2), 82/8–86]; myrobalan or *Therminalia chebula* (*a ru ra*), which is the main ingredient of the "bone-theriac" (*rus pa dar yak an*) [*'Chi med bdud rtsi bum* pa' (1), 81v/6–84r/6; 'Chi *med bdud rtsi bum pa* (2), 79–82/7]; *Chrysosplenium carnosum H.* (*gsha' g.ya'; lha mo g.ya', g.ya' kyi ma*), a key ingredient of blood-theriac (*khag dar yak an*) [*'Chi med bdud rtsi bum pa* (1), 50v/1–56r/6; *'Chi med bdud rtsi bum pa* (2), 93–101/1]. On *Chrysosplenium carnosum* see Dga' ba rdo rje, *'Khrungs dpe dri med shel gyi me long*, 283.

109 On consecrated nectars see Garrett, "The Alchemy of Accomplishing Medicine," 300–26.

beings; in particular, each of the nine heroes is associated with a specific Buddha's manifestation.[110]

In order to achieve invulnerability, the nine substances must be eaten with food and used to prepare a magical unguent. The text instructs one to intake, or literally to "thrust into the body" (*nang zug gu gzud*),[111] these substances in order to protect the organs. The medicinal powder, once amalgamated with animal fat or butter, becomes an unguent used to anoint the eight important points of the body (*gnas brgyad*), precluding them from demonic forces. Inserted in the amulets, the powders cast out demons.

The *Vase of Amṛta* conforms to the model of the "Khyung texts" of the *Mahāyogatantra* literature, which can be compared with other tantric medical literatures centered on the cult of the Garuḍa and connected to the knowledge of poisons and their herbal and ritual healing methods.[112] It prescribes the practitioner to visualize himself as a powerful bird-of-prey deity, the transcendent emanation (*sprul ba'i ye shes*) of the wrathful "Great Noble Lord of the Secrets" or Guhyapati (*gsang bdag rje bstun chen po*) Vajrapāṇi, who is unified with Hayagrīva, the "resplendent subjugator" of evil beings. The Khyung should be envisioned while churning the primordial ocean with his "blazing meteoric beak and claws" (*gnam lcags 'bar ba'i mchu sder*) and devouring the serpent spirits that cause *nyenné* and *rimné*. The visualization is animated by theomorphic figures which represent the wheel of life: eagles and ravens, wild boars, and poisonous and medicinal snakes (*dug sbrul dang sman sbrul*).[113]

While absorbed in this non-dual state of profound and indissoluble communion with the real divine nature,[114] the officiant is able to draw down the virtues of divine intelligences. One is then instructed to impart them upon, or better yet, infuse them into the images and diagrams inscribed with magical formulas by reciting the incantations and empowering the medical powders

110 *'Chi med bdud rtsi bum pa* (1), 40r/5–6; 41v/2–3: [...] *sman so so rang rang gi// lha bskyed de de'i steng du ye shes sems pa spyan drengs la// mchos stod bskur bsol bar gdab bar bya*; [...] *sman lha a ru ra gu ru yab yum sman chen gla ba// thugs rje chen po shu dag// manju shri gi wang//gsang bdag gu gul// rta mgrin shin kun//bdud rtsi khyil ba mu zi// sgrol ma chig skyes//*.

111 See *'Chi med bdud rtsi bum pa* (2), 24/16–20; *'Chi med bdud rtsi bum pa* (1), 91v/3; provides a different spelling: [...] *phru gu 'jug//*.

112 Gregory Hillis, "The Khyung Texts in the *Rnying ma'i Rgyud 'Bum*," in The *Many Canons of Tibetan Buddhism*, ed. H. Eimer and D. Germano (Leiden: Brill, 2002), 313–32. For references on Garuḍa medicine, see Michael Slouber, *Early Tantric Medicine: Snakebite, Mantras, and Healing in the Garuda Tantras* (Oxford: Oxford University Press, 2017).

113 *'Chi ned bdud rtsi bum pa* (2), 71/9–22.

114 *'Chi med bdud rtsi bum pa* (1), 12v/6; *'Chi med bdud rtsi bum pa* (2), 25/5: [...] *mi rtogs stong ba'i ngang nyis las// lha'i nga rgyal ma brel ba//*.

and pills. The texts recommend preparing the amulets at auspicious times to attune them astrologically to the planets and constellations,[115] and to use specific writing supports (black sheets of paper, fabric, or bark), material such as inks made of gold, cinnabar, or black Chinese ink mixed with precious substances, and envelopes made from five-colored silk, all of which need to be consecrated.

Textual amulets are illustrated with powerful iconic elements: the three figures of Vajrapāṇi, the Khyung, and the black wild boar (*phag nag*), which accomplish the function of devourer of evil *nyen* and snake-demons,[116] are decorated with their specific mantras in order to bestow them with magical efficacy. The "Khyung remedy" (*gnyen po khyung*) or "condensed protective diagram" (*sgril ba'i srung 'khor*), represents the sophisticated union of the diverse divine figures and their mantras. This textual amulet is a *maṇḍala* diagram, which replicates the primordial universe within six concentric circles (*mu khyu*) drawn at the center of the Khyung's body. As with every magical wheel, this diagram is characterized by a specific orientation determined by sacred geometrical and geographical elements and also by the orientation of the Khyung's head. The Khyung's shoulders should be marked with the mother and father cakras representing the two lineages and smeared respectively with bezoar and saffron (representing the male and female sexual fluids); and his head can be oriented towards one of the two wheels overpowering the specific lineage or look at front in order to potentiate the practitioner. All of the circular patterns should contain a mantra and, each part of the Khyung body should be marked with mantras and smeared with empowered fragrant medical substances.[117]

During the consecration ritual the lunar and solar *cakras* written on the palms of the sacred Khyung should be joined and the *Essence of Interdependence Mantra* (*rten 'brel snying po*) should be written on the back of the paper sheet. These final actions embody the nonduality of reality through its symbols (union of the solar and lunar cakras) and mantra, which condenses the ontological ground of the magical act. The mantras and the magical formula will be not analyzed here; however, it should be said that its general meaning refers

115 *'Chi med bdud rtsi bum pa* (2), 68/8: [...] *zla stod rgyal dang rta chen brgyad//*. *'Chi med bdud rtsi bum pa* (2), 73/ 6–7: [...] *dus tshod gza' skar gyi gnad rang gi bla gza' bla skar bla nyi ma dang po 'o.*

116 This interpretation of the boar is substantiated by other sections of the *'Chi med bdud rtsi bum pa*, such as the cited *Reversal Suppressant* [*Ritual*] *of Sucking* [*the Infection*] *with the Adamantine Sow's Tongue* (*log gnon phag mo'i ljags 'jibs*). *'Chi med bdud rtsi bum pa* (1), 110r/1; *'Chi med bdud rtsi bum pa* (2), 152/11.

117 *'Chi med bdud rtsi bum pa* (1), 117r/3–117v/6; *'Chi med bdud rtsi bum pa* (2), 64/21.

to the annihilation of any evil forces, adjuring the demons by the name of the afflictions they cause (*rims thams cad la svāhā*), and bestowing a powerful protection on the "holder" (*'chang ba po* = Skt. *dhara*, the one who mastered the magical formula) from all kinds of poisons emerged from the prime *kālakūṭa* poison (*ha la ha la*).[118]

Finally, the textual amulets should be rolled up and wrapped in colored silk, ready to be bound to the body of the patient (worn around the neck or arm, or tied in the hair). The amulets are considered to be also effective against any kind of sorcery or negative astral influence, misfortune, or natural calamity. They also protect children from ghosts' assaults (*chung sri*), and they can even bestow fortitude (*dpa' la 'dzangs*) and fecundity (*gshin la 'dzangs*).[119] The magical diagrams and unguents can also be used to protect residences by applying them on the door lintels (*sgo ltag*), and they are used during extensive ritual to protect the entire land from the outbreak of pestilences or to stop their spreading.[120]

These magico-alchemical sections allow us to restate some considerations about the composite structure and the contents of the *Vase of Amṛta*. This corpus is rooted in the religious discerning of epidemics and communicable diseases. Indeed, due to the apocalyptical and prophetical frame of this literature, the diffusion of the diseases reflects the eruption of evil and corruption in the human world: communicable diseases originate in invisible entities, which are conceptualized as demonic. Therefore, apotropaic rituals are the ultimate methods to tear away the disease from the body. The threefold subdivision of the *Vase of Amṛta*, claimed by the various titles attributed to it (see the introduction), mirrors a specific conception of medical knowledge as a tripartite system (diagnosis, therapeutics, and rituals), and operative forms of knowledge, such as alchemy and the art of amulets, are considered essential.

5 Conclusion

The contents of the *Vase of Amṛta* reveal an intricate web of connections, with diverse historical and literary traditions. The wide array of topics associated with epidemiology, such as channel examination and the techniques for divinatory prognosis insert the *Vase of Amṛta* in the context of *Seminal Essence* literature, alongside magical and apotropaic procedures that relate it to the broader literature of *Mahāyogatantra*. As we have seen there are several

118 *'Chi med bdud rtsi bum pa* (2), 25/21–26/19.

119 *'Chi med bdud rtsi bum pa* (2), 69/16–70/5.

120 *'Chi med bdud rtsi bum pa* (1), 15r/1–15v/1; and *'Chi med bdud rtsi bum pa* (2), 27/9–28/1.

important correspondences between the contents of important medical sources such as the *Ultimate Tantra* and other sources, including the *Vase of Amṛta*. In particular the connections regard the body physiology, the taxonomy, and the etiological models of *nyen* and *rim* diseases. The title of the *Quintessential Scripture* (*yang thig gces*) defines not only to the esoteric nature of this corpus but also refers to the interrelation of different theoretical models deriving from Āyurveda, tantric alchemy, and demonology within this source.

In the history of Tibetan medical thought, the *Vase of Amṛta* represents a refined attempt to codify and systematize medical theories and practices in a coherent and comprehensive body of knowledge. The structure of the *Vase of Amṛta* reflects a clear authorial intent of keeping the secrecy of teachings, a methodology akin to the principle of "dispersed knowledge" we find in other alchemical traditions.[121] The language is often metaphorical and the information is scattered here and there, disseminated in main sections and ancillary explanatory scrolls and chapters, which clarify the main ritual and alchemical sections. The explanatory sections are called "strengths" (*gyad*), which might refer both to the mastering of magic-alchemical arts and to the effective application of this power to the opus. Another term for referring to these sections is "keys" (*lde'u mig*), which disclose the real and deep meanings of the scriptures.[122] This terminology, which has ancient origins, in this context means "commentarial" or "interpretative" and could refer to the hermetical tradition based on the precious contribution of the transmitters of the text.[123] According to Deumar's analysis of this corpus, these keys are the "filial texts" (*bu yig*) included in the *Vase of Amṛta*, which proceed from the main "maternal texts" (*ma yig*), and are a medium (*them ltar*, lit. "door threshold" or even "ladder") for ascending to a deeper understanding of medical knowledge.[124]

Despite its mysterious origin, the history of the transmission of the *Vase of Amṛta* appears to be connected to important medical collections. In the fourteenth century, physicians culled fragments or entire sections from the rituals and the pharmacopeia of the *Vase of Amṛta*, which was considered an

121 See for example, Lawrence Principe, *The Aspiring Adept: Robert Boyle and His Alchemical Quest Including Boyle's "Lost" Dialogue on the Transmutation of Metal* (Princeton, NJ: Princeton University Press, 2000), 143 and passim.

122 The complete series of "keys" and "strength" can be found in *'Chi med bdud rtsi bum pa* (2), 33–34; 38–39; 53–55; 55–58; 58–61; 79–112; and 135–42. These sections are also complemented by two groups of minor scrolls: *'Chi med bdud rtsi bum pa* (2), 149–53; 154–59; and 163–93.

123 See Michael Walter's comparison of Tibetan alchemical tradition and Gnosticism in Michael Walter, *The Role of Alchemy and Medicine in Indo-Tibetan Tantrism* (Bloomington, IN: Doctoral Dissertation at Indiana University, 1980), 13–27.

124 De'u dmar bstan'dzin phun tshogs, *Gso rig gces btus*, 94/19–95/12.

authoritative recipe source and a repository of an ancient magical and alchemical lore. At the turn of the seventeenth century, the hermetical corpus of the *Vase of Amṛta* was examined in exegetical literatures and served along with other apocryphal writings as extensive treatises on nosology. However, further and more detailed research on the contents of the *Vase of Amṛta* and its intertextual legacy might allow us to better understand the historical connection between the "accomplishing medicine" literature of the Nyingma tradition and canonical medical sources.

References

Tibetan-language Sources

Byams pa 'phrin las. *Gangs ljongs gso rig bstan pa'i nyin byed rim byon gyi rnam thar phyogs bsgrigs*. Beijing: Mi rigs dpe skrun khang, 2000.

Byams pa 'phrin las and Bod rang skyong ljongs sman rtsis khang, eds. *Bod lugs gso rig tshig mdzod chen mo*. Beijing: Mi rigs dpe skrun khang, 2006.

De'u dmar btan'dzin phun tshogs. *Gso rig gces btus rin chen phreng ba*. Xining: Mtsho sgnon mi rigs dpe skrun khang, 1993. BDRC W21588.

De'u dmar btan'dzin phun tshogs. *Lag len gces rigs sdus pa'i sman kun bcud du sgrub pa'i las gyi cho ga kun gsal snang mdzod ces bya ba bzhugs so*. In *Dri med shel gong dang dri med shel phreng dang lag len gces bsdus*. Leh: Tashigang S. W., 463–590. BDRC W23762

Dga' ba rdo rje. *'Khrungs dpe dri med shel gyi me long*. Beijing: Mi rigs dpe skrun khang, 1995.

Dpal ldan rgyal mtshan. *Brang ti lha rje'i rim brgyud kyi man ngag gser bre chen mo*. Lhasa: Bod ljongs mi dmangs dpe skrun khang, 2005.

G.yu thog snying thig zhes bya ba gzgugs so. Beijing: Mi rigs dpe skrun khang, 2007.

'Jam mgon kong sprul blo sgros mtha' yas. *Gter ston brgya rtsa'i rnam thar*. Lhasa: Bod ljongs mi dmangs dpe skrun khang, 2007. BDRC W1PD83972.

Lha btsun Rin chen rgya mtsho. *'Brong tse be'u bum dkar po*. Beijing: Mi rigs dpe skrun khang, 2005. BDRC W1PD2.

Ngag dbang blo bzang rgya mtsho. *Zab pa dang rgya che ba'i dam chos kyi yig gang ga'i chu rgyun*. In *Gsung 'bum*, vol. 1 (*Gsan yig ka*). Gangthok: Sikkim Research Institute of Tibetology, 1991–95. BDRC W294.

Nyi zla kha sbyor chen mo gsang ba'i rgyud. In *Rnying ma rgyud bcu bdun* (*A 'Dzom par ma*). Dpal yul rdzong: A 'dzom chos sgar par khang, 2000. BDRC W1KG11703.

Pha khol (Vāgbhaṭa). *Yan lag brgyad pa'i snying po'i bsdus*. In *Sbyor ba brgya pa dang yan lag brgyad pa'i snying po bsdus pa sogs*. Beijing: Mi rigs dpe skrun khang, 2005.

Phags pa klu sgrub (Nāgārjuna), Hashang Ma hā ya na, and Vairocana (Bai ro tsa na) (transl.). *Sman dpyad zla ba'i rgyal po: The Somarājabhaisajyasādhanā, an Indian Medical Work by Nāgārjuna in Its Tibetan Translation by Hashang Ma hā ya na and Vairocana.* Leh: T. Y. Tashigang, 1989. BDRC W29577.

Phags pa klu sgrub (Nāgārjuna), Hashang Ma hā ya na, and Vairocana (Bai ro tsa na). *Rtsa yig cha nyi zer sgron ma*. In *Slob dpon klu sgrub kyi sman yig gces btus*. Beijing: Mi rigs dpe skrun khang, 2008.

Phags pa klu sgrub (Nāgārjuna), Hashang Ma hā ya na, and Vairocana (Bai ro tsa na). *Mdze rigs bco brgyad kyi rtags rdo rje bde khros kyi dgongs pa las*. In *Slob dpon klu sgrub kyi sman yig gces btus*. Beijing: Mi rigs dpe skrun khang, 2008.

Sangs rgyas rgya mtsho. *Gso ba rig pa'i bstan bcos sman bla'i dgongs rgyan rgyud bzhi'i gsal byed baidurya sngon po'i mallika*. Lhasa: Bod ljongs mi dmangs dpe skrun khang, 1982. BDRC W2DB4602.

Sangs rgyas rgya mtsho. *Man ngag gi yon tan rgyud gi lhan thabs*. Xining: Mtsho mi rigs dpe skrung khang, 1991.

Slop dpon pad ma 'byung gnas. *'Chi med bdud rtsi bum pa. In Rin chen gter mdzod* vol. 46. Paro: Stod lung mtsur phu'i par khang, 1980.

Slop dpon pad ma 'byung gnas. *'Chi med bdud rtsi bum pa*. In *Slob dpon pad 'byung gi sman yig gces btus*. Beijing: Mi rigs dpe skrung khang, 2006.

G.yu thog yon tan mgon po. *Bdud rtsi snying po yan lag brgyad pa gsang ba man ngag gi rgyud*. Lhasa: Bod ljongs mi dmangs dpe skrun khang, 1982. BDRC W1KG1315.

G.yu thog yon tan mgon po. *Bu don ma*. Beijing: Mi rigs dpe skrung khang, 2009.

Zhang zhung snyan rgyud las sgron me drug gi gdams pa. In *Zhang zhung snyang rgyud kyi gsung pod* (Sde dge par ma). Lun grub steng: Sde dge par khang, [n.d.]; BDRC W00EG1016835.

Zur mkhar ba mnyams nyid rdo rje. *Man ngag bye ba ring bsrelpod chung rab 'byams gsal ba'i sgron me*. Lanzhou: Kan su'u mi rigs dpe skrun khang, 1993.

European-language Sources

Akosay, Anna, and Ronit Yoeli-Tlalim. "Along the Musk Routes: Exchanges Between Tibet and the Islamic World." *Asian Medicine: Tradition and Modernity* 3 (2007): 217–40.

Beckwith, Christopher I. "The Introduction of Greek Medicine into Tibet in the Seventh and Eighth Centuries." *Journal of the American Oriental Society* 99, no. 2 (1979): 297–313.

Beyer, Stephan. *The Cult of Tara: Magic and Ritual in Tibet*. Delhi: Motilal Banarsiddass, 2001.

Bhayro, Siam, and Catherine Rider, eds. *Demons and Illness from Antiquity to the Early-Modern Period*. Brill: Leiden, 2017.

Bühnemann, Gudrun. "Maṇḍala, Yantras and Cakra: Some Observations." In *Maṇḍalas and Yantras in the Hindu Traditions*, edited by Gudrun Bühnemann, 13–56. Leiden: Brill, 2003.

Cantwell, Cathy. "The Medicinal Accomplishment (*sman sgrub*) Practice in the Dudjom Meteoric Iron Razor (*gnam lcags spu gri*) Tradition: Reflections on the Ritual and Meditative Practice at a Monastery in Southern Bhutan." *Journal of the Oxford Centre for Buddhist Studies* 8 (2015): 49–95.

Crisciani, Chiara, and Michela Pereira. "Black Death and Golden Remedies: Some Remarks on Alchemy and the Plague." In *The Regulation of Evil: Social and Cultural Attitudes to Epidemics in Late Middles Ages*, edited by Agostino Paravicini Bagliani and Francesco Santi, 7–40. Firenze: Sismel-Edizioni del Galluzzo, 1998.

Cuevas, Bryan J. "'The Calf's Nipple' (*Be'u bum*) of Ju Mipham (*'Ju mi pham*): A Handbook of Tibetan Ritual Magic." In *Tibetan Ritual*, edited by José Ignacio Cabezón, 165–86. Oxford: Oxford University Press, 2010.

Cunningham, Andrew. "Epidemics, Pandemics and the Doomsday Scenario." *Historically Speaking* 7 (2008): 29–31.

Czaja, Olaf. "The Substitution of *Materia Medica* in Tibetan Medicine: An Inquiry into Traditional Tibetan Treatises." *East Asian Science, Technology and Medicine* 46 (2017): 119–212.

Czaja, Olaf. "*The Four Tantras* and the Global Market: Changing Epistemologies of *Drä* (*'bras*) versus Cancer." In *Medicine Between Science and Religion: Explorations on Tibetan Grounds*, edited by V. Adams, M. Schrempf, and S. Craig, 265–96. New York, NY: Berghahn Books, 2011.

Davidson, Ronald M. *Tibetan Renaissance: Tantric Buddhism in the Rebirth of Tibetan Culture* New York, NY: Columbia University Press, 2005.

de Nebesky-Wojkowitz, René. *Oracles and Demons of Tibet: The Cult and Iconography of the Tibetan Protective Deities*. Delhi: Book Faith India, 1993.

Garrett, Francis. "The Alchemy of Accomplishing Medicine (*sman sgrub*): Situating the *Yuthok Heart Essence* Ritual Tradition." *Journal of Indian Philosophy* 37, no. 3 (2009): 207–30.

Garrett, Francis. "Tapping the Body Nectar: Gastronomy and Incorporation in Tibetan Literature." *Journal of the History of Religions* 49, no. 3 (2010): 300–26.

Gerke, Barbara. "Treating Essence with Essence: Re-inventing *bcud len* as Vitalising Dietary Supplements in Contemporary Tibetan Medicine." *Asian Medicine: Tradition and Modernity* 7, no. 1 (2012): 196–224.

Gerke, Barbara. "Treating the Aged and Maintaining the Health: Locating *bcud len* Practices in the *Four Medical Tantras*." *Journal of International Buddhist Studies* 35, nos. 1–2 (2012): 329–62.

Hillis, Gregory. "The Khyung Texts in the *Rnying ma'i Rgyud 'Bum*." In *The Many Canons of Tibetan Buddhism. PIATS 2000: Proceedings of the Ninth Seminar of The*

International Association of Tibetan Studies, Leiden 2000, edited by H. Eimer and D. Germano, 313–32. Leiden: Brill, 2002.

Gyatso, Janet. *Being Human in a Buddhist World: An Intellectual History of Medicine in Early Modern Tibet*. New York, NY: Columbia University Press, 2015.

Jouanna, Jacques. *Disease as Aggression in Hippocratic Corpus and Greek Tragedy: Wild and Devouring Diseases*. In *Greek Medicine from Hippocrates to Galen*. Selected Papers by Jacques Jouanna translated by Neil Allias, edited with a preface by Philips van der Eijk. Leiden-Boston: Brill, 2012: 81–96.

Kilty, Gavin, trans. *Mirror of Beryl: A Historical Introduction to Tibetan Medicine*. Boston, MA: Wisdom Publications, 2009.

Martin, Dan. "An Early Tibetan History of Indian Medicine." In *Soundings in Tibetan Medicine: Anthropological and Historical Perspectives. Proceedings of the 10th Seminar of the International Association of Tibetan Studies*, edited by Mona Schrempf, 307–25. Leiden: Brill, 2007.

Martin, Dan. "Greek and Islamic Medicines' Historical Contact with Tibet." In *Islam and Tibet: Interactions along the Musk Routes*, edited by Anna Akasoy, Charles S. F. Burnett, and Ronit Yoeli-Tlalim, 117–44. Burlington, VT: Ashgate Publishing Company, 2011.

McGrath, William. "Vessel Examination in the *Medicine of the Moon King*." In *Buddhism and Medicine: An Anthology of Premodern Sources*, edited by C. Pierce Salguero, 501–13. New York, NY: Columbia University Press, 2017.

McGrath, William. *Buddhism and Medicine in Tibet: Origins, Ethics, and Tradition*. Charlottesville, VA: Doctoral Dissertation at the University of Virginia, 2017.

Orofino, Giacomella, *Sacred Tibetan Teachings on Death and Liberation*. Bridport, Dorset: Prims-Unity Press, 1990.

Principe, Lawrence. *The Aspiring Adept: Robert Boyle and His Alchemical Quest Including Boyle's "Lost" Dialogue on the Transmutation of Metals*. Princeton, NJ: Princeton University Press, 2000.

Scheiddeger, Daniel. "Lamps in the Leaping Over." *Revue d'Etudes Tibétaines* 8, no. 10 (2005): 40–64.

Scheiddeger, Daniel. "The First Four Themes of Klong chen pa's Tsig don bcu gcig pa." *Revue d'Etudes Tibétaines* 16, no. 3 (2009): 43–73.

Sharma, Prayavrat. *Carakasaṃhitā* (Text with English Translation). Varanasi: Chaukhambha Orientalia, 2014.

Simioli, Carmen. "The 'Brilliant Moon Theriac' (*Zla zil dar ya kan*): A Preliminary Study of Mercury Processing according to the *Vase of Amrita of Immortality* (*'Chi med bdud rtsi bum pa*) and Its Influence on Tibetan Pharmacological Literature." *Revue d'Etudes Tibétaines* 37 (2016): 391–419.

Simioli, Carmen. "Alchemical Gold and the Pursuit of the Alchemical Elixir." *Asian Medicine: Tradition and Modernity* 8, no. 1 (2013): 43–77.

Skemer, Don C. *Binding Words Textual Amultes in the Middle Ages*. Philadelphia, PA: Pennsylvania University Press, 2006.

Slouber, Michael. *Early Tantric Medicine: Snakebite, Mantras, and Healing in the Garuda Tantras*. Oxford: Oxford University Press, 2017.

Tucci, Giuseppe. *Le Religioni del Tibet*. Roma: Edizioni Mediterranee, 1996.

Van Kooij, Karel R. "Protective Covering (*Kavaca*)." In *Selected Studies on Ritual in the Indian Religions*, edited by Ria Kloppenborg, 118–29. Leiden: Brill, 1983.

Lo, Vivienne, and Sylvia Schroer. "Deviant Airs in Traditional Chinese Medicine." In *Asian Medicine and Globalisation*, edited by Joseph S. Alter, 46–66. Philadelphia, PA: University of Pennsylvania Press, 2005.

Wallace, Vesna A. "Medicine and Astrology in the Healing Arts of the *Kālacakratantra*." In *As Long as Space Endures: Essays on the Kālacakra Tantra in Honor of H. H. The Dalai Lama*, edited by Edward A. Arnold, 179–91. Ithaca, NY: Snow Lion Publications, 2009.

Walter, Michael L. *The Role of Alchemy and Medicine in Indo-Tibetan Tantrism*. Bloomington, IN: Doctoral Dissertation at the University of Indiana, 1980.

Wujastyk, Dagmar. "Acts of Improvement: On the Use of Tonics and Elixirs in Sanskrit Medical and Alchemical Literature." *History of Science in South Asia* 5, no. 2 (2017): 1–36.

Wujastyk, Dominik. *The Roots of Āyurveda: Selections from Sanskrit Medical Writings*. London: Penguin Books, 2001.

Yoeli-Tlalim, Ronit. "A Tibetan Image of Divination: Some Contextual Remarks." In *Imagining Chinese Medicine*, edited by Vivienne Lo and Penelope Barrett, 429–40. Sir Herry Wellcome Asiane Series, vol. 8. Leiden: Brill 2018.

Yoeli-Tlalim, Ronit. "Between Medicine and Ritual: Tibetan 'Medical Ritual' from Dunhuang." In *Tibetan and Himalayan Healing: An Anthology for Anthony Aris*, edited by Charles Ramble and Ulrike Roesler, 739–46. Kathmandu: Vajra Publications, 2015.

Yoeli-Tlalim, Ronit. "Central Asian Mélange: Early Tibetan Medicine from Dunhunag." In *Scribes, Texts, and Rituals in Early Tibet and Dunhuang*, edited by Brandon Dotson, Kazushi Iwao, and Tsuguhito Takeuchi, 53–60. Wiesbaden: Reichert-Verlag, 2013.

Yoeli-Tlalim, Ronit. "On Urine Analysis and Tibetan Medicine's Connections with the West." In *Studies of Medical Pluralism in Tibetan History and Society*, edited by Sienna Craig, Mingji Cuomu, Frances Garrett, and Mona Schrempf, 195–211. Halle: International Institute for Tibetan and Buddhist Studies GmbH, 2010.

Yoeli-Tlalim, Ronit. "Re-visiting 'Galen in Tibet.'" *Medical History* 56, no. 3 (2012): 355–65.

Zahara, Kulsoom et al. "A Review of Therapeutic Potential of Saussurea lappa: An Endangered Plant from Himalaya." *Asian Pacific Journal of Tropical Medicine* 7, no. 1 (2014): 60–69.

Zhen Yan. "*rTsa* in the Tibetan Manuscripts from Dunhuang." Translated by Vivienne Lo. *Asian Medicine* 3 (2007): 296–307.

CHAPTER 8

Tantric Divination and Empirical Diagnosis: a Genealogy of Channel *Prasenā* Rituals in the Tibetan Medical Tradition

William A. McGrath

> The twenty-one sages imparted upon Nāgārjuna, master of the five fields [of knowledge], the attainments of medicine. With this supreme [mode of] healing, one shall master all medical practices. With these methods for achieving the clairvoyance of the sages, one shall be able to diagnose disease without examining the channels, fluids, or other external objects. Even without *mo* divination or other calculations, one will be able to identify demons with the point of a finger. Even without the precedents of the tantras, scriptures, or [other] instructions, one will know all medical formulae without exception. Even without practical and experiential accounts, one will know the practices of phlebotomy and cauterization. Pray, sages, bestow upon me these holy instructions for attainments.[1]
>
> —Excerpt form a channel *prasenā* ritual[2]

1 The present study is based on the comparison of five different editions of instructions for channel *prasenā* rituals. Not all editions agree who the "me" (*bdag*) is here, but several have notes indicating that it is Nāgārjuna: Bod rang skyong ljongs sman rtsis khang, ed., *Brang ti lha rje'i rim brgyud kyi man ngag gser bre chen mo* (Lha sa: Bod ljongs mi dmangs dpe skrun khang, 2005), 1; A ru ra, ed., *Man ngag gser bre ma dang dngul bre ma*, Bod kyi gso ba rig pa'i gna' dpe phyogs bsgrigs dpe tshogs, vol. 6 (Beijing: Mi rigs dpe skrun khang, 2004), 1. Such a note does not appear in *Reg pa rtsa'i spra sgrub klu sgrub gyis mdzad pa bzhugs s.ho*, in *Krung go'i bod lugs gso rig rtsa che'i dpe rnying kun btus: Pho brang po ta la'i gsung rab gter mdzod las btus* [Zhongguo yiyao yingyin guji zhenben 中国藏医药影印古籍珍本; China's Traditional Tibetan Medical Texts: A Treasury of Scriptures from the Potala Palace], ed. Bod ljongs bod lugs gso rig slob grwa chen mo (Lha sa: Bod ljongs mi dmangs dpe skrun khang, 2014), vol. 1, text 10, p. 53 (f. 2a); *Gser khri* [=*bre*] *rgyas pa zhes bya ba bzhugs so*, in *Krung go'i bod lugs gso rig rtsa che'i dpe rnying kun btus*, vol. 18, text 13, p. 198 (f. 2a; note that folios are out of order); or A ru ra, ed., *G.yu thog snying thig*, Bod kyi gso ba rig pa'i gna' dpe phyogs bsgrigs dpe tshogs, vol. 43 (Beijing: Mi rigs dpe skrun khang, 2007), 620. I read the verb in the final line (*phul*, "bestow") as imperative rather than indicative.

2 As indicated in the previous note, instructions for the *Evocation Ritual of the Yellow Sage Kapila and His Two Sons* (*drang srong ser skya spun gsum gyi sgrub thabs*) cited here, as well as the other rituals examined below, currently exist in many different editions. For the *Yellow Sage*, the present study will primary focus on the edition found in a recently published manuscript,

 | DOI:10.1163/9789004404441_009

∴

The expressions of the body elude immediate understanding.[3] As a result, medical traditions have relied on diagnostic techniques in order to identify and interpret empirical signs. Each method of observation—the visual examination of the tongue, the olfactory examination of the urine, or the haptic examination of the channels—may involve a different sense faculty, resulting in a diverse array of potential diagnostic methods for the trained physician. Sometimes even different observations of the same object, such as the haptic observation of the same channels of the same patient, will result in different understandings of disease, particularly if these pulsations are observed by different physicians trained in different diagnostic traditions. As these observations were named, systematized, and incorporated within larger intellectual systems for understanding the body, health, and illness, the physicians trained in such traditions gained repertoires of possible resources with which he or she might diagnose and treat disease.[4] The diagnostic system of the Tibetan medical tradition is one such repertoire of resources, including loosely related or even contradictory instructions, such as the empirical observation of symptoms alongside divinatory methods for the attainment of clairvoyance and communication with the divine.

The Tibetan medical tradition has long been celebrated as being grounded in both scholastic learning and empirical observation. For a majority of the last millennium, physicians have trained in its formative texts, such as the *Four Tantras* (*rgyud bzhi*) and its associated exegetical literature, and implemented

---

entitled the *Prasenā Divination Ritual of Channel Palpation*, attributed to Nāgārjuna, with notable discrepancies indicated. See *Reg pa rtsa'i spra sgrub klu sgrub gyis mdzad pa bzhugs s.ho*, in *Krung go'i bod lugs gso rig rtsa che'i dpe rnying kun btus*, vol. 1, text 10, p. 53 (ff. 1b–2a): *gnas lnga dag la mkhas pa'i klu sgrub la// drang srong nyi shu rtsa gcig gis// sman gyi dngos grub byin nas su// gso ba'i mchog tu gyur pa yis// sman spyad kun la mkhas bya'i phyir// drang srong mngon shes sgrub pa'i thabs// rtsa dang chu dang phyi'i yul// kun la ma ltos nad ngos 'dzin// mo dang rtsis la ma ltos par// gdon ngos 'jug* [=*mdzub*] *tshugs 'dzin pa dang // rgyud gzhung man ngag dpe la ma ltos par// sman sbyor ma lus shes pa dang // lag len nyams la ma ltos par// gtar bsregs dpyad rnams shes pa yis// sgrub pa'i man ngag dam pa 'di// drang srong rnams kyis bdag la phul//.*

3 The phrase "expressions of the body" alludes, of course, to Shigehisa Kuriyama, *The Expressiveness of the Body and the Divergence of Greek and Chinese Medicine* (New York, NY: Zone Books, 1999).

4 For an analysis of such "repertoires" in religious traditions, see Robert F. Campany, "On the Very Idea of Religions (In the Modern West and in Early Medieval China)," *History of Religions* 42, no. 4 (2003): 287–319.

these instructions to both diagnose and treat disease.[5] Ever since the establishment of Tibetan medical lineages and schools in the eleventh and twelfth centuries, medical knowledge has been refined, reinterpreted, and expanded in scholastic summaries, commentaries, and instructional collections, potentially even on the basis of empirical investigation.[6] Non-empirical approaches to the diagnosis and treatment of disease—such as the divinatory identification of disease, the therapeutic recitation of spells, and the exorcism of pathogenic demons—can also be found throughout the texts of the Tibetan medical tradition, even if such ritual methods are rare in the *Four Tantras* itself.[7] In the opening evocation of the instructions for a diagnostic ritual cited above, for example, physicians are instructed to renounce both scholastic learning and empirical observation, the cornerstones of Tibetan medicine, and to seek the clairvoyance of the sages. In light of the seeming contradiction between medical healing on the one hand and ritual healing on the other, how did these opposing modes of diagnosis and divination come to be transmitted together? And how were these contradictions of empirical observation and divine

5 On the notion of formative texts, see Moshe Halbertal, *People of the Book: Canon, Meaning, and Authority* (Cambridge, MA: Harvard University Press, 1997), 94: "a formative text is one in which progress in the field is made through interpretation of the text itself. A text-centered culture that has formative texts proceeds in that mode; its achievements are interpretative." Cited in Georges Dreyfus, *The Sound of Two Hands Clapping: The Education of a Tibetan Buddhist Monk* (Berkeley, CA: University of California Press, 2003), 100. Regarding the importance of scriptural authority and scholastic learning in the sixteenth- and seventeenth-century Tibetan medical tradition, see Kurtis R. Schaeffer, "Textual Scholarship, Medical Tradition, and Mahāyāna Buddhist Ideals in Tibet," *Journal of Indian Philosophy* 31 (2003): 621–41.

6 On the relationship between empiricism and scriptural authority in the theories and practical instructions of the Tibetan medical tradition, see Janet Gyatso, "The Authority of Empiricism and the Empiricism of Authority: Medicine and Buddhism in Tibet on the Eve of Modernity," *Comparative Studies of South Asia, Africa and the Middle East* 24, no. 2 (2004): 83–96; which was republished as "Experience, Empiricism and the Fortunes of Authority: Tibetan Medicine and Buddhism on the Eve of Modernity," in the *Tibetan History Reader*, ed. Gray Tuttle and Kurtis R. Schaeffer (New York, NY: Columbia University Press, 2013), 363–85; and reformulated as the so-called "medical mentality" in *Being Human in a Buddhist World: An Intellectual History of Medicine in Early Modern Tibet* (New York, NY: Columbia University Press, 2015), 18: "It is more important to recognize that certain medical theorists were *reaching toward* empirical accountability than to judge, from the vantage of the twenty-first century, whether they actually attained it or not. [...] But the medical impulse to heed direct perception over scriptural authority nonetheless had the potential to reshape the entire epistemic matrix in ways that Dreyfus [cited in previous note] judges to be missing in scholastic debate culture."

7 Gyatso, *Being Human in a Buddhist World*, 422–23, n. 95: "But all of these statements on ritual means of healing taken together occupy less than 10 pages, scattered through a work of more than 660 pages."

revelation ultimately reconciled in the orthodox teachings of the Tibetan medical tradition?

Unlike the empirical methods for observation promoted in channel examination, instructions for *prasenā* divination promise the divine revelation of past, present, and future actions and events.[8] A specific genre of *prasenā* divination rituals instructs the practitioner to supplicate either sages or goddesses in order to predict the lifespan of a patient, see pathogenic demons with the aid of divine sight, and intuitively sense the appropriate methods for treatment. These sets of instructions are collectively called "channel *prasenā* rituals" (*rtsa'i pra sgrub*), and have been repeatedly redacted and transmitted together in Tibet from at least the twelfth century onward. They can be found alongside commentaries on the *Four Tantras* in the *Eighteen Auxiliary Branches* collection,[9] as well as other ritual instructions in the *Golden Measure* of the Drangti lineage,[10] and the *Essential Nucleus of Yutok* of the Yutok school.[11] Thus, despite the demonstrated centrality of empirical observation in the *Four Tantras*, an oracular approach to diagnostics promoted in these channel *prasenā* rituals also remained popular in the Tibetan medical tradition for nearly an entire millennium.[12] By tracing a genealogy of the transmission and transformation of channel *prasenā* rituals and other related methods, we can begin to construct a nuanced history for the Tibetan medical tradition, identifying the processes by which specific diagnostic methods were actively

8 *Prasenā* divination, *pra se na* in Tibetan (or, often, just *pra*, *spra*, or *kra*), refers to a diverse set of divinatory instructions and practices. See below for a full discussion.

9 See *Rtsa'i pra sgrub med thabs med pa*, in *Cha lag bco brgyad*, ed. A ru ra, Bod kyi gso ba rig pa'i gna' dpe phyogs bsgrigs dpe tshogs, vol. 25 (Beijing: Mi rigs dpe skrun khang, 2005), 492–94.

10 See *Gsang ba man ngag gi skor*, in *Man ngag gser bre ma dang dngul bre ma*, ed. A ru ra, Bod kyi gso ba rig pa'i gna' dpe phyogs bsgrigs dpe tshogs, vol. 6 (Beijing: Mi rigs dpe skrun khang, 2004), 1–12. This Arura edition is inferior to the Mentsikhang edition due to several lacunae throughout the instructions: *Brang ti lha rje'i rim brgyud kyi man ngag gser bre chen mo* (Lhasa: Bod ljongs mi dmangs dpe skrun khang, 2005). Below manuscript editions are also used.

11 See *Dngul bre las* [sic] *drang srong ser skya'i sgrub thabs*, in *G.yu thog snying thig*, ed. A ru ra, Bod kyi gso ba rig pa'i gna' dpe phyogs bsgrigs dpe tshogs, vol. 43 (Beijing: Mi rigs dpe skrun khang, 2007), 619–23.

12 As I was preparing the final version of this essay in the summer of 2017, it came to my attention that Dr. Nida Chenagtsang of Sorig Khang International would soon be offering the "Empowerment for the Rishis and Dakinis of Medicine," an "extremely rare and precious empowerment from the Yuthok Nyingthig tradition," in Boulder, CO. Thus, channel *prasenā* rituals continue to be transmitted to this day, even in North America.

assimilated and adapted, even across diverse intellectual contexts.[13] Finally, this genealogy of divination and diagnosis in Tibetan medical instructions illuminates the composite nature of the instructional anthologies and classical texts of Tibetan medicine, creating space for a reevaluation of the *Four Tantras* and its place in the history of the Tibetan medical tradition as a whole.

1 *Prasenā* Divination and the Divine Revelation of the Past, Present, and Future

It is difficult to know the precise circumstances of the origins, transmission, and performance of instructions in intellectual traditions,[14] and the instructions analyzed here are no exception. Indeed, practices cannot themselves be transmitted in a tradition, even if descriptions of and instructions for such practices can be recorded.[15] As a result, we must continually remember the stark disparity between prescriptive instructions and descriptive accounts when studying the practices of both religious and medical traditions, particularly those that derive from cosmopolitan contexts.[16] If a particular set of practical instructions were translated into Tibetan from Sanskrit, for example, how do we know if these cosmopolitan instructions were not transformed in the process of vernacular performance? Lacking other instructions or descriptions from within this tradition, the answer to this question is that we simply cannot. If further sets of related instructions still exist, however, and if these

13 The language of "genealogy" and its emphasis on "descent" (*Herkunft*) and "emergence" (*Entstehung*) over "origins" (*Ursprung*) primarily derives from the work of Nietzsche and Foucault. See, for example, Michel Foucault, "Nietzsche, Genealogy, History," in *Language, Counter-Memory, Practice: Selected Essays and Interviews*, ed. Donald F. Bouchard (Ithaca, NY: Cornell University Press, 1977), 139–64.

14 On the philosophical assumptions and philological methods associated with a "quest for origins," see the previous note, as well as José Ignacio Cabezón, "Buddhist Studies as a Discipline and the Role of Theory," *Journal of the International Association of Buddhist Studies* 18 (1995): 231–68, especially 245–47.

15 Edward Shils, *Tradition* (Chicago, IL: University of Chicago Press, 1981), 12: "In the case of practices and institutions made up of human actions, it is not the particular concrete actions which are transmitted; that is impossible. An action ceases to exist once it is performed. Human actions are the most evanescent of things. [...] What particular actions and complexes and sequences of actions leave behind are the conditions for subsequent actions, images in memory and documents of what they were when they happened and, under certain conditions, normative precedents or prescriptions for future actions."

16 For the relationship between the vernacular and the cosmopolitan in a South Asian context, see Sheldon Pollock, "The Cosmopolitan Vernacular," *The Journal of Asian Studies* 51, no. 1 (1998): 6–37.

instructions can be ordered chronologically—that is, if multiple and distinct instances of historical emergence can be determined—a genealogical account of instructional transmissions can be created, from which we may deduce the historical vicissitudes of interpretation and performance.

Despite the ubiquitousness of *prasenā* divination in Tibetan literature, there have been relatively few studies of this particular technique. Throughout English-language secondary literature, Tibetan-language instructions for *prasenā* have generally been described as some kind of "mirror divination."[17] Such an understanding is by no means incorrect but, as we shall see in the case of channel *prasenā* divination below, the divine revelation of past, present, and future events through *prasenā* divination can come through the medium of not only mirrors, but also thumbnails, butter lamps, young children, and even the palpation of the channels. *Prasenā* refers to a mode of inquiry, a ritual process through which a practitioner may communicate with the divine, either directly by means of spontaneous visions and voices, or indirectly by means of a prepubescent ritual assistant. In both direct and indirect forms of *prasenā* divination, the revelation of past, present, and future actions (*karma*) is described as a form of extrasensory knowledge or a visionary sign that usually requires further interpretation. Although the instructions for the performance of *prasenā* divination throughout Tibetan literature are generally quite precise, descriptions of the results of such practices are often ambiguous, if they are even described at all. Thus, *prasenā* divination is best thought of as a diverse body of oracular practices that can be performed to evoke the divine revelation of past, present, and future actions and events.

17 See, for example, Giacomella Orofino, "Divination with Mirrors: Observations on a Simile Found in the Kālacakra Literature," in *Tibetan Studies: Proceedings of the 6th Seminar of the International Association for Tibetan Studies, Fagernes 1992*, ed. Per Kvaerne (Oslo: Institute for Comparative Research in Human Culture, 1994), 612–28; Hildegard Diemberger, "Female Oracles in Modern Tibet," in *Women in Tibet*, ed. Janet Gyatso and Hanna Havnevik (New York, NY: Columbia University Press, 2005), 113–68, especially 133–36; and Hildegard Diemberger, "Padmasambhava's Unfinished Job: The Subjugation of Local Deities as Described in the *dBa' bzhed* in Light of Contemporary Practices of Spirit Possession," in *Pramāṇakīrtiḥ: Papers Dedicated to Ernst Steinkellner on the Occasion of his 70th Birthday*, ed. Birgit Kellner et al. (Vienna: Arbeitskreis für Tibetische und Buddhistische studien Universität Wien, 2007), 85–93.

2 Cosmopolitan Instructions for *Prasenā* in Tibetan Canonical Literature

The *locus classicus* of *prasenā* divination in the Tibetan language is the early seventh-century action tantra (*bya rgyud* = Skt. *kriyātantra*), the *Questions of Subāhu* (Skt. *subāhuparipṛcchā*).[18] As far as I am aware, the work is no longer extant in Sanskrit,[19] but is available in both Tibetan- and Chinese-language translations,[20] along with three distinct Tibetan-language

18 *'Phags pa dpung bzang gis zhus pa zhes bya ba'i rgyud*, in *Bka' 'gyur dpe bsdur ma*, ed. Krung go'i bod rig pa zhib 'jug ste gnas kyi bka' bstan dpe sdur khang (Beijing: Krung go'i bod rig pa dpe skrun khang, 2006–2009), text 0835, vol. 96 (*wa*), pp. 434–508. On the interpretation of early action tantras, including the *Questions of Subāhu*, as ritual manuals, see Jacob Dalton, "How Dhāraṇīs WERE Proto-Tantric: Liturgies, Ritual Manuals, and the Origins of the Tantras," in *Tantric Traditions in Transmission and Translation*, ed. David B. Gray and Ryan Richard Overbey (Oxford: Oxford University Press, 2016), 199–229.

19 For a discussion of the *Questions of Subāhu Tantra* and *prasenā* divination in South Asian sources, see Frederick M. Smith, *The Self Possessed: Deity and Spirit Possession in South Asian Literature and Civilization* (New York, NY: Columbia University Press, 2006), 421–27.

20 For an introduction to *prasenā* divination (Chi. *bosina* 鉢私那 or *botian* 鉢天) in Chinese religious traditions, see Michel Strickmann, *Chinese Magical Medicine*, ed. Bernard Faure (Stanford, CA: Stanford University Press, 2002), 210–14. There are actually two extant Chinese-language translations of the *Questions of Subāhu Tantra*, one of which has two editions: the *Sipohu tongzi qingwen jing* 蘇婆呼童子請問經 (T18no895; trans. ca. 724) and *Miaobi pusa suowen jing* 妙臂菩薩所問經 (T18no896; trans. 10th c.?). There are two texts listed under the title of *Sipohu tongzi qingwen jing* in the Chinese Buddhist Canon, which appear to be distinct but related translations (a twelve-chapter T18no895a and a thirteen-chapter T18no895b). Only T18no895b lists Śubhakarasiṃha (Shan Wuwei 善無畏; 637–735) as the translator in its colophon (CBETA pp. 16–17): "Translated by Master Śubhakarasiṃha, from the west of the Central Kingdom of the Great Tang (and a group of *śrāmaṇa* monks). Redacted by Master Da Gu on the first day of the third month of the third year of the Cheng era. It was offered [to the emperor] and received with respect" (右大唐中天竺國二藏輸波迦羅[唐云善無畏]譯[沙門一行筆] 承曆三年三月一日於大谷阿闍梨御　房奉受了). The *Nanjio Catalog* lists this edition as having been translated in 724 with the help of Yixing 一行 (683–727): Bunyiu Nanjio, *A Catalogue of the Chinese Translation of the Buddhist Tripitaka: The Sacred Canon of the Buddhits in China and Japan* (Oxford: Clarendon Press, 1883), 122–23 (#531). On the role of Śubhakarasiṃha in the establishment of esoteric Buddhism in China see, for example, Charles D. Orzech, "The 'Great Teaching of Yoga' the Chinese Appropriation of the Tantras, and the Question of Esoteric Buddhism," *Journal of Chinese Religions* 34 (2006): 29–78. Regarding the twelve-chapter *Miaobi pusa suowen jing* 妙臂菩薩所問經 (T18no896), the colophon does not mention Dharmadeva (Fa Tian 法天; d. 1001), but the Nanjio Catalog attributes the work to him: Bunyiu Nanjio, *A Catalogue of the Chinese Translation of the Buddhist Tripitaka*, 189 (#822). On the life and works of Dharmadeva, see Tansen Sen, "The Revival and Failure of Buddhist Translations During the Song Dynasty," *T'oung Pao* 88 (2002): 27–80; and Charles D. Orzech, "Translation of Tantras and Other

commentaries.[21] Despite the fact that the *Questions of Subāhu* contains instructions for rituals that might be termed *prasenā* divination in its seventh chapter, the term *prasenā* (*pra se na*) can only be found in one of the anonymous commentaries and not in the root text itself. The first mention of *prasenā* is used to describe revelatory appearances found in ritual implements:

> [Potential ritual implements:] One's thumb, a mirror, a sword, water, a crystal, a butter lamp, earth, iron, the sky, a begging bowl, or a jewel in firelight. Clear revelations of the past, present, and future **shall always arise** [in these]. One shall understand the clear and timeless revelations of all the virtuous and non-virtuous actions of the higher realms and those on the earth—those of not only humans, but also the gods and demigods.[22]
>
> **Shall always arise:** Such implements are the grounds for *prasenā* revelation, the capacity for visions.[23]

Esoteric Buddhist Scriptures," in *Esoteric Buddhism and the Tantras in East Asia*, ed. Charles D. Orzech, Henrik H. Sørensen, and Richard K. Payne (Leiden: Brill, 2011), 439–50.

21 Only one of the commentaries mentions an author, Master Buddhaguhya (*slob dpon sangs rgyas gsang ba*, fl. early 8th c.): *Dpung bzangs kyis zhus pa'i rgyud kyi bsdus pa'i don*, in *Bstan 'gyur dpe bsdur ma*, ed. Krung go'i bod rig pa zhib 'jug ste gnas kyi bka' bstan dpe sdur khang (Beijing: Krung go'i bod rig pa dpe skrun khang, 2006–2009), *rgyud*, text 1578, vol. 36 (*thu* [71]), pp. 102–49 (full text), 119–23 (ch. 7). Chapter Seven of Buddhaguhya's commentary is effectively just an abridged retelling of the root text with very little added information. The first anonymous commentary is: *'Phags pa dpung bzangs kyis zhus pa'i rgyud kyi tshig gi don bshad pa'i brjed byang*, in *Bstan 'gyur dpe bsdur ma, rgyud*, text 1579, vol. 36 (*thu* [71]), pp. 150–273 (full text), 212–20 (ch. 7). Chapter Seven of this commentary is rich in detail and adds much information for the study of *prasenā* divination. The second anonymous commentary on the *Questions of Subāhu Tantra* does not treat the seventh chapter: *'Phags pa dpung bzangs kyis zhus pa'i rgyud kyi bsdus pa'i don dgrol ba'i brjed byang*, in *Bstan 'gyur dpe bsdur ma, rgyud*, text 1580, vol. 36 (*thu* [71]), pp. 274–319 (full text). Therefore, only the first anonymous commentary will be considered below. For more on the *Questions of Subāhu Tantra* and its connection to early *yoginī tantras*, see Ronald M. Davidson, *Indian Esoteric Buddhism: A Social History of the Tantric Movement* (New York, NY: Columbia University Press, 2002), 203–204.

22 *'Phags pa dpung bzang gis zhus pa zhes bya ba'i rgyud*, in *Bka' 'gyur dpe bsdur ma, rgyud 'bum*, text 0835, vol. 96 (*wa*), 467: *mthe bong me long ral gri chu dang shel// mar me sa gzhi lcags dang nam mkha' dang// lhung bzed nor bu dag dang me 'bar ba// 'di la gsal bar ston pa rtag tu 'byung // 'das pa dang ni ma 'ongs da ltar byung // mtho ris sa steng dus dang mi ldan yang // lha dang lha min dge dang mi dge ba'i// las rnams thams cad gsal bar ston par rtogs//.*

23 Bold font and indented passages indicate quotations from the anonymous commentary cited above: *'Phags pa dpung bzangs kyis zhus pa'i rgyud kyi tshig gi don bshad pa'i brjed byang*, in *Bstan 'gyur dpe bsdur ma, rgyud*, text 1579, vol. 36 (*thu* [71]), 216: *rtag tu 'byung*

In this commentary the phrase, "grounds for *prasenā* revelation" (*pra se na ston pa'i gzhi*), is placed in apposition with the "capacity for visions" (*snang tu btub*) inherent in such reflective surfaces and other media. This reading is also supported by the *Mahāvyutpatti*, which glosses *prasenaṃ* with "bright appearance" or "clear vision" (*gsal snang*).[24] Thus, despite indications in the Chinese-language editions of the *Questions of Subāhu* that the word *prasenā* may be the name of a deity,[25] in the Tibetan-language exegetical materials, the term *prasenā* refers not to the deity responsible for such a vision, but to the revelatory appearance itself.

Although the above quotation presents *prasenā* as a spontaneous vision found in reflective surfaces and other such media, subsequent instructions included in the *Questions of Subāhu* elaborate upon these instructions with two further possible methods. Instead of instructing the ritual master to stare into a mirror, a butter lamp, or the sky and witness a vision oneself, sequent instructions involve the incorporation of a young child (*byis pa gzhon nu* or *bus pa gzhon nu*) into the ritual practice. One is instructed to clean and dress the child in white clothes, reciting mantras and encouraging him or her to look into a mirror wiped with ashes. The child will come to "see the past, present, and future with divine eyes,"[26] which the anonymous commentary explains as "seeing the visual form of things or the indication of meaning with written syllables; and some have said that [the child] will even hear the sound of an explanation."[27] Here the ritual master is no longer directly privy to divine revelation, but instead can only access knowledge of the three times by the indirect means of his ritual assistant. Thus, within the *Questions of Subāhu*, separate but related cycles of ritual instructions have been placed together in the same text: one in which the ritual master seeks a spontaneous vision of

---

zhes bya ba ni rdzas de rnams pra se na ston pa'i gzhi yin te/ snang tu btub ces bya ba'i tha tshig go/.

24 *Bye brag tu rtogs par byed pa*, in *Bstan 'gyur dpe bsdur ma, sna tshogs*, text 3590, vol. 115 (*co* [219]), 135.

25 See the discussion in Strickmann, *Chinese Magical Medicine*, 210–14.

26 *'Phags pa dpung bzang gis zhus pa zhes bya ba'i rgyud*, in *Bka' 'gyur dpe bsdur ma, rgyud 'bum*, text 0835, vol. 96 (*wa*), 468: *me long thal ba gtsang mas lan bdun nam// brgyad dam yang na bcur ni phyis nas su// rtse gcig sems kyis gsang sngags zlos bzhin du// bus pa gzhon nu nub tu kha bstan nas// lha yi mig gis bltas na 'das pa dang // da ltar dang ni ma 'ongs mthong bar 'gyur//.*

27 *'Phags pa dpung bzangs kyis zhus pa'i rgyud kyi tshig gi don bshad pa'i brjed byang*, in *Bstan 'gyur dpe bsdur ma, rgyud*, text 1579, vol. 36 (*thu* [71]), 217: *mthong bar gyur zhes bya ba ni dngos po rnams gzugs su mthong ba 'am/ yi ge'i 'bras bus kyang brda sprod par byed do// kha cig na re gzhi bsnyen na sgrar yang grag ce'o//.*

the past, present, and future, and another in which one induces a child to have such a vision.

In a third cycle of ritual instructions found in Chapter Seven of the *Questions of Subāhu*, the child is described as a "vessel of descent" (*dbab pa'i snod*) and, instead of inducing the child to have a vision, the ritual master is instructed to call a spirit to descend into the child so that he may interrogate it: "What manner of deity are you? Pray, what must I [do] in the three times? Please consider this carefully and tell me."[28] In this third mode of *prasenā* divination, which involves a spirit-possessed child as the medium instead of a reflective instrument, the practitioner is no longer interpreting divine revelations by means of direct sight or indirect assistance, but is instead able to directly communicate with the divine through the speech of a possessed child. Thus, in sum, *prasenā* in the *Questions of Subāhu Tantra* refers to at least three distinct but related methods for divination: one in which the ritual master communicates with the divine through the medium of visionary implements, a second in which an assistant communicates with the divine through the medium of visionary implements, and a third in which the ritual master communicates with the divine through the medium of a spirit-possessed child.

Although the instructions for *prasenā* divination prescribed in Chapter Seven of the *Questions of Subāhu Tantra* include diverse media and methods, the promised results remain the same: the divine revelation of past, present, and future actions (*karma*). The interpretation of the *Questions of Subāhu Tantra* as a miscellaneous compilation of distinct but related ritual instructions, organized into chapters that each promise similar attainments, supports Jacob Dalton's proposition that early action tantras are best understood as meta-collections of disparate ritual manuals.[29] The miscellaneous nature of these ritual instructions, paired with a consistent promise of clairvoyant attainments (*sgrub pa* = Skt. *siddhi*), continues throughout the vernacular expression of *prasenā* divination in Tibetan literature.

---

28 *'Phags pa dpung bzang gis zhus pa zhes bya ba'i rgyud*, in *Bka' 'gyur dpe bsdur ma, rgyud 'bum*, text 0835, vol. 96 (*wa*), 468: *phyag 'tshal nas ni lha phyogs gang yin dri// dus gsum dag gi bdag gi dgos pa gang // de ni legs par dgongs la bka' stsol cig//*.

29 Dalton, "How Dhāraṇīs WERE Proto-Tantric," 216 *et passim*.

3 Vernacular Expressions of *Prasenā* in Early Tibetan Instructional Literature

As evinced by their inclusion in the Denkarma/Lhenkarma (*ldan/lhan kar ma*) and Pangtangma (*'phang thang ma*) catalogues, the *Questions of Subāhu Tantra* and its three commentaries had been translated into Tibetan by the beginning of the ninth century at the latest. The former catalogue lists the *Questions of Subāhu* (*dpung bzangs kyis zhus pa*) and "its commentar(ies)" (*de'i 'grel pa*),[30] while the latter lists each of the three aforementioned commentaries separately.[31] The Tibetan translation of these tantric instructions at such an early stage,[32] paired with the multiple Chinese-language translations that took place between the eighth and ninth centuries, indicates that the instructions for *prasenā* divination were disseminated throughout the cosmopolitan networks of East and Central Asia. Finally, vernacular instructions for and descriptions of *prasenā* divination indicate that *prasenā* divination was not only included in the official translations of the Tibetan Buddhist canon, but also in early Tibetan ritual manuals and historical literature.

The emergence of vernacular instructions and descriptions are, of course, not indicative of actual events. However, when there is evidence that a specific author recorded ritual instructions at a specific time and in a specific place, presumably for the sake of performing the prescribed ritual practices, such instances do indicate the *transmission* of these instructions. The tenth-century ritual manual of Bhikṣu Prajñāprabhā (*b-ig kru prad nya pra ba '-i no pyi ka* = Skt. [*sādha*]*naupayika*?; IOL Tib J 401) found in the Library cave at Dunhuang, for example, was a ritual manual written by an otherwise unknown Bhikṣu

30 Adelheid Herrmann-Pfandt, ed., *Die Lhan Kar Ma: Ein früher Katalog der in Tibetische übersetzten buddhistischen Texte* (Wien: Verlag der Österreichischen Akademie der Wissenschaften, 2008), 178–79 (#325–26).

31 Georgios T. Halkias, "Tibetan Buddhism Registered: A Catalogue from the Imperial Court of 'Phang Thang," *The Eastern Buddhist* 36, nos. 1–2 (2004): 97 (#905–908).

32 Matthew T. Kapstein, *The Tibetan Assimilation of Buddhism: Conversion, Contestation, and Memory* (Oxford: Oxford University Press, 2000), 61: "It is furthermore important to recall in this connection that the Tibetan court appears to have been very restrained in its commitment to the esoteric traditions of tantric Buddhism. The circulation of the tantras was restricted by order of the court, and permission to translate and to transmit them strictly controlled." In note 60 (p. 231), Kapstein cites the proscription of Tantric translation purportedly issued by Tri Songdetsen to support this point. See Mie Ishikawa, *A Critical Edition of the Sgra sbyor bam po gnyis pa, An Old and Basic Commentary on the Mahāvyutpatti*, Studia Tibetica 18 (Tokyo: Toyo Bunko, 1990), 4.

Prajñāprabhā.[33] Among many other ritual procedures, the ritual manual of Bhikṣu Prajñāprabhā includes one set of instructions for the "Ritual of the Sky Soarer" (*nam ka lding gi cho ga*), which adapts *prasenā* divination to an evocation of the sky-soaring bird spirit, the Garuḍa (*khyung*). Although references to the "Lord of the Birds" are not found in the other ritual instructions of IOL Tib J 401, the centrality of the Garuḍa in this particular ritual may be enough to associate the ritual manual with the *Gāruḍa Tantras*, further blurring the ritual boundaries between the Buddhist Bhikṣu and the Śaiva Gāruḍika.[34]

A note at the beginning of the "Ritual of the Sky Soarer" assures us, "if one wishes to see *prasenā*, one should engage in this meditative method."[35] The association of *prasenā* with seeing (*mthong*) is significant here, particularly in light of the diverse modes of divine revelation described in the *Questions of Subāhu*. Again, not unlike the *Questions of Subāhu*, Bhikṣu Prajñāprabhā's ritual manual also provides instructions for the performance of *prasenā* both with and without the help of a child assistant. The first ritual cycle begins with the visualization of oneself sitting upon a white lotus in the middle of an ocean, the creation of a mandala, the performance of mudras, and the recitation of mantras. Without specifying to whom, the practitioner is also instructed to provide the five kinds of offerings and make prayers, such that one might arouse divine blessings. Finally, not unlike a consecration ritual,[36] one is also instructed to invite the unnamed spirit into a vase, and then the mirror or other reflective surface, followed by an inspection of the *prasenā* vision.[37] This use of the full word *prasenā* (*pra se na*)—as opposed to the abbreviated

---

33 Jacob Dalton and Sam van Schaik, eds., *Tibetan Tantric Manuscripts from Dunhuang: A Descriptive Catalogue of the Stein Collection at the British Library* (Leiden: Brill, 2006), 136–42. See also Cathy Cantwell and Robert Mayer, *Early Tibetan Documents on Phur pa from Dunhuang* (Wien: Verlag der Österreichischen Akademie der Wissenchaften, 2008), 201–203; and Sam van Schaik, "A Tibetan Book of Spells," *Early Tibet* (19 February 2009), <earlytibet.com/2009/02/19/a-tibetan-book-of-spells/>.

34 On the *Gāruḍa Tantras* and their relationship with medicine, see Michael Slouber, *Early Tantric Medicine: Snakebite, Mantras, and Healing in the Gāruḍa Tantras* (Oxford: Oxford University Press, 2017). For a brief analysis of a Garuḍa ritual in Chinese-language sources, see Rolf W. Giebel, "A Śaiva Text in Chinese Garb? An Annotated Translation of the *Suji liyan Moxishouluo tian shuo aweishe fa*," in *Esoteric Buddhism in Mediaeval Maritime Asia: Networks of Masters, Texts, Icons*, ed. Andrea Acri (Singapore: ISEAS Publishing, 2016), 381–88. Building upon the foundational work of Slouber, a more thorough analysis of the *Gāruḍa Tantras* in early Tibet remains a desideratum.

35 IOL Tib J 401, 12v.7: *pra se na mthong bar 'dod na bsgom ba'i thabs 'di ltar bya 'o.*

36 See Yael Bentor, "On the Symbolism of the Mirror in Indo-Tibetan Consecration Rituals," *Journal of Indian Philosophy* 23 (1995): 57–71; particularly pages 58 and 61–64.

37 IOL Tib J 401, 12v.2–4: *sngar bum pa'i nang du spyan drang / de'i 'og du mye long la bstsogs pa'i nang du spyan drang ba dang / dgug par bya ste/ pra se na blta 'o//.*

[*s*]*pra*—is rather rare in Tibetan-language vernacular instructions, and its reference to a reflected vision is in line with the presentation in the *Questions of Subāhu* explored above.

This first ritual cycle is then followed by an obeisance to the Garuḍa, Lord of Birds (*bya rje* = Skt. *vipati*),[38] beginning a more explicit association of these rituals with the *gārudika*. This second ritual cycle also begins with a visualization of oneself sitting upon a white lotus in the middle of an ocean, with interlinear notes instructing the practitioner to enter the "concentration of the Sky Soarer," and to "fly, soaring in the sky" with the "blessings of the Sky Soarer."[39] Having identified with the Garuḍa, the practitioner is then instructed to recite either a six- or eleven-syllable mantra,[40] apply oil to the thumb of the child assistant, and ask questions.[41] In a subsequent variation, one is instructed to urge the child to look into a mirror and "whatever one's thoughts and questions might be, they shall clearly appear from within the mirror."[42] Finally, in yet another variation, one is instructed to ask, "Where will I be reborn? What about others? What has been done? What will come to be?"[43] Then, "all events of the three times shall appear."[44] Instructions for the use of other glossy ritual instruments follow,[45] along with detailed instructions for the mantric consecration of one's

38 IOL Tib J 401, 12v.6: *bya rje khyung la phyag 'tshal lo/.*

39 IOL Tib J 401, 13r.2–13r.4: *nam ka lding gi ltar byin kyis brlab/* [...] *bdag nyid nam ka lding gi ti nge 'dzin du zhugs* [...] *bdag nyid nam ka lding du 'phur*. This visualization is similar to, but not identical with, the descriptions found in Slouber, *Early Tantric Medicine*, 57–77. An important distinction is the lack of Bhairava in IOL Tib J 401.

40 IOL Tib J 401, 13r.3–5: *yi ge 'bru drug pa'-i sngags la/ khkho khkho rda*[ ]*na hum phaṭ/ 'bru bcu gcig pa'i sngags la/* [...]*ōṃ dha ba khrom na ma khkho khkho rdan khuṃ phaṭ/.*

41 IOL Tib J 401, 13r.5–7: *lag pa'i mthe bo la bskus nas/ yi ge 'bru bcu gcig gi sngags kyis btab c-ing / byis pa la byug/ ci yin ba'i gtam dri 'o//.*

42 IOL Tib J 401, 13v.2–3: *yid la bsam shing dri ba'i rnams kyang / mye long gi nang nas gsal rab du snang ngo /.*

43 IOL Tib J 401, 13v.9 and 14r.2: *bdag dang gzhan cir skye ci byas ci byed pa* (interlinear note).

44 IOL Tib J 401, 13v.8 and 14r.1: *der ni dus gsuṃ du bya ba thams cad snang ngo /.*

45 Instructions are provided for the use of a quality sword (*ral g*[*r*]*i bzang po*)—in which "what one needs [to do]" will appear (*dgos pa bzhin du snang ngo*)—as well as other instruments, including a moist trumpet (*dung chen po gsher bag*), a lacquered skull (*thod pa'i phral bar bskus*), and about three cubits of quality white wood (*shing dkar po bzang po khru gsum tsam*). These, along with the mirror, are "the five rituals for seeing." IOL Tib J 401, 14v.2–3: *de ltar blta ba'i cho ga rnaṃ pa lnga ste/.*

hand.[46] This section of Bhikṣu Prajñāprabhā's manual ends with a single line: "such is the inspection of *prasenā*."[47]

Like a dim reflection in the mirror of *prasenā* divination, Bhikṣu Prajñāprabhā's ritual manual provides some insight into the ritual climate of tenth-century Dunhuang. Regardless of whether Bhikṣu Prajñāprabhā is best understood as a monk, tantric priest, or *gāruḍika*, his ritual manual demonstrates that the instructions for *prasenā* divination were not only translated in the canonical tantras of eighth- or early ninth-century Tibet, but also reformulated in the vernacular manuals of tenth-century Tibetan ritualists. Looking beyond the imbrication of both Śaiva and Buddhist tantric instructions in this early period, a phenomenon that has been widely observed in secondary literature,[48] in Bhikṣu Prajñāprabhā's ritual manual we also find the imbrication of *prasenā* divination with healing rituals. Indeed, despite the fact that *prasenā* lacks an explicitly diagnostic role in the "Ritual of the Sky Soarer," the other rituals found in the manual include methods for healing illnesses and exorcising pathogenic demons.[49] With such a repertoire of rituals, one might imagine Bhikṣu Prajñāprabhā using *prasenā* divination to identify the demon that is possessing an ill patient, calling out the demon, and binding it with an oath. Indeed, such is the method that Padmasambhava used when he exorcized the demons of Tibet.

4 Descriptions of *Prasenā* in Early Tibetan Historical Literature

If *prasenā* divination is only implicitly related to ritual modes of healing in Bhikṣu Prajñāprabhā's tenth-century manual, by the eleventh and

---

46 Mantric syllables are to be visualized on the limbs (*yan lag*), middle finger (*gung mo*), thumb (*mthe bo*), index finger (*'dzub mo*), ring finger (*srin sag*), little finger (*mthe 'u cung*), and two palms (*lag mthil gnyis*). IOL Tib J 401, 14v.4–8: *'di rnams kyi sngags ni/ yi ge 'bru bcu gcig pa ste 'di dag go/ kshaṃ/ yan lag du yi ge bsngo ba ni 'og ma 'di dag go / swi* [?] */ swōṃ swem sw-īṃ swuṃ swaṃ swa swoṃ ni gung mo la/ swaṃ ni mthe bo la/ swiṃ ni 'dzub mo la/ swuṃ ni srin lag la/ swaṃ ni mthe 'u cung la/ swa ni lag mthil gnyis su bsam/ yang swoṃ ni snying kar/ sweṃ ni rkang pa la/ swiṃ mdze la/ swuṃ ni lte bar/ swaṃ ni khar/ swa ni skye bor bsam/ swa swa ni dus su/ brkya sca brgyad du bzlas par bya 'o/*. Although the syllables differ, this process of hand consecration is nearly identical to that which is described in Slouber, *Early Tantric Medicine*, 65–67.

47 IOL Tib J 401, 14v.8: *di yan cad ni pra sen na blta ba 'o/*.

48 For a particularly provocative account, see Alexis Sanderson, "Vajrayāna: Origin and Function," in *Buddhism: Critical Concepts in Religious Studies*, ed. Paul Williams (New York, NY: Routledge 2005), vol. 6, 392–408.

49 For a list and general description, see van Schaik, "A Tibetan Book of Spells."

twelfth centuries these associations become more explicit. In the pre-twelfth-century *Testament of Wa* (*dba'*[*/sba/rba*] *bzhed*),[50] for example, Emperor Tri Songdetsen called upon the tantric master Padmasambhava to subdue the gods and demons responsible for the flooding at the palace in Pangtang, the fire at the castle in Lhasa, and the epidemics among the people and livestock. Petty ministers had interpreted these calamities as the demonic consequences of the introduction of Buddhism to Tibet, and the monk Śāntarakṣita was sent away to Nepal in order to prevent further damage. Before his departure, however, Śāntarakṣita promised to return with a master of mantra, Padmasambhava, explaining that he would use the *prasenā* divination of the Four Great Kings to identify and subdue the wicked deities and demons responsible for such calamities:

> After the *pra*[*senā*] of the Four Great Kings descends, this master of mantras [Padmasambhava] will ask, "Who are the dark deities and wicked serpent spirits that caused the [calamities] that occurred last year—such as the great flood in Pangtang, the great fire in the royal castle of Lhasa, and so forth—prohibiting the emperor from propagating the doctrine?" He will examine the *prasenā*, call the wicked deities and common serpent spirits to come to his presence, and bind them with an oath. [Padmasambhava] is the kind of mantric master that is capable of commanding and disciplining [these demons], causing the land to become peaceful, and allowing for the future practice of the holy [Buddhist] doctrine.[51]

Although Padmasambhava's subjugation of the demons of Tibet is a tale that has been told repeatedly throughout the Tibetan historical tradition, the central role of *prasenā* divination in his identification of these demons was generally

50 On the complex question of dating the *Testament of Wa*, see Per Sørensen, "Preface," in *Dba' bzhed: The Royal Narrative Concerning the Bringing of the Buddha's Doctrine to Tibet*, trans. Pasang Wangdu and Hildegard Diemberger (Wien: Österreichischen Akademie der Wissenschaften, 2000), *ix–xv*.

51 *Rba bzhed phyogs bsgrigs* (Beijing: Mi rigs dpe skrun khang, 2009), 253: *sngags mkhan 'dis ni na ning 'phang thang du chu bo che byung ba dang lha sa'i sku mkhar mes tshig pa la sogs te/ lha klu gnag cing mi srun pa rnams kyis btsan po'i zha snga nas chos mdzad du mi ster ba gang lags pa rgyal po chen po bzhi'i pra phab ste dri ba dang / pra se na lta ba dang / lha klu mi srun pa phal ba gnad* [*=gnas*] *la dbab cing dam 'og tu stsal cing mna' bsgag pa dang / bsgo zing nan tur bgyis na yul zhi ste slan chad lha chos mdzad par sngags mkhan 'dis rngo thog na de ltar mdzad pa'i rigs/*. Translated in consultation with Wangdu and Diemberger, *Dba' bzhed*, 17 (summary), 54 (translation), and f. 11b (Tibetan); but with some important differences in interpretation.

elided from later renditions.[52] Instead of the omniscient Second Buddha of later tradition,[53] here Padmasambhava is a tantric master that relies upon the divine eye of the Four Great Kings in order to identify the demons that had tormented the palace, livestock, and people of Tibet. By learning their identities through *prasenā* divination, Padmasambhava was able to call the demons to his presence and bind them with an oath, thereby resolving any obstacles to the promotion of Buddhism in Tibet.

Unlike later accounts, the identification and naming of demonic forces remains central in the eleventh-century (?) *Testament of Wa*. According to the tale, Padmasambhava did indeed perform the *prasenā* divination of the Four Great Kings, thereby "grasping the given names and clan names of the wicked ones that had caused the previous great flood in Pangtang, the great fire in the royal castle of Lhasa, the famine, and the plagues among the people and cattle. He then summoned them to appear in reality."[54] Thus, it is this process of naming the demons responsible for the calamities that allowed him to identify, conjure, and subdue them. This triad of identifying, conjuring, and subduing is not unlike the stages of medical diagnosis, wherein a physician identifies, names, and treats the opaque illness of a patient.[55] Indeed, in the case of Padmasambhava's exorcism, the object of identification is not the illness of a single patient, but plagues that were affecting the people and livestock of Tibet. Regardless of whether this illustrious exorcism *really* happened or not, it is *prasenā* divination that was depicted as the means for identifying the demons of Tibet in the *Testament of Wa*, allowing Padmasambhava to heal and open the spiritual landscape of Tibet for the propagation of Buddhism.

---

52 See, for example, Per Sørensen, *Tibetan Buddhist Historiography: The Mirror Illuminating the Royal Genealogies, an Annotated Translation of the XIVth Century Tibetan Chronicle: rGyal-rabs gsal-ba'i me-long* (Wiesbaden: Harrassowitz Verlag, 1994), 368.

53 For a similar observation regarding the presentation of Padmasambhava in the *Testament of Wa* and his subsequent apotheosis, see Kapstein, *The Tibetan Assimilation of Buddhism*, 155–60.

54 *Rba bzhed phyogs bsgrigs*, 254: *rgyal po chen po bzhi pra'i phab ste smrar stsal/ gzhe ni 'phang thang du cho bo che 'bebs pa dang / ra sa'i* [*sku*] *mkhar mes tshig par byed pa dang / mi nad phyugs nad dang mu ge gtong ba'i rgyu bgyid pa'i lha klu gang lags rmas nas/ mi srun pa kun gyi ming rus bzung nas dngos su bkug ste/*. Translated in consultation with Wangdu and Diemberger, *Dba' bzhed*, 55.

55 For a relevant differentiation of illness and disease, see Arthur Kleinman, *The Illness Narratives: Suffering, Healing and the Human Condition* (New York, NY: Basic Books, 1988), 3–5: "Illness refers to how the sick person and the members of the family or wider social network perceive, live with, and respond to symptoms and disability.... Disease is the problem from the practitioner's perspective."

5 Channel *Prasenā* Rituals in the Early Yutok School

By the eleventh or twelfth century, *prasenā* divination had come to be explicitly associated with channel examination. In line with the miscellaneous nature of the *prasenā* divination rituals examined above, these early instructions for channel *prasenā* divination rituals (*rtsa'i pra*) call for the involvement of an effigy instead of a child medium, the examination of a messenger instead of a ritual implement, and the visual, auditory, and mental revelation of diagnosis instead of an all-encompassing clairvoyance. Although a similar diversity of prescribed ritual methods is common to all of the early *prasenā* instructions examined above, the central involvement of an effigy, a messenger, and the narrow range of promised results—reducing knowledge of any and all events of the past, present, and future to the identification of pathogenic demons and the prediction of the patient's time of death—are specific to the instructions for channel *prasenā* rituals. Thus, the specific medical contexts of channel *prasenā* rituals represent a move toward specification within the larger genealogy of *prasenā* rituals in Tibet, a reactionary development that may have been spurred by the introduction of channel examination during this early period.

As far as I am aware, there are five unique sets of instructions for channel *prasenā* rituals, each of which evokes either goddesses of medicine (*sman gyi lha mo*) or sages (*drang srong*) of South Asian inspiration. The earliest extant instructions for channel *prasenā* divination are dedicated to the former, and can be found in the *Three Indispensable Rituals* (*med thabs med pa'i 'phyong gsum*) subcollection of the *Eighteen Auxiliary Branches* (*cha lag bco brgyad*).[56] As described in the opening section of one recently published manuscript witness:

> The teachings of the *Three Indispensable Rituals* are the precious oral instructions transmitted from the King of Tantras, the *Essence of Ambrosia*. Because it demonstrates reasons for faith, the *Account of Transmission* is indispensable. For examining the seven wonder channels, the *Channel Prasenā Rituals* is indispensable. For healing children, the *Instructions for Pediatrics* is indispensable.[57]

---

56 Again, see *Rtsa'i pra sgrub med thabs med pa*, in *Cha lag bco brgyad*, 492–94.

57 *Med thabs med pa'i mchong* [='*phyong*] *gsum*, in *Krung go'i bod lugs gso rig rtsa che'i dpe rnying kun btus*, vol. 3, text 3, p. 257 (f. 1b): *rgyud rgyal bdud rtsi snying po las// snyan* [*b*] *rgyud man ngag gces pa'i mchong* [='*phyong*] *// med thabs med pa rnams gsum bstan// yid ches pa'i khungs bstan phyir// rgyud pa'i rnam thar med thabs med// ngo mtshar rtsa bdun brtag pa la// rtsa'i pra sgrub med thabs med// byis pa nyer spyod gso ba la// sri'u gso ba med thabs med//*.

This opening, absent from other editions,[58] presents the instructions for channel *prasenā* rituals, along with the famed *Indispensable Account of Transmission*, as the "oral instructions" deriving from the "King of Tantras, the *Essence of Ambrosia*." The *Essence of Ambrosia* (*bdud rtsi snying po*) is, of course, part of the full title of the *Four Tantras* (*rgyud bzhi*), the *Secret Essence of Ambrosia in Eight Branches: An Instructional Tantra*, as well as the so-called *Little Tantra* (*rgyud chung*), the *Secret Essence of Ambrosia: An Instructional Tantra*.[59] Although it is difficult to determine the precise identity of the *Essence of Ambrosia* from this allusion alone, both the *Four Tantras* and the *Little Tantra* were important texts for the early Yutok school (*g.yu thog lugs*) of the Tibetan medical tradition, indicating an institutional context in which these early channel *prasenā* rituals were transmitted.

Further information for the early transmission of channel *prasenā* rituals can be found in the colophons for these instructions. The earliest layers of these colophons can be found in the aforementioned *Three Indispensable Rituals* collection:

> The *Channel Divination of the Three Goddess Sisters of Medicine*:
> [Colophon:] Master Vairocana translated this work in the land of China. It was the personal commitment of Drapa Ngönshé.[60]
>
> The *Channel Evocation of the Black-lipped Brahminess*:
> [Colophon:] This *Channel Evocation of the Brahmin* was translated by Master Vairocana in the land of China. It was the personal commitment of Drapa Ngönshé. This *Lamp Illuminating the Seven Wonder Channels*, taught in the tantras, was appended to the [*Four*?] *Tantras* by Vairocana.[61]

58 On the seventeenth-century publication of the *Eighteen Auxiliary Branches* (*cha lag bco brgyad*; therein called the *Eighteen Pieces from Yutok*), see Gyatso, *Being Human in a Buddhist World*, 119. This opening is also absent from another manuscript of the *Three Indispensable Rituals* subcollection published in the *Krung go'i bod lugs gso rig rtsa che'i dpe rnying kun btus* collection. See *Rtsa'i spra sgrub med thabs med pa* (vol. 10, text 5).

59 Compare *Bdud rtsi snying po yan lag brgyad pa gsang ba man ngag gi rgyud* with *Bdud rtsi snying po gsang ba man ngag gi rgyud*, respectively. As demonstrated by Yang Ga, these works display an intimate degree of intertextuality. See Yang Ga, *Sources for the Writing of the Rgyud bzhi* (Cambridge, MA: Harvard University Doctoral Dissertation, 2010).

60 *Med thabs med pa'i mchong* [='*phyong*] *gsum*, in *Krung go'i bod lugs gso rig rtsa che'i dpe rnying kun btus*, vol. 3, text 3, p. 259 (f. 5a): *slob dpon be ro tsa nas rgya nag yul nas sgyur/ gra pa mngon shes kyis thugs dam lags so//.*

61 *Med thabs med pa'i mchong* [='*phyong*] *gsum*, in *Krung go'i bod lugs gso rig rtsa che'i dpe rnying kun btus*, vol. 3, text 3, p. 260 (f. 5b): *bram ze'i rtsa sgrub 'di// slob dpon bai ro tsa na*

As these early colophons for the *Three Goddess Sisters* and the *Black-lipped Brahminess* channel *prasenā* rituals indicate (again, redacted within the *Three Indispensable Rituals* collection; see Fig. 8.1), both are said to derive from the "land of China" (*rgya nag yul*), translated into Tibetan by Master Vairocana (*slob dpon be ro tsa na*), and transmitted by Drapa Ngönshé (*gra pa mngon shes*, 1012–1090; literally the "Clairvoyant One from Dra[nang]"). This short account in the colophons translated above is one of the earliest references to Drapa Ngönshé in a medical work and, considering the inclusion of the *Indispensable Account of Transmission* in the *Three Indispensable Rituals*, may help to explain his purported role in the transmission of the *Four Tantras*.[62] The paired transmission of these two channel *prasenā* rituals—particularly in combination with the otherwise unattested title, the *Lamp Illuminating the Seven Wonder Channels*—also implies that these channel *prasenā* rituals were transmitted independently prior to their inclusion in the *Three Indispensable Rituals* and *Eighteen Auxiliary Branches*, potentially even predating the *Four Tantras* itself.

Unlike the instructions for *prasenā* divination described in the *Questions of Subāhu* or the ritual manual of Bhikṣu Prajñāprabhā examined above, the instructions for channel *prasenā* rituals found in the *Three Goddess Sisters* and the *Black-lipped Brahminess* each call for the creation of a child effigy out of birchwood (*stag pa la byas pa'i bu chung*) instead of the involvement of a real

---

yis// rgya nag yul nas bsgyur ba yin// gra pa mngon shes thugs dam mo// rgyud nang [g?] sung pa'i ngo mtshar gyi rtsa bdun [~~ston par 'byung~~] gsal bar byed pa'i sgron ma 'dis/ be ro tsa nas rgyud kyi btsas su bzhag pa'o/ rdzogs s.ho//.

62 The *Indispensable Account of Transmission* (*brgyud pa'i rnam thar med thabs med pa*, ca. 1174?)—attributed to Sumtön Yeshé Zung (*sum ston ye shes gzungs*, fl. late 12th c.?), a student of Yutok Gönpo—is probably the earliest history of the transmission of the *Four Tantras*. On this work, see Gyatso, *Being Human in a Buddhist World*, 132 *et passim* (therein called the *Crucial Lineage Biography*); and my translation, "Origin Narratives of the Tibetan Medical Tradition: History, Legend, and Myth," *Asian Medicine* 12, nos. 1–2 (2017): 295–316. It is also the first work to name Drapa Ngönshé as a treasure revealer involved in the transmission of the *Four Tantras*. *Med thabs med pa'i mchong [='phy-ong] gsum*, in *Krung go'i bod lugs gso rig rtsa che'i dpe rnying kun btus*, vol. 3, text 3, pp. 257–58 (ff. 2a–2b): "The Sovereign Tri Songdetsen concealed [the *Four Tantras*] in a pillar in the center of the upper chapel of the Three Families at Samyé monastery. After three days in the heavens of the desire realm [300 years on earth], Drapa Ngönshé revealed them, and became the master of the world" (*mnga' bdag khri [b]srong lde btsan des/ bsam yas dbu rtse rigs gsum gyi/ bar khang ka ba'i nang du sbas/ de nas 'dod lha'i zhag gsum nas/ grwa ba mngon shes can gyis bton/ 'dzam bu gling gi bdag por gyur/*). For one expression of the confusion regarding Drapa Ngönshe's involvement in the Tibetan medical tradition, see Ronald M. Davidson, *Tibetan Renaissance: Tantric Buddhism in the Rebirth of Tibetan Culture* (New York, NY: Columbia University Press, 2005), 105.

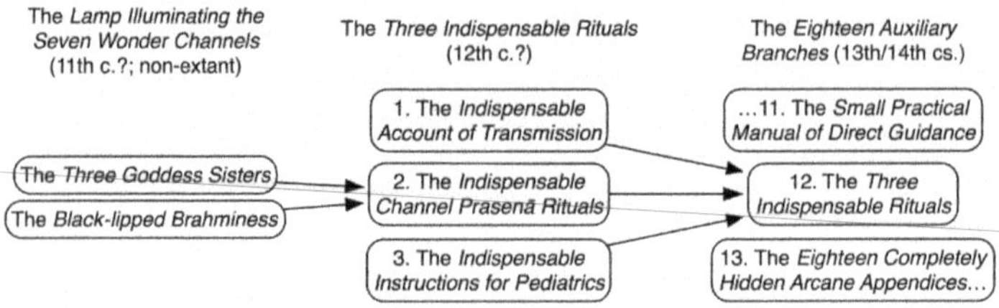

FIGURE 8.1 The redaction and transmission of channel *prasenā* rituals in the Yutok school

child medium. Although the instructions for *prasenā* examined above do not generally mention the creation of a statue, the use of a birchwood effigy in this ritual instead of an actual child or reflective ritual implement is not unprecedented. The Chinese-language Śubhakarasiṃha translation of the *Questions of Subāhu*, for example, suggests a statue as an appropriate vessel for the descent of the Prasenā deity (Bosina 鉢私那), while the Dharmadeva Chinese-language and Tibetan-language editions do not.[63] Thus, this emphasis on a birchwood effigy may indeed be interpreted as a relic of an early Chinese or Central Asian (that is, Chinese-language) *prasenā* tradition rooted in the Śubhakarasiṃha edition of the *Questions of Subāhu*, as opposed to the Tibetan-language translation that was made during the Tibetan empire.

Following these ritual preparations, one is instructed to visualize three white goddesses of medicine, each of which are holding a golden myrobalan fruit. After thousands of mantra recitations—interspersed with supplications like "descend!" (*phob*); "tell all that exists!" (*srid pa shod*); and "reveal all that exists!" (*srid pa ston*)—one should make the following requests: "Tell me what to do! Tell me the causes and conditions of disease! Tell me in a clear voice! As soon as I grasp the channels of the wrist of the messenger, reveal to me all of the classifications of the diseases of sentient beings."[64] After reciting further mantras, one will come to know whatever any worldly being (*'jig rten pa*) is thinking. After more recitations, "Regardless of whether one examines the

63 Compare the *Sipohu tongzi qingwen jing* 蘇婆呼童子請問經 (T18n0895) translated by Śubhakarasiṃha and the *Miaobi pusa suowen jing* 妙臂菩薩所問經 (T18n0896) translated by Dharmadeva. For a translation and discussion of these instructions, see Strickmann, *Chinese Magical Medicine*, 210–14.

64 *Med thabs med pa'i mchong* [='phyong] *gsum*, in *Krung go'i bod lugs gso rig rtsa che'i dpe rnying kun btus*, vol. 3, text 3, pp. 259 (f. 4b): *nga yi ci bya zer ba dang / nad kyi rgyu dang rkyen 'di yin zer ba dang // sgra lhang lhang po'ang // de byang pa dang / sems can rnams kyis nad kyis rigs su gyur pa thams cad bdag gi bang chen pa'i lag pa'i rtsa la bzungs pa tsam gyis shes par ston gcig ces brjod de/.*

channels or performs *mo* divination, one will come to recall with one's mind and hear with one's ears."[65] All of the above instructions are for preparatory rituals that are to be performed before meeting the patient or, as mentioned above, a messenger (*bang chen*) of the patient. "When examining the channels" of the messenger, we are told,

> one should shave off a little myrobalan fruit and roast it on a smokeless fire. Reciting the twenty-one mantras, one should mentally request, "Reveal the one hundred wonder channels—that of the messenger, that of the parent and the child, that of the husband and wife, and so forth—as well as the etiology, the prognosis, indications, and contraindications!" And so they all shall be revealed.[66]

Unlike channel examination, wherein the channels of the sick patient are to be empirically observed by a physician, these ritual instructions explicitly name the object of examination as not the patient, but the patient's "messenger." Indeed, the attainments of the *Three Goddess Sisters* ritual are described as being the revelation of the "hundred wonder channels"—which are described as being that of the "messenger," that of the "parent and the child," that of the "husband and wife," and so forth—as well as the "etiology" (*nad bzhi* [=*gzhi*], lit. "the basis of the disease"), the "prognosis" (*sos mi sos*, lit. "whether they can be healed or not"), "indications" (*ci phan*, lit. "what will benefit them"), and contraindications (*ci snod* [=*gnod*], lit. "what will harm them"). Thus, the proper performance of the *Three Goddess Sisters* promises the so-called "one hundred wonder channels" (*ngo mtshar gyi rtsa brgya*)—which may be a scribal error for the "eight wonder channels" (*ngo mtshar gyi rtsa brgyad*)[67]—representing the oracular revelation of all desired medical knowledge. We shall return to the wonder channels again below, but for now it should suffice to say that the wonder channels represent a diagnostic technique in which the messenger of

---

65 *Med thabs med pa'i mchong* [=*'phyong*] *gsum*, in *Krung go'i bod lugs gso rig rtsa che'i dpe rnying kun btus*, vol. 3, text 3, pp. 259 (f. 4b): *rtsa lta ba dang // mo 'debs pa gang byed kyang // snying gis dran pa dang // rna bas thos te 'ong ngo //.*

66 *Med thabs med pa'i mchong* [=*'phyong*] *gsum*, in *Krung go'i bod lugs gso rig rtsa che'i dpe rnying kun btus*, vol. 3, text 3, pp. 259 (f. 4b): *rtsa lta ba'i dus su/ a ru ra la bag tsam re bzhar la mes du ba med pa la bsreg/ sngags nyi shu rtsa gcig bzlas la// bang chen pa dang // pha ma bu tsha dang // khyo dang chung ma la sogs pa/ ngo mtshar gyi rtsa brgya dang / nad bzhi* [=*gzhi*] *gang yin pa dang / sos mi sos dang / ci phan ci snod* [=*gnod*] *thams cad ston gcig/ ces yid la bya'o//.*

67 For another instance where the numbers "one hundred" (*brgya*) and "eight" (*brgyad*) have been confused, see Jacob Dalton, *The Gathering of Intentions: A History of a Tibetan Tantra* (New York, NY: Columbia University Press, 2016), 158–59, n. 34.

a patient—be it their relative or their spouse—can be examined in lieu of the actual sick person. The divinatory examination of a messenger (*dūta*) instead of the diagnostic examination of a patient has parallels in the Gāruḍika traditions of South Asia,[68] and in the context of the lofty mountains and vast plains of Central Tibet, such ritual technology must have proved convenient.

Like the *Three Goddess Sisters* ritual, the *Brahminess* ritual involves neither a reflective implement nor a child medium, but does involve an effigy. Unlike the *Three Goddess Sisters* ritual, however, the *Brahminess* ritual does not call for the effigy of a child, but "a foot-tall figure of the Brahminess with vibrant black-blue lips," composed of meat and clay.[69] One is then instructed to make offerings and prepare ritual substances, reciting mantras and exhort the Brahminess to "take these water-blister eyes and reveal sights of the divine realm!"[70] After five days of recitation, signs (*rtags*) should appear, and after seven days, the goddess will come to manifest in reality (*dngos su 'ong*).[71] "When examining the channels," again we are told,

> one should recite the mantra seven times and then perform the examination with the six fingers [on the messenger]. Thus [the diagnosis] shall be revealed in one's ears, and shall suddenly and clearly come to mind. Thus the disease, the demon, and the seven wonder channels shall come to be revealed.[72]

Like the *Three Goddess Sisters* described above, the instructions for the *Black-lipped Brahminess* ritual involve an ornate ritual setting, the creation of an effigy, and divine revelation by means of the wonder channels. Unlike the

68 See Slouber, *Early Tantric Medicine*, 126, 148–49.

69 *Med thabs med pa'i mchong* [='phyong] *gsum*, in *Krung go'i bod lugs gso rig rtsa che'i dpe rnying kun btus*, vol. 3, text 3, p. 259 (f. 5a): *gsang pa yid kyi rtsa sgrub/ gsang rten du rta bra nag gi rnga ma g.yas skor byas la rna lag g.yas su rtags/ sgrub rdzas la chen po bzhi'i sha//* [*bse dri can bzhi'i sha/*] *khams pas mgo bsdus la/ bram ze mo'i gzugs chags* [*gang*] *pa// mchu sngo yal ba le ba gcig byas la//.*

70 *Med thabs med pa'i mchong* [='phyong] *gsum*, in *Krung go'i bod lugs gso rig rtsa che'i dpe rnying kun btus*, vol. 3, text 3, p. 259 (f. 5a): *chu bur dmig gi go sol/ mthong pa lha'i yul ston//.*

71 Interestingly, later editions add the caveat that "For middling practitioners, she will come in a dream. For inferior practitioners, she will come to appear in the mind" (*'bring rmi lam du 'ong / tha ma yid snang du 'ong ngo //*). See *Brang ti lha rje'i rim brgyud kyi man ngag gser bre chen mo*, 13.

72 *Med thabs med pa'i mchong* [='phyong] *gsum*, in *Krung go'i bod lugs gso rig rtsa che'i dpe rnying kun btus*, vol. 3, text 3, pp. 259–60 (ff. 5a–5b): *rtsa lta ba'i dus su/ so mo drug po la sngags bdun btab nas ltas pas/ rna bar ston pa dang / yid la wal gyis gsal btang ngo // nad dang gdon dang ngo mtshar gyi rtsa bdun ston par 'gyur ro//.*

Three Goddess Sisters, however, the attainment described in the *Black-lipped Brahminess* is neither the eight nor the one hundred wonder channels, but the seven wonder channels (*ngo mtshar gyi rtsa bdun*). These seven wonder channels are revealed in connection with the disease and the demon causing the disease, such that the practitioner might exorcise the ultimate source of his patient's suffering. Thus, the instructions for both the *Three Goddess Sisters* and the *Black-lipped Brahminess* include many similar elements—such as the centrality of the effigy, the evocation of a goddess (or three), the examination of a messenger, and the divine revelation of the seven, eight, or one hundred wonder channels—which indicates that they were part of the same teaching cycle even before being redacted together in the *Three Indispensable Rituals*.

Taking all of the aforementioned variations of practical instructions into account, *prasenā* divination in Tibet emerges as a means for explicit inquiry and divine revelation. From their cosmopolitan beginnings in the *Questions of Subāhu Tantra* to their early vernacular expression in the ritual manual of Bhikṣu Prajñāprabhā, the instructions for *prasenā* divination have long encompassed a family of diverse but related divinatory techniques, each promising the divine revelation of the past, present, and future. By the time the general instructions for *prasenā* divination were adapted to the specific contexts of medical practice in the channel *prasenā* rituals, the methods for divination and their promised results also took on a quasi-clinical character: the general methods for all-encompassing clairvoyance transformed into the specific examination of a messenger for particular predications about an ill patient. After three centuries of transmission in Tibet with relatively minor adaptations, in the eleventh century *prasenā* divination appears to have transformed from a nebulous set of oracular practices into a specific repertoire for clinical divination. Examining the genealogy of the wonder channels in the Tibetan medical tradition reveals that, by the eleventh century, *prasenā* divination had come into competition with a new set of diagnostic practices that were based not on divine revelation, but on empirical observation of the patient, resulting in a dialogue of these two prominent practices.

6 Channel Examination, *Prasenā* Divination, and the Seven Wonder Channels

Not unlike the instructions for *prasenā* divination, the introduction and transmission of cosmopolitan instructions for channel examination led to significant developments and vernacular transformations in Tibet over the centuries. Despite the centrality of channel examination in the recent history of the

Tibetan medical tradition, there are no extant Tibetan-language instructions for channel examination prior to the eleventh or twelfth century.[73] While it is entirely possible that Tibetan physicians were practicing channel examination in the ninth and tenth centuries, they would have probably learned and transmitted such methods using Chinese.[74] "Literary silence is real, and it can be broken," Sheldon Pollock asserts, "and when it is broken, something truly consequential in history is taking place."[75] With the adaptation of channel examination to the Tibetan language in the eleventh, twelfth, and thirteenth centuries, the proponents of empirical observation came into dialogue with the ritual practitioners of *prasenā* divination, resulting in a method for remote divination performed in conjunction with empirical observation.

Channel examination (*rtsa la brtag pa* = Chi. *mai zhen* 脈診)—also known as pulse diagnosis or sphygmology—involves the haptic observation of the pulsations of a patient, usually felt by the physician at three points along each wrist of a patient in the Tibetan tradition.[76] According to the *Four Tantras*, a physician should observe the qualities of a patient's pulsations—such as quantitative characteristics like frequency and intensity, but also qualitative characteristics like fullness, rigidity, and texture—to determine the nature of a

73 On the lack of Tibetan-language instructions for channel examination found at Dunhuang, see Zhen Yan, "*rTsa* in the Tibetan Manuscripts from Dunhuang," trans. Vivienne Lo, *Asian Medicine* 3 (2007): 296–307; and Zhen Yan and Cai Jingfeng, "Tibetan and Chinese Pulse Diagnostics: A Comparison—With Special Reference to Locations for Pulse Taking," in *Soundings in Tibetan Medicine: Anthropological and Historical Perspectives. Proceedings of the 10th Seminar of the International Association of Tibetan Studies*, ed. Mona Schrempf (Leiden: Brill, 2007), 327–43.

74 For more on Chinese-language channel examination at Dunhuang (including some problematic speculations regarding its relation to the Tibetan tradition), see Elisabeth Hsu, "A Hybrid Body Technique: Does the Pulse Diagnostic *cun guan chi* Method Have Chinese-Tibetan Origins?" *Gesnerus* 65, nos. 1–2 (2008): 5–29; and, more recently, "Le diagnostic du pouls dans la chine mediévale d'apres les manuscrits de Dunhuang (with notes on P2115, P3106, P3287, P3477, P3481, P3655, P4093, S79, S181, S202, S5614, S6245, S8289, plus index)," in *Médecine, religion et société dans la Chine médiévale: Étude de manuscrits chinois de Dunhuang et de Turfan*, ed. C. Despeux (Paris: College de France, Institut des Haute Etudes Chinoises, 2010), book 1, pp. 107–84.

75 Sheldon Pollock, *The Language of the Gods in the World of Men: Sanskrit, Culture, and Power in Premodern India* (Berkeley, CA: University of California Press, 2006), 296–97.

76 Here I use the term "channel" to translate the Tibetan term *rtsa*, which denotes both the obvious vessels and sinews, as well as the non-obvious tracts of wind and breath that traverse the human body. I also use the verbal noun, "pulsation," instead of the more familiar "pulse" due to the connotations of diastolic and systolic phases inherent in the latter term, which are inappropriate for the present context. For a parallel distinction in the terms of the Chinese and Greek traditions, see Kuriyama, *The Expressiveness of the Body and the Divergence of Greek and Chinese Medicine*.

humoral imbalance, thermal disease, visceral disease, demonic possession, or even the patient's time of death.[77] In the chapter of the *Root Tantra* dedicated to the diagnosis of disease (*ngos 'dzin rtags*), the sage Rikpé Yeshé (*rig pa' ye shes*, lit. Gnostic Awareness) provides the sage Yilé Kyé (*yid las skyes*, lit. Mind Born) with a brief introduction to channel examination. Therein he introduces basic symptoms that can be observed either visually or haptically, as well as those that indicate humoral imbalances in the tongue, urine, and channels. Regarding the channels, he states:

> Channels that are floating, empty, and halt sporadically [indicate] wind. Channels that are rapid, bulky, and beat tautly [indicate] bile. Channels that are submerged, waning, and ponderous [indicate] phlegm.[78]

In these summarized instructions for channel examination, disease is primarily expressed in terms of the three humors—unambiguously defined as wind, bile, and phlegm—without any mention of their relationship with the five inner viscera, the six outer viscera, or thermal imbalances. Thus, with the systematization of channel examination in the *Four Tantras*, the specific characteristics of the pulsations come to be primarily interpreted in terms of the three humors of South and/or Central Asian inspiration.

Unlike this synthetic account found in the opening chapters of the *Four Tantras*, however, when instructions for channel examination were first recorded in the Tibetan language, the primary organizing principle for channel examination was not the humors, but the viscera. The *Medicine of the Moon King* (*sman dpyad zla ba'i rgyal po*, redacted in ca. 11th c.), for example, includes the most extensive and probably the earliest instructions for channel examination.[79] The chapters are generally organized according to the five inner

---

77 For a summary of channel examination according to the tradition of the *Four Tantras*, see Yuri Parfionovitch, Feranand Meyer, and Gyurme Dorje, eds., *Tibetan Medical Paintings: Illustrations to the Blue Beryl Treatise of Sangye Gyamtso (1653–1705)* (New York, NY: Harry N. Abrams, 1992), vol. 1, pp. 123–40 (plates 54–62).

78 Rje bstan 'dzin don grub, ed., *Dpal ldan rgyud bzhi dpe bsdur ma* (Chengdu: Si khron dpe skrun khang, 2010), vol. 1, 39–40: *rlung gi rtsa ni rkyal stong skabs su sdod// mkhris pa'i rtsa ni mgyogs rgyas grims par 'phar// bad kan rtsa ni bying rgud dal ba 'o//*. For an alternative translation and analysis of these same lines, see R. E. Emmerick, "Some Remarks on Tibetan Sphygmology," in *Medical Literature Form India, Sri Lanka and Tibet*, ed. G. Jan Meulenbeld (Leiden: Brill, 1991), 66–71.

79 See Sgrol dkar skyabs, "Zla rgyal dang rgyud bzhi'i rtsa brtag thad la cung tsam bsdur te dpyad pa" [Comparative Studies on Pulsology in the Texts: King of Moon and rGyu-Zhi (sic)], *Krung go'i bod kyi gso rig* [Tibetan Medicine in China] 7, no. 3 (2008): 103–110; and Yang Ga, *Sources for the Writing of the Rgyud bzhi*, 243: "It seems to me that these sections

viscera (*don lnga* = Chi. *wuzang* 五臟), with one chapter dedicated to the examination of the channels of each of the five inner viscera: the heart, liver, kidneys, lungs, and spleen.[80] The instructions for the examination of the channels also derives from this system of the five inner viscera, for each of the three sites along the wrist of the patient—that is, the *tsön*-inch (*tshon* < Chi. *cun* 寸), the *gan*-gate (*kan* < Chi. *guan* 關), and the *chak*-foot (*chag* < Chi. *chi* 尺) openings—corresponds to the viscera of either the upper, middle, or lower section of the body:

> The physician should examine the characteristics of heat and cold in the surfaces and depths of the six openings. If, at the patient's two *tsön*-inch openings, the physician's middle fingers detect repletion, depletion, emptiness, strength, weakness, and so forth, this corresponds to the area between the diaphragm and the head of the patient. If, at the patient's two *gan*-gate openings, the physician's forefingers detect powerful pulsations and so forth, this corresponds to the area between the diaphragm and the navel of the patient. Pulsations detected by the physician's ring fingers at the patient's two *chak*-foot openings correspond to the area from below the navel [down to the soles of the patient's feet]. Thus the physician should examine the channels for strength or weakness—that is, for heat or cold.[81]

Elsewhere in the text these correspondences are made even more explicit: the points that are closest to the creases on the patient's wrists, the *tsön*-inch

---

in the [*Four Tantras*] chapter actually are summaries of what we see in [the *Moon King*]. However, we also can see that other sections in this chapter are not from [the *Moon King*]." For excerpts from my translations of these chapters, see William A. McGrath, "Vessel Examination in the *Medicine of the Moon King*," in *Buddhism and Medicine: An Anthology of Premodern Sources*, ed. C. Pierce Salguero (New York, NY: Columbia University Press, 2017), 501–513.

80 The channel examination section of the *Moon King* is organized into ten chapters (chs. 15–24), five of which each treat the diagnosis of imbalances in a single viscus (chs. 16–20). See A ru ra, ed., *Sman dpyad zla ba'i rgyal po*, Bod kyi gso rig pa'i gna' dpe phyogs bsgrigs dpe tshogs, vol. 33 (Beijing: Mi rigs dpe skrun khang, 2005), 60–85.

81 *Sman dpyad zla ba'i rgyal po*, in *Krung go'i bod lugs gso rig rtsa che'i dpe rnying kun btus*, vol. 5, text 1, p. 23 (f. 34b): *tsha grang dag gi khyad par ste// stod smad sor mo drug la 'o// kan* [=*tshon*] *gnyis lhag chad stong pa ste// drag zhan dag kyang de bzhin no// mchin dri 'go'i* [=*mgo'i*] *bar dag go/ tshon* [=*kan*] *gnyis drag tu 'phar ba na// mchin dri lte ba'i bar dag ste// chag gnyis lte ba man chad smad//* [*rkang pa'i mthil ni yan chad do//*] *drag zhan tsha grang brtag par bya'o//*. The Degé print edition found in A ru ra, ed., *Sman dpyad zla ba'i rgyal po*, 61; has many different readings, the most significant of which have been noted in [square brackets] above.

openings, correspond to the uppermost viscera, the heart and lungs. The middle points, the *gan*-gate openings, correspond to the liver and spleen, and the points furthest from the wrist, the *chak*-foot openings, correspond to the kidneys. Importantly, disorders of the five inner viscera, as well as the six outer viscera (*snod drug* = Chi. *liufu* 六腑), that can be found in the three sections of the body are described in terms of heat and cold (*tsha grang*), not wind, bile, and phlegm.

Although the three humors do not act as the central paradigm in the above-cited paragraph, they still play a supporting role in the *Moon King*. Indeed, the triad of wind, bile, and phlegm do appear together throughout the ten channel examination chapters of the *Moon King*, often in association with a fourth humor of blood (*khrag*) or hepatic blood (*mchin khrag*).[82] Wind also appears alongside disorders of heat and cold,[83] indicating an early correspondence of bile with heat and phlegm with cold.[84] Throughout the ten channel examination chapters of the *Moon King*, disorders of wind, bile, and phlegm, as well as heat, cold, and blood, all should be understood as localized within the viscera for, as we have seen in the citation above, imbalances detected in the pulsations of the patient's wrists correspond to the three sections of the body, as well as the viscera located therein. Combining these details, we find a set of instructions in the *Moon King* for palpating six specific points on the wrists

82 *Sman dpyad zla ba'i rgyal po*, in *Krung go'i bod lugs gso rig rtsa che'i dpe rnying kun btus*, vol. 5, text 1, p. 24 (f. 36a): "[If the pulsations are] strong and rough, there is hepatic blood. [If the pulsations are] twisted and fast, there is bile. [If the pulsations are] large and slow, there is phlegm. [If the pulsations are] empty and solid, there is wind" (*drag cing rtsub na mchin khrag ste// grims shing myur ba mkhris pa ste// che la bul ba bad kan no// stong la mkhrang ba gang na rlung //*). Although orthodox presentations of the humors (*nyes pa*) in the Tibetan medical tradition often only include wind, bile, and phlegm, sets of four humors including blood (*khrag*) are also not unattested. See Dan Martin, "Greek and Islamic Medicines' Historical Contact with Tibet: A Reassessment in View of Recently Available but Relatively Early Sources on Tibetan Medical Eclecticism," in *Islam and Tibet: Interactions along the Musk Routes*, ed. Anna Akasoy, Charles Burnett, Ronit Yoeli-Tlalim (Burlington, VT: Ashgate, 2011), 132, n. 41. See also Henk Blezer's "A New Sense of (Dark) Humor in Tibet: Brown Phlegm and Black Bile," in the present volume.

83 *Sman dpyad zla ba'i rgyal po*, in *Krung go'i bod lugs gso rig rtsa che'i dpe rnying kun btus*, vol. 5, text 1, p. 24 (f. 35b): "Weak, strangulated, submerged, slow, and fragile [pulsations indicate] cold. Solid, replete, twisted, and strong [pulsations indicate] heat. Floating and empty [pulsations indicate] wind" (*zhan dang 'khyig pa bying ba dang // dal ba [g.yung ba] ghung pa grang ba 'o// mkhrang ba rgyas pa 'phril ba dang // drag pa dag ni tsha ba 'o// rkyal ba stong pa rlung yin te//*).

84 For a similar correspondence in Chinese-language translations, see Chen Ming, "The Transmission of Indian Ayurvedic Doctrines in Medieval China: A Case Study of *Aṣṭāṅga* and *Tridoṣa* Fragments from the Silk Road," *Annual Report of The International Research Institute for Advanced Buddhology at Soka University* 9 (2006): 201–30.

of a patient, used to determine the thermal and humoral imbalances in corresponding visceral sites on the body.

Does a rapid and powerful pulsation at the site one inch from the crease of the patient's right wrist (the *tsön*-inch opening) indicate heat, bile disease, heart disease, or just hypertension? Regardless of the interpretation, the haptic observation of a rapid pulsation can be quantified (in beats per breath or, more reproducibly, beats per second) just as a powerful pulsation can be qualified (according to the experience and training of the physician). These observations are real, even if their interpretations are various. And even if each of these interpretations may be mutually exclusive, such a range of interpretations allows the physician to adapt his or her observations according to his or her abilities and the availability of different treatments. Humoral imbalances are often treated using *materia medica*, for example, while visceral imbalances are treated with acu-phlebotomy and moxa-cauterization. Thus, not unlike Padmasambhava interpreting the spontaneous visions of *prasenā* divination to name the demons of Central Tibet, the physician of the Tibetan medical tradition can select from this diagnostic repertoire to interpret the haptic signs observed in the channels of a patient and transform his or her illness into a treatable disease.

7 Channel Examination as *Prasenā* Divination

With the introduction of cosmopolitan instructions for channel examination to Tibet in the eleventh- or twelfth-century *Moon King*, there was a subsequent proliferation of small sets of vernacular instructions in which the methods for and interpretations of channel examination were expanded to fit local sensibilities. One way that channel examination was transformed following its introduction to Tibet was by means of comparison with *prasenā* divination. "Guiding instructions for channel *prasenā* divination" (*rtsa yi pra khrid*) or, more generally, "guiding instructions for *prasenā* divination" (*pra khrid*) appear in some of the earliest literature on channel examination, which was most probably composed under the influence of the instructions found in the *Moon King*. Although there are few features of these guiding instructions on channel *prasenā* that resemble canonical forms of *prasenā* that we saw above, the nebulousness of the very concept of *prasenā* itself may have allowed its practitioners to be some of the first figures to take up foreign practices like channel examination. Thus, following the introduction of channel examination to Tibet, physicians came to incorporate a modified *prasenā* divination into their repertoires, just as tantric diviners had also adapted the semblance of channel examination for their predictions in channel *prasenā* rituals.

Most descriptions of channel *prasenā* divination appear in works attributed to Nāgārjuna, the illustrious Indian sage and mythological redactor of the *Moon King*. Distinct cycles of medical teachings attributed to Nāgārjuna number in the dozens, with a majority of these works including at least a small section on channel examination.[85] One such work, the *Lamp of Sunbeams: A Channel Manual* (*rtsa yig nyi zer sgron me*) attributed to Nāgārjuna, includes a chapter entitled "Guiding Instructions for Channel *Prasenā* Divination," which includes not the three humors of Āyurvedic provenance, but five—blood (*khrag*), bile (*mkhris pa*), wind (*rlung*), brown phlegm (*bad kan smug po*), and yellow phlegm (*bad kan skya bo*)—as well as many other common descriptions of disease.[86] The *Lamp of Sunbeams* also involves terminology for the three fingers/sites of palpation that is found in the *Moon King* and clearly derives from the Chinese language—that is, the *tsön*-inch, *kan*-gate, and *chak*-foot openings, located along the radial artery of the patient. After a brief explication of observable haptic phenomena and their corresponding disorders, the *Lamp* assures us: "Having understood the above [correspondences] thusly, one should then diagnose individual diseases."[87] Thus, the *Lamp of Sunbeams* provides instructions for the observation and interpretation of a patient's channels according to a humoral conception of disease and, with the exception of the label of *prasenā* and an expanded repertoire of interpretations, these instructions for channel examination found in the *Lamp of Sunbeams* resemble those found in the *Moon King*.

This labelling of channel examination as *prasenā* divination continues in an early collection of instructions attributed to Yutok Gönpo (*g.yu thog mgon po*, 12th c.), the *Thousand-session Tutorial on the Channels* (*rtsa'i stong thun*).[88] The genre of the "thousand-session tutorial" (*stong thun*) is not

---

85 For an anthology of such works, see A ru ra, ed., *Slob dpon klu sgrub kyi sman yig gces btus*, Bod kyi gso ba rig pa'i gna' dpe phyogs bsgrigs dpe tshogs, vol. 73 (Beijing: Mi rigs dpe skrun khang, 2008).

86 *Rtsa yig nyi zer sgron me*, in *Slob dpon klu sgrub kyi sman yig gces btus*, 365–66. See also Blezer, "A New Sense of (Dark) Humor in Tibet," in the present volume.

87 *Rtsa yig nyi zer sgron me*, in *Slob dpon klu sgrub kyi sman yig gces btus*, 365: *yin par gong ma dag gis shes// de ltar so sor nad ngos bzung //.*

88 Sumtön Yeshé Zung names thousand-session tutorials among the few compositions of Yutok Gönpo in *Med thabs med pa'i mchong* [='*phyong*] *gsum*, in *Krung go'i bod lugs gso rig rtsa che'i dpe rnying kun btus*, vol. 3, text 3, p. 257 (f. 2b): "The Sage Yutok Gönpo composed the *Thousand-session Tutorials* that arrange the contents of the topics [of medical practice], outlined the abridged topics in the scriptures, composed the small lexical

limited to the literature of medicine, and refers to the experiential knowledge that derives from one thousand (*stong*) repetitions or sessions (*thun*) of any particular practice.[89] Individual manuscript witnesses of several medical tutorials have recently come to light, as well as one complete collection of the *Eleven Cycles of Thousand-session Tutorials* (*skor tshoms stong thun bcu gcig*) that also includes the *Thousand-session Tutorial on the Channels*.[90] Although these medical instructions may indeed derive from the twelfth century, polemics found at the end of the *Thousand-session Tutorial on the Fluids* (*chu'i stong thun*) reveals the role of the Drangti family in the redaction of the tutorials.[91]

---

commentary on the collection of [meanings that are] difficult [to understand]. He elided that which was incomplete and redacted that which was clear. He also was committed to not disseminating these teachings to others and achieved fame throughout the world" (*drang srong g.yu thog mgon po yis/ don gyi khog dbubs tongs* [*=stong*] *thun mdzad/ bsdus don gzhung las sa mtshams phye/ rka 'phrang* [*dka' 'phreng*] *'bru 'grel yig chung bkod/ ma tshang gab 'khrugs gsal bar bsdebs/ gzhan la ma spel yi dam mdzad/ 'dzam bu gling du grags pa thob/*).

89 See, for example, José Cabezón's *A Dose of Emptiness: An Annotated Translation of the sTong thun chen mo of mKhas grub dGe legs dpal bzang* (Albany, NY: State University of New York Press, 1992). Perhaps due to the subject of Khedrup Jé's tutorial, Cabezón appears to have been led into thinking that the word *stong* refers to "emptiness" (*stong pa nyid*) instead of the number one thousand (*stong*). I opt to include the word "tutorial" in the translation because the thousand-session genre is didactic in nature, with the effect of imparting the aforementioned experiential knowledge on to the student.

90 In the *Krung go'i bod lugs gso rig rtsa che'i dpe rnying kun btus*, see the following works: *Skor tshoms stong thun bcu gcig las dang po rtsa'i stong thun*, vol. 3, text 5; *Rtsa chu'i stong thun g.yu thog gi bzhed pa*, vol. 3, text 7; *Grang ba'i stong thun*, vol. 3, text 9; *Grang ba'i stong thun*, vol. 14, text 4; *Bad kan smug po'i stong thun*, vol. 14, text 5; *Skor tshoms stong thun bcu gcig*, vol. 14, text 3.

91 *Skor tshoms stong thun bcu gcig*, in *Krung go'i bod lugs gso rig rtsa che'i dpe rnying kun btus*, vol. 14, text 4, p. 22 (8b): "May Master Yutok Gönpo bless us! *Mangalam!* I am the retainer of this textual tradition. Although there are many others that claim to understand [this tradition], what can they do other than find the section on the practical instructions or the section on the measurements in the text? These days here in the Snowy Land of Tibet, although there are many people who claim to be physicians, other than Master Drangti and his students, there are no others that I would consider to be healers. A 'physician' once claimed that only practices are important, and had long abandoned the commentaries. But, if the discussion of essential meanings is important, professing doctrines with no textual basis is laughable. Similarly, for a physician who does not understand textual meanings to understand practices would be like a star appearing in daylight. Ha ha!" (*mkhas pa g.yu thog mgon po'i byin gyi brlobs// mang gha lam// gzhung lugs 'di la kho bo'i yongs 'dzin 'khas* [*=mkhas*]*// bzhan* [*=gzhan*] *dag shes par rlom pa mang yod kyang // bzhung* [*=gzhung*] *gdams lag len gang gi phyogs la yang // tshod tsam phyogs tsam ma gtogs ci byar yod// ding sang kha ba can gyi ljongs 'di na// sman par rlom pa'i skye bo rab mang mod// brang ti mkhas pa slob mar bcas ma gtogs// mtsho* [*='tsho*] *byed yin snyam bdag gi*

Thus, regardless of their ultimate origins, the instructions found in the *Eleven Cycles of Thousand-session Tutorials* were probably first redacted during the life of Drangti Jampel Zangpo (ca. 1276–1335) or his son Drangti Penden Tsojé (ca. 1310–1380),[92] and were then included as a sub-collection in the *Eighteen Auxiliary Branches* by the middle of the fourteenth century.[93]

The *Thousand-session Tutorial on the Channels* also has a section on channel *prasenā*, but rather than use *prasenā* as a general rubric for the interpretation of channel examination, like in the *Lamp of Sunbeams*, the author of the *Thousand-session Tutorial* assigns channel *prasenā* the specific function of "identifying pathogenic demons."[94] As we have seen, channel examination involves the diagnostic interpretation of haptic signs observed in the channels of the patient, and one possible interpretation found in nearly all instructions for channel examination is that of pathogenic demons.[95] In the case of the *Thousand-session Tutorial on the Channels*, pathogenic demons can be identified by pulsations that are "halting, intermittent, and turbulent, with intensities that are uneven, like a lasso that has caught a wild horse."[96] If such

---

sems la med// sman pa kha cig lag len kho na tso [=gtso]// ces smras 'grel trig [=tī ka] ring du spong pa yod// 'o na mtshan nyid pa la sgro [=bgro] gleng tso [=gtso]// gzhung don med pa'i chos gtam gzhad [=bzhad] dgad gnas// de bzhin sman pa gzhung don mi shes pa'i// lag len shes rlom nyin mo'i rgyu skar lags// he he//). The colophon notes that this work is within the system of Yutok Gönpo, but is also the special teaching of Lharjé Sanggyé Pelrin (*mkhas pa g.yu thog mgon po'i lugs so// lha rje sangs rgyas dpal rin gyis khad nor yin//*). See p. 40 (f. 35b). The Degé colophon states that this work is the special teaching of Yutok Gönpo (*mkhas pa g.yu thog yon tan mgon po'i khyad chos lags so*). See *Skor tshoms stong thun bcu gcig*, in *Cha lag bco brgyad*, 386.

92 In his commentary on the *Small Practical Manual*, Drangti Jampel Zangpo directs his readers to the *Thousand-session Tutorials on Channels and Fluids* (and not the *Four Tantras*). See *Lag len spod chung gyi 'brel [='grel] pa*, in *Krung go'i bod lugs gso rig rtsa che'i dpe rnying kun btus*, vol. 3, text 2, p. 231 (f. 2b): *rtsa chu gnyis bstong [=stong] thun du gsal lo/*. This may indicate that the *Eleven Cycles of Thousand-session Tutorials* were an orthodox source for channel and fluid examination as late as the thirteenth century.

93 For the Degé edition of the *Eleven Cycles of Thousand-session Tutorials* found in the *Eighteen Auxiliary Branches* collection, see *Skor tshoms stong thun bcu gcig*, in *Cha lag bco brgyad*, 243–386.

94 *Skor tshoms stong thun bcu gcig*, in *Krung go'i bod lugs gso rig rtsa che'i dpe rnying kun btus*, vol. 14, text 3, pp. 19–20 (ff. 5a–5b): *log [g]non gyi gdon ngos bzung pa/*.

95 See, for example, translated excerpts from the chapter on "Pathogenic Demon Channels" (*gnod pa'i gdon rtsa*) in the *Moon King* in McGrath, "Vessel Examination in the *Medicine of the Moon King*," 508–509.

96 *Skor tshoms stong thun bcu gcig*, in *Krung go'i bod lugs gso rig rtsa che'i dpe rnying kun btus*, vol. 14, text 3, p. 20 (f. 5b): *zhag gcig gi gsu[m?] bcod [=gcod] sdod dang / 'thsub dang / che chung mi snyom par rta rgod zhags kyis btab pa lta bu byung na gdon gyis rtsa'o//*.

pulsations are detected at the heart channel, it indicates a god or spirit haunting an image; if they are at the liver channel, it indicates an earth-lord spirit; if they are at the left kidney, it indicates an earth-worm spirit or serpent-worm spirit; and so forth.[97] Further specifications are provided if such pulsations are observed in combination with diseases—such as madness (*smyo nad*), contagious disease (*rims nad*), liver disease (*mchin nad*), painful disease (*gzer nad*), and fluid disease (*chu nad*)—resulting in precise instructions for the identification of specific pathogenic demons.[98]

Although the relative chronology of these early instructions for channel examination, attributed to Nāgārjuna and Yutok Gönpo, is not clear, the general association of Nāgārjuna with the *Moon King* (redacted 11th c.?) and the *Thousand-session Tutorials* with the Drangti family (redacted 14th c.?) indicates that the *Lamp of Sunbeams* probably predates the *Thousand-session Tutorial on the Channels*. If such is indeed the case, it would seem that the "Guiding Instructions for Channel *Prasenā* Divination" (*rtsa yi pra khrid*) found in the *Lamp of Sunbeams* represents an early vernacular expression of channel examination in the Tibetan language, in which the diagnostic interpretation of haptic signs is implicitly likened to the oracular interpretation of spontaneous visions in *prasenā* divination. By the time of the *Thousand-session Tutorials*, however, "Guiding Instructions for *Prasenā* Divination" (*pra khrid*) in the context of channel examination came to refer only to the identification of pathogenic demons by means of channel palpation. In light of the fact that *prasenā* divination was also used to identify pathogenic demons in the channel *prasenā* rituals (*rtsa'i pra sgrub*) analyzed above, the competitive tone evident in the epigraph cited at the beginning of this essay probably derives from the professional struggle between the physician proponents of empirical diagnosis and the tantric proponents of divine revelation.[99]

---

97 *Skor tshoms stong thun bcu gcig*, in *Krung go'i bod lugs gso rig rtsa che'i dpe rnying kun btus*, vol. 14, text 3, p. 20 (f. 5b): *de yang khyad par snying rtsa 'tshub na/ rang rten pa'i lha'am dkor bdag gnod/ mchin rtsa la sa bdag mkhal ma g.yon la sa srin klu srin/ glo rtsa la klu bdud drag* [=*brag*] [*b*]*tsan/ mcher rtsa la dri* [=*gre*] *pho dri* [=*gre*] *mo/ mkhal ma g.yas la klu bdud drag* [=*brag*] *bdud/*.

98 On such demons and their role in conceptualizing madness, see Susannah Deane, "Madness and the Spirits: Examining the Role of Spirits in Mental Illness in the Tibetan Communities of Darjeeling," in the present volume.

99 For further evidence on the separation of such spheres of professional specialization, see Tsering Samdrup, "The *Nine-fold Magical Cord Cycle*: Investigating *'Phrul gyi the gu brgu skor*, a Wartime Medical Manual," in the present volume.

8 The Wonder Channels, Messengers, and the Interpretation of Empirical Observation

A professional struggle between the Tibetan physicians and tantric diviners of the eleventh and twelfth centuries is evinced in their defining of terms. For the scholar primarily concerned with Indian provenance, *prasenā* referred to the spontaneous visions seen in a reflective implement, with or without the aid of a child assistant, as described in the *Questions of Subāhu Tantra*. For the tantric diviner with potential connections to Central Asian traditions, *prasenā* referred to a much wider body of oracular practices in which a goddess or some other deity reveals knowledge of the past, present, and future. For the early physician of the Tibetan medical tradition, *prasenā* referred to either the general practice of channel examination, or the more specific identification of pathogenic demons by means of palpating the channels. Despite general agreement regarding the result of *prasenā* divination—that is, clairvoyant knowledge of some kind—there was general disagreement regarding the actual procedure by which *prasenā* divination should be performed. Central to this disagreement was the question of whether this knowledge had to derive from the interpretation of an observed object, or whether it could arise as the result of ritual evocation and divine revelation. Turning now to the wonder channels, we find a similar struggle over the meaning of a polysemous term.

As we have already seen in the different editions of the *Three Goddess Sisters* and the *Black-lipped Brahminess*, the wonder channels have been variously expressed as set of seven (*bdun*), eight (*brgyad*), or one hundred (*brgya*). We have also already noted that the latter can probably be explained as a scribal error for the number eight, which is further supported by another set of eight wonder channels that can be found in the aforementioned work on channel examination attributed to Nāgārjuna, the *Lamp of Sunbeams*. There the eight wonder channels (*ngo mtshar can gyi rtsa brgyad*) are listed as:

[1.] The three diseases exist in relation to the three poisons; understanding this from the channels is truly wondrous!

[2.] Understanding the diseases of the body using surgical instruments is extremely wondrous!

[3.] Bile induces heat; corroborating this using one's sense faculties and understanding this from the [patient's] channels is truly wondrous!

[4.] Phlegm induces stupidity;[100] understanding the channels as being polluted and obscured is truly wondrous!

100 Although the phrase *gti mug bad kan bskyed pa* seems to indicate that stupidity induces phlegm, the parallel structure of the previous and subsequent passages supports the reading that phlegm induces stupidity instead.

TABLE 8.1 Systematic correspondences between the humors, the poisons, and diseases in the *Lamp of Sunbeams*

[Four humors]	Three poisons (*dug gsum po*)	Three diseases (*nad gsum*)
Bile (*mkhris pa*)		Heat (*tsha ba*)
Phlegm (*bad kan*)	Stupidity (*gti mug*)	
Wind (*rlung*)	Desire (*'dod chags*)	Cold (*grang ba*)
Fluids (*chu*)	Envy (*phrag dog*)	Lymph (*chu ser*)

[5.] Wind induces desire and cold; regardless of whatever [qualities there are in the] channels that one encounters, understanding this from the channels is truly wondrous!

[6.] Understanding how to heal empty [fevers] and prevent their expansion from the channels is truly wondrous!

[7.] The fluids induce envy and lymph; corroborating this using the sense faculties and understanding this from the channels is truly wondrous!

[8.] To understand the prognoses of both life and death from the channels, conquering demons without error, is truly wondrous![101]

This set of eight stanzas is primarily dedicated to an expression of wonder (*ngo mtshar che*) at the ability to assess the relationship between the three diseases (heat, cold, and lymph), the three poisons (stupidity, desire, and envy), and, implicitly, the four humors (bile, phlegm, wind, and the fluids [blood?]). This set of correspondences contrasts with the respective equation of wind, bile, and phlegm with desire, hatred (*zhe sdang*), and stupidity found in the *Root Tantra* (*rtsa rgyud*), wherein the triad of the so-called "three diseases" is expanded to the four hundred and four diseases.[102] Also, envy is not mentioned

101 *Rtsa yig nyi zer sgron me*, in *Slob dpon klu sgrub kyi sman yig gces btus*, 372–73: *dug gsum po la nad gsum yod// rtsa yi shes pa ngo mtshar che// 'thur* [=*thur*] *ma'i sgo nas lus kyi nad// shes pa shin tu ngo mtshar che// mkhris pa'i tsha ba bskyed pa yin// dbang po'i sgo nas 'grigs pa ste// rtsa yi shes pa ngo mtshar che// gti mug bad kan bskyed pa ste// dbang po'i sgo nas 'grib cing 'thib// rtsa yi shes pa ngo mtshar che// 'dod chags grang ba rlung gis bskyed// rtsa ni gang phrod* [*'phrod*] *'gyur ba ste// rtsa yi shes pa ngo mtshar che// stong ba gso zhing rgyas pa gsod// rtsa yi shes pa ngo mtshar che// phrag dog chu ser chu yis bskyed// dbang po'i sgo nas 'grib* [=*'grigs*] *pa de// rtsa yi shes pa ngo mtshar che// 'tsho 'chi gnyis kyi bye brag rnams// ma nor skye bre* [=*'dre?*] *rgyal ba ni// rtsa yi shes pa ngo mtshar che//.*

102 Rje bstan 'dzin don grub, ed., *Dpal ldan rgyud bzhi dpe bsdur ma*, vol. 1, 35: *de la 'dod chags zhe sdang gtig mug gsum// rlung mkhris bad kan rim pas skyed pa'i rgyud//.*

in relation to the humors or classes of disease in the *Four Tantras*. Thus, not unlike its use of *prasenā* seen above, the *Lamp of Sunbeams* provides an unorthodox presentation of systematic correspondences in which the relationships between corresponding parts are ambiguous and seemingly open. In addition to this haphazard set of relationships, the passage cited above also wonders at the ability "to understand the prognoses of both life and death from the channels, conquering demons without error." Indeed, it is only this eighth wonder channel, concerning the oracular ability to diagnose and predict the patient's time of death, that corresponds at all to the wonder channels found in the channel *prasenā* rituals examined above.

An important characteristic of the wonder channels that is explicitly described in the *Three Goddess Sisters* and implicitly noted in the *Black-lipped Brahminess*, but missing from this list found in the *Lamp of Sunbeams*, is the ability to diagnose a patient by means of a messenger. Again, relative chronologies are difficult to establish, but it would seem that the notion of the eight wonder channels was probably introduced in the *Lamp of Sunbeams*, redefined as *prasenā* divination by means of a messenger in the *Three Goddess Sisters*, and rendered as the seven wonder channels in the *Black-lipped Brahminess*. By the time that the instructions for channel examination were systematized in the *Subsequent Tantra*, the wonder channels would have been a term of ambiguous meaning and disputed numeration. It comes as no surprise, then, that the channel examination chapter of the *Subsequent Tantra* definitively delineates the "seven wonder channels" (*ngo mtshar rtsa bdun*) as a set, describing each one in detail.

According to the *Subsequent Tantra*, the seven wonder channels include: family divination (*khyim phywa*), guest divination (*mgron phywa*), enemy divination (*dgra phywa*), fortune divination (*grogs* [=*grog*] *phywa*), demon divination (*gdon phywa*), the reversal of fire and water (*me chu go ldog*), and the pregnancy channel (*bu rtsa*).[103] Family divination, the first of the seven classes of wonder channels, associates predictions of future events with pulsation characteristics—like pain (*mya ngan*) with sluggish and obscure pulsations, terror (*bred dngangs*) with torrential and faint pulsations, suffering (*sdug bsngal*) with prickly and thorny pulsations, defamation (*mi kha*) with boiling pulsations, and a loss of wealth (*nor god*) with intermittent pulsations.[104] This

103 For descriptions and illustrations of the seven wonder channels, see Parfionovitch, Meyer, and Gyurme Dorje, eds., *Tibetan Medical Paintings*, 127–34 (plates 56–59).

104 Rje bstan 'dzin don grub, ed., *Dpal ldan rgyud bzhi dpe bsdur ma*, vol. 3, 23–24: *dang po bying zhing 'thibs na mi gtsang rtsa// rmugs shing 'thibs na mya ngan 'ong ba'i rtsa// 'brub cing brgyal na bred dngangs 'ong ba'i rtsa// skyer tsher 'dra na sdug bsngal thar med rtsa// chu tshan khol 'dra mi kha 'ong ba'i rtsa// me lce chad 'dra nor god 'ong ba'i rtsa//.*

technique is called family divination because, the predicted fate depends upon not just the characteristics of the pulsation, but also the channel in which the pulsation occurs:

> Regarding these [predictions], when the "self" channel [that corresponds to the current season] flourishes, whatever [prediction] emerges in the "self" channel will happen to oneself. If it is in the mother channel, then it will happen to the mother or maternal uncle. If it is in the child channel, then it will happen to one's child, nephew, or grandson. If it is in the friend channel, then it will happen to one's livestock. If it is in the enemy channel, then it will happen to one's enemies.[105]

The self, mother, child, friend, and enemy channels can be determined according to the systematic correspondence of elemental astrology (*'byung rtsis*),[106] in which the "self" channel corresponds to the viscus of the same element as the current season (the liver [wood] in the spring [wood], for example), the mother corresponds to the viscus of the previous element (the kidney [water] in the spring [wood]), the child corresponds to the viscus of the subsequent element (the heart [fire] in the spring [wood]), the friend corresponds to the viscus of the element after next (the spleen [earth] in the spring [wood]), and the enemy corresponds to the viscus of the element before last (the lung [metal] in the spring [wood]). Thus, the family divination wonder channel technique provides a means for the physician to foretell future pains and losses for a patient and his or her family members.

Similarly, the guest divination wonder channel reveals whether a guest is still at home (*gzhi la yod*), is on the road (*lam du zhugs pa*), has almost arrived (*nye bar sleb*), is about to leave (*phyin la khad pa*), or if an enemy of the traveler is coming (*'gron dgra 'ong ba*) based on the emergence of a fierce (*drag pa*) pulsation in the self, mother, child, friend, or enemy channels. Thus, guest divination is performed to determine whether a guest will successfully arrive or not.[107] The enemy divination wonder channel predicts one's fate in battle,

105 Rje bstan 'dzin don grub, ed., *Dpal ldan rgyud bzhi dpe bsdur ma*, vol. 3, 24: *de dag gang yang rang rtsa dar dus su// rang gi rtsa la gang byung rang la 'ong // ma rtsa ma zhang bu rtsa bu tsha la// grogs rtsa nor la dgra rtsa dgra la 'ong //.*

106 For a description of the elements and their relationships, see Philippe Cornu, *Tibetan Astrology* (Boston, MA: Shambhala, 2002), 52–63 *et passim*. For the notion of "systematic correspondences" in the Chinese medical tradition, see Paul Unschuld, *Huang Di nei jing su wen: Nature, Knowledge, Imagery in an Ancient Chinese Medical Text* (Berkeley, CA: University of California Press, 2003), 99–124 *et passim.*

107 Rje bstan 'dzin don grub, ed., *Dpal ldan rgyud bzhi dpe bsdur ma*, vol. 3, 24.

both when attacking (*phar rgol*) and defending (*tshur rgol*).[108] The fortune divination wonder channel relates to one's fortune in terms of wealth and livestock (*nor*).[109] The similarity between between the Tibetan words for "fortune" (*grog*) and "friend" (*grogs*) caused these two terms to be used interchangeably, but because the instructions are for the prediction of either the gain or loss of wealth, this technique should be called the "fortune divination" (*grog phywa*) rather than the more common phonetic equivalent, "friend divination" (*grogs phywa*).

The latter three types of wonder channel examination are more medically oriented than the first four: identifying demons, death, and pregnancy. The demon divination wonder channel helps the physician identify the pathogenic demons that have come to afflict his or her patients. Not unlike the instructions found in the *Thousand-session Tutorial on the Channels*, distinct pulsations found in specific channels indicate specific pathogenic demons, such as a *nyen* demon (*gnyan*), a king spirit (*rgyal po*), and so forth. Less typical demons are different classes of ghosts (*'dre*), including the ghost of a child haunting its parents (*pha ma'i chags 'dre*), the ghost of a child's maternal uncle (*bu tsha'i zhang 'dre*), the ghost of an enemy's curse (*dgra bos rbad 'dre*), the ghost of lost (?) livestock (*nor gyi phyi 'dre*), and the ghost of a contaminated friend (*grogs kyi 'gos dre*).[110] While the former classifications of possession refer to generally afflictive demons that are common causes of disease in the Tibetan imaginary, the latter classes of spirits refer to ghosts that derive from specific family members, social transgressions, and undesirable events.

The so-called "reversal of fire and water" divination refers to the examination of a relative in the place of a patient. For example, if a father is ill, the physician could examine the son (*pha na bu la blta*) and determine whether or not the disease is terminal (*'chi*) or not (*mi 'chi*). The same is true that if a son is ill, the physician could examine the channels of the father (*bu na pha yi rtsa la bltas pa*), or if a mother is ill, one could also examine her daughter (*ma dang bu mo'i rtsa yang de ltar blta*), or if a husband is ill, one could examine his wife (*khyo na chung ma'i rtsa la bltas pa*), and vice versa.[111] In sum, the "reversal of fire and water" refers to the prognosis of distant patients by means of a messenger, not unlike the description of the wonder channels found in the *Three Goddess Sisters* ritual examined above. The seventh wonder channel

108 Rje bstan 'dzin don grub, ed., *Dpal ldan rgyud bzhi dpe bsdur ma*, vol. 3, 24–25.

109 The very term for wealth used here (*nor*) also has the connotation of livestock. Thus, the gain or loss of wealth also implies the gain or loss of livestock. See Rje bstan 'dzin don grub, ed., *Dpal ldan rgyud bzhi dpe bsdur ma*, vol. 3, 25.

110 Rje bstan 'dzin don grub, ed., *Dpal ldan rgyud bzhi dpe bsdur ma*, vol. 3, 25.

111 Rje bstan 'dzin don grub, ed., *Dpal ldan rgyud bzhi dpe bsdur ma*, vol. 3, 25–26.

divination, the pregnancy channel (*sbrum ma'i rtsa*), provides the means for predicting the gender of the child in utero, as well as the ease (*sla*) or difficulty (*dka'*) for the mother during postpartum recovery (*btsas nas gso*).[112] Thus, these final three modes of demon identification, remote prognosis, and pregnancy predictions have the most obvious practical implications for the physician of medicine, while the former four appear to be the tools of the generic soothsayer.

Despite their differences, the eight wonder channels listed above in the *Lamp of Sunbeams* and the seven wonder channels listed in the *Subsequent Tantra* each provides the physician with tools for creatively interpreting the pulsations in the channels of his or her patients. In the case of the former, the eight wonder channels remain grounded in the conception of the humors—listed as bile, phlegm, wind, and the fluids—and, depending on whichever humor is dominant, it also provides some information regarding predominant diseases and afflictive emotions (Table 1). The instructions are vague, however, and other comments regarding the use of surgical tools and the use of the channels to prognosticate the life and death of patients are also lauded as wondrous. Thus, the *Lamp of Sunbeams* appears to represent an early example of the wonder channels in which the instructions for the practice—if this short passage can even be considered an independent practice—remain incomplete and imprecise. The instructions in the *Subsequent Tantra*, by contrast, are totally explicit and consummately described, even if they overlap with the more detailed instructions found in the "Death Channels" (*'chi rtsa*) and "Demonic Channels" (*gdon rtsa*) subsections of the *Subsequent Tantra*. Thus, despite the differences in their textual instantiations, the wonder channels generally refer to a set of diagnostic practices through which the physician can creatively interpret the haptic characteristics of a patient or a patient's relative to determine future fortunes and misfortunes.

Tracing the genealogy of the instructions found in the *Subsequent Tantra* reveals that this fourth book of the *Four Tantras* is neither the primordial scripture of the Master of Medicine nor the twelfth-century teaching of a single author. Instead, the instructions for channel examination found in the *Subsequent Tantra* represent the culmination of several centuries of assimilation and adaptation, resulting in the transformation of imprecise vernacular expressions into a systematic cosmopolitan instruction (Figure 8.2). Following the introduction of channel examination to Tibet around the eleventh century by means of works like the *Medicine of the Moon King*, these instructions were reformulated and labeled as a form of *prasenā* divination in Nāgārjuna's *Lamp*

112 Rje bstan 'dzin don grub, ed., *Dpal ldan rgyud bzhi dpe bsdur ma*, vol. 3, 26.

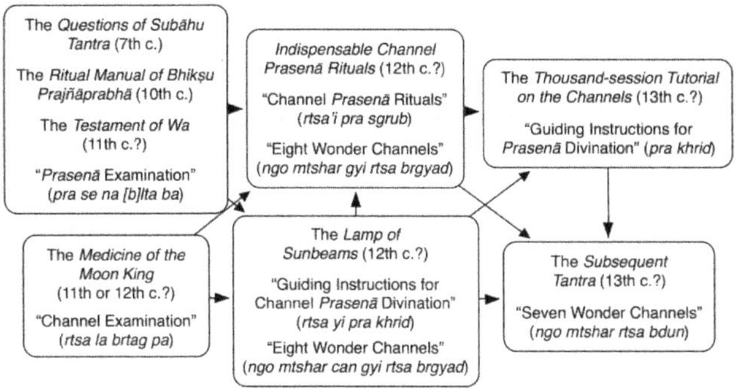

FIGURE 8.2 A genealogy of *prasenā* rituals, channel examination, and the wonder channels

of Sunbeams. By the thirteenth century, channel *prasenā* divination had come to refer solely to the identification of pathogenic demons, as represented by the instructions found in the *Thousand-session Tutorial on the Channels* of the Yutok school. Perhaps in response to the success of channel examination and its propinquity to the medical uses of *prasenā* divination, eleventh- and twelfth-century tantric ritualists in Drapa Ngönshé's lineage reappropriated the notion of channel *prasenā* divination, leading to the tradition of channel *prasenā* rituals centered around the divine revelation of diagnostic and prognostic information. Throughout this process, the wonder channels passed from being a general description of corresponding interpretations of haptic observation in the *Lamp of Sunbeams*, to the remote diagnosis of a patient by means of a messenger in the *Three Goddess Sisters* and *Black-lipped Brahminess*, and finally back to a more sophisticated hermeneutic of systematic correspondences in the *Subsequent Tantra*. Although in the *Subsequent Tantra* the wonder channels were fixed at seven (instead of eight) and definitively delineated as the divinatory interpretation of haptic observations, effectively deemphasizing *prasenā* divination and its associated methods for divine revelation, instructions for channel *prasenā* rituals continued to be transmitted alongside the *Four Tantras* in the *Eighteen Auxiliary Branches* collection and beyond.

9 Conclusions: Subsequent Transmissions and the Repertoire of the Tibetan Medical Tradition

For approximately seven hundred years, the *Subsequent Tantra* and its exegetical literature have served as the orthodox sources for instructions on channel examination in the Tibetan medical tradition. Prior to its systematization in the thirteenth and fourteenth centuries, however, the field of instructions regarding channel examination in the Tibetan language remained vast and diverse, including the interpretation of specific haptic observations to indicate the diagnosis of humoral imbalance, the prognosis of impending death, or even the identification of demonic possession. It was the latter interpretive capacity that ultimately led the early proponents of empirical diagnosis in Tibet to enter into conflict with the long-established tantric practitioners of *prasenā* divination. Although these tantric practitioners offered a means to diagnose patients remotely, by means of divine revelation and under the rubric of the wonder channels, the physicians responsible for the systematization of the *Subsequent Tantra* effectively adapted the capacity for remote diagnosis and incorporated the wonder channels back within the realm of empirical interpretation. Despite the standardization of these techniques in the *Four Tantras*, the fourteenth-century scions of the Drangti family and generations of other medical lineages continued to transmit and elaborate upon the channel *prasenā* rituals that came to be included in the *Eighteen Auxiliary Branches*.

Drangti Penden Tsojé (*brang ti dpal ldan 'tsho byed*, ca. 1310–1380) is primarily responsible for our present understandings of both the divine revelations of channel *prasenā* rituals and the instructions for empirical diagnosis in the *Subsequent Tantra*. It was he who first determined the contents of the *Eighteen Auxiliary Branches* in his *Expanded Elucidation of Knowledge* (*shes bya rab gsal rgyas pa*, ca. 1372), indicating his involvement in the redaction of the *Eighteen Auxiliary Branches* as a definite corpus of texts. It was also he who transmitted the instructions for channel *prasenā* rituals to his nephew, Drangti Penden Gyentsen (*brang ti dpal ldan rgyal mtshan*), who then went on to redact them in the *Gold Measure* collection.[113] Finally, it was he who composed the first commentary on any part of the *Subsequent Tantra*,[114] thereby promoting the *Four Tantras* as an orthodox source of instructions for channel examination. The

113 The colophon of each channel divination ritual mentions both figures, among other scions of the Drangti clan, indicating the fact that each teaching may have once been redacted by Drangti Penden Gyentsen on the basis of Penden Tsojé's teachings. See, for example, *Reg pa rtsa'i spra sgrub klu sgrub gyis mdzad pa bzhugs s.ho*, in *Krung go'i bod lugs gso rig rtsa che'i dpe rnying kun btus*, vol. 1, text 10, p. 57 (f. 10b): "I, Drangti Penden Gyentsen, requested this [work] from the exact teachings and practices of Drangti Penden Tsojé" (*brang ti dpal ldan 'tsho byed kyi gsung ngag phyag len ji bzhin du/ brang ti dpal ldan rgyal mtshan bdag gis zhus pa'o//*).

114 Brang ti dpal ldan 'tsho byed, *Rtsa mdo'i 'grel pa nyi ma'i 'od zer*, in *Krung go'i bod lugs gso rig rtsa che'i dpe rnying kun btus*, vol. 1, text 14, pp. 207–16 (ff. 1–19). Although other commentaries on the *Explanatory Tantra* predate this work, this is one of the earliest commentaries on (or even mentions of) the *Subsequent Tantra*.

colophons of the *Gold Measure* collection also promote the channel *prasenā* rituals as the teachings of Yutok Gönpo,[115] a trend that continues in the subsequent *Essential Nucleus of Yutok* collection,[116] which became even more popular following the apotheosis of Yutok Gönpo in the seventeenth century.[117]

By attempting to contextualize an instruction in a time and in a place—that is, by describing the genealogy of channel *prasenā* rituals as the product of centuries of human agency—we are able to read that instruction, in the words of Arnaldo Momigliano, "as if it were not a document, but an actual event of past life," representative of "men and institutions, ideas, beliefs, emotions, and the needs of individuals who no longer exist."[118] Regarding the past lives responsible for the dialogue of empirical diagnosis and divine revelation within the early Tibetan medical tradition, we have few reliable notions of time, space, and agency, for all documents have been recast as the primordial teachings of the Emanated Sage Rikpé Yeshé, the Indian Sage Nāgārjuna, or the Tibetan Sage Yutok Yönten Gönpo. By analyzing the emergence of specific terminology like *prasenā* and the wonder channels, however, we can begin to tease out the historical processes by which the instructional repertoire of the Tibetan medical tradition was created. As we have seen above, by the fourteenth century the physician trained in the orthodox teachings of the *Four Tantras* and its ancillary teachings of the *Eighteen Auxiliary Branches* could choose to practice both the instructions for empirical diagnosis found in the first chapter of the *Subsequent Tantra* and those for divine revelation found in the *Three Indispensable Rituals*, despite their apparent contradictions.

In contrast to the contrarian supplication found in the epigraph above, an homage to Drangti Penden Tsojé that is found in the very same text reaffirms

---

115 Mentions of Yutok Gönpo are absent from the colophons of all other manuscript witnesses of the *Three Indispensable Rituals* and xylographic editions of the *Eighteen Auxiliary Branches*. See, respectively, *Rtsa'i spra sgrub med thabs med pa*, in *Krung go'i bod lugs gso rig rtsa che'i dpe rnying kun btus*, vol. 10, text 5, pp. 198–99; and *Rtsa'i pra sgrub med thabs med pa*, in *Cha lag bco brgyad*, 492–94.

116 See *Dngul bre las* [sic] *drang srong ser skya'i sgrub thabs*, in *G.yu thog snying thig*, 619–23. Note that the title of these channel *prasenā* rituals found in the *Essential Nucleus of Yutok* collection explicitly pay homage to the *Silver Measure* (*dngul bre*) collection of the Drangti clan (even if it should be the *Gold Measure*!).

117 On the *Essential Nucleus of Yutok* in the seventeenth century (therein called the *Yutok Heart Essence*), see Stacey Van Vleet, "Medicine as Impartial Knowledge: The Fifth Dalai Lama, the Tsarong School, and Debates of Tibetan Medical Orthodoxy," in *The Tenth Karmapa and Tibet's Turbulent Seventeenth Century*, ed. Karl Debreczeny and Gray Tuttle (Chicago, IL: Serindia Publications, 2016), 263–91.

118 Arnaldo Momigliano, "The Rules of the Game in the Study of Ancient History," trans. Kenneth W. Yu, *History and Theory* 55 (2016): 45.

both the clairvoyance of the sages as well as diagnostic knowledge derived from observation and textual study:

> To the blessed lineage extending from the sages,
> To the mandala of texts, instructions, and knowledge,
> To he whose intellect understands objects just as they are, whose eyes are open,
> At the feet of Drangti Penden Tsojé, I pay homage.[119]

With conflicting instructions for tantric divination, empirical diagnosis, and prognosis, it is the prerogative of the physician trained in such instructions to decide how they will actually perform their practices. Indeed, the physicians of the Drangti family would have learned to palpate the wrist of a patient—haptically seeking empirical evidence of either thermal, humoral, or visceral diseases—as well as to evoke the divine revelation of the goddesses. As this genealogy has shown, although each of these methods for conceptualizing illness entails a distinct historical provenance and approach to healing, their inclusion in the same practical repertoire provides the physician with the power to choose between them. Indeed, when unresolved conflicts are embedded within the accretive repertoires of medical traditions, each performance of learned instructions is a momentary resolution of such conflicts. It is the capaciousness of diagnostic techniques in the Tibetan medical tradition—the diverse methods for observing and interpreting the body—that allows the trained physician to see, hear, and intuit the many expressions of the body, even when each of these expressions appears to contradict the others.

Acknowledgements

This research was assisted by a fellowship from The Robert H. N. Ho Family Foundation Program in Buddhist Studies administered by the American Council of Learned Societies.

119 *Reg pa rtsa'i spra sgrub klu sgrub gyis mdzad pa*, in *Krung go'i bod lugs gso rig rtsa che'i dpe rnying kun btus*, vol. 1, text 10, p. 53 (f. 1b): *drang srong brgyud pas rgyud la byin brlabs shing / lung rigs man ngag shes bya'i dkyil 'khor la/ ji bzhin rtogs pa'i blo gros spyan yangs pa/ brang sti* [=*ti*] *dpal ldan mtsho* [='*tsho*] *byed zhabs la gus phyag mtshal* [='*tshal*]//.

Bibliography

Tibetan-language Sources

A ru ra, ed. *Cha lag bco brgyad*, Bod kyi gso ba rig pa'i gna' dpe phyogs bsgrigs dpe tshogs, vol. 25. Beijing: Mi rigs dpe skrun khang, 2005.

A ru ra, ed. *G.yu thog snying thig*. Bod kyi gso ba rig pa'i gna' dpe phyogs bsgrigs dpe tshogs, vol. 43. Beijing: Mi rigs dpe skrun khang, 2007.

A ru ra, ed., *Man ngag gser bre ma dang dngul bre ma*. Bod kyi gso ba rig pa'i gna' dpe phyogs bsgrigs dpe tshogs, vol. 6. Beijing: Mi rigs dpe skrun khang, 2004.

A ru ra, ed. *Slob dpon klu sgrub kyi sman yig gces btus*. Bod kyi gso ba rig pa'i gna' dpe phyogs bsgrigs dpe tshogs, vol. 73. Beijing: Mi rigs dpe skrun khang, 2008.

A ru ra, ed. *Sman dpyad zla ba'i rgyal po*. Bod kyi gso rig pa'i gna' dpe phyogs bsgrigs dpe tshogs, vol. 33. Beijing: Mi rigs dpe skrun khang, 2005.

Bod ljongs bod lugs gso rig slob grwa chen mo, ed. *Krung go'i bod lugs gso rig rtsa che'i dpe rnying kun btus: Pho brang po ta la'i gsung rab gter mdzod las btus* [Zhongguo yiyao yingyin guji zhenben 中国藏医药影印古籍珍本; China's Traditional Tibetan Medical Texts: A Treasury of Scriptures from the Potala Palace]. Lha sa: Bod ljongs mi dmangs dpe skrun khang, 2014.

Bad kan smug po'i stong thun (vol. 14, text 5).

Grang ba'i stong thun (vol. 3, text 9).

Grang ba'i stong thun (vol. 14, text 4).

Gser khri [=*bre*] *rgyas pa zhes bya ba bzhugs so* (vol. 18, text 13).

Lag len spod chung gyi 'brel [=*'grel*] *pa* (vol. 3, text 2).

Med thabs med pa'i mchong [=*'phyong*] *gsum* (vol. 3, text 3).

Reg pa rtsa'i spra sgrub klu sgrub gyis mdzad pa bzhugs s.ho (vol. 1, text 10).

Rtsa chu'i stong thun g.yu thog gi bzhed pa (vol. 3, text 7).

Rtsa mdo'i 'grel pa nyi ma'i 'od zer (vol. 1, text 14).

Rtsa'i spra sgrub med thabs med pa (vol. 10, text 5).

Skor tshoms stong thun bcu gcig (vol. 14, text 3).

Skor tshoms stong thun bcu gcig las dang po rtsa'i stong thun (vol. 3, text 5).

Sman dpyad zla ba'i rgyal po (vol. 5, text 1).

Sman dpyad zla ba'i rgyal po (vol. 5, text 2).

Bod rang skyong ljongs sman rtsis khang, ed. *Brang ti lha rje'i rim brgyud kyi man ngag gser bre chen mo*. Lha sa: Bod ljongs mi dmangs dpe skrun khang, 2005.

Bye brag tu rtogs par byed pa. In *Bstan 'gyur dpe bsdur ma*, edited by Krung go'i bod rig pa zhib 'jug ste gnas kyi bka' bstan dpe sdur khang, *sna tshogs*, text 3590, vol. 115 (*co* [219]). Beijing: Krung go'i bod rig pa dpe skrun khang, 2006–2009.

Dpung bzangs kyis zhus pa'i rgyud kyi bsdus pa'i don. In *Bstan 'gyur dpe bsdur ma*, edited by Krung go'i bod rig pa zhib 'jug ste gnas kyi bka' bstan dpe sdur khang, *rgyud*, text

1578, vol. 36 (*thu* [71]), pp. 102–49. Beijing: Krung go'i bod rig pa dpe skrun khang, 2006–2009.

'Phags pa dpung bzang gis zhus pa zhes bya ba'i rgyud. In *Bka' 'gyur dpe bsdur ma*, edited by Krung go'i bod rig pa zhib 'jug ste gnas kyi bka' bstan dpe sdur khang, text 0835, vol. 96 (*wa*), pp. 434–508. Beijing: Krung go'i bod rig pa dpe skrun khang, 2006–2009.

'Phags pa dpung bzangs kyis zhus pa'i rgyud kyi tshig gi don bshad pa'i brjed byang. In *Bstan 'gyur dpe bsdur ma, rgyud*, text 1579, vol. 36 (*thu* [71]), pp. 150–273

'Phags pa dpung bzangs kyis zhus pa'i rgyud kyi bsdus pa'i don dgrol ba'i brjed byang. In *Bstan 'gyur dpe bsdur ma, rgyud*, text 1580, vol. 36 (*thu* [71]), pp. 274–319.

Rba bzhed phyogs bsgrigs. Beijing: Mi rigs dpe skrun khang, 2009.

Sgrol dkar skyabs. "Zla rgyal dang rgyud bzhi'i rtsa brtag thad la cung tsam bsdur te dpyad pa [Comparative Studies on Pulsology in the Texts: King of Moon and rGyu-Zhi (sic)]." *Krung go'i bod kyi gso rig* [Tibetan Medicine in China] 7, no. 3 (2008): 103–110.

European-language Sources

Bentor, Yael. "On the Symbolism of the Mirror in Indo-Tibetan Consecration Rituals." *Journal of Indian Philosophy* 23 (1995): 57–71.

Cabezón, José Ignacio. "Buddhist Studies as a Discipline and the Role of Theory." *Journal of the International Association of Buddhist Studies* 18 (1995): 231–68.

Cabezón, José Ignacio. *A Dose of Emptiness: An Annotated Translation of the sTong thun chen mo of mKhas grub dGe legs dpal bzang*. Albany, NY: State University of New York Press, 1992.

Cantwell, Cathy, and Robert Mayer. *Early Tibetan Documents on Phur pa from Dunhuang*. Wien: Verlag der Österreichischen Akademie der Wissenchaften, 2008.

Campany, Robert F. "On the Very Idea of Religions (In the Modern West and in Early Medieval China)." *History of Religions* 42, no. 4 (2003): 287–319.

Chen Ming. "The Transmission of Indian Ayurvedic Doctrines in Medieval China: A Case Study of *Aṣṭāṅga* and *Tridoṣa* Fragments from the Silk Road." *Annual Report of The International Research Institute for Advanced Buddhology at Soka University* 9 (2006): 201–30.

Cornu, Philippe. *Tibetan Astrology*. Boston, MA: Shambhala, 2002.

Dalton, Jacob. *The Gathering of Intentions: A History of a Tibetan Tantra*. New York, NY: Columbia University Press, 2016.

Dalton, Jacob. "How Dhāraṇīs WERE Proto-Tantric: Liturgies, Ritual Manuals, and the Origins of the Tantras." In *Tantric Traditions in Transmission and Translation*, edited by David B. Gray and Ryan Richard Overbey, 199–229. Oxford: Oxford University Press, 2016.

Dalton, Jacob, and Sam van Schaik, eds. *Tibetan Tantric Manuscripts from Dunhuang: A Descriptive Catalogue of the Stein Collection at the British Library*. Leiden: Brill, 2006.

Davidson, Ronald M. *Indian Esoteric Buddhism: A Social History of the Tantric Movement*. New York, NY: Columbia University Press, 2002.

Davidson, Ronald M. *Tibetan Renaissance: Tantric Buddhism in the Rebirth of Tibetan Culture*. New York, NY: Columbia University Press, 2005.

Diemberger, Hildegard. "Female Oracles in Modern Tibet." In *Women in Tibet*, edited by Janet Gyatso and Hanna Havnevik, 113–68. New York, NY: Columbia University Press, 2005.

Diemberger, Hildegard. "Padmasambhava's Unfinished Job: The Subjugation of Local Deities as Described in the *dBa' bzhed* in Light of Contemporary Practices of Spirit Possession." In *Pramāṇakīrtiḥ: Papers Dedicated to Ernst Steinkellner on the Occasion of his 70th Birthday*, edited by Birgit Kellner et al., 85–93. Vienna: Arbeitskreis für Tibetische und Buddhistische studien Universität Wien, 2007.

Dreyfus, Georges. *The Sound of Two Hands Clapping: The Education of a Tibetan Buddhist Monk*. Berkeley, CA: University of California Press, 2003.

Emmerick, R. E. "Some Remarks on Tibetan Sphygmology." In *Medical Literature Form India, Sri Lanka and Tibet*, edited by G. Jan Meulenbeld, 66–71. Leiden: Brill, 1991.

Foucault, Michel. "Nietzsche, Genealogy, History." In *Language, Counter-Memory, Practice: Selected Essays and Interviews*, translated by Donald F. Bouchard and Sherry Simon, and edited by Donald F. Bouchard, 139–64. Ithaca, NY: Cornell University Press, 1977.

Giebel, Rolf W. "A Śaiva Text in Chinese Garb? An Annotated Translation of the *Suji liyan Moxishouluo tian shuo aweishe fa*." In *Esoteric Buddhism in Mediaeval Maritime Asia: Networks of Masters, Texts, Icons*, edited by Andrea Acri, 381–88. Singapore: ISEAS Publishing, 2016.

Gyatso, Janet. "The Authority of Empiricism and the Empiricism of Authority: Medicine and Buddhism in Tibet on the Eve of Modernity." *Comparative Studies of South Asia, Africa and the Middle East* 24, no. 2 (2004): 83–96.

Gyatso, Janet. *Being Human in a Buddhist World: An Intellectual History of Medicine in Early Modern Tibet*. New York, NY: Columbia University Press, 2015.

Gyatso, Janet. "Experience, Empiricism and the Fortunes of Authority: Tibetan Medicine and Buddhism on the Eve of Modernity." In the *Tibetan History Reader*, edited by Gray Tuttle and Kurtis R. Schaeffer, 363–85. New York, NY: Columbia University Press, 2013.

Halbertal, Moshe. *People of the Book: Canon, Meaning, and Authority*. Cambridge, MA: Harvard University Press, 1997.

Halkias, Georgios T. "Tibetan Buddhism Registered: A Catalogue from the Imperial Court of 'Phang Thang." *The Eastern Buddhist* 36, nos. 1–2 (2004): 46–105.

Herrmann-Pfandt, Adelheid, ed. *Die Lhan Kar Ma: Ein früher Katalog der in Tibetische übersetzten buddhistischen Texte*. Wien: Verlag der Österreichischen Akademie der Wissenschaften, 2008.

Hodge, Stephen. *The Maha-Vairocana-Abhisambodhi Tantra: With Buddhaguhya's Commentary*. New York, NY: Routledge, 2003.

Hsu, Elisabeth. "A Hybrid Body Technique: Does the Pulse Diagnostic *cun guan chi* Method Have Chinese-Tibetan Origins?" *Gesnerus* 65, nos. 1–2 (2008): 5–29

Hsu, Elisabeth. "Le diagnostic du pouls dans la chine mediévale d'apres les manuscrits de Dunhuang (with notes on P2115, P3106, P3287, P3477, P3481, P3655, P4093, S79, S181, S202, S5614, S6245, S8289, plus index)." In *Médecine, religion et société dans la Chine médiévale : Étude de manuscrits chinois de Dunhuang et de Turfan*, edited by C. Despeux, book 1, pp. 107–84. Paris: College de France, Institut des Haute Etudes Chinoises, 2010.

Ishikawa, Mie. *A Critical Edition of the Sgra sbyor bam po gnyis pa, An Old and Basic Commentary on the Mahāvyutpatti*. Studia Tibetica 18. Tokyo: Toyo Bunko, 1990.

Kapstein, Matthew T. *The Tibetan Assimilation of Buddhism: Conversion, Contestation, and Memory*. Oxford: Oxford University Press, 2000.

Kleinman, Arthur. *The Illness Narratives: Suffering, Healing and the Human Condition*. New York, NY: Basic Books, 1988.

Kuriyama, Shigehisa. *The Expressiveness of the Body and the Divergence of Greek and Chinese Medicine*. New York, NY: Zone Books, 1999).

Martin, Dan. "Greek and Islamic Medicines' Historical Contact with Tibet: A Reassessment in View of Recently Available but Relatively Early Sources on Tibetan Medical Eclecticism." In *Islam and Tibet: Interactions along the Musk Routes*, edited by Anna Akasoy, Charles Burnett, and Ronit Yoeli-Tlalim. Burlington, VT: Ashgate, 2011.

McGrath, William A. "Origin Narratives of the Tibetan Medical Tradition: History, Legend, and Myth." *Asian Medicine* 12, nos. 1–2 (2017): 295–316.

McGrath, William A. "Vessel Examination in the *Medicine of the Moon King*." In *Buddhism and Medicine: An Anthology of Premodern Sources*, edited by C. Pierce Salguero, 501–513. New York, NY: Columbia University Press, 2017.

Momigliano, Arnaldo. "The Rules of the Game in the Study of Ancient History." Translated by Kenneth W. Yu. *History and Theory* 55 (2016): 39–45.

Nanjio, Bunyiu. *A Catalogue of the Chinese Translation of the Buddhist Tripitaka: The Sacred Canon of the Buddhists in China and Japan*. Oxford: Clarendon Press, 1883.

Orofino, Giacomella. "Divination with Mirrors: Observations on a Simile Found in the Kālacakra Literature." In *Tibetan Studies: Proceedings of the 6th Seminar of the International Association for Tibetan Studies, Fagernes 1992*, edited by Per Kværne, 612–28. Oslo: Institute for Comparative Research in Human Culture, 1994.

Orzech, Charles D. "The 'Great Teaching of Yoga' the Chinese Appropriation of the Tantras, and the Question of Esoteric Buddhism." *Journal of Chinese Religions* 34 (2006): 29–78.

Orzech, Charles D. "Translation of Tantras and Other Esoteric Buddhist Scriptures." In *Esoteric Buddhism and the Tantras in East Asia*, edited by Charles D. Orzech, Henrik H. Sørensen, and Richard K. Payne, 439–50. Leiden: Brill, 2011.

Parfionovitch, Yuri, Feranand Meyer, and Gyurme Dorje, eds. *Tibetan Medical Paintings: Illustrations to the Blue Beryl Treatise of Sangye Gyamtso (1653–1705)*. New York, NY: Harry N. Abrams, 1992. 2 vols.

Pasang Wangdu and Hildegard Diemberger, trans. *Dba' bzhed: The Royal Narrative Concerning the Bringing of the Buddha's Doctrine to Tibet*. Wien: Österreichischen Akademie der Wissenschaften, 2000.

Pollock, Sheldon. "The Cosmopolitan Vernacular." *The Journal of Asian Studies* 51, no. 1 (1998): 6–37.

Pollock, Sheldon. *The Language of the Gods in the World of Men: Sanskrit, Culture, and Power in Premodern India*. Berkeley, CA: University of California Press, 2006.

Sanderson, Alexis. "Vajrayāna: Origin and Function." In *Buddhism: Critical Concepts in Religious Studies*, ed. Paul Williams, vol. 6, 392–408. New York, NY: Routledge 2005.

Schaeffer, Kurtis R. "Textual Scholarship, Medical Tradition, and Mahāyāna Buddhist Ideals in Tibet." *Journal of Indian Philosophy* 31 (2003): 621–41.

Sen, Tansen. "The Revival and Failure of Buddhist Translations During the Song Dynasty." *T'oung Pao* 88 (2002): 27–80.

Shils, Edward. *Tradition*. Chicago, IL: University of Chicago Press, 1981.

Slouber, Michael. *Early Tantric Medicine: Snakebite, Mantras, and Healing in the Gāruḍa Tantras*. Oxford: Oxford University Press, 2017.

Smith, Frederick M. *The Self Possessed: Deity and Spirit Possession in South Asian Literature and Civilization*. New York, NY: Columbia University Press, 2006.

Sørensen, Per K. *Tibetan Buddhist Historiography: The Mirror Illuminating the Royal Genealogies, an Annotated Translation of the XIVth Century Tibetan Chronicle: rGyal-rabs gsal-ba'i me-long*. Wiesbaden: Harrassowitz Verlag, 1994.

Strickmann, Michel. *Chinese Magical Medicine*, edited by Bernard Faure. Stanford, CA: Stanford University Press, 2002.

Unschuld, Paul. *Huang Di nei jing su wen: Nature, Knowledge, Imagery in an Ancient Chinese Medical Text*. Berkeley, CA: University of California Press, 2003.

van Schaik, Sam. "A Tibetan Book of Spells." *Early Tibet*. 19 February 2009. <earlytibet.com/2009/02/19/a-tibetan-book-of-spells/>.

Van Vleet, Stacey. "Medicine as Impartial Knowledge: The Fifth Dalai Lama, the Tsarong School, and Debates of Tibetan Medical Orthodoxy." In *The Tenth Karmapa and*

Tibet's Turbulent Seventeenth Century, edited by Karl Debreczeny and Gray Tuttle, 263–91. Chicago, IL: Serindia Publications, 2016.

Yang Ga. *Sources for the Writing of the Rgyud bzhi.* Cambridge, MA: Harvard University Doctoral Dissertation, 2010.

Zhen Yan. "*rTsa* in the Tibetan Manuscripts from Dunhuang." Translated by Vivienne Lo. *Asian Medicine* 3 (2007): 296–307.

Zhen Yan and Cai Jingfeng. "Tibetan and Chinese Pulse Diagnostics: A Comparison—With Special Reference to Locations for Pulse Taking." In *Soundings in Tibetan Medicine: Anthropological and Historical Perspectives. Proceedings of the 10th Seminar of the International Association of Tibetan Studies*, edited by Mona Schrempf, 327–43. Leiden: Brill, 2007.

CHAPTER 9

Madness and the Spirits: Examining the Role of Spirits in Mental Illness in the Tibetan Communities of Darjeeling

Susannah Deane

1 Introduction

There are several ways in which spirits may be involved in mental illness in ethnically Tibetan contexts,[1] some of which are described in the seminal Tibetan medical text, the *Four Tantras* (*rgyud bzhi*), and others of which we find included in contemporary Tibetan discourses about mental health and illness. Afflictions may or may not involve possession, and may involve one or more of a diverse array of spirits and/or deities, with conditions ranging from afflictions related to "spirits that cause madness" (*smyo byed kyi gdon*), to periods of "madness" (*smyo nad*) preceding an individual's recognition as a spirit-medium. Such explanations highlight the fundamental role which spirits and deities play in everyday life for many Tibetans, and in Darjeeling, northeast India, where I conducted research exploring Tibetan approaches to mental health, illness, and healing. A diverse array of non-human entities was discussed by Tibetan informants, particularly in relation to certain forms of mental illness. Here, spirit-related explanations of health and illness often sat alongside Tibetan medical and biomedical explanatory frameworks in an area home to a diversity of medical and healing facilities, including biomedical clinics and hospitals, Ayurvedic clinics, and Tibetan Sowa Rigpa medical clinics.[2] However, what was evident during my time here, was that in cases of suspected spirit-caused illness, many people

---

1 I use the term "ethnically Tibetan contexts" to refer to Tibetan cultural areas of the Himalayan region, stretching from Ladakh in northwest India, across the contested border with the People's Republic of China (PRC) and Chinese-controlled Tibet, to Bhutan in the east and Nepal in the south.

2 In Darjeeling there were two Tibetan Sowa Rigpa medical clinics: the Chagpori Tibetan Medical Institute (CTMI; http://chagpori.org) clinic, and the Darjeeling branch clinic of the Tibetan government-in-exile-affiliated Men-Tsee-Khang (MTK). These "branch clinics" of the MTK Tibetan Medical and Astrological Institute are administered and funded by the Tibetan Department of Health in Dharamsala. Today there are approximately fifty branch clinics across India staffed by both lay and monastic, male and female practitioners—a list of these can be found on the MTK website: http://www.men-tsee-khang.org/branch/main.htm.

 | DOI:10.1163/9789004404441_010

described *religious* practitioners—monks, Tibetan or Nepali spirit-mediums (*lha pa* and *jhānkri/mataji*, respectively), and/or *ngakpas* (*sngags pa*; "mantra healers")—as the most appropriate practitioners to consult for such afflictions.

In this article, I will explore some Tibetan perspectives on the role of spirits and deities in different forms of "mental illness"—usually referred to in Tibetan as "*semné*" (*sems nad*, "illness of the mind"). In doing so, I will demonstrate how such understandings reflect broader Tibetan notions about the place of spirits in society, and the relationships between these non-human entities, lay Tibetans, religious specialists, and medical practitioners. A picture will emerge of the continuing importance of such non-human entities in contemporary Tibetan communities, and the discourses and health-seeking behaviours which may arise when such narratives sit alongside a plethora of diverse explanatory frameworks within a medically- and culturally-pluralistic community. I will first describe two narratives of spirit-caused mental illness which I encountered in Darjeeling,[3] where I conducted ethnographic fieldwork as part of my doctoral research project in 2011 and 2012.[4] I will then turn to examine some Tibetan perspectives on spirits and deities more broadly, delineating descriptions of spirit affliction in the main medical text, the *Four Tantras* (*rgyud bzhi*), and the perspectives of Tibetan medical practitioners, known as *amchi* (*am chi*).

Darjeeling is home to a sizeable Tibetan exile community, residing both within the town itself and at the Tibetan Refugee Self-Help Centre (TRSHC), a two-mile walk from the Darjeeling town square. However, the population of around four to five thousand first-, second-, and third-generation exiles[5] lives within a culturally- and medically-pluralistic area, home to the majority Nepali

3 All names and identifying details of informants—other than those specialists interviewed in their official capacity—and those described by them have been changed to protect anonymity.

4 This research—part-funded by Cardiff University School of History, Archaeology and Religion, and for which the fieldwork was kindly funded by grants from Cardiff University School of History, Archaeology and Religion, and Body, Health and Religion Research Group (BAHAR), and the Wellcome Trust—was completed in 2015 and is described in more detail elsewhere (see Susannah Deane, *Tibetan Medicine, Buddhism and Psychiatry: Mental Health and Healing in a Tibetan Exile Community* [Durham, NC: Carolina Academic Press, 2018]).

5 This figure was estimated by the Tibetan Settlement Office accountant, Tsering Dhondup, while I was there in 2011, with the caveat that it was difficult to give any kind of definitive figure due to the significant number of Tibetans working and studying outside of the area. In 1998, a demographic survey of Tibetans in India and Nepal conducted by the Central Tibetan Administration (CTA) counted 2,455 Tibetans living in Darjeeling (Barbara Gerke, *Long Lives and Untimely Deaths: Life-span Concepts and Longevity Practices among Tibetans in the Darjeeling Hills, India* [Leiden: Brill, 2012], 56–57).

and Indian populations in a town spread across the steep hillside. As a result of this plurality, individuals have access to a broad range of explanatory models of illness, and I interviewed lay Tibetans alongside medical and religious specialists, examining a number of different mental health diagnoses, aetiologies, and treatments. Here, however, I will focus my attention on conditions related to the action of spirits and deities—usually referred to as *dön* (*gdon*) and *lha* respectively—entities which may be implicated in a range of psychiatric diagnoses, and which were discussed quite frequently in Darjeeling.

We find spirit-caused illnesses included in the Tibetan Sowa Rigpa medical tradition which, despite its Tibetan history, was officially legalized and recognized by the Indian government as a "system of Indian medicine" (alongside Ayurveda, Siddha, Yoga, Unani, Naturopathy, and Homeopathy) in 2010, affording it a certain amount of protection and availability across India.[6] In fact, the term "Sowa Rigpa" (*gso ba rig pa*; lit. "knowledge/science of healing") refers to a number of diverse healing traditions and practices across ethnically Tibetan areas in the Himalayan region and beyond. Known in different regions as "Tibetan medicine," *Bömen* (*bod sman*; lit. "Tibetan medicine"), "*amchi* medicine," "Mongolian medicine," and "Buddhist medicine," practices often vary significantly between the different regions of the Tibetan cultural context.[7] However, across these related traditions, the four-volume, twelfth-century *Four Tantras* medical text is often held up as the "root" medical text,[8] used in teaching across the Tibetan plateau.[9] Perhaps unsurprisingly then, much of the previous research on health, illness, and medicine in Tibetan contexts has tended to focus on this text,[10] and its description of the three *nyepa* (*nyes pa*, "factors" or "humors") of *loong* (*rlung*, "wind"), *tripa* (*mkhris*

6 See the Government of India's Ministry of Ayurveda, Yoga and Naturopathy, Unani, Siddha and Homeopathy (AYUSH, previously known as the Department of Indian System of Medicine and Homeopathy [ISM&H]) website for more on this: ayush.gov.in.

7 Stephan Kloos, *Tibetan Medicine in Exile: The Ethics, Politics and Science of Cultural Survival* (Berkeley, CA: PhD Dissertation, University of California, Berkeley, 2010), 16.

8 The full title of this text is often given as *Bdud rtsi snying po yan lag brgyad pa gsang ba man ngag gi rgyud*, although in practice the title varies somewhat between different editions. See Janet Gyatso's *Being Human in a Buddhist World: An Intellectual History of Medicine in Early Modern Tibet* (New York, NY: Columbia University Press, 2015) for a very comprehensive exploration of the development of medical theory in Tibet in the twelfth to eighteenth centuries.

9 Yang Ga, *The Sources for the Writing of the Rgyud bZhi, Tibetan Medical Classic* (Cambridge, MA: PhD dissertation, Harvard University, 2010), 1–2.

10 See, for example, work by Barry Clark, trans., *The Quintessence Tantras of Tibetan Medicine* (Ithaca, NY: Snow Lion Publications, 1995); and Ferdinand Meyer "The History and Foundations of Tibetan Medicine," in *The Buddha's Art of Healing: Tibetan Paintings Rediscovered*, ed. by John Avedon (New York, NY: Rizzoli, 1998), 21–31.

pa, "bile"), and *béken* (*bad kan*, "phlegm"),[11] which form much of the basis of the Sowa Rigpa understanding of physiology.[12] In particular, there has been much attention paid to the wind "current" by researchers examining mental illness in this context—in both textual and ethnographic studies. In fact, any one of these three *nyepa* can be related to mental and/or physical illness, but it is the wind which is most often linked to *mental* illness, due to the close relationship it is understood to have with consciousness.[13] Indeed, it is often said that the mind rides on the wind as a man rides a horse,[14] meaning that any "disturbance" in the various wind "currents" or the channels (*rtsa*) in which they reside can lead to symptoms such as dizziness, anger, sadness, confusion, or insomnia. Conditions related to wind disturbances include those likened to biomedical categories of "depression" and "anxiety"—a comparison drawn by both Tibetan and non-Tibetan practitioners and researchers.[15] In fact, the term

11 See Chapter One of this volume for an exploration of "brown phlegm" and its relation to Greek medical conceptions of melancholia: Henk Blezer, "A New Sense of (Dark) Humor in Tibet: Brown Phlegm and Black Bile," in the present volume.

12 These three bodily "humors" of wind, bile, and phlegm are integral to both Tibetan and Ayurvedic medical theory. However, whilst the Tibetan term *nyes pa* is a direct translation of the Sanskrit *doṣa*, and is usually translated into English as "humor," there are significant problems with this translation. *Nyes pa* actually translates literally into the English terms "fault" or "weakness" (Geoffrey Samuel "Tibetan Medicine in Contemporary India: Theory and Practice," in *Healing Powers and Modernity: Traditional Medicine, Shamanism, and Science in Asian Studies*, ed. Linda H. Connor and Geoffrey Samuel [Westport and London: Bergin and Garvey, 2001], 247–68, 255), and has more recently been translated as "defective energies" by some *amchi* (Kloos, *Tibetan Medicine in Exile*, 17, n. 20).

13 Indeed, Amchi Sonam Dolma (at that time head of the MTK Translation Department in Dharamsala), whom I interviewed in August 2012, suggested that, "the principle cause of all mental problems is *rlung*. And then along with the *rlung* … there could be other associating factors, like, there could also be *mkhris pa*, there could be *bad kan*." For an overview of the role of *rlung* in mental health and illness, see Mark Epstein and Sonam Topgay, "Mind and Mental Disorders in Tibetan Medicine," *ReVision: A Journal of Consciousness and Change* 9 no. 1 (1982): 67–79.

14 Colin Millard, "Tibetan Medicine and the Classification and Treatment of Mental Illness," in *Soundings in Tibetan Medicine: Historical and Anthropological Perspectives*, ed. Mona Schrempf (Leiden: Brill, 2007), 265–66. In fact, others go further, describing the mind as a *lame* rider on the *blind* horse of the winds. Wangyal explains, "[w]ithout the mind, the *prana* [wind] has no direction. Without the *prana*, the mind has no capacity to move. They function as a unity" (Tenzin Wangyal and Mark Dahlby, *Healing with Form, Energy and Light: The Five Elements in Tibetan Shamanism, Tantra, and Dzogchen* [Ithaca, NY: Snow Lion Publications, 2002], 82). See also Tsering Thakchoe Drungtso, *Tibetan Medicine: The Healing Science of Tibet* (Dharamsala: Drungtso Publications, 2004), 88.

15 See, for example, Pema Dorjee, *The Spiritual Medicine of Tibet: Heal Your Spirit, Heal Yourself* (London: Watkins Publishing, 2005), 167; Eric Emil Jacobson, "Panic Attack in a Context of Comorbid Anxiety and Depression in a Tibetan Refugee," *Culture, Medicine*

"wind" itself is often used alone to denote conditions related to its disturbance, heard in expressions such as "She has high wind today," indicating a high level of anxiety and/or worry. Treatment for such conditions often starts with the consultation of a Sowa Rigpa practitioner who will likely prescribe appropriate herbal medicines, and perhaps also some form of physical therapy (such as massage, moxibustion, or cupping), depending on his/her medical skills and experience.

However, in Darjeeling it was apparent that in narratives of more severe cases of mental illness—particularly those where a patient may be described as suffering from "madness"—*nyoné* (*smyo nad*; usually translated as "madness" or "psychosis")—there was actually often far less focus on the role of wind (or either of the other *nyepa*), or even the role of Sowa Rigpa as a whole, in terms of diagnosis and treatment. Here, I encountered a variety of explanations of causation, such as those related to certain behaviours or emotions including "worry," "stress," and particular religious behaviours perceived to be problematic,[16] but a number of conditions were attributed to the action of one or more spirits or deities, either through possession or non-possession afflictions. Here, treatment was often seen to predominantly come under the jurisdiction of a religious specialist of some kind. Indeed, many informants described such practitioners as the best individuals to deal with these afflictions. What became clear, however, was that these specialists were not necessarily accessible for many and, in reality, other practitioners—such as biomedical doctors—were sometimes consulted by patients and their families. The narratives below thus highlight two facets of life in contemporary Darjeeling: the salience of long-standing perceptions about spirits and their relationships to humans through the notion of "spiritual power"—ideas fundamental not only in the sphere of health and illness, but also foundational to many Tibetan conceptions of the world—and the lack of Tibetan spirit-mediums now in the area—a topic raised by many of my informants.

---

and Psychiatry 26, no. 2 (2002): 259–79; Eric Emil Jacobson, "Life-wind Illness in Tibetan Medicine: Depression, Generalised Anxiety, and Panic Attack," in *Soundings in Tibetan medicine: Historical and Anthropological Perspectives*, ed. Mona Schrempf (Leiden: Brill, 2007), 225–46.

16 Susannah Deane, "Madness in a Tibetan Context: A Comparison of Tibetan Textual and Lay Perceptions of '*smyo nad*' (Madness) among Tibetans Living in North India," *PJMH: The Postgraduate Journal of Medical Humanities* 1 (2014): 24–49.

2 Lhakpa

One of the people I got to know quite well during my time in Darjeeling was Lhamo, a forty-five-year-old second-generation Tibetan exile who worked as a biomedical nurse in Darjeeling town. In one of our discussions about mental health and illness, Lhamo related the story of Lhakpa, a young woman and first-generation exile of twenty-six, whom she knew from the TRSHC. Lhakpa, Lhamo told me, had been very ill around two years previously, becoming afflicted by a spirit not long after arriving in India from Tibet. Fluent in English, Lhamo described Lhakpa's condition as she remembered it as follows:

> [Lhakpa] came down to the toilet.... She felt giddiness ... and she fell outside the toilet.... Then everyone helped her up [but] she was not herself, she was completely strange.... She felt something black closing over her ... then maybe she lost consciousness.... Then, all of a sudden, she became conscious, and then she started speaking whatnot [nonsensical things].... [We thought that] maybe a spirit might have got her.... We [took her to and] kept her in the hospital [in Darjeeling]—they said she might have some problem with her brain and all, [but] medicine's not working.... Then we took her down to Siliguri.[17] In the hospital the same thing ... she became very violent and all. This was a *dön* [spirit] or something ... *shindré* [spirit/ghost] or something.

I heard several similar descriptions of possession by *dön* in Darjeeling, with a combination of psychological and physical symptoms, unusual behaviour, and garbled speech described. Lhamo proceeded to recount what had happened when Lhakpa's childhood friend, a young monk of around the same age from a local Tibetan Buddhist Sakya monastery, had come to try and help her while she was in hospital, conducting rituals in an attempt to control the spirit. She described how the young monk came and did some "*puja*" [Skt. *pūjā*, "ritual"], explaining that, "We have different lamas.... The ordinary lama cannot do *all* the *pujas*. You need special powers to do that." However, because of his concern for his friend, "maybe he wanted to do it himself." Lhamo described how Lhakpa had recovered after a few days, but the monk himself had died: "He did

17 This city, three to four hours' drive south of Darjeeling, was home to several large hospitals, described to me by many lay Tibetans in Darjeeling as significantly superior to those in Darjeeling.

some sacrifice ... maybe the spirit was stronger than him.... he had to give up his life."

Thus Lhamo's narrative described how, whilst Lhakpa's spirit affliction had been successfully treated by her friend's rituals, due to his lack of experience and low level of "spiritual power" (*dbang thang*), this young lama had been unable to sufficiently control the offending spirit, and he had died as a result of his interaction with it. Whilst Lhakpa's condition was now said to be good, with no further episodes, Lhamo noted that some people unfortunately blamed Lhakpa for her young friend's death.

Lhamo's narrative illustrates a number of key concepts which recurred in many of the discussions I had about spirits and mental illness in Darjeeling. The main focus of this narrative is of course the spirit cause of the affliction, and the differing levels of spiritual "power" of the individuals involved. Indeed, in discussions on mental illness in Darjeeling, a number of Tibetan informants talked of *dön* ("spirit") or *shindré* ("spirit," "ghost") possession, relating cases they had seen, or stories they had heard about others in the community. This was particularly the case when I asked questions about "madness." For example, Tsering (59 years old) explained that "some [*shindré*] are very powerful" and may enter a person's consciousness, leading them to become "mad," suicidal, and/or violent. He told me that such "madness" initially comes and goes, saying that those afflicted should go to a lama or Tibetan spirit-medium (*lha pa*) for treatment. And when I discussed this topic with Jampa (25 years old), a young monk from Dali Gönpa, he described how the possessing spirit might start to talk through the affected person (indicted by a change in the sound of the voice and/or the topic[s] of conversation), and he/she may become unusually aggressive, perhaps throwing objects and/or behaving abnormally in some other way. Such recurring "episodes," Jampa explained, tend to be intermittent, usually lasting fifteen to thirty minutes, with the person affected having no memory of the episode afterwards.

Evident in Lhamo's narrative is the importance placed on "spiritual power," described here by Lhamo as "special powers," and referencing the hierarchy of spiritual power inherent in Tibetan Buddhist notions of the relationships between humans and spirits/deities. Indeed, there is a clear illustration here of the "power" of the spirit involved—greater than that of a lay person (hence its ability to affect Lhakpa), but also greater than that of a young lama. Thus the "inexperienced" lama's spiritual power is described as strong enough to subdue the spirit and help—or, indeed, cure—his friend, but unfortunately *not* powerful enough to completely overpower the spirit, tragically leading, we are told, to his own death. This is a clear illustration, then, of the dangers posed by even "low-level" spirits such as *dön* and *shindré* (i.e. spirits understood to have a low level of spiritual power, as compared to more powerful local deities such as *gyelpo* or *tsen*)—entities which can pose a danger to all but the most experienced of monastic practitioners and spirit-mediums.

As Lhamo described this case, there was no suggestion that any Sowa Rigpa practitioner was consulted in this instance—indeed, Lhamo explained to me that for cases of spirit affliction, "the only option is [to visit] a lama." However, as we read here, Lhakpa was in fact initially taken to biomedical practitioners, and when these interventions did not help her, then it seems that religious intervention was conducted. In fact, we do not know from Lhamo's narrative whether Lhakpa's condition was immediately understood to have a spirit cause, or whether the very failure of the biomedical treatment suggested this to her family. However, this course of events perhaps hints at some general perspectives on "western" and "traditional" medicine which I encountered in Darjeeling. Here, I often heard biomedicine described by Tibetan informants as good for "treating the symptoms" of an illness. This, I was told on several occasions, contrasts with Sowa Rigpa, which is said to "cut the roots of disease."[18] In addition, biomedicine is also often said to work quickly, and therefore frequently said to be useful for "acute" conditions (such as medical emergencies), with Sowa Rigpa preferable for "chronic" conditions. Reading Lhamo's description of Lhakpa's illness then, perhaps we should not be surprised by the initial resort to biomedicine; such an episode was likely very distressing—and perhaps frightening—for her and her family. In such a situation, treatment expected to manage or "calm down" Lhakpa's severe symptoms might in fact be an obvious resort.

3 Mikmar

The second narrative of spirit-caused mental illness I will describe here is the case of a young man of nineteen named Mikmar, described to me by Sönam (21 years old), a second-generation Tibetan exile and student at a local college, who was a neighbor of Mikmar's and was fluent in English. In a general

18 The delineation of "traditional" versus "western" medicine in Tibetan contexts in this way has also been reported by others (see, for example, Geoffrey Samuel in Dalhousie, "Religion, Health and Suffering Among Contemporary Tibetans," in *Religion, Health and Suffering*, ed. John R. Hinnells and Roy Porter [Abingdon and New York: Routledge, 2009], 85–110; Jurme Wangda, *Health Seeking Behaviours of Tibetan Refugee Community in Dharamsala, India* [Kingston, ON: MSc dissertation, Queen's University, 1996]).

discussion about mental health and illness, Sönam mentioned Mikmar, initially describing him as having become “a little crazy” around two years previously. He related how Mikmar had apparently stopped sleeping, had begun singing and crying all day and night, and had started behaving very unlike himself, including being unusually verbally abusive, arguing with classmates, and occasionally even becoming violent, throwing things inside his house. Sönam described how Mikmar had started to wear large numbers of prayer beads around his neck, day and night. Moreover, he had apparently started to dance every time he heard any drumming and, on one occasion, Mikmar had apparently suddenly started doing *'cham* (Tibetan masked religious dance, usually practised only by monks).

Mikmar's family had taken him to a biomedical psychiatrist who had prescribed medication which, Sönam explained, had helped significantly. However, not long after, Mikmar had stopped taking this on the advice of a local Nepali spirit-medium (*jhānkri*), leading, Sönam said, to a recurrence of his symptoms. Mikmar's family then took him to a high-level Tibetan Buddhist lama in Kurseong (a few hours' drive away), who conducted blessings and a ritual, leading to some limited improvement in his condition. However, Mikmar was still not himself, and another *jhānkri* consulted by his family explained that the problems were the result of a spirit affliction, with a particular spirit having taken a “liking” to him. Sönam explained that after the *jhānkri* had performed the appropriate rituals, Mikmar was (and remained) “90% better.”

Here again we hear that the family of the afflicted individual consulted both biomedical and religious practitioners—both Tibetan Buddhist and Nepali Hindu—but *not* Sowa Rigpa practitioners. In addition, this narrative of Mikmar's condition highlights some difficulties which may arise when dealing with multiple healing modalities in a culturally- and medically-pluralistic context such as this, each with its own explanatory framework and treatment strategies. Here, we hear that Mikmar received conflicting advice from different practitioners, which led him to cease one treatment, which was apparently working to at least some extent. For patients and their families such conflicts may further complicate an already difficult and often distressing situation, as they attempt to navigate a path through the various explanatory models and their suggested treatments.

It is interesting to note that Mikmar and his family consulted two Nepali spirit-mediums for assistance. This highlights a fundamental aspect of life in contemporary Darjeeling: whilst many of my Tibetan informants told me that the best practitioner to consult in cases of spirit affliction was a Tibetan spirit-medium, the reality in 2011 and 2012 was that there were in fact no longer any Tibetan spirit-mediums in the area, the last known practitioner (residing in

Mirik, around two hours' drive away) having passed away a few years previously. There were, however, a number of Nepali spirit-mediums in the area, some of whom were particularly well-regarded and held regular rituals for spirit afflictions. Under such circumstances, several of the Tibetans I spoke to expressed the view that Nepali spirit-mediums could be consulted in such cases. Others, however, argued that as the majority of these Nepali practitioners are "Hindu," they would be unlikely to be able to help in Tibetan cases of spirit affliction.

The two narratives I have described above echo the views of many of the Tibetans I interviewed in Darjeeling. In discussing "madness" in particular, spirit affliction was often mentioned, and the consultation of religious practitioners was frequently described as preferable. Such narratives highlight the salience of long-standing Tibetan notions of spirits and their continued place in Tibetan society. Indeed, in Darjeeling, many people described encounters with spirits and/or deities, and the Tibetan Buddhist understandings of "spiritual power" referenced above are fundamental to understanding these explanations. Next, I will give a brief overview of this notion of "spiritual power" in relation to these entities, before turning to examine their role in illness causation.

4 Spirits and Deities in Tibetan Life

Descriptions of the wide variety of non-human entities of the Tibetan pantheon differ within both Tibetan and non-Tibetan works, where we find descriptions of entities ranging from powerful protective deities down to local spirits residing in water courses, trees, and mountaintops.[19] Whilst these entities are frequently "categorized" into different groups, as Samuel has argued, the boundaries between the different categories is not entirely clear-cut.[20] What is important to note, however, is that these kinds of spirits and deities are *unenlightened*: as "worldly" beings, they are subject to worldly emotions (such as

19 One of the first English-language accounts of Tibetan spirits and deities was Réne de Nebesky-Wojkowitz's *Oracles and Demons of Tibet* (The Hague: Mouton, 1956). More recent research has examined these entities in more detail (see, for example, Anne-Marie Blondeau, ed., *Tibetan Mountain Dities, Their Cults and Representations: Papers Presented at a Panel of the 7th Seminar of the International Association for Tibetan Studies, Graz, 1995* [Graz: Austrian Academy of Sciences Press, 1998]).

20 Geoffrey Samuel, *Civilized Shamans: Buddhism in Tibetan Societies* (Washington, DC: Smithsonian Institution Press, 1993), 166–67.

anger, jealousy, and pride), just as humans are. Thus, as Calkowski notes, much like humans, these spirits and deities may be both "easily offended and readily appeased."[21] Indeed, some deities are even well-known for their arrogance and pride—particularly the class of spirits known as *gyelpo* (*rgyal po*)—and may even be wrathful in nature.

These non-human entities may interfere in humans' lives in numerous ways: for example, causing misfortune or illness, affecting the weather, or sometimes, protecting humans against harm from other (less powerful) spirits. However, bearing in mind their rather unpredictable "worldly" nature, it is wise to take a certain amount of care when dealing with them. People will often make offerings to shrines associated with particular local deities, and frequently take care not to pollute or damage the natural environment in which spirits are understood to live (for example, advising children not to urinate into a water course, or avoiding unnecessary tree felling when constructing a new building). In addition, as I have described in more detail elsewhere, spirits' ability to harm humans is also sometimes ascribed to factors such as the "relationship" or "connection" (*'drel ba*) between them, or humans' "faith" (*dad pa*) or "belief" (*yid ches*) in the entity involved.[22] However, there is a significant difference between the manner in which lay Tibetans and experienced religious practitioners deal with these entities, due to the differential levels of "spiritual power," which different individuals are understood to hold (or at least, *have access to*, due to their Buddhist practice). Indeed, there is a clear hierarchy in terms of power between humans and spirits/deities, a concept underscored by a key Tibetan narrative about the history of Tibet and the role of Buddhism in shaping its people and landscape.

Many of these deities (who are said to pre-date Buddhism's arrival into Tibet in the seventh century) are said to have originally been opponents of Buddhism. Many of these deities were "tamed," however, when faced with the superior spiritual power of the Tantric Buddhist teacher Guru Rinpoché—whose power is understood to be stronger than all other forms of (non-Buddhist) spiritual power—during his travels around Tibet in the eighth century. Not only were they converted to Buddhism, but some of them even became protectors of Buddhism and its teachings. Despite their conversion, however, these entities have remained "worldly" (*'jig rten pa*, i.e. unenlightened), and as a result they

21 Marcia Calkowski, *Power, Charisma, and Ritual Curing in a Tibetan Community in India* (Vancouver, BC: PhD Dissertation, University of British Columbia, 1985), 70.

22 Susannah Deane, "'There is Power in Belief': Creating Space for Psychiatric Illness and Healing in the Tibetan Context," *SHARE: Studies in History, Archaeology, Religion and Conservation* 1, no. 1 (2014): 43–45.

are understood to hold *more* spiritual power than lay humans, but *less* power than advanced Buddhist monastic and Tantric practitioners. As a consequence of these differential levels of spiritual power, lay Tibetans must negotiate with these spirits and deities from a position of inferiority—they can only politely request their assistance, and hope for acquiescence. In contrast, Tibetan Buddhist lamas, whose greater spiritual power is provided by their Tantric Buddhist accomplishments, can negotiate with even more powerful deities from a position of superiority, able to compel the deities to assist them when necessary,[23] and often ritually inducing them to be helpful and to prevent misfortune.[24] Different again is the spirit-medium, who gains his/her power by becoming possessed by an unenlightened deity—a deity which has more power than a low level spirit such as a *dön* or *dré*. Thus, this kind of practitioner has access to more power than a lay person, but less than a Tantric practitioner who gains his/her power from an enlightened deity. And, as we saw in Lhamo's narrative about Lhakpa and her friend, attempting to deal with a spirit when the practitioner does not have enough spiritual power may lead to problems—sometimes with terrible consequences, as we are told here.

When it comes to the role of spirits in health and illness, an examination of the *Four Tantras* finds five classes of spirits described in the *Oral Instruction Tantra* (*man ngag rgyud*), which may cause mental and/or physical illnesses:

- Chapter 77: "Elemental Spirits" (*'byung po'i gdon*)
- Chapter 78: "Spirits That Cause Madness" (*smyo byed kyi gdon*)
- Chapter 79: "Spirits That Cause Forgetfulness or Epilepsy" (*brjed byed kyi gdon*)
- Chapter 80: "Planetary Spirits That Cause Strokes or Partial Paralysis" (*gza'yi gdon*)
- Chapter 81: "Serpent Spirits" (*klu'i gdon*)

Indeed, these five chapters are often held up in English-language publications on the topic as the definitive chapters on spirit-caused illness in the Tibetan context,[25] and we find these five classes of spirits described in some detail by a number of Tibetan *amchi*, including Donden and Drungtso.[26] However, these

23 Geoffrey Samuel, *Introducing Tibetan Buddhism* (Abingdon: Routledge 2012), 170–71.

24 Samuel, *Civilized Shamans*, 161.

25 See, for example, Terry Clifford's *The Diamond Healing: Tibetan Buddhist Medicine and Psychiatry* (Irthlingborough: Crucible, The Aquarian Press, 1989).

26 Yeshi Donden, *Health Through Balance: An Introduction to Tibetan Medicine* (Delhi: Motilal Banarsidass, 1997), 101–102, 233; Drungtso, *Tibetan Medicine*, 53. Indeed, Pasang Y. Arya discusses "Tibetan Buddhist psychology and psychotherapy" on his "Tibetan Medicine Education Centre" website, where he references these five categories in describing the

spirits actually take up proportionally little space in the *Four Tantras*,[27] and in fact, *amchi* may be more or less familiar with these sections of the text, depending on their medical training and experience. This certainly seemed to be the case in Darjeeling, where I interviewed Amchi Lozang Tupten, the resident *amchi* at the Men-Tsee-Khang (MTK) branch clinic. When I asked him about these spirits, he told me that he was rather unfamiliar with these chapters of the *Four Tantras*. Similarly, conducting research in the area in the 1990s, Jacobson reported several Tibetan *amchi* telling him that they did not understand some of these verses well, because "they are not really practiced anymore."[28] Indeed, Samuel argues that the *Oral Instruction Tantra* is the one volume of the *Four Tantras* not necessarily learned by heart by student *amchi* at the MTK medical colleges in India.[29] However, it is not only in this Third Tantra that we find information on spirits. Chapters One and Two of the *Subsequent Tantra* (*phyi ma'i rgyud*), which describe traditional methods of pulse and urine diagnosis, include descriptions of the characteristics of the pulse and urine which may indicate spirit causation.[30] Indeed, Donden has described what we might call a "spirit pulse" which indicates spirit affliction: an "uneven" pulse which changes suddenly, "sometimes pausing, sometimes jerky, and sometimes double;"[31] similarly, Dorjee has described the "distinct irregularity" felt within this "spirit" pulse.[32] It may even be possible to determine *which* specific entity is involved through pulse analysis.[33]

Nonetheless, as we see from the narratives above from Darjeeling, in cases of suspected spirit affliction, Sowa Rigpa practitioners may not actually be consulted by patients and their families, who instead may consult a religious practitioner or biomedical doctor in the first instance. Others too have encountered this situation: Samuel notes for example, that in many Tibetan communities, in reality, spirit afflictions are less often even diagnosed by *amchi*, and more often via divination by a religious specialist,[34] with the list of spirits given in Chapters 77–81 actually rather unrelated to contemporary spirit diagnoses.[35] Indeed, in Darjeeling, whilst "epilepsy" and "spirits that cause forgetfulness"

"five major, mild and aggressive mental disorders" that are related to possession by these classes of spirits.

27 Samuel, "Tibetan Medicine in Contemporary India", 262.

28 Eric Emil Jacobson, *Situated Knowledge in Classical Tibetan Medicine: Psychiatric Aspects* (Cambridge, MA: PhD dissertation, Harvard University, 2000), 116.

29 Samuel, "Tibetan Medicine in Contemporary India," 258.

30 See Donden, *Health Through Balance*, 126–30; and Millard, "Tibetan Medicine and the Classification and Treatment of Mental Illness," 260.

31 Donden, *Health Through Balance*, 101–102.

32 Dorjee, *The Spiritual Medicine of Tibet*, 41.

33 Donden, *Health Through Balance*, 88–89, 101–105; Drungtso, Tibetan Medicine, 295–97.

34 Samuel, "Religion, Health and Suffering Among Contemporary Tibetans," 93.

35 Samuel, "Tibetan Medicine in Contemporary India," 259–60.

were occasionally included in discussions of "mental illness" with lay Tibetans, I found that in reality, narratives here (involving both possession and non-possession afflictions) were predominantly focused simply on descriptions of *dön* (*gdon*) and (*shin*)*dré* ([*shi*] *'dre*). These terms were sometimes used interchangeably to refer to low-level spirits or entities we might describe as "ghosts," while *tsen* (*btsan*) and *gyelpo* (*rgyal po*) were often described (in English) as specific classes of "local deities."

These entities were implicated in conditions ranging in severity from atypical "restlessness" to "psychosis," by both lay Tibetans and *amchi*, and it was in stories of "madness" that I found spirit causes most frequently invoked. As mentioned above, all such entities are "worldly" and unenlightened, and thus they may be offended either intentionally or unintentionally by the behavior of humans. Behaviors understood to cause "offense" include activities such as polluting the water or ground in which these spirits and deities reside, or neglecting any regular offerings traditionally made to them. Any such "offense" can lead to a variety of problems for the human(s) involved if the affected entities cause harm in response. In Darjeeling, people described "harms" including car accidents and illnesses, ranging from minor skin rashes to full-blown "madness." This harm may sometimes be unintentional, however, even for the deities—as Donden explains, sometimes spirits may *inadvertently* cause harm to humans, by becoming attracted to and involved with them,[36] as we saw in the case of Mikmar above.

4.1 *Possession and Non-possession Afflictions*

With regard to these categories of spirits and deities, in Darjeeling I encountered a broad delineation between those involved in possession and non-possession afflictions. Thus, when discussing conditions including psychological symptoms arising from spirit *possession*, Tibetans generally talked of "*dön*" and "*shindré*," reflecting at least to some extent the textual categorisation of "spirits that cause madness" mentioned above. In cases like these, the symptoms may be quite clear: for example, when discussing possession with Amchi Lozang Tupten at the MTK clinic, he described an array of possible symptoms including aggression, restlessness, an inability to sit still, sweating, talking non-stop, and sudden behavior change. Similarly, Amchi Teinlay Trogawa explained that, with illnesses caused by *dön*, the afflicted individual's symptoms will likely be extremely changeable—indeed, in severe cases the patient will be very unlike him/herself, perhaps even having the "habit" of the particular spirit involved, thus making the spirit cause "very clear." In contrast, cases of *non*-possession

36 Donden, *Health Through Balance*, 103.

spirit/deity affliction were more often related to the (usually inadvertent) offense of a deity such as a *tsen* or *gyelpo*. It was explained that such afflictions were more likely to manifest in a slow escalation of diverse symptoms related to the mind, such as confusion and/or nonsensical conversation. Because these symptoms are less specific, the spirit cause may not initially be so clear.

I came across several narratives of mental illness involving these spirits and deities during my time in Darjeeling; and others too have reported spirit and deity afflictions as fairly commonplace: in Ladakh, for example, Day found numerous illnesses attributed to "local gods, lu, tsan and a host of other figures" who were understood to be angered by the neglect of usual rituals or the pollution of their area, or "greedy for people's food or wealth." And these figures are often particularly relevant in mental illness: for example, Day reported that many cases of "madness" were attributed to *gson 'dre* (so-called "living demons"),[37] and in Dhorpatan, Nepal, Millard reported that *all* of the cases of mental illness he encountered were related in some way to spirits.[38]

In addition, in some cases, a spirit-caused "mental illness" may be the first indication that the afflicted individual is actually on a path towards becoming a spirit-medium—usually referred to as a *lha bzhugs mkhan, lha pa* (male), or *lha mo* (female).[39] For a working spirit-medium, of course, possession by a particular deity is actively induced—often through ritual and in the service of the wider community through healing rituals of various forms. But for such individuals, the first indicator of this is often an unsolicited possession manifesting in psychological symptoms: a kind of spirit-caused "madness." Rösing has explored this phenomenon amongst spirit-mediums in Ladakh, northwest India, describing how an afflicted individual may initially be viewed as "mad," until it gradually becomes clear that they are, in fact, suffering from a "shamanic illness," rather than any "normal" form of madness. Their condition is said to be caused by a struggle between a god, which is attempting to possess the person's body, and the spirits.[40] In Nepal too, Berglie has described a Tibetan "hero" (*dpa' bo*) medium as seeming "just like a 'madman' (Tib. *smyon pa*)."[41]

---

37 Sophie Day, *Embodying Spirits: Village Oracles and Possession Rituals in Ladakh, North India* (London: PhD dissertation, London School of Economics and Political Science [University of London], 1989), 278.

38 Millard, "Tibetan Medicine and the Classification and Treatment of Mental Illness," 259.

39 In fact, there are many terms to refer to such practitioners in ethnically Tibetan communities, but in Darjeeling, these were the only terms I heard, and they were used interchangeably.

40 Ina Rösing, *Shamanic Trance and Amnesia: Traditional Healing in Ladakh* (New Delhi: Concept Publishing Company, 2006), 114.

41 Per-Arne Berglie, "Preliminary Remarks on Some Tibetan 'Spirit-mediums' in Nepal," *Kailash* 4, no. 1 (1976): 85–108, 89. This phenomenon is not unique to Tibetan contexts—this "journey" from apparent mental illness to recognition as a spirit-medium is common

Rösing argues that this kind of "madness" frequently plays a fundamental role on an individual's path towards shamanism, and describes symptoms including: "erratic roaming around," "vivid dreams," "visions and hallucinations," and "indecent or nonsensical behaviour."[42] Indeed, in Darjeeling I met one such individual—Dechen—who had had this kind of experience.

Dechen's father (a first-generation exile from east Tibet) described to me how his daughter had initially become possessed by a *lha* at the age of three. Rituals conducted by a Tibetan *ngakpa* (*sngags pa*) had been successful in subduing the deity for some time, but when Dechen was fifteen, the *ngakpa* had passed away, and she had again been possessed by the deity. Dechen and her family described symptoms at that time including her "falling down ... senseless" [unconscious] at school, and being confined to her bed, very weak, and vomiting. Whilst neighbours had told her that she "must be dying," she had thought that perhaps she was going mad. Told by biomedical doctors at a local hospital that there was nothing wrong with her, her condition had finally been diagnosed by a Tibetan spirit-medium whom she and her father had travelled to see in Dharamsala, who had ascertained (through ritual) that Dechen was in fact a spirit-medium, affected by a *yul lha*—a local protector deity from her father's hometown in Tibet.[43]

Thus, we find a diversity of psychological (and sometimes also physical) symptoms caused by different forms of spirit and/or deity affliction in ethnically Tibetan contexts, only some of which seem to be delineated in the main medical text. However, spirit affliction is rarely the sole cause for such conditions, frequently co-occurring in relation to one or more other factors in the causation of illness, such as a person's "spiritual power" (*dbang thang*; as mentioned above),[44] "luck" (*rlung rta*), "life force" (*bla*), and/or (Buddhist) "merit" (*bsod nams*). Thus if, for example, a person's life force or merit is "low" or "weak," it is said that a spirit may be able to "come in and take over [the consciousness]."[45] In Darjeeling, Purbu (50 years old) explained to me that when an individual's luck has "broken" or "run out," he is more likely to see

---

across many cultural contexts. There is unfortunately not space to explore this more widely here, but for further descriptions of such phenomena in the Himalayan region, see work by Day (*Embodying Spirits*); Hildegard Diemberger ("Female Oracles in Modern Tibet," in *Women in Tibet*, ed. Janet Gyatso and Hanna Havnevik, [London: Hurst and Company, 2005], 113–68); and Kim Gutschow ("A Study of 'Wind Disorder' or Madness in Zangskar, Northwest India," in *Recent Research on Ladakh*, ed. Thierry Dodin and Hanz Räther [Kröning: Asanger Verlag, 1997], 177–202).

42 Rösing, *Shamanic Trance and Amnesia*, 128–29, 114.

43 I have described this case in more detail elsewhere (Deane, *Tibetan Medicine, Buddhism and Psychiatry*).

44 Calkowski, *Power, Charisma, and Ritual Curing in a Tibetan Community in India*, 219–21.

45 Donden, *Health Through Balance*, 103.

spirits and/or ghosts. Drölma (31 years old) agreed, telling me that *dön* may attack someone when their luck has broken, and/or their life force is "weak." In contrast, if an individual possesses a certain amount of luck, this may offer her some protection against spirit affliction.[46]

Indeed, in Tibetan explanations of illness of any kind, there are often several "causes" (*rgyu*) and "conditions" (*rkyen*). Similarly, in discussing madness Rapgay describes cases of madness as "primarily due to harmful spirit," but also notes the interaction of several possible factors, explaining that sometimes, a spirit may act as a "helping agent": the "immediate external factor that precipitates the changes in consciousness" which acts together with the predisposing causes.[47] Thus it is not *only* the action of a spirit which causes illness, but one or more other "causes" or "conditions" can also act in conjunction with it. Rapgay specifically discusses the role of the wind "currents" and the "channels" (*rtsa*) in which these currents reside here, explaining that spirits or deities may force entry into the wind current, known as the "life channel" (*srog rtsa*). He describes this as similar to "two people forcefully living together in one room": now, the affected person's mind does not "bear its original nature," but neither has the afflicted person totally "lost his mind."[48]

This is not to suggest that there were no discussions around the validity of spirit explanations of illness (or of spirits and deities in general) amongst Tibetans in Darjeeling—this was particularly in relation to increasing knowledge of contemporary biomedical understandings of mind, body, health, and illness. For example, I discussed the case of Dechen with Gyentsen (28 years old), who had introduced me to her. Having previously told me very clearly that he did not believe in "spirits and all these things," after talking to Dechen, he reflected that in fact it was "very difficult" to understand the process of possession, questioning how this might happen in terms of the biology of the brain, and concluding that "*maybe*" Dechen was being possessed by a *lha*, but that he was unsure.

Another informant, Dorjé (49 years old), suggested that a family's desire to avoid the "stigma" of "mental illness" might encourage them to focus instead on an explanation of spirit affliction, whilst others—perhaps reflecting a more biomedical approach—suggested that a belief in having seen spirits could simply be a *symptom* of a mental illness of some kind. For example, Orgyen (39 years old), a first-generation exile from Central Tibet, who had lived in

---

46 Calkowski, *Power, Charisma, and Ritual Curing in a Tibetan Community in India*, 220.

47 Lobsang Rapgay, *Tibetan Medicine: A Holistic Approach to Better Health* (New Delhi: Sona Printers, 1985), 48–51.

48 Rapgay, *Tibetan Medicine*, 48–49.

India for twenty years, argued that in Tibet "many people" reported seeing spirits, but he believed that they were in fact suffering from "some psychological problem … the mind becomes disordered and you see things that aren't there." Indeed, Orgyen told me that he used to believe in these things—"but I was westernized by coming to India!" However, it was notable that while several of those I interviewed debated the validity of spirit explanations in relation to specific cases, only a handful of Tibetans I discussed this topic with expressed doubt over the actual existence of such entities, with the majority of informants describing spirits and deities in very real terms.

Thus, we see that from a Tibetan perspective, a variety of spirits and deities may be involved in everyday life in multiple ways, including in the causation of various forms of mental illness. Whilst some of these entities are delineated in the *Four Tantras*, others were more commonly discussed by Tibetan medical and religious practitioners and lay Tibetans in Darjeeling. In addition, an illness including some kind of spirit affliction may also involve one or more contributory causes or conditions, suggesting the need for a multi-pronged approach to address these diverse factors in terms of any treatment of the resulting illness. In the next section, I will explore treatment approaches to spirit-caused mental illness as they were discussed in Darjeeling, in comparison to what we can see in the *Four Tantras*.

4.2 *Treating Spirit-Caused Mental Illness*

In the *Four Tantras* we find descriptions of herbal medical preparations suitable for the treatment of mental and physical illnesses, including those related to the action of spirits. On a visit to the Men-Tsee-Khang's Museum in Dharamsala in 2012, I saw displays of some of concoctions, the ingredients of which included precious stones such as agate, tiger's eye, and quartz—each labelled for use in the treatment of "disorders caused by naga [*klu*] spirits," "elemental spirits," and "demonic possession." In addition, herbs such as *acorus calamus* (sweet flag), *sinapis alba* (white mustard), and *commiphora mukul* (Indian bdellium-tree) have been described by Sowa Rigpa practitioners for the treatment of "provocations"[49] and "madness."[50] However, as we

49 "Provocation" is a fairly common translation of *gdon* in some of the contemporary English-language literature on this topic, perhaps indicating a discomfort with some of the more traditional translations, such as "spirits" or "demons," which we saw in older works.

50 See Aleksandr Arbuzov, "Pharmacology in TTM Psychiatry," paper presented at the International Academy of Traditional Tibetan Medicine (IATTM) 2nd International Congress on Traditional Tibetan Medicine, Innsbruck, September 2013.

have seen, in such cases, it seems that in some communities at least, afflicted individuals and their families may not in fact even consult a Sowa Rigpa practitioner. Moreover, Sowa Rigpa practitioners themselves may emphasise the importance of religious intervention—perhaps alongside prescribed herbal medicines to address any other underlying factors, such as a disturbance in one of the *nyepa*. For example, in Darjeeling, Amchi Lozang Tupten explained to me that while most cases of spirit affliction co-occur with disturbance in the wind, sometimes there may be a disturbance in the bile. In such cases, herbal medicines that treat this *nyepa* disturbance should be prescribed alongside any treatment aimed at the spirit affliction. At the Chagpori Tibetan Medical Institute clinic, Amchi Teinlay Trogawa described to me the importance of religious intervention for spirit-caused illness, explaining that in some cases, both medicine and religious intervention are necessary: "sometimes, for some patients, only with blessings [from a lama] will they get well." For Trogawa, the best option for a spirit affliction was to visit a lama (rather than any other religious practitioner, such as a spirit-medium). He explained that "treatment from the spiritual side" must be done by lamas then, "from the medical aspect," it is possible for doctors to treat the patient, but he was clear that "medicines alone will not work on the patient."

Such suggestions echo the perspectives of other Sowa Rigpa practitioners too: Dorjee suggests that in cases of spirit affliction, any pharmacological treatment would "always be accompanied by specific spiritual practices,"[51] and Donden stresses the importance of religious activities in treating such conditions, arguing that any such activities should be conducted *before* any medicines are taken—otherwise, he tells us, no medicine will be effective.[52] In addition, where factors such as "luck," "merit," or the "life-force" are understood to be involved in a case of illness, these must be addressed by particular Buddhist activities, such as monastic or Tantric ritual(s), blessings, or personal Buddhist practices, such as recitation of certain prayers.

Thus, we see that treatment for spirit affliction frequently straddles the religious and medical spheres. In some communities, practitioners' work may also span both spheres, with practitioners prescribing herbal medicines and conducting ritual treatments for patients: for example, in Spiti, northwest India, Besch described several *amchi* who were also renowned ritual specialists.[53] In others, as Millard found in Dhorpatan, Nepal—and as I saw in Darjeeling—there

51 Dorjee, *The Spiritual Medicine of Tibet*, 41.

52 Donden, *Health Through Balance*, 103.

53 Nils Florian Besch, *Tibetan Medicine off the Roads: Modernizing the Work of the Amchi in Spiti* (Heidelberg: PhD dissertation, Universität Heidelberg, 2006), 156–61.

may be a clear division between local *amchi*(s), who focus on herbal medicines and external therapies, and the religious practitioner(s), who focus on ritual intervention.[54] Indeed, in Darjeeling, for many informants, the focus in discussions on spirit affliction was often on religious intervention, rather than Sowa Rigpa. Here, in conversations on "madness" in particular, many Tibetans I interviewed suggested spirit causation and described ritual intervention as the best treatment.

There are a variety of monastic and lay religious specialists who may be called upon to manage and treat spirit afflictions in Tibetan communities. The most well-known, perhaps, are the spirit-mediums, and several lay informants in Darjeeling named such practitioners as the best people to consult for such conditions. Having learnt to induce and control their possession by a powerful higher-level (although unenlightened) deity (with the possession usually induced through ritual), these practitioners utilise the power of this deity to subjugate less powerful entities such as *dön, dré, tsen*, or *gyelpo*.[55] These activities again illustrate the Tibetan Buddhist understanding of "spiritual power" which I described above. Here, with the spirit-medium's access to the spiritual power of the possessing deity—a deity understood to have more such power than both humans and less powerful spirits like *dön* and *dré*—it is possible to subjugate these less powerful spirits. Rösing has described several such practitioners—who may be "monastic oracles" or "village shamanic healers"—in Ladakh in detail,[56] and although she describes some monastic practitioners here, such spirit-mediums are often lay individuals. Nonetheless, in contemporary Tibetan societies, these lay practitioners are often integrated into the Buddhist system,[57] and may in fact come under the auspices of a local monastery, and/or have a local lama's blessing for their work.[58] However, it is important to remember that such Tibetan spirit-mediums only have access to a certain amount of spiritual power—as Amchi Teinlay Trogawa explained, such practitioners can only help to a certain extent, due to the fact that the power which they access through possession by a deity is that of a *worldly*

54 Millard, "Tibetan Medicine and the Classification and Treatment of Mental Illness," 260.

55 See, for example, descriptions of such practitioners by Day (*Embodying Spirits*) in Ladakh; Diemberger ("Female Oracles in Modern Tibet") in Tibet; Gutschow in Zangskar ("A Study of 'Wind Disorder' or Madness in Zangskar, Northwest India") and Berglie (within a Tibetan refugee community) in Nepal ("Preliminary Remarks on Some Tibetan 'Spirit-mediums' in Nepal").

56 Rösing, *Shamanic Trance and Amnesia*. These practitioners may have particular areas of speciality, for example, divination, exorcism, physical healing practices (such as sucking illness out of a patient's body), or the recalling of a wandering "spirit," "soul," or "life force" (*bla*).

57 Samuel, *Civilized Shamans*, 194.

58 Berglie, "Preliminary Remarks on Some Tibetan 'Spirit-mediums' in Nepal," 93.

entity—one which remains within Samsara. In contrast, of course, a Tibetan Buddhist Tantric specialist has access to greater spiritual power than does a spirit-medium, through his/her Tantric Buddhist practice, which deals with *enlightened* deities. Again, the notion of differential levels of spiritual power—conferred by the non-human entities with which the practitioner is engaged with through ritual—is fundamental here.

Although many people described a preference for rituals conducted by spirit-mediums in Darjeeling, the reality was that, as I mentioned above, there were no longer any working Tibetan spirit-mediums in the area when I was there in 2011 and 2012. Indeed, I was told that as older practitioners had passed away, there had been no younger practitioners taking their place. This is a result of numerous factors, not least the emigration of many young people due to the decades' long political troubles in Darjeeling,[59] with many young Tibetans moving away to study and/or work, often financially supporting older relatives back in Darjeeling.[60] However, in contrast to this notable lack of Tibetan spirit-mediums, as I noted above, in Darjeeling and the surrounding area there was in fact a thriving Nepali spirit-medium tradition, and several of the Tibetans I interviewed there had utilized the services of these practitioners—known as *jhānkri* (male) and *mata-ji* (female)—in cases of spirit affliction. Whilst some lay Tibetan informants described these practitioners as following a very similar tradition to that of the Tibetan spirit-mediums, others disagreed, arguing that the Nepali *jhānkri* and *mata-ji* could be of no use in dealing with Tibetan spirits.

In this context, with no spirit-mediums any longer in Darjeeling, but a plethora of Tibetan Buddhist monasteries and Nepali spirit-mediums around the town, for many lay Tibetans I spoke to, it was preferable to commission rituals to be conducted by ritual specialists at local Tibetan Buddhist monasteries, and I encountered several people who had indeed done this. As the largest monastery in the area, the Druk Sangngak Chöling Monastery (known locally as "Dali Gönpa," a few miles outside of the main town) was a popular choice, and I attended two rituals there which had been commissioned by

59 I refer here to the ongoing campaign for independence from the state of West Bengal, whereby many in the Nepali community are calling for an independent "Gorkhaland" state. The campaign has led to violence and significant disruption over the last few decades particularly. See, for example, Atis Dasgupta, "Ethnic Problems and Movements for Autonomy in Darjeeling," *Social Scientist* 27, nos. 11–12 (1999): 47–68.

60 Whilst this emigration was clearly an issue for various communities in Darjeeling, I would argue that the situation was particularly acute for Tibetans in the area, for many of whom the financial situation has remained precarious after generations of exile.

local families to deal with spirit problems. Such rituals usually last one or two days, with a suggested donation dependant on the length and complexity of the ritual commissioned. Other religious practitioners consulted in relation to spirit afflictions included ritual healers such as *ngakpa*. One such practitioner was allied with a smaller Tibetan Buddhist monastery near Darjeeling, and described to me a recent ritual he had conducted for a local Tibetan family after their relative had died suddenly, thought to have been killed by a particularly dangerous kind of spirit known as a *sri*.

In addition to any rituals performed by such specialists, a medical or religious practitioner may also recommend particular religious activities to be conducted by the afflicted individual (if this is possible), or by members of their family and/or community. For example, Amchi Lozang Tupten described the efficacy of certain personal Buddhist practices, suggesting that in some cases, an afflicted individual's family should recite Medicine Buddha prayers for a condition caused by spirits. Furthermore, different kinds of blessings from high lamas, and the making of offerings at monasteries were often felt to be generally helpful in cases of mental illness (as they often were too for physical illnesses), whether or not they involved spirits or deities of any kind.

In my interviews with lay Tibetan informants, several people described biomedicine as generally unable to treat spirit affliction—not least, I was told, because biomedical doctors may be unaware of the spirit cause of an illness. Nyima (35 years old), for example, related the story of a neighbour of his, whom he explained had suffered from an affliction related to Nepali Rai spirits,[61] after inadvertently offending them, leading her to become "very quickly mad." Nyima described how the biomedical doctors who were consulted—unaware of the spirit cause—were unable to treat her, and she had sadly died from her illness, again highlighting the significant dangers of involvement with spirits, be they Tibetan or non-Tibetan. I would argue that whilst the majority of informants expressed a fairly pessimistic view of biomedicine's ability to treat cases of spirit affliction in theory, in practice, when faced with an acute case of illness, some afflicted individuals and their families do in fact consult a biomedical practitioner, as part of their broad-ranging efforts to manage this very difficult situation, as we saw above.

For many of the Tibetans I spoke to then, preferred treatment choices were not necessarily accessible, particularly in relation to Tibetan spirit-mediums: with no such practitioners in the area, afflicted individuals and their families

---

61 Nyima explained that due to the Rai tradition of burying the dead in their farmland, it was dangerous to damage the ground in which the spirits of the dead reside, which Nyima's neighbour had inadvertently done.

had to choose from the other available treatment options. Thus, as we saw in Lhamo's narrative, whilst the focus was on a religious explanation for Lhakpa's condition—indeed, it was the only explanation offered by Lhamo—a rather pragmatic approach to this episode of illness was evident, with Lhakpa taken to two biomedical hospitals, whilst also receiving Tibetan Buddhist rituals from a rather inexperienced lama in attempts to treat her. Perhaps in the absence of an appropriate religious specialist, this seemed like the best combination of available treatments.

Similarly, for Mikmar, his family consulted a combination of Nepali spirit-mediums and biomedical practitioners, leading to some contradictions in terms of treatment advice. Indeed, this pragmatic approach was typical of a number of narratives of mental illness I encountered in Darjeeling, where patients and their families often consulted a diversity of medical and/or religious practitioners simultaneously. In fact, with many cases of illness—including those related to the action of spirits—often understood to have multiple contributing causes and conditions, as we saw above, it perhaps makes sense to utilize a diversity of healing modalities.

What is notable here, however, is that in some cases, such as Lhakpa's, some of these modalities (such as biomedicine) were not clearly related to the perceived cause. Of course, issues of treatment availability are not unique to Darjeeling—indeed, in many cultural contexts, treatment options are often limited by factors such as resources, time, and/or accessibility. What is interesting in these narratives is the very clear implications for such problems: in one case, a man—unqualified to perform ritual treatment that he is nevertheless keen to provide—dies; in another, two treatment protocols clash, leading to confusion and difficulty in treating the afflicted individual's condition. Thus, whilst it is not unusual in many cultural contexts to witness such pluralism in health-seeking behaviour, what is particularly interesting here is the notable adherence to long-standing explanations of spirit causation coupled with a reality devoid of related treatment options.

5 Conclusion

Thus, we find some contrast between the information in the *Four Tantras*, with its singular category of "spirits that cause madness," and lay Tibetans' descriptions of mental illness related to entities such as *dön*, (*shin*)*dré*, *tsen*, and *gyelpo*. Similarly, there is a clear distinction between the listed herbal medicines for spirit afflictions in the *Four Tantras*, and the way in which many Tibetans actually approach such conditions when they occur, as evidenced in

Darjeeling and elsewhere. As we have seen, both *amchi* and lay Tibetans often describe religious intervention as a preferable option, with some *amchi* themselves less familiar with these sections of the medical text, and not often seeing patients for such conditions. Moreover, we can see in these narratives the reality of contemporary life in this Tibetan community, where preferred practitioners such as spirit-mediums may no longer be present, leading afflicted individuals and their families to choose instead from a range of other treatment modalities in this culturally and medically pluralistic context.

In some contemporary Tibetan communities then, long-standing notions about spirits and their role in health and illness remain predominant, and my findings in Darjeeling reflect those of other researchers in other ethnically Tibetan communities across the Himalayan region in this respect (see, for example, work by Day, Millard, Rösing, and others, mentioned above). In a medically and culturally pluralistic community such as Darjeeling, where diverse religious and medical explanatory frameworks of mental illness may "compete" for attention, I encountered only a small handful of lay Tibetans who denied the existence of spirits and deities, and the possibility of illness caused by them. However, there may be questions about how such explanations referencing spirits "fit in" with other notions of causation and treatment, and the contemporary relevance of these Tibetan understandings, as with Gyentsen's discussion on how spirit affliction might occur in relation to his biomedical understandings of anatomy and the brain, or Orgyen's suggestion that a belief in seeing spirits is itself an indicator of psychological illness. In addition, we encounter some common perceptions about the utility of biomedicine and Sowa Rigpa in relation to the management and treatment or "acute" and "chronic" conditions respectively, which I would argue also play a part in treatment choices here.

Within this context, Lhamo's and Mikmar's narratives illustrate a number of key factors: not only the endurance of long-standing Tibetan ideas about the role of spirits and deities in causation of mental illness, but also of Tibetan notions of spiritual power and the continued involvement of spirits and deities in the everyday lives of Tibetan people. In addition, these narratives illustrate some quite specific concerns in the everyday reality in a contemporary Tibetan community. Here, the preferred practitioners for certain forms of illness may simply not be available, and patients may have to be pragmatic in their health-seeking behavior, utilizing a range of different treatment modalities. So, for example, whilst an individual or their family might feel that the best course of action in a case of suspected spirit affliction is to consult a spirit-medium with expertise in dealing with such problems, in contemporary Darjeeling, they may have to consult other practitioners out of necessity. Thus, we hear of Lhakpa receiving treatment from both a biomedical doctor and her lama friend, and Mikmar's family consulting a biomedical practitioner, two Nepali spirit-mediums, and a lama. In the first case, the resolution is understood to have come ultimately from the lama's rituals—but to have come at high cost to the lama himself; in the second, the consultation of practitioners from diverse traditions leads to conflicting treatment advice, highlighting some of the consequences of cultural and medical pluralism, where multiple explanatory models offer a plethora of treatment options.

In both cases, textual descriptions of spirit affliction as they are set out in the *Four Tantras* appear somewhat irrelevant in terms of both diagnosis and treatment. Whilst the spirits understood to be involved here may perhaps fall under the *Four Tantras* categorization of the "spirits that cause madness," there is no diagnosis sought from Sowa Rigpa practitioners. Perhaps this is unsurprising when we hear such practitioners also recommending the consultation of religious specialists in such cases. Instead, these narratives highlight the enduring notion of "spiritual power" amongst many in this community—an understanding that underlies Tibetan conceptions of the hierarchical relationship between humans and different types of spirits and deities. Thus, in the narrative of Lhakpa's spirit-caused illness, we are told of a limited success: the patient herself has been successfully treated, but her friend's demise serves as a stark reminder of the dangers of spirits, and the importance of Tantric Buddhist expertise and power in successfully managing entities such as this. In contrast, a combination of Nepali spirit-mediums' practices, biomedicine, and blessings and ritual intervention from a lama seems to have been successful in treating Mikmar.

In Darjeeling, I encountered a number of narratives of mental illness similar to those told here—particularly in cases of madness, where discussion often focused around the intervention of spirits and deities and the resulting ritual treatments. These perspectives highlight the endurance of these long-standing Tibetan understandings of spirits and deities and their relationship to humans. However, as we saw here too, such perspectives increasingly come up against alternative explanatory models, leading to questions from some about the validity of these traditional notions of spirits, alongside a utilization of diverse medical and healing modalities in dealing with such afflictions in contemporary Tibetan societies.

References

Arbuzov, Aleksandr. "Pharmacology in TTM Psychiatry." Paper presented at the International Academy of Traditional Tibetan Medicine (IATTM) 2nd International Congress on Traditional Tibetan Medicine, Innsbruck, September 2013. <http://attm-austria.at/download/kongress2013/DrArbuzov_TTMIC2013.pdf>.

Arya, Pasang Y. "Tibetan Buddhist Psychology and Psychotherapy." *Tibetan Medicine Education Centre*. <http://www.tibetanmedicine-edu.org/index.php/psychology-and-psychotherapy>.

Berglie, Per-Arne. "Preliminary Remarks on Some Tibetan 'Spirit-mediums' in Nepal." *Kailash* 4, no. 1 (1976): 85–108.

Besch, Nils Florian. *Tibetan Medicine Off the Roads: Modernizing the Work of the Amchi in Spiti*. Heidelberg: PhD dissertation at the Universität Heidelberg, 2006.

Blondeau, Anne-Marie, ed. *Tibetan Mountain Deities, Their Cults and Representations: Papers Presented at a Panel of the 7th Seminar of the International Association for Tibetan Studies, Graz, 1995*. Graz: Austrian Academy of Sciences Press, 1998.

Calkowski, Marcia. *Power, Charisma, and Ritual Curing in a Tibetan Community in India*. Vancouver, BC: PhD dissertation at the University of British Columbia, 1985.

Clark, Barry, trans. *The Quintessence Tantras of Tibetan Medicine*. Ithaca, NY: Snow Lion Publications, 1995.

Clifford, Terry. *Tibetan Buddhist Medicine and Psychiatry: The Diamond Healing*. Irthlingborough: Crucible, The Aquarian Press, 1989.

Dasgupta, Atis. "Ethnic Problems and Movements for Autonomy in Darjeeling." *Social Scientist* 27, nos. 11–12 (1999): 47–68.

Day, Sophie. *Embodying Spirits: Village Oracles and Possession Rituals in Ladakh, North India*. London: PhD dissertation at the London School of Economics and Political Science (University of London), 1989.

Deane, Susannah. "Madness in a Tibetan Context A Comparison of Tibetan Textual and Lay Perceptions of '*smyo nad*' (Madness) among Tibetans Living in North India." In *PJMH: The Postgraduate Journal of Medical Humanities* 1 (2014): 24–49.

Deane, Susannah. "'There is Power in Belief': Creating Space for Psychiatric Illness and Healing in the Tibetan Context." *SHARE: Studies in History, Archaeology, Religion and Conservation* 1, no. 1 (2014): 40–48.

Deane, Susannah. *Tibetan Medicine, Buddhism and Psychiatry: Mental Health and Healing in a Tibetan Exile Community*. Durham, NC: Carolina Academic Press, 2018.

Diemberger, Hildegard. "Female Oracles in Modern Tibet." In *Women in Tibet*, edited by Janet Gyatso and Hanna Havnevik, 113–68. London: Hurst and Company, 2005.

Donden, Yeshe. *Health Through Balance: An Introduction to Tibetan Medicine*. Delhi: Motilal Banarsidass, 1997.

Dorjee, Pema. *The Spiritual Medicine of Tibet: Heal Your Spirit, Heal Yourself.* London: Watkins Publishing, 2005.

Drungtso, Tsering Thakchoe. *Tibetan Medicine: The Healing Science of Tibet.* Dharamsala: Drungtso Publications, 2004.

Epstein, Mark and Sonam Topgay. "Mind and Mental Disorders in Tibetan Medicine." *ReVision: A Journal of Consciousness and Change* 9 no. 1 (1982): 67–79.

Ga, Yang. *The Sources for the Writing of the Rgyud bZhi, Tibetan Medical Classic.* Cambridge, MA: PhD dissertation at Harvard University, 2010.

Gerke, Barbara. *Long Lives and Untimely Deaths: Life-span Concepts and Longevity Practices among Tibetans in the Darjeeling Hills, India.* Leiden: Brill, 2012.

Gutschow, Kim. "A Study of 'Wind Disorder' or Madness in Zangskar, Northwest India." In *Recent Research on Ladakh: Proceedings of the 7th Colloquium of the International Association for Ladakh Studies, Bonn/Sankt Augustin, June 1995*, edited by T. Dodin and H. Räther, 177–202. Kröning: Asanger Verlag, 1997.

Gyatso, Janet. *Being Human in a Buddhist World: An Intellectual History of Medicine in Early Modern Tibet.* New York, NY: Columbia University Press, 2015.

Jacobson, Eric Emil. *Situated Knowledge in Classical Tibetan Medicine: Psychiatric Aspects.* Cambridge, MA: PhD dissertation at Harvard University, 2000.

Jacobson, Eric. "Panic Attack in a Context of Comorbid Anxiety and Depression in a Tibetan Refugee." *Culture, Medicine and Psychiatry* 26, no. 2 (2002): 259–79.

Jacobson, Eric. "Life-wind Illness in Tibetan Medicine: Depression, Generalised Anxiety, and Panic Attack." In *Soundings in Tibetan medicine: Historical and Anthropological Perspectives. Proceedings of the Tenth Seminar of the International Association of Tibetan Studies (PIATS), Oxford, 2003*, edited by Mona Schrempf, 225–46. Leiden: Brill, 2007.

Kloos, Stephan. *Tibetan Medicine in Exile: The Ethics, Politics and Science of Cultural Survival.* San Francisco, CA: PhD dissertation at the University of California, San Francisco, in association with the University of California, Berkeley, 2010.

Meyer, Ferdinand. "The History and Foundations of Tibetan Medicine." In *The Buddha's Art of Healing: Tibetan Paintings Rediscovered*, edited by John Avedon, 21–31. New York, NY: Rizzoli, 1998.

Millard, Colin. "Tibetan Medicine and the Classification and Treatment of Mental Illness." In *Soundings in Tibetan Medicine: Historical and Anthropological Perspectives. Proceedings of the Tenth Seminar of the International Association of Tibetan Studies (PIATS), Oxford, 2003*, edited by Mona Schrempf, 247–82. Leiden: Brill, 2007.

de Nebesky-Wojkowitz, Réne. *Oracles and Demons of Tibet: The Cult and Iconography of the Tibetan Protective Deities.* The Hague: Mouton, 1956.

Rapgay, Lobsang. *Tibetan Medicine: A Holistic Approach to Better Health.* New Delhi: Sona Printers, 1985.

Rösing, Ina. *Shamanic Trance and Amnesia: Traditional Healing in Ladakh*. New Delhi: Concept Publishing Company, 2006.

Samuel, Geoffrey. *Civilized Shamans: Buddhism in Tibetan Societies*. Washington, DC: Smithsonian Institution Press, 1993.

Samuel, Geoffrey. "Tibetan Medicine in Contemporary India: Theory and Practice." In *Healing Powers and Modernity: Traditional Medicine, Shamanism, and Science in Asian Studies*, edited by Linda H. Connor and Geoffrey Samuel, 247–68. Westport and London: Bergin and Garvey, 2001.

Samuel, Geoffrey. "Religion, Health and Suffering Among Contemporary Tibetans." In *Religion, Health and Suffering*, edited by John R. Hinnells and Roy Porter, 85–110. Abingdon and New York: Routledge, 2009.

Samuel, Geoffrey. *Introducing Tibetan Buddhism*. Abingdon: Routledge, 2012

Wangda, Jurme. *Health Seeking Behaviours of Tibetan Refugee Community in Dharamsala, India*. Kingston, ON: MSc dissertation at Queen's University, 1996.

Wangyal, Tenzin and Mark Dahlby. *Healing with Form, Energy and Light: The Five Elements in Tibetan Shamanism, Tantra, and Dzogchen*. Ithaca, NY: Snow Lion Publications, 2002.

CHAPTER 10

Material Presentations and Cultural Drug Translations of Contemporary Tibetan Precious Pills

Barbara Gerke

1 Introduction

Along the shopping roads of Lhasa, a pharmacy-cum-gift shop (Fig. 10.1) sells multi-colored sachets of Tibetan precious pills (*rin chen ril bu*) made at the Shong Bala Chu pharmaceutical company, which is located outside the city. In Central Lhasa, the Mentsikhang's shop sells seven types of precious pills made by the TAR Tibetan Pharmaceutical Factory.[1] Gift packs are labeled in Tibetan, Chinese, and English, while smaller, less expensive sachets (Fig. 10.2) are labeled only in Tibetan and Chinese. The package descriptions promise a cure for acute and chronic illnesses and other severe diseases. Each package has a registration number.

The packages are adorned with Tibetan ornamental symbols, some of which resemble the Eight Auspicious Signs of Tibetan Buddhism. The logo of the Tibetan Autonomous Region (TAR) Tibetan Pharmaceutical Factory (Fig. 10.2) depicts three rivers, apparently symbolizing the Tibetan, Indian, and Chinese influences on the "science of healing" or Sowa Rigpa (*gso ba rig pa*), their essence accumulating into a nectar lake represented by a chebulic myrobalan fruit.[2] Myrobalan is a popular medicinal ingredient but also a cultural symbol of healing, since in Tibetan Buddhism the Medicine Buddha is portrayed holding a myrobalan branch in his right hand. The top right of this package also depicts the colors of the five elements, fundamental to Tibetan Buddhism and Sowa Rigpa physiology.

1 The Mentsikhang was founded in 1916 under the auspices of the Thirteenth Dalai Lama as the first secular Tibetan medical institute in Lhasa.

2 *Terminalia chebula* Retz. (Fam. Combretaceae), or *arura* (*a ru ra*) in Tibetan. Theresia Hofer, personal communication October 2017.

 | DOI:10.1163/9789004404441_011

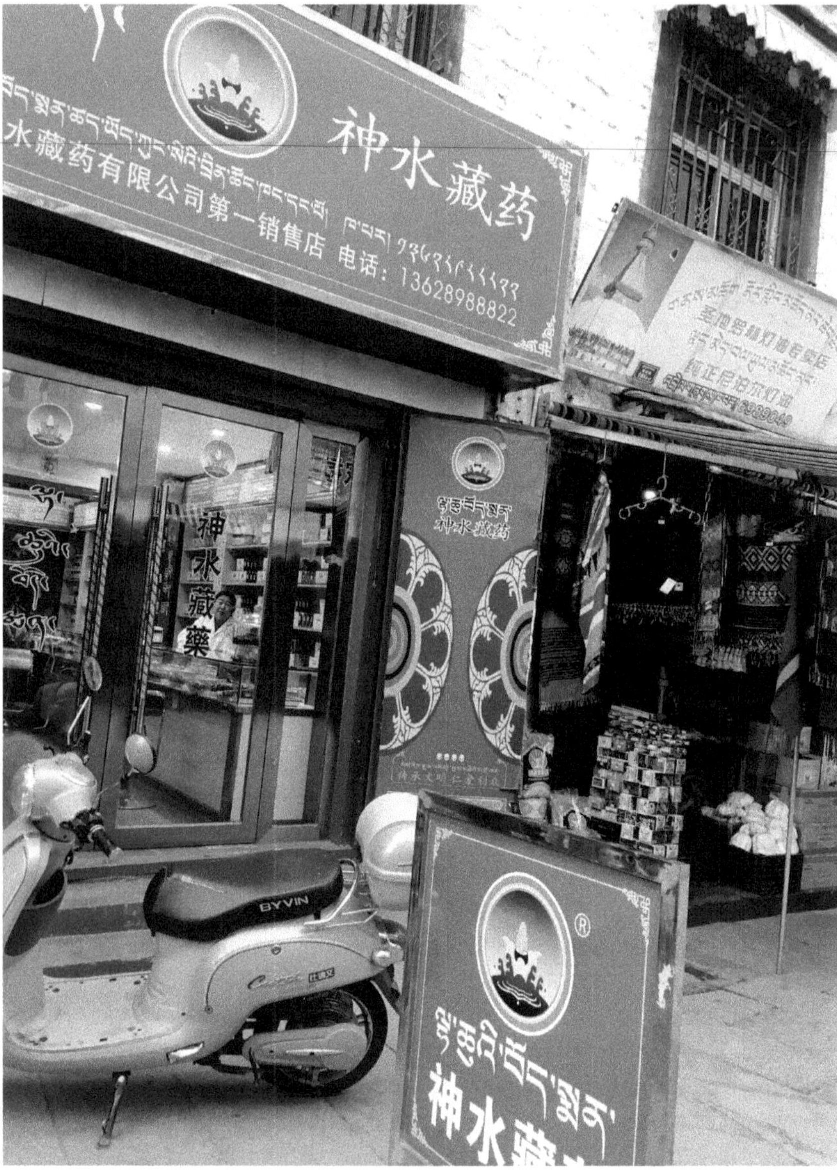

FIGURE 10.1 A shop selling precious pills in Lhasa
PHOTO CREDIT: THERESIA HOFER. ALL OTHER PHOTOS WERE TAKEN BY THE AUTHOR.

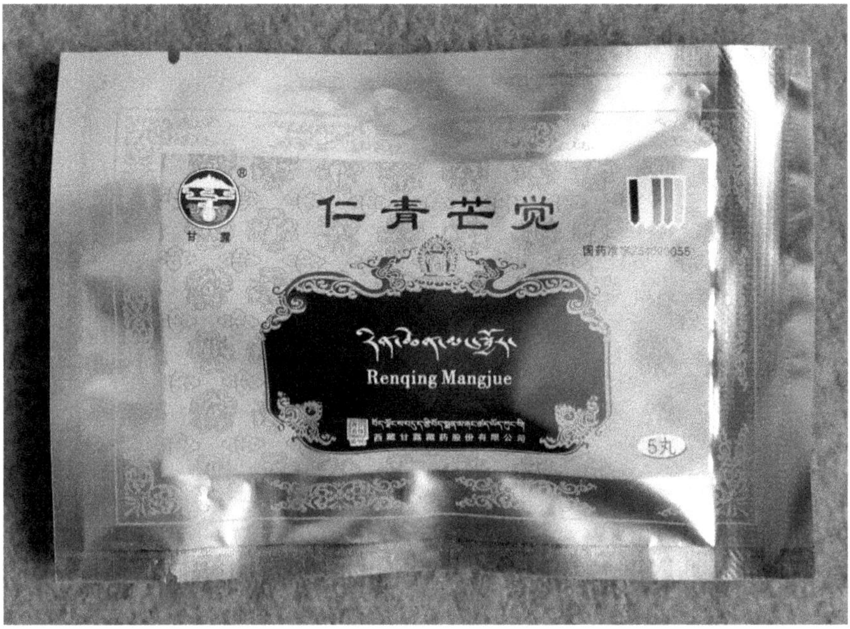

FIGURE 10.2 A packaged precious pill from the TAR Tibetan Pharmaceutical Factory, labeled in Chinese and Tibetan

What do these visual and textual representations of precious pills tell us about their commodification?[3] This chapter explores how the pharmaceuticalization of Sowa Rigpa has affected the material representations of precious pills.[4] With the example of a translated leaflet of the precious pill, "Jikmé's

3 Mark and Mimi Nichter have defined health commodification as "the tendency to treat health as a state which one can obtain through the consumption of commodities, namely, medicine" (Mark and Mimi Nichter, *Anthropology and International Health: Asian Case Studies* [London: Routledge, 2003], 272). They argue that the appeal of medicines as a commodity is not simply the result of pharmaceutical marketing campaign, but has to be seen within broader cultural contexts and practices (p. 274). On the commodification in contemporary Ayurveda see, for example, Madhulika Banerjee, *Power, Knowledge, Medicine: Ayurvedic Pharmaceuticals at Home and in the World* (Hyderabad: Orient Black Swan, 2009); Maarten Bode, *Taking Traditional Knowledge to the Market: The Modern Image of the Ayurvedic and Unani Industry 1980–2000* (Hyderabad: Orient Longman Private Limited, 2008); Nazrul Islam, "Indigenous Medicine as Commodity: Local Reach of Ayurveda in Modern India," *Current Sociology* 58, no. 5 (2010): 777–98; Laurent Pordié, "Pervious Drugs," *Asian Medicine* 9, nos. 1–2 (2014): 49–76; and Laurent Pordié and Jean-Paul Gaudillière, "The Reformulation Regime in Drug Discovery: Revisiting Polyherbals and Property Rights in the Ayurvedic Industry," *East Asian Science, Technology and Society* 8, no. 1 (2014): 57–79.

4 Pharmaceuticalization here is different from commercialization in that is refers to a process that often includes the commodification of knowledge and is thus political in nature.

Old Turquoise-70" (*'jigs med g.yu rnying bdun cu*),[5] made in the People's Republic of China (PRC), I analyze how the current trend towards an expanding pharmaceuticalization of precious pills reflects in their material representation and specific instructions offered in bi- or tri-lingual leaflets. I show that in the PRC Sowa Rigpa's specific terminology and disease etiologies are largely sidelined while catering to a Chinese-speaking patient and consumer clientele, whereas in India we find elements from Buddhism and Tibetan identity integrated in the presentation and packaging of precious pills. Each serves the commodification of precious pills, but in different ways. I also point to the potential dangers of precious pill sales as over-the-counter medicines (OTCs) and how these are dealt with on leaflets.

Precious pills or *rinchen rilbu* are multi-compound formulations that contain between twenty-five and approximately one hundred and fifty ingredients of herbal, mineral, metal, and animal origins, including precious and semi-precious stones (turquoise, sapphire, lapis, coral, pearl, and so forth). They have undergone very complex manufacturing processes, and some of their formulas go back to the twelfth century.[6] Overall, they are considered the pinnacle of Tibetan medicine, especially when they contain the multi-compound mercury-sulfide ash called *tsotel* (*btso thal*), which is difficult to produce.[7] They have been used as prescription medicines for specific and severe diseases, as well as amulets and tonics taken on auspicious dates. These practices have been popular among Tibetans for centuries.[8]

Banerjee defines it as "a development of the pharmacological products from any medical system, irrespective of the autonomous world-view on health, illness, and disease, such that the drugs prescribed by the system acquire a salience detached from the fundamental tenets of the system itself" (Banerjee, *Power, Knowledge, Medicine*, 13). Thanks to Harilal Madhavan for pointing this out.

5 Pronounced *jikmé yunying dünchu*.

6 For a translation on the chapter on precious substances in the *Four Tantras* see: Barbara Gerke and Florian Ploberger, "Jewels in Medicines: On the Processing and Efficacy of Precious Pills According to the *Four Treatises*," in *Buddhism and Medicine: An Anthology*, ed. Pierce Salguero (New York, NY: Columbia University Press, 2017).

7 See, for example, Barbara Gerke, "The Social Life of *Tsotel*: Processing Mercury in Contemporary Tibetan Medicine," *Asian Medicine* 8, no. 1 (2013): 120–52; and Barbara Gerke, "Buddhist Healing and Taming in Tibet," in *The Oxford Handbook of Contemporary Buddhism*, ed. Michael Jerryson (Oxford: Oxford University Press, 2016).

8 On the use of precious pills as tonics see Olaf Czaja, "The Administration of Tibetan Precious Pills: Efficacy in Historical and Ritual Contexts," *Asian Medicine* 10, nos. 1–2 (2015): 36–89; and Barbara Gerke, "Tibetan Precious Pills as Therapeutics and Rejuvenating Longevity Tonics," *History of Science in South Asia* 5, no. 2 (2017): 216–17.

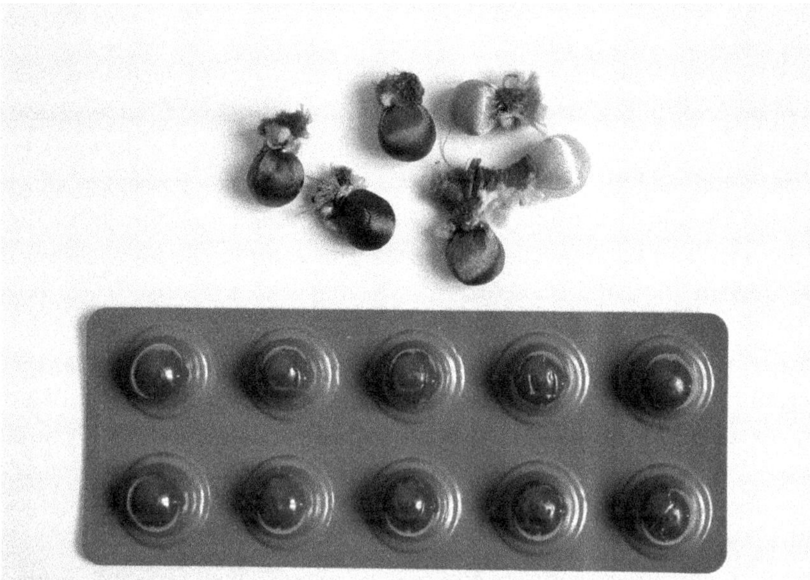

FIGURE 10.3 Precious pills from the Khangkar Memorial Clinic (above) and a blister pack of precious pills from the Men-Tsee-Khang (below), both produced in the Dharamsala area

Their commodification as over-the-counter drugs in the PRC has been described as a showcase for a "developing" and "living" Tibetan medical culture.[9] In the PRC they are regulated in a similar fashion to Traditional Chinese Medicine (TCM).[10] Their pharmaceuticalization has turned them into valuable commodities expressing "Tibetanness," driving a "moral economy," further discussed below.[11] In Dharamsala, India, where many Tibetans have settled in exile, the largest Tibetan medical institute, the Men-Tsee-Khang, produces eight types of precious pills as prescription drugs. Other smaller, private clinics in the area use their own packaging style, but rarely sell them over the counter. For example, the Khangkar Memorial Clinic sells them as OTCs, wrapped in colored silk cloth, tied with a five-colored thread representing the five elements, and a wax seal embossed with a Buddhist emblem (Fig. 10.3).

9 Theresia Hofer, "Socio-Economic Dimensions of Tibetan Medicine in the Tibet Autonomous Region, China—Part One," *Asian Medicine* 4, no. 1 (2008): 177.

10 Mona Schrempf, "Cultural Translations and Shifting Identities of Tibetan Medicine(s) in China: An Ethnographic Case Study," *East Asian Science, Technology and Society: An International Journal* (forthcoming).

11 Martin Saxer, *Manufacturing Tibetan Medicine: The Creation of an Industry and the Moral Economy of Tibetanness* (Oxford, New York: Berghahn Books, 2013).

2 The Commodification of Precious Pills in the PRC

Below, I explore what material presentations tell us about the commodification of precious pills in the PRC and in India. Their commodification as over-the-counter drugs in the TAR has been described by Hofer as a showcase for a "developing" and "living" Tibetan medical culture, in the process of which they have "become what many urban Tibetans, Chinese, and foreign visitors to Tibet view as Tibetan medicine *per se.*"[12] This contributes to a widespread misunderstanding that precious pills form a homogenous group of special pills within a homogenous system called "Tibetan Medicine." I have explained elsewhere why precious pills comprise heterogeneous Sowa Rigpa formulas that emerged from different histories, contexts, and sources and should, at least textually and historically, not be treated as a homogenous group.[13] Only more recently, largely with the onset of the pharmaceuticalization of Tibetan medical products beginning in the 1990s, have they been presented as a cohesive group of medicines.

Precious pills are expensive to produce and often difficult for common people to afford. In the 1990s, some Tibetan pharmacies in the PRC were able to counteract the increase in prices by manufacturing *tsotel* and precious pills by themselves instead of buying them readymade and more expensive from larger pharmacies elsewhere. For example, in August 1991 the Lhokha Tibetan Pharmaceutical Factory, south of Lhasa, made *tsotel* under the guidance of Karma Chömpel (*kar ma chos 'phel*) and Jamyang Lhündrup (*'jam dbyangs lhun grub*).[14] Within five years of establishing the Mentsikhang at Lhokha, they were able to make *tsotel*. In 1991, it took them two months with a group of seven physicians and assistants to prepare around ten to fifteen kilograms of *tsotel* and three types of precious pills (Rinchen Dranjor, Rinchen Mangjor, and Tsodru Dashel).[15] Jamyang Lhündrup notes that the expenditure was cut by a third through producing *tsotel* locally instead of buying *tsotel*-containing

12 See Hofer, "Socio-Economic Dimensions of Tibetan Medicine," 177.

13 Barbara Gerke, "Tibetan Precious Pills as Therapeutics and Rejuvenating Longevity Tonics," *History of Science in South Asia* 5, no. 2 (2017): 216–17.

14 Both physicians had been imprisoned at Powo Tramo and were first trained during the 1977 *tsotel* event by Tenzin Chödrak. On this story, see Barbara Gerke, "Biographies and Knowledge Transmission of Mercury Processing in Twentieth Century Tibet," *Asiatische Studien/Etudes Asiatiques* 69, no. 4 (2015): 867–99. They gained more *tsotel* experience later at the Lhasa Mentsikhang, where Troru Tsenam was actively teaching. Personal communication, Yeshe Gelek, Men-Tsee-Khang, Dharamsala, October 2012.

15 Personal communication, Yeshe Gelek, Men-Tsee-Khang, Dharamsala, October 2012. He himself was trained at the event in Lhokha in 1991.

medicines from outside. The medicine now costs sixty *yuan* per *zho* (3.125 grams = approximately one pill), and it was sold to farmers and nomads for only thirty *yuan* per *zho* (approximately four Euros per pill), eighty percent less than the previous price.[16] This *tsotel* manufacturing event clearly led to the production of more affordable medicines for rural Tibetans in Lhokha and serves as an example of precious pill production development by smaller-scale factories in the 1990s.

Beginning in the mid-1990s and culminating in 2001 with the introduction of the Tibetan Drug Administration Law, the Sowa Rigpa industry entered a new phase of commodification in the PRC, initiating Good Manufacturing Practices (GMP), drug registration, and the commercialization of Tibetan hospitals and pharmacies.[17] Since then Sowa Rigpa enterprises have emerged as important players of the "social market economy" on a larger platform of industrialized production.[18] Kloos recently approached this trans-national "pharmaceutical"[19] development through the theoretical framework of a "pharmaceutical assemblage."[20] Kloos' argument is that the emerging Sowa Rigpa industry cannot be understood simply through gathering statistics and figures on production and market values, but requires an approach that encompasses its ongoing development in "real time" to get to the larger picture of this development within global and national contexts within Asia.[21] This theoretical approach, according to Kloos, will enable multidisciplinary researchers to put together "seemingly unconnected phenomena" of the industry's development across Asia to understand the various levels of its "assemblage" as what it is: "an emerging transnational entity greater than, and different from, simply the sum of its heterogeneous parts."[22] This will require ongoing and substantial

16 'Jam dbyangs lhun grub, No title [Untitled Tibetan Text on the Making of Tsotel in Lokha, Southern Tibet, in 1991] (No date), 6/12–22.

17 Saxer, *Manufacturing Tibetan Medicine*, 35–37.

18 Saxer, *Manufacturing Tibetan Medicine*, 35–37.

19 Here, I follow Kloos' definition of using "pharmaceutical" "to refer to the science and technique of preparing and dispensing drugs in the most general sense." See Stephan Kloos, "The Pharmaceutical Assemblage: Rethinking Sowa Rigpa and the Herbal Pharmaceutical Industry in Asia," *Current Anthropology* 58, no. 6 (2017): 694. In Sowa Rigpa the making of medicines is more aptly called *menjor rikpa* (*sman sbyor rig pa*), a large field of knowledge comprising the study of *materia medica* (pharmacognosy), as well as the compounding of medicine or *menjor*.

20 Kloos, "The Pharmaceutical Assemblage."

21 Kloos, "The Pharmaceutical Assemblage," 703–704.

22 Kloos, "The Pharmaceutical Assemblage," 704.

ethnographic research on the ground in several countries were Sowa Rigpa industries are being established.[23]

Martin Saxer ethnographically documented examples of the emerging competition among PRC-based Tibetan pharmacies in the 2000s. *Tsotel* itself was first patented in 1992 by the Lhasa Mentsikhang, and it was also included in the PRC Intangible Cultural Heritage List in 2006.[24] Another strategy has been to register certain precious pills as "national heritage drugs," which has translated into a practice in which only a limited number of pharmacies are allowed to produce them "under the pretext of safeguarding a national trade secret."[25] Several companies applied for so-called "protection certificates," which was meant to safeguard the knowledge of traditional Chinese medicines produced within a certain territory. Two companies (the Arura Group in Xining and the Lhasa Mentsikhang) applied for such "protection certificates" in the 1990s and received exclusive permission to produce the three precious pills, Rinchen Drangjor, Rinchen Mangjor, and Rinchen Ratna Samphel, between 1998/99 and 2011. After that, "protection certificates" could not be extended.[26] These two companies held the monopoly on precious pill production for many years, leading to limited supplies and the curtailing of other pharmacies from being able to produce their own precious pills.

Saxer describes in detail how these "protection" practices led to legal disputes between Jikmé Püntsok's company, Jiumei Tibetan Medicine Co. Ltd. (the company who makes the precious pill further discussed below), and the Arura Group in Xining. Jikmé has argued that the knowledge of making precious pills belongs to all Tibetans, that many physicians were already able to make them across Tibet, and that they should not be barred from doing so. Regardless, the Arura group has insisted on safeguarding protected medical knowledge, since the precious pills in question were "national heritage drugs." They won the case, and Jikmé's precious pills were considered "counterfeit pills." The case reveals the paradox of how governmental efforts to protect "traditional medical knowledge" in practice caused the actual holders of that knowledge to be stripped of the right to make their medicines.[27] It also highlights the economic value of precious pills as profitable commodities worthy of competition. The players on this stage are large pharmaceutical companies since many small-scale Tibetan clinics with manufacturing units became unable to make

23 Kloos' current ERC project on the Sowa Rigpa pharmaceutical industry covers developments in India, Nepal, Mongolia, and the PRC.

24 Saxer, *Manufacturing Tibetan Medicine*, 74.

25 Saxer, *Manufacturing Tibetan Medicine*, 74, 147.

26 They were issued only twice, for a maximum of seven years each.

27 Saxer, *Manufacturing Tibetan Medicine*, 147–48.

their medicines because complying to GMP regulation made it too expensive for them. Packaged for tourists and rich clienteles, precious pills became expensive and often unaffordable for rural Tibetans. During her visit to Lhasa in 2006/2007, Hofer observed precious pill boxes in Lhasa's souvenir shops as described above. Their extensive TV advertisements and sales amongst tourists made her raise questions of whether *rinchen rilbu* were only "for the rich?"[28]

While many Tibetan physicians and their companies have been barred from producing precious pills, "Tibetanness" nevertheless continues to be the key element in how precious pills are depicted and presented to a largely Chinese-speaking clientele across the PRC and elsewhere. Despite this emphasis on the Tibetanness of precious pills, now their therapeutic indications are often presented in terms of biomedical and TCM-related terminology, further discussed below. Schrempf has described this form of Tibetanness as an integral part of the companies' corporate "culture" (*wenhua*); it is linked to the "pure" *materia medica* resources of the Tibetan high plateau coupled with the "ancient" and thus "authentic" knowledge of Tibetan medical formulas.[29] Some of this kind of Tibetanness is depicted in the metaphors and symbols used on the packaging shown above (Fig. 10.2). Saxer presents this corporate culture as a "moral economy of Tibetanness." He views this "re-enchantment" of Tibetanness as a part of the industry's strategy, in which "authentic Tibetanness" emerges as the key economic factor in a non-localized "moral economy."[30] This entire economy is also embedded in the morality of Buddhism and Tibet's presence within China at large.

Saxer devotes an entire chapter to the aesthetic enterprise of presenting Tibetan medicines to the public. Relying on Alfred Gell's work on the "technology of enchantment," he illustrates how the ritual consecration of Tibetan pills becomes a strategy of production by evoking "magic" as an "ideal technology."[31] Saxer's examples of the "heterogeneity of aesthetics found within the industry" are the rituals performed to consecrate Tibetan pills, the aesthetics of a vegetarian spa center, and the Arura museum in Xining with the largest *thangka* on display.[32] His point is that in "the context of industrial production, the ritual

28 Hofer, "Socio-Economic Dimensions of Tibetan Medicine," 177. Their high price is actually not a new development. Also in the past, precious pills were rare and unaffordable for common people, but for different reasons. For a description of their use among the elites in pre-1959 Lhasa, see Tubten Khétsun, *Memories of Life in Lhasa under Chinese Rule*, trans. Matthew Akester (New York, NY: Columbia University Press, 2008), 80–81.

29 Schrempf, "Cultural Translations."

30 Saxer, *Manufacturing Tibetan Medicine*, chapter 7.

31 Saxer, *Manufacturing Tibetan Medicine*, 247.

32 Saxer, *Manufacturing Tibetan Medicine*, 198.

automatically acquires an additional layer of meaning, as it endows—or re-enchants—the industry with the aesthetics and power of tantric Buddhism."[33] Applied to the context of this paper, the art of packaging precious pills, using specific Buddhist or Tibetan symbols, and listing certain potent substances (turquoise, musk, mercury, bear's bile; see below), re-enchants the commodification of the pills with an additional efficacy of "authentic" Tibetan *materia medica*. In Saxer's words: "The images and things produced in this context, the aesthetic output of Tibetan medicine enterprises, are part of an aesthetic enterprise writ large: the remaking of Sowa Rigpa ties in with the remaking of Tibet."[34] Below we shall see how in the context of precious pills this "remaking of Sowa Rigpa" often sidelines its own epistemologies.

Paralleling the re-enchantment of Tibetanness in the presentation and advertisement of pills in the PRC, we find at the same time a form of disenchantment when it comes to the leaflets accompanying Tibetan precious pills. Chinese-speaking patients and consumers as well as many TCM-trained physicians describing these pills do not understand the Sowa Rigpa epistemologies that lie at the heart of these multicompound formulas. This epistemology is complex, has its own terminology, and does not fit the advertising strategies. As my translated leaflet example below shows, Sowa Rigpa terminology and epistemology remains largely limited to the Tibetan version of the leaflet, while the Chinese and English versions promote biomedical and Traditional Chinese Medicine (TCM) terminology. This can be explained in part by the fact that in the PRC precious pills, like most Tibetan formulas, are regulated in a similar fashion to Traditional Chinese Medicine drugs.[35] Thus, the Chinese descriptions on the leaflets provide the only legally binding information; the English translation is aimed at foreigners, based on the Chinese, and generally done poorly (often through official translation offices who rely on electronic translation programs). The Tibetan descriptions retain some of the textual terminology of key Tibetan compendia, but are insignificant from the point of view of industry regulations.[36] Tibetanness thus remains an aesthetic strategy for commodifying precious pills, sidelining their complex histories and indigenous understandings of how and why they are therapeutically considered efficacious. The sale of potentially strong medicines as OTCs in China also raises

33 Saxer, *Manufacturing Tibetan Medicine*, 170.

34 Saxer, *Manufacturing Tibetan Medicine*, 198.

35 Schrempf, "Cultural Translations."

36 Thanks to Mona Schrempf, who was able to ask Jikmé Püntsok directly about these leaflets during a Sowa Rigpa conference. Mona Schrempf, e-mail communication, 26 October, 2017. See also her forthcoming work.

various questions on their safety, which Schrempf will discuss in her forthcoming work.[37]

3 The Material Culture of Precious Pills in the Indian Diaspora

In Dharamsala, India, where many Tibetans have settled in exile and one of my long-term field sites, the Sowa Rigpa industry still remains largely uncontrolled.[38] Precious pills are manufactured by medium- and small-scale cottage industries (with or without *tsotel*).[39] The Men-Tsee-Khang produces eight types of precious pills as prescription drugs.[40] The demand remains much higher than the production; therefore the prescription of precious pills remains limited to patients visiting Men-Tsee-Khang clinics and local Tibetans, who receive a regulated monthly supply.[41] Among the smaller private clinics-cum-pharmacies in the area that make precious pills, only the Khangkar Memorial Clinic sells them as OTCs. Others produce limited amounts (usually without *tsotel*) for their own patients or Tibetan physicians working privately.

In 2009, the Men-Tsee-Khang in Dharamsala replaced traditional wrapping with machine-made blister-packs, emphasizing Good Manufacturing Practices (GMP).[42] The packaging (Figs. 10.4 and 10.5) demonstrates a purposeful integration of Buddhism and medicine in the aesthetic presentation of precious pills. First, the packages' transparent background depicts *materia medica* images from Tibetan medical paintings of the seventeenth century, when the Fifth Dalai Lama's Gelukpa-oriented government in Lhasa promoted the state-sponsored

37 Mona Schrempf, *Transnational Tibetan Medicine—Formulation Regimes, Therapeutic Networks and Styles of Practice in China and Europe* (In preparation).

38 Sowa Rigpa received official government recognition under the Ministry of AYUSH (Ayurveda, Yoga and Naturopathy, Unani, Siddha, Sowa Rigpa, and Homoeopathy) only in 2010, and first efforts to standardize and control its practice are focusing on medical education.

39 I discuss this in my forthcoming book. Barbara Gerke, *Taming the Poisonous: Mercury, Toxicity and Safety in Tibetan Medical Practice* (Heidelberg: Heidelberg University Publishing, forthcoming).

40 I introduce these pills and discuss what makes them "precious" (*rinchen*) in Gerke, "Tibetan Precious Pills."

41 In 2016/17 this supply was limited to ten precious pills per type available per month, a total of 80 pills per month per local Tibetan. In 2018, this was further reduced to five precious pills of two types per month, a total of 10 pills per month per person. This does not mean that every Tibetan actually takes all these precious pills every month. They are also used as gifts, amulets, and are often traded.

42 See <www.men-tsee-khang.org/announcement/eng-rinchen.htm>. Last accessed October 3, 2017.

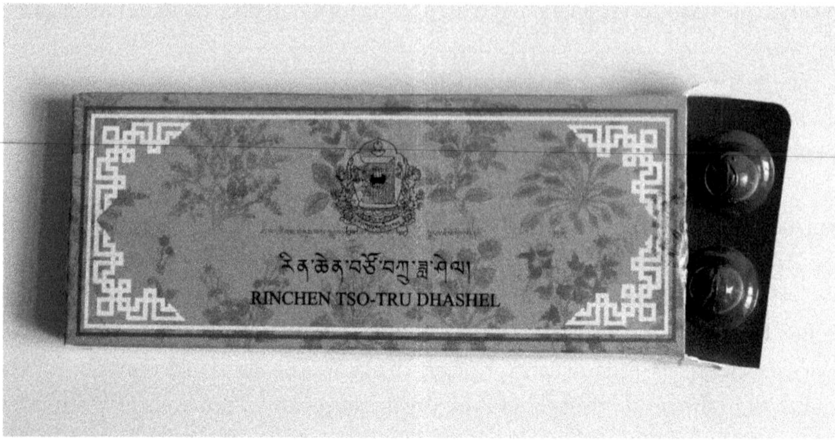

FIGURE 10.4 Contemporary packaging of precious pills by the Men-Tsee-Khang, Dharamsala

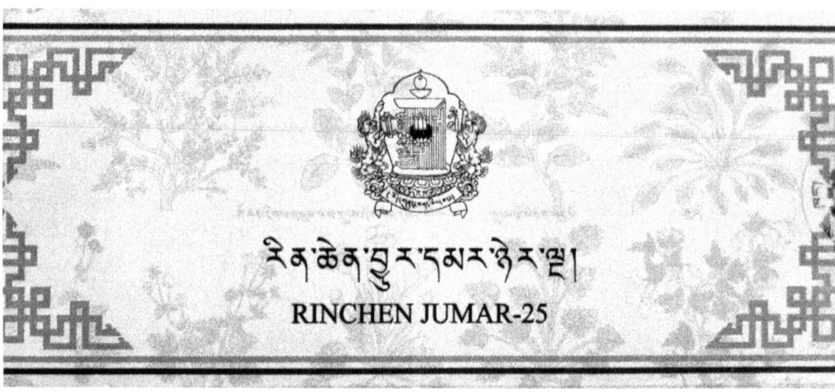

FIGURE 10.5 The Men-Tsee-Khang logo with medical paintings in the background on a package of Rinchen Jumar-25

systematization of Buddhism and medicine.[43] Second, the logo (Fig. 10.5) centers around the sacred syllable of the Buddhist Kālacakra Tantra,[44] framed by

43 See Kurtis R. Schaeffer, "Textual Scholarship, Medical Tradition, and Mahayana Buddhist Ideals in Tibet," *Journal of Indian Philosophy* 31 (2003): 621–41; and Janet Gyatso, *Being Human in a Buddhist World: An Intellectual History of Medicine in Early Modern Tibet* (New York, NY: Columbia University Press, 2015).

44 The Kālacakra Tantra is the last Buddhist tantra that came from India to Tibet in the eleventh century. The Dalai Lama frequently gives the Kālacakra initiation for World Peace and is thus associated with this sign.

two standing snow lions, which mirror the snow lions on the Tibetan national flag of 1916 to 1959, now used only in exile.

These aesthetics demonstrate the desire to highlight the important relationship between medicine, Buddhism, and Tibetan national identity. The Men-Tsee-Khang's presentation of precious pills can be seen as a visual and material identifier of Tibetan cultural knowledge in exile, which has often been encapsulated in a "narrative of preservation and loss."[45] In this narrative, according to Kloos, Tibetan medicines are viewed as the "material essence of an 'authentic'—yet threatened—Tibetan culture. In this role, they are considered not only pharmaceutically but also politically effective in the struggle for 'Free Tibet.'"[46] Moreover, the blessings of the Dalai Lama are incorporated into precious pills by adding special "Dharma nectar medicine" called *dütsi chömen* (*bdud rtsi chos sman*). These small-sized multi-compounds are manufactured by the Men-Tsee-Khang and then consecrated at the Dalai Lama's temple to be added in small amounts during the manufacturing of precious pills back at the Men-Tsee-Khang pharmacy. Consequently, precious pills from Dharamsala are collectively viewed as especially efficacious because of the Dalai Lama's vicinity and his "blessings," or *jinlap* (*byin rlabs*), and are therefore especially valued among the Tibetans who visit Dharamsala from the PRC.[47]

The Men-Tsee-Khang's bi-lingual leaflets (English and Tibetan) describe the pill's (incomplete) formula and indications. There are currently no regulations or standardization practices in place that would compel the Men-Tsee-Khang to print the list of ingredients on their packages. Instructions on how to take the pills are followed by the Medicine Buddha mantra.[48] In the past, Buddhist rituals played a significant role during the administration of precious pills.[49] Spiritual practice still underlines their preciousness and is believed to increase their efficacy, even though most patients taking Tibetan medicine in India today are non-Buddhists, but within their largely Indian and Hindu cultural contexts are familiar with mantra recitations.

To sum up, Sowa Rigpa pharmacies both in exile and in the PRC use Buddhist symbolism in their marketing of precious pills, but with different emphases. For obvious political reasons, nationalism and identity aspects are more prominent in the diaspora than in the PRC, where images linked to Tibet's

---

45 Kloos, "The Pharmaceutical Assemblage," 135.

46 Kloos, "The Pharmaceutical Assemblage," 197.

47 Gerke, "Tibetan Precious Pills," 205–206.

48 See English leaflets online: <www.men-tsee-khang.org/medicine/pills.htm>. Last date of access October 3, 2017.

49 See Czaja, "The Administration of Precious Pills."

independence would not be permitted. In the PRC Buddhist symbols relate to the Sowa Rigpa as a *minzu* ethnic cultural heritage.[50]

4 The Leaflet of the Precious Pill "Jikmé's Old Turquoise-70"

In this section, I explore the leaflet of "Jikmé's Old Turquoise-70," produced by the Jiumei Tibetan Medicine Company in Xining (capital of Qinghai Province, PRC). This formula with seventy ingredients is not included in *The Standard Tibetan Pharmacopeia of 1998*,[51] nor is it found among the 335 formulas of the Lhasa Mentsikhang list,[52] or in Lhakpa Tsering and Wangtop's *Catalogue of Everyday Tibetan Medicines* of 2008.[53] I also have not seen it in other classical Tibetan formula texts. It could be an extensive reformulation, or Jikmé Püntsok's own creation.[54]

---

50 See Mona Schrempf, "Contested Issues of Efficacy and Safety between Transnational Formulation Regimes of Tibetan Medicines in China and Europe," *Asian Medicine* 10, nos. 1–2 (2015), 279, n. 20; on the term *minzu*, which refers to a specific medical system of an ethnic minority which at the same time is part of China's cultural heritage.

51 Ministry of Health (PRC), *Krung hwa mi dmangs spyi mthun rgyal khab 'phrod bsten pu'u'i sman rigs tshad gzhi. Bod sman. Deb dang po.* [Standard Tibetan Pharmacopeia of the Ministry of Health, People's Republic of China. Tibetan Medicine, Volume 1] (Beijing: Ministry of Health, PRC, 1998).

52 Bsod nams don grub, *Bod sman sbyor sde chen mo* [The Great Book of Tibetan Medicine Compounding] (Lhasa: Bod ljongs mi dmangs dpe skrun khang, 2006).

53 Lhag pa tshe ring and Dbang stobs, eds. *Rgyun spyod bod sman dkar chag* [Catalogue of Everyday Tibetan Medicines] (Lhasa: Bod ljongs mi dmangs dpe skrun khang, 2008).

54 Several formulas circulate under the name of "Old Turquoise." The most well-known precious pill is "Old Turquoise-25" (*g.yu rnying nyer lnga*), which has twenty-five ingredients. This formula is discussed in Barbara Gerke, "The Signature of Recipes: Authorship, Intertextuality and the Epistemic Genre of Tibetan Formulas," *Revue d'Etudes Tibétaines* 45 (2018): 178–220. This formula is also listed, for example, in: Zla ba ri brag, *Bod kyi gso ba rig pa las sman rdzas sbyor bzo'i lag len gsang sgo 'byed pa'i lde mig* (Delhi: Rig Drag Publications, 2003), 202; Lhag pa tshe ring and Dbang stobs, *Rgyun spod bod sman dkar chag*, 20, 140; and Bsod nams don grub, *Bod sman sbyor sde chen mo*, 700. "Old Turquoise" formulas with fewer ingredients are "Old Turquoise-7," "Old Turquoise-9," and "Old Turquoise-16," all listed in Bsod nams don grub, *Bod sman sbyor sde chen mo*, 699. "Old Turquoise-7" and "Old Turquoise-16" are also found in Zla ba ri brag, *Bod kyi gso ba rig pa las sman rdzas sbyor bzo'i lag len gsang sgo 'byed pa'i lde mig*, 65, 202. *The Standard Tibetan Pharmacopeia* of 1998 also mentions an "Old Turquoise Powder" (*g.yu rnying cur nyis*[*sic*] *nis*) with eight ingredients (Ministry of Health, *Krung hwa mi dmangs spyi mthun rgyal khab 'phrod bsten pu'u'i sman rigs tshad gzhi*, 389), which is also listed under the category of "powders" (*phye ma'i rigs*) in Lhag pa tshe ring and Dbang stobs, *Rgyun spod bod sman dkar chag*, 28, 157.

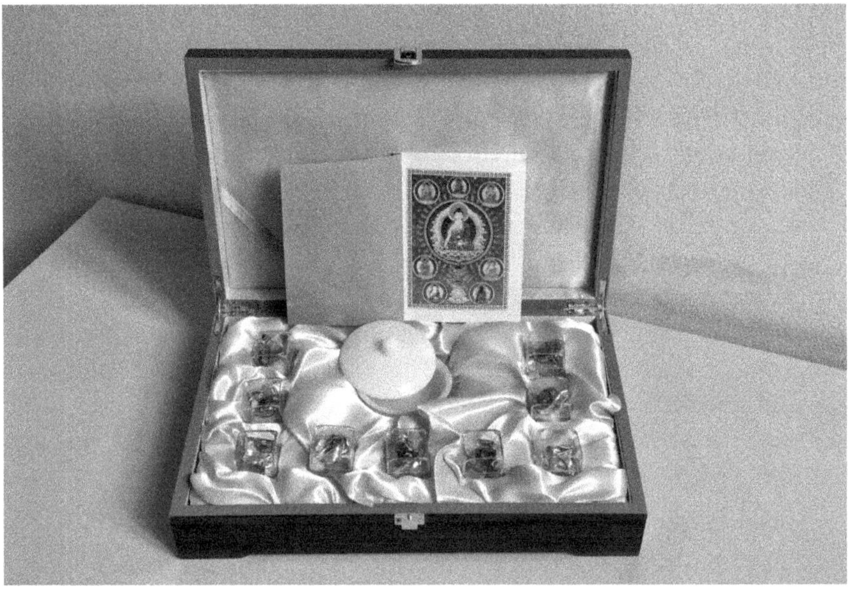

FIGURE 10.6 A gift-box of the pills "Jikmé's Old Turquoise-70"; the box includes a prayer book to consecrate the pills and a bowl to soak them overnight before consumption.

Nine individually packed pills are placed in a wooden gold-color scripted gift box with artificial silk lining (Fig. 10.6). A plastic bowl is included for soaking the pills in warm water overnight, one of the ways of administering a precious pill.[55] A prayer booklet includes a photo of the Medicine Buddha and recitations in Tibetan and Chinese for those wanting to consecrate their pills. The pills are, among twelve other drugs, also sold online on the company's website, though with a different packaging and under the category of "Chinese Medicine" (probably for legal reasons),[56] while the company presents itself as "Jiumei Tibetan Medicine" on its opening page.[57]

The pharmacy's owner Jikmé Püntsok told the anthropologist Mona Schrempf in an interview: "I have studied the way in which Chinese medicinal herbs are produced for the market and copied that, using Tibetan

55 See Czaja, "The Administration of Tibetan Precious Pills"; on different techniques and rituals on how to administer precious pills based on historical texts.

56 <www.jmtm.com.cn/JM/en/productshow.php?cid=63&id=315>. Last accessed April 26, 2018. Not anymore online.

57 <www.jmtm.com.cn/JM/en/index.php>. Last accessed April 26, 2018. See also: <www.xyzyw.cn/gandanxitong/qishiweisongshiwan_jiumei_.html>. Last accessed May 8, 2018. Not anymore online.

formulas."[58] This approach is apparent in the leaflet. It illustrates what is at stake in this form of cultural drug translation, which reveals what Schrempf describes as "arbitrary hybrid biomedical and TCM-related terminologies of symptoms, syndromes and diseases, indicating an adjustment of language and conceptions for their new Chinese TCM and/or biomedical professionals and Chinese-speaking patient-customers."[59]

Recently, Jikmé Püntsok himself explained to Mona Schrempf that only the Chinese part of the leaflet is legally binding and important for the authorities. As mentioned above, the English is mainly based on the Chinese version, typically commissioned to a translation company, mixing Tibetan, TCM, and biomedical disease names, while the Tibetan terms remain largely based on classical medical texts. The following analysis thus has to be understood in the context of what is legally binding for PRC-based companies producing and marketing Sowa Rigpa formulas.

When I translated the Tibetan leaflet of "Jikmé's Old Turquoise-70" (Fig. 10.7) and compared it with its available printed English version, three key issues became apparent, which illustrate the cultural translation of precious pills in the PRC. While I am not analyzing the Chinese part of the leaflet in detail, for the point I wish to make the translation of the Tibetan section juxtaposed with the English version suffices, since it demonstrates fundamental characteristics of the expanding pharmaceuticalization of precious pills in the PRC. Below I present translated excerpts from the leaflet to highlight each of the key issues. The complete translation of the Tibetan leaflet can be found at the end of the chapter.

4.1 *Only Twelve Ingredients are Given on the Tibetan Leaflet, Whereas a List of All Seventy Ingredients are Provided in English* (*Based on the Chinese*)

The Tibetan version of the leaflet lists the following twelve substances under the heading of "medicinal compound" (*sman sbyor*):

> Old turquoise (*g.yu rnying*), pearl (*mu tig*), musk (*gla rtsi*), the salt *kharutsa* (*kha ru tshwa*),[60] man-made bezoar (*mi'i bzos gi wang*),[61] bear's

58 Schrempf, "Cultural Translations."

59 Schrempf, "Cultural Translations." See also Schrempf, "Contested Issues of Efficacy and Safety."

60 *Kharutsa* refers to black salt (primarily sodium chloride [NaCl] with high sulfur content and greigite) derived from halite mines. Thanks to Tawni Tidwell for this identification.

61 This is the solidified bile of an animal. "Man-made" possibly refers to its being sourced from domesticated cattle. The English leaflet refers to it as "natural."

> bile (*dom mkhris*), a yellow type of corydalis called *sumi serpo* (*su mi ser bo* [*po*]),[62] costus root known as *ruta* (*ru rta*),[63] [preprocessed, artificial] cinnabar (*cog la*),[64] mercury (*dngul chu*),[65] an *Aristolochia* species known as *baleka* (*ba le ka*), blue poppy (*utpal sngon po*),[66] a type of fern called *rerel* (*re ral*), [and] seventy kinds of medicine [substances] to complete [the formula].

It is difficult to say what led to listing these particular ingredients in the leaflet and not others. Some of the substances listed are known to Tibetans as particularly potent, valuable, and precious, such as turquoise, pearl, musk, bear's bile, and processed forms of mercury/cinnabar. However, the use of mercury and *Aristolochia* are also controversial. *Aristolochia* is known to the biomedical community as a dangerous TCM drug that is banned in many countries, including Germany, the UK, Belgium, Japan, the USA, Canada, Australia, and New Zealand. A detailed cautionary advice is given in the English, and only partially in the Tibetan version (see point 4.3 below).

The list of ingredients in the English version is complete (see full English leaflet text at the end of this article). The names reveal a mix of Latin botanical names, English names (such as natural ox gallstone and golden ash), pharmacopeia names instead of botanical names (for example, *Semen myristicae* instead of *Myristica fragrans* for nutmeg), and anglicized spellings of Chinese terms (such as *zogta*, an anglicized rendering of the Chinese term *zuotai*, meaning *tsotel*).

The tri-lingual presentation of ingredient names raises questions concerning the translation, identification, and standardization of Tibetan *materia medica* terms, for which there are often several possible botanical identifications, considering possible (sub)types and spatio-temporal variations.[67] The accuracy of existing attempts to standardize ingredient names, especially the identification of Tibetan medicinal plants, is problematic for both practitio-

62 Identified as *Corydalis yanhusuo W. T. Wang* in many works (listed in Czaja, "The Administration of Tibetan Precious Pills," 53, n. 50).

63 Identified as *Saussurea costus* and *Saussurea lappa* (Decne.) Sch. Bip. See Jan van der Valk, *Alternative Pharmaceuticals: The Technoscientific Becomings of Tibetan Medicines in-between India and Switzerland* (Canterbury: PhD thesis, University of Kent, 2017), 48.

64 Also found as *choklama* (*cog la ma*).

65 *Ngülchu* (*dngul chu*) translates as "silver water" or quicksilver in unprocessed form. Its most complex processed form is called *tsotel* (*btso thal*) in Tibetan and *zuotai* in Chinese. In the English leaflet it is called *zogta*, an anglicized rendering of *zuotai*.

66 A Meconopsis species.

67 See van der Valk, *Alternative Pharmaceuticals*, 62; on the problems of idealized identification, naming, and classification practices in Sowa Rigpa.

ners of Sowa Rigpa and scholars. Jan van der Valk has argued that such "acts of translation are fraught with misrepresentation, instability, and concealed ambiguity."[68]

4.2 *In the Tibetan Version, Disease Names Rely Largely on Classical Sowa Rigpa Categories; in the English Version Biomedical and* TCM *Disease Categories Predominate*

The naming of traditional formulas commodified as TCM drugs in China, as well as the translation of related disease categories, is a significant issue in the reformulation and pharmaceuticalization of Sowa Rigpa formulas. Schrempf and Czaja recently studied in detail Sowa Rigpa drug-naming practices in the PRC.[69] With regard to renaming Tibetan drugs, Czaja offers examples of three different methods applied by companies producing Sowa Rigpa formulas in the PRC,[70] each of which I shall illustrate below. The first refers to a more "literal" translation.[71] An example here is Eaglewood-8 (*a gar brgyad pa*), which has been translated into Chinese as the "Eaglewood-8 Pill" (*bawei chenxiang wan* 八味沉香丸). The second is based on the phonetic transcription of the Tibetan name. For example, the drug "Saffron Garuḍa" (*gur khyung*),[72] is simply phoneticized in Chinese as Guer Qiong 古尔琼. In the third method a known ingredient is highlighted in the name instead of translating or transcribing the Tibetan name into Chinese. An example here is the Tibetan drug, "Garuḍa-5"

68 van der Valk calls this process "commensuration" and warns that "These identifications constitute a process of standardisation along modern scientific lines in disguise, a standardisation which solidifies the multiplicity of Tibetan medical plant knowledges into unsuitably narrow and rigid categories while sometimes unintentionally universalising this flawed simplification as the one and only correct identification" (van der Valk, *Alternative Pharmaceuticals*, 42).

69 Schrempf, "Cultural Translations"; and Olaf Czaja, "Adapting Tibetan Drugs to the Chinese Market. A Textual Study of Pomegranate and Eaglewood Formulas and Their Indications," *East Asian Science, Technology and Society: An International Journal* (forthcoming).

70 Czaja, "Adapting Tibetan Drugs."

71 I use "literal" here reluctantly considering the many levels involved in the complex processes that impact acts of translation. Anthropologists have been cautious to speak of a "single definite translation," which has the danger of evoking dichotomies between the "literal" and "metaphorical," but instead emphasize the "open-endedness of translation" as a precondition to mutual intelligibility. William F. Hanks and Carlo Severi, "Translating Worlds: The Epistemological Space of Translation," *HAU: Journal of Ethnographic Theory* 4, no. 2 (2014): 12.

72 *Garuḍa* is a mythical bird of large size that offered its body as medicine. See Thinley Gyatso and Chris Hakim, *Essentials of Tibetan Traditional Medicine* (Berkeley, CA: North Atlantic Books, 2010), 317. Quoted in van der Valk, *Alternative Pharmaceuticals*, 213–14.

(*khyung lnga*),[73] which in Chinese is renamed as the "Musk-5 Pill" (*wuwei shexiang wan* 五味麝香丸), highlighting musk as one of the five ingredients. The motivation for choosing a certain method is not always clear and would require detailed ethnographic research with the companies that are manufacturing and labeling these formulas.

In the example discussed here, Jikmé's company re-named the "Old Turquoise-70" pill into the "Seventy Flavors Rammel Pill," which is based on the Chinese name, "Turquoise-70 Pill" (*qishiwei songshi wan* 七十味松石丸), and not the Tibetan name. Rammel is a rarely used English term for turquoise (it also means broken stone), and was possibly taken from an online translation program without considering the widely-used English term "turquoise," which is already a part of many translated Tibetan formula names containing this semi-precious gemstone. Similarly, "flavor" is a translation of the Chinese term, *wei* 味, which is used here as a measure word referring to the number of ingredients in a formula. Taken together, the English name of the precious pill is just a poor translation of the Chinese; as I said above, the English version is not the legally binding part of the naming/packaging and consequently did not get the attention it might deserve.

As for the translation of disease categories, when comparing the Tibetan with the English version, they appear quite different from each other. The Tibetan section on "benefits" (*phan nus*) translates as follows:

> [This medicine] is beneficial for old and new liver heat (*mchin tshad gsar rnying*), a poison-like liver disease known as "liver *duktap*" (*mchin pa dug thabs*),[74] liver swelling (*mchin sbangs*), inflammation of the gallbladder called "*tripa* heat" (*mkhris tshad*),[75] a poison-like stomach disease called "stomach *duktap*" (*pho ba dug thabs*), a type of gut-liver metabolic disorder called "brown stomach" (*pho ba smug po*), etc. Specifically, it is very beneficial for "*tripa* heat," a nutritional essences metabolic disruption related to blood conditioned by the liver (*mchin khrag dwangs ma ma zhu*

73 According to the myth, each of the *garuḍa* bird's body parts metaphorically corresponds to one of the drug's ingredients. For a more detailed discussion of its ingredients and contemporary use in India see van der Valk, *Alternative Pharmaceuticals*, 212–17.

74 This refers to one of the eighteen liver diseases listed in the *Four Tantras* (*Instructional Tantra*, chapter 36).

75 *Tripa* is one of the three principle parameters of Sowa Rigpa physiology, dominated by the fire element. It is one of the three basic physiological principles (*nyes pa*), which are explained in numerous works of secondary literature on Tibetan medicine. "*Tripa* heat" is a polysemous term and here refers to the inflammation of the gallbladder (*snod mkhris*).

> *ba*),[76] and for types of fluid accumulation (e.g. edema, ascites) secondary to hardening of the liver (*mchin pa sra 'gyur chu zags kyi nad*).[77]

The English leaflet for "Old Turquoise-70" lists the following benefits (with errors as appearing in print):

> [Functions and indications:] comfort gallbladder and cured silt pain. It's used for chest pain which caused by liver stagnation, thermal resistance, and vomiting. Hiccups. Loss of appetite. Acute and chronic hepatitis etc.

"Liver stagnation" refers to "liver depression and *qi* stagnation" (*ganyu qizhi* 肝郁气滞) in the Chinese version of the leaflet, which is a technical term from TCM practice; it does not have a Tibetan "equivalent" as such since the medical thinking is based on different epistemologies. "Silt pain" and "thermal resistance" are obscure English translations of the Chinese. "Silt pain" probably refers to the Chinese term, *lidan* 利胆, which translates as "benefits the gallbladder." "Thermal resistance" appears to be an attempt at rendering the TCM illness category of "damp heat" (*shihan* 湿热) comprehensible to an English-reading audience. "Acute and chronic hepatitis" refer to biomedical liver diseases; the Chinese term for "acute and chronic" (*jimanxing* 急慢性) is a neologism, using the premodern terms "slow" (慢), "quick" (急), and "nature" (性).[78] What we find here is the conflation of TCM and biomedical terminology through the use of polysemous Chinese terms in an attempt to market a Tibetan formula to a contemporary, non-Tibetan clientele in the PRC.

Clearly, the English section of the leaflet is a bad translation of the Chinese and not a translation of the Tibetan. This is in line with other leaflets from Jikmé Püntsok's company that were studied by Czaja. Analyzing therapeutic indications in Chinese on other leaflets, Czaja concludes, "his Chinese indications are a new creation which one can hardly call a translation [from the Tibetan]."[79] It is only in the Tibetan version of the leaflet that the technical disease terms based on authentic Tibetan medical texts appear. Understanding these terms requires a deeper training in Sowa Rigpa medical epistemology and the *Four Tantras*, which for the most part neither Chinese nor English speaking sellers or consumers of this pill will have.

---

76 This is related to a vast group of diseases in Tibetan medicine where the nutritional essence is not properly produced due to metabolic disruptions in the gut that affects liver function and associated development of proper qualities in the blood.

77 See left column of Fig. 10.7 for Tibetan version.

78 Thanks to William McGrath for his support with the Chinese translations.

79 Czaja, "Adapting Tibetan Drugs."

4.3 *Specific Cautionary Advice Given in English is Not Found in Detail in the Tibetan Version*

The Tibetan cautionary advice translates as: "Not only should you read the leaflet clearly, it is [also] necessary to follow the guidance of a physician."[80] This statement makes clear that this medicine should not be sold as an OTC but as a prescription drug, which is not put into practice. The Tibetan section on "precautions" (*'dzem bya*) translates as:

> [This pill is] unsuitable to be taken by those with weakened liver and kidney functions, and illnesses of the blood production system, [as well as] newborns, pregnant and breastfeeding women, etc.[81]

The "weakened liver and kidney functions" appears contradictory to the liver-related indications of the pill's benefits listed above, but should be understood as a general warning that the administration of precious pills is complex, should be done under a physician's supervision, and should be avoided when kidney and liver functions are weak. These precautions might be overlooked during the OTC (mis)use of precious pills.

In contrast, the English leaflet pays attention to the existing toxicity debates concerning the use of mercury and *Aristolochia* in Asian medicines. It reads:

> [Cautions:] 1. The product contains Cinnabaris, Zogta,[82] and Fructus Aristolochine and long term use is not suitable. The probuct [sic] is a prescription drug and doctor's advice should be followed.
>
> 2. During the drug administration, Hg concentration In [sic] blood and urine should be tested regularly. The product should be withdrawn when hepatic and renal functions exceed the defined limit.
>
> 3. The product is notable [sic, not suitable] to children and elderly.

The toxicity of the plant *Aristolochia fructus*, in Tibetan *baleka*, has been debated largely in TCM.[83] It is also used in Sowa Rigpa formulas. Tibetan physicians in

80 "Old Turquoise-70 Leaflet": *khyod kyis gsal bshad yi ge gsal bor klog dgos pa ma zad/ sman pa'i mdzud [mdzub] ston 'og tu bsten dgos.*

81 "Old Turquoise-70 Leaflet": *mchin pa dang mkhal ma'i nus ma zhan pa/ khrag bzo ma lag la nad yod pa/ byis pa btsas rung/ sbrum ma dang byis par 'o ma ster ba'i bud med sogs kyo bsten mi rung.*

82 This refers to the Chinese term *zuotai*, which is a phonetic transcription of the Tibetan term *tsotel*.

83 On the dangers of renal toxicity and carcinogenicity of the *Aristolochia* species in Chinese medicines see, for example: M. J. Martena, et al., "Enforcement of the Ban on Aristolochic

India who are aware of the controversy avoid using *baleka* in their medicines.[84] The dangers of prolonged exposure to certain forms of mercury are well-known.[85] Consumed in the processed form of *tsotel* (mostly mercury-sulfide) it is less toxic since mercury-sulfide is largely insoluble; thus mercury-sulfide is unlikely to contribute to elevated levels of mercury in blood and urine.[86] Elevated mercury levels might rather point to an inaccurate or incomplete processing of *tsotel*. To date only a few studies, largely Chinese, address the potential toxicity of *tsotel*.[87] The cautionary advice on the leaflet has to be understood in the context of safety concerns surrounding precious pills being sold as OTC drugs in the PRC.[88] The English leaflet indicates more clearly that this is a prescription drug. However, precious pills largely remain OTC products in the PRC.

5 Discussion and Conclusion

In both India and the PRC, Tibetan authenticity and identity have been used strategically to advance local and global economies of precious pills. The "Tibet" image is utilized in various ways both in the PRC and in the diaspora to present precious pills as "authentic" Tibetan culture. Their commodification could well lead to a dis-enchantment of the potential therapeutic benefits they might be able to offer suffering patients.

Acids in Chinese Traditional Herbal Preparations on the Dutch Market," *Analytical and Bioanalytical Chemistry* 389, no. 1 (2007): 263–75; and Lan Wu, et al., "An Integrated System for Identifying the Hidden Assassins in Traditional Medicines Containing Aristolochic Acids," *Scientific Reports* 5 (2015): 113–18.

84 Personal communication, Dr. Namgyal Qusar, Sidhbari, June 2016.

85 Ki-Hyun Kim, Ehsanul Kabir, and Shamin Ara Jahan, "A Review on the Distribution of Hg in the Environment and its Human Health Impacts," *Journal of Hazardous Materials* 306 (2016): 376–85; and Kern L. Nuttall, "Interpreting Mercury in Blood and Urine of Individual Patients," *Annals of Clinical and Laboratory Science* 34, no. 3 (2004): 235–50.

86 Jie Liu, et al., "Mercury in Traditional Medicines: Is Cinnabar Toxicologically Similar to Common Mercurials?" *Experimental Biology and Medicine* 233, no. 7 (2008): 810–17.

87 *Tsotel* studies in Chinese published before 2013 are listed in Gerke, "The Social Life of *Tsotel*," 151–52. The Men-Tsee-Khang in Dharamsala carried out two preliminary toxicity studies: Sarah Sallon, et al., "Mercury in Tibetan Medicine—Panacea or Problem?" *Human Experimental Toxicology* 25, no. 7 (2006): 405–12; and Sarah Sallon, et al., "Is Mercury in Tibetan Medicine Toxic? Clinical, Neurocognitive and Biochemical Results of an Initial Cross-Sectional Study," *Experimental Biology and Medicine* 242, no. 3 (2017): 316–32.

88 Personal communication, Mona Schrempf, December 2017. Mona Schrempf has done fieldwork on this topic and will discuss results in her forthcoming publications.

The leaflet example above points to certain dangers of OTC sales of precious pills. Even though the tri-lingual leaflet has its translation flaws, it is clear from the few cautionary remarks that precious pills are actually prescription drugs and should be taken with caution. Even as tonics they are typically taken only once a month on an auspicious day.[89]

The commodification and OTC-sales of precious pills, found largely in the PRC but also at certain clinics in India, can easily lead to their misuse, especially if they are sold in shops that do not have trained personnel to caution consumers. Wrong dosage and too frequent intake might not only cause side-effects but also negatively affect the reputation of Sowa Rigpa. On the one hand, the idealized image of "Tibet" is used to present and market the "authenticity" of the pills. On the other hand, the way information is presented on the precious pill leaflets in the PRC leads to an underrepresentation of Sowa Rigpa epistemologies, undermining a deeper understanding of the therapeutic benefits that these pills might have if they were prescribed by a trained Sowa Rigpa physician.

The leaflet example above also raises broader questions on the control and OTC sales of Asian medicines in general. The move from prescription drug to OTCs is characteristic of the emerging global Asian pharmaceutical industry,[90] where a "reformulation regime" has become an integral part of the "social lives" of commodified medicines.[91] Social scientists have pointed out that in the commodification process the epistemology of the medical system often gets subjugated, and new forms of health and body ideologies emerge, sometimes even contradicting the actual medical principles from which the formula was initially derived.[92] To give an example from Ayurveda in India:

89 Gerke, "Tibetan Precious Pills," 214.

90 An exception here is Pordié's study on PartySmart, which moved from a proprietary OTC product to a prescription drug. In India, where it received negative connotations as a lifestyle drug linked to the consumption of alcohol, it could be marketed better when medicalized as a prescription drug. See Laurent Pordié, "Hangover Free! The Social and Material Trajectories of PartySmart," *Anthropology and Medicine* 22, no. 1 (2015): 34–48.

91 Pordié and Gaudillière, "The Reformulation Regime." See also Laurent Pordié and Anita Hardon, eds. "Special Issue on Asian Industrial Medicines," *Anthropology and Medicine* 22, no. 1 (2015).

92 There are plenty of examples on Ayurvedic commodification in the literature. For example: Ayurvedic female beauty and health products are discussed by Nazrul Islam, "Indigenous Medicine as Commodity"; and the Ayurvedic Cyavanaprāsh tonic is analyzed in Maarten Bode, "Assembling Cyavanaprāsh, Ayurveda's Best-Selling Medicine," *Anthropology and Medicine* 22, no. 1 (2015): 23–33. For an interesting example of how a Sowa Rigpa formula (Samphel Norbu) has repositioned itself in the emerging industry, see Calum Blaikie, "Wish-Fulfilling Jewel Pills: Tibetan Medicines from Exclusivity to Ubiquity," *Anthropology and Medicine* 22, no. 1 (2015): 7–22.

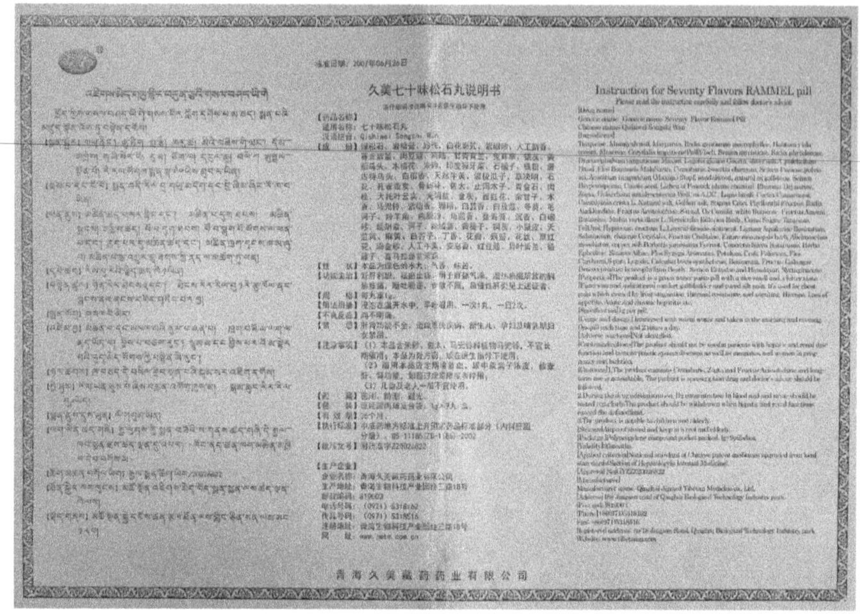
久美七十味松石丸说明书

Instruction for Seventy Flavors RAMMEL pill

青海久美藏药药业有限公司

FIGURE 10.7 The tri-lingual leaflet of "Jikmé's Old Turquoise-70"

Maarten Bode points out that lenient government legislation supports the development of OTCs since "manufactures can choose if they want to market their goods straight to consumers as OTC-products or as 'ethical' Ayurvedic medicines—carrying the label 'for the use by registered physicians only'—to medical practitioners."[93] Consequently, Ayurvedic OTCs, and not Ayurvedic prescription drugs, are responsible for almost ninety percent of the industry's growth.[94] This is financially attractive for companies but not necessarily safe for patients.

To get back to my example from the PRC, the cautionary advice on leaflets, even if translated more accurately, or in the Tibetan version, explained more elaborately, does not prevent the large-scale sale and potential misuse of precious pills as OTCs, whose sale in the PRC is steered by extensive advertising, packaging, and the marketing of an "authentic Tibet." The recent and unprecedented large-scale production and sale of precious pills also raises questions regarding the sustainability of precious substances and related *materia medica* resources. In this paper, my main concern has been to show that the commodification of precious pills with financial gain as the main strategy undercuts the

93 Bode, "Assembling Cyavanaprāsh," 24.

94 Bode, "Assembling Cyavanaprāsh," 29.

therapeutic purpose of precious pills as potent medicines and tends to lead to their overuse. Uninformed consumers outside the Tibetan cultural context, who buy OTC precious pill products as tonics, supplements, or when self medicating, can easily underestimate their effects.

6 Translation of the Tibetan Part of the Leaflet of "Jikmé's Old Turquoise-70"

Explanatory Leaflet of "Jikmé's Old Turquoise-70"
Not only should you read the leaflet clearly, it is [also] necessary to follow the guidance of a physician.[95]
Medicinal Compound: Old turquoise, pearl, musk, *kharutsa*, man-made bezoar, bear's bile, a yellow type of corydalis, costus, [preprocessed, artificial] cinnabar, mercury, an *Aristolochia* species, blue poppy, a type of fern, [and] seventy kinds of medicine [substances] to complete [the formula].
Type and Nature: This medicine is a pill with the color of turquoise,[96] a fragrant smell, and a bitter taste.[97]
Benefit: [This medicine] is beneficial for old and new liver heat (*mchin tshad gsar rnying*), a poison-like liver disease known as "liver *duktap*" (*mchin pa dug thabs*), liver swelling (*mchin sbangs*), inflammation of the gallbladder called "*tripa* heat" (*mkhris tshad*), a poison-like stomach disease called "stomach *duktap*" (*pho ba dug thabs*), a type of gut-liver metabolic disorder called "brown stomach" (*pho ba smug po*), etc. Specifically, it is very beneficial for "*tripa* heat," a nutritional essences metabolic disruption related to blood conditioned by the liver (*mchin khrag dwangs ma ma zhu ba*), and for types of fluid accumulation (e.g. edema, ascites) secondary to hardening of the liver (*mchin pa sra 'gyur chu zags kyi nad*).
Normal Size: Each pill weighs one gram.
Way of Administering: Twice per day, one pill per dose; after soaking [the pill] in boiled water, take [it] in the morning and at night.
Adverse Reaction: Not clearly provided.

95 "Old Turquoise-70 Leaflet": *khyod kyis gsal bshad yi ge gsal bor klog dgos pa ma zad/sman pa'i mdzud [mdzub] ston 'og tu bsten dgos*. This statement makes clear that this medicine should not be sold as an OTC but as a prescription drug, which is not put into practice.

96 We should read this as a symbolic acknowledgement of the beautiful ascetics of the turquoise color, rather than describing the actual pill's color, which is blackish. In general, turquoise stones lose their color during pre-processing before being added to precious pills (Dr. Choelothar, personal communication, June 2017).

97 "Old Turquoise-70 Leaflet": *sman 'di ril bu g.yu mdog dang dri zhim zhing ro kha ba yin*.

Precautions: [This pill is] unsuitable to be taken by those with weakened liver and kidney functions, and illnesses of the blood production system, [as well as] newborns, pregnant and breastfeeding women, etc.
Storage: It is imperative to keep [the pills] in a dry, cool, and covered [place].
Packaging: In a sealed polypropylene moisture-protective pouch.[98] Nine pills in each box.
Shelf Life:[99] It is three years.
Applied Criteria:[100] National Standard of Medicines upgraded from the local criteria of manufacturing traditional Chinese medicines. Booked in the Liver-Gallbladder Division of the Internal Medicine Department.[101]
Authorization Letter: National Medicine Approval Number:[102] 20026822.
Production Department: Qinghai Jikmé Tibetan Medicine Pharmaceutical Company[103]
Address: 18 Jingsan Road, Qinghai Biological Technology Industry Park

7 Original English Version of the Leaflet (Not Corrected)

Instructions for Seventy Flavors RAMMEL pill
Please read the instruction carefully and follow doctor's advice
[Drug name]
Generic name: Generic name: Seventy Flavor Rommel Pill
Chinese name: Qishiwei Songshi Wan
[Ingredients]
Turquoise, Mumiyahrasil, Margarita, Radix gentianae macrophyllae, Halitum viola ceoum, Muscone, Corydalis impatiens(Pall)Fisch. Semen myristicae. Radix phytolaccae. Dracocephahum tanguticum Maxim. Lagotis glauca Gaertn, sliver ash. A .pulchellum Hand ,Flos Bombacis Malabarici, Cinnabaris,

98 The Tibetan *lig yan cus pe zhis* refers to the Chinese for "sealed polypropylene" (*liuyan jubingxi* 流延聚丙烯).

99 The Tibetan *sman nus dus yun* refers to the "duration of the medicinal potency."

100 "Old Turquoise-70 Leaflet": *lag len tshad gzhi. Lag len* usually refers to "practice" but here it is a technical legal term and means "applied."

101 "Old Turquoise-70 Leaflet": *rgya lugs kyi sman bzo'i sa gnas tshad gzhi de rgyal khab sman rdzas tshad ldan du 'phar/ khong nad tshan khag mchin mkhris deb bgos ma.*

102 The Chinese version uses the term "national medicine" (*guo yao* 国药), which should be understood as "Traditional Chinese Medicine." The Tibetan version uses the term "national medicine" (*rgyal sman*), which also generally refers to TCM. Note that Tibetan medicine is subsumed under TCM in China.

103 "Old Turquoise-70 Leaflet": *sman las tshad ldan khe las*, "a standard factory of medicine activity," which I translate as "pharmaceutical company."

Swertia chirayita, Semen Punicae, pulvis aci. Aconitum tanguticum (Maxim.) Stapf, sandalwood, natural ox gallstone, Semen Herpetospermi, Cassin seed, Lichen of Peacock plume charcoal. Rhizoma Drynariae, Zogta,[104] Holarrhena antidysenterica Wall. ex A.DC., Lapis lazuli, Cortex Cinnamomi, Caesalpinia crista L.Natural salt, Golden ash, Stigma Croci, Phyllanthi Fructus, Radix Aucklandiae, Fructus Aristolochine, Santal, Os Corallii, white Rutaceae, Fructus Amomi Rotundus, Malva verticillata L., Terminalia Billerica Roxb., Comu Saigne Tataricae, FelUrsi, Hypecoum erectum L., Linariifolioside ointment, Lignum Aquilariae Resinatum, Salmiacum, rhizome Corydalis, Fructus Chebulae, Entire meconopsis herb, Abelmosehus moschatus, copper ash, Berberis jamesiana Forrest, Concretio Silcea Bambusae, Herba Ephedrae, Sinapis Albae, Flos Syzygii Aromatici, Petalum, Crab, Faliment, Flos Carthami, Spora Lygodii, Calculus bovis syntheticus, Benzonum, Fructus Galangae, Dracocephalum heterophyllum Benth., Semen Entadae and Himalayan Nyctaginaceae.

[Properties]The product is a green water paste pill with a nice smell and a bitter taste.

[Functions and indications] comfort gallbladder and cured silt pain. It's used for chest pain which caused by liver stagnation, thermal resistance, and vomiting. Hiccups. Loss of appetite. Acute and chronic hepatitis etc.

[Specification]1g per pill.

[Usage and dosage] Immersed with warm water and taken in the morning and evening. One pill each time and 2 times a day.

[Adverse reactions] Not identified.

[Contraindications]The product should not be used in patients with hepatic and renal dysfunction and hematopoietic system diseases as well as meonates, and women in pregnancy and lachtion[sic. lactation].

[Cautions]1. The product contains Cinnabaris, Zogta,[105] and Fructus Aristolochine and long term use is not suitable. The probuct [sic.] is a prescription drug and doctor's advice should be followed.

2. During the drug administration, Hg concentration In blood and urine should be tested regularly. The product should be withdrawn when hepatic and renal functions exceed the defined limit.

3. The product is notable [sic, not suitable] to children and elderly.

[Storage]Airproof stored and keep in a cool and elderly.

[Package]Polypropylene compound pocket packed. 1g x 9pills/box

[Validity]36months.

104 This refers to the Chinese term *zuotai*.

105 This refers to the Chinese term *zuotai*.

[Applied criterion]National standard of Chinese patent medicines upgraded from local standards (Section of Hepatology of Internal Medicine).
[Approval No]GYZZZ20026822
[Manufacturer]
Manufacturer name: Qinghai Jikmé Tibetan Medicine co., Ltd.
[Address]18# Jingsan road of Qinghai Biological Technology Industry park.
[Post code]810003
Phone]+86(971)5318162
Fax:+86(971)5318516
Registered address: no:18 Jingsan Road. Qinghai Biological Technology Industry park
Website: www.tibetanm.com

Acknowledgements

The research and writing of this chapter were carried out during the Lise-Meitner senior research fellowship M1870-G28, and was completed during the FWF project P30804-G24, both funded by the Austrian Science Fund (FWF) through the University of Vienna. I thank Mona Schrempf, Olaf Czaja, Theresia Hofer, Florian Ploberger, Tawni Tidwell, and Jan van der Valk for their useful comments on this chapter. Special thanks to Tawni Tidwell for explaining difficult-to-translate polysemous Tibetan technical terms and to William McGrath for his help in understanding the Chinese terminology. I also thank Theresia Hofer, Stephan Kloos, and Katharina Sabernig for providing samples of precious pills from the PRC and Mona Schrempf and Olaf Czaja for sharing their unpublished papers with me.

References

Banerjee, Madhulika. *Power, Knowledge, Medicine: Ayurvedic Pharmaceuticals at Home and in the World*. Hyderabad: Orient Black Swan, 2009.

Blaikie, Calum. "Wish-Fulfilling Jewel Pills: Tibetan Medicines from Exclusivity to Ubiquity." *Anthropology and Medicine* 22, no. 1 (2015): 7–22.

Bode, Maarten. "Assembling Cyavanaprāsh, Ayurveda's Best-Selling Medicine." *Anthropology and Medicine* 22, no. 1 (2015): 23–33.

Bode, Maarten. *Taking Traditional Knowledge to the Market: The Modern Image of the Ayurvedic and Unani Industry 1980–2000*. Hyderabad: Orient Longman Private Limited, 2008.

Bsod nams don grub and Bod rang skyong ljongs sman rtsis khang. *Bod sman sbyor sde chen mo*. Lhasa: Bod ljongs mi dmangs dpe skrun khang, 2006.
Czaja, Olaf. "Adapting Tibetan Drugs to the Chinese Market. A Textual Study of Pomegranate and Eaglewood Formulas and Their Indications." *East Asian Science, Technology and Society: An International Journal* (forthcoming).
Czaja, Olaf. "The Administration of Tibetan Precious Pills: Efficacy in Historical and Ritual Contexts." *Asian Medicine* 10, nos. 1–2 (2015): 36–89.
Gerke, Barbara. "Biographies and Knowledge Transmission of Mercury Processing in Twentieth Century Tibet." *Histories of Mercury in Medicine Across Asia and Beyond. Special issue, edited by Dagmar Wujastyk, Asiatische Studien/Etudes Asiatiques* 69, no. 4 (2015): 867–99.
Gerke, Barbara. "Buddhist Healing and Taming in Tibet." In *The Oxford Handbook of Contemporary Buddhism*, edited by Michael Jerryson. Oxford: Oxford University Press, 2016.
Gerke, Barbara. "The Signature of Recipes: Authorship, Intertextuality and the Epistemic Genre of Tibetan Formulas." *Revue d'Etudes Tibétaines* 45 (2018): 178–220.
Gerke, Barbara. *Taming the Poisonous: Mercury, Toxicity and Safety in Tibetan Medical Practice*. Heidelberg Studies on Transculturality. Heidelberg: Heidelberg University Publishing, forthcoming.
Gerke, Barbara. "Tibetan Precious Pills as Therapeutics and Rejuvenating Longevity Tonics." *History of Science in South Asia [Proceedings of AyurYog Workshop, Rejuvenation, Longevity, Immortality. Perspectives on rasāyana, kāyakalpa and bcud len practices, Vienna 2016]* 5, no. 2 (2017): 204–33.
Gerke, Barbara. "The Social Life of *Tsotel*: Processing Mercury in Contemporary Tibetan Medicine." *Asian Medicine (Special Issue on Mercury in Ayurveda and Tibetan Medicine)* 8, no. 1 (2013): 120–52.
Gerke, Barbara, and Florian Ploberger. "Jewels in Medicines: On the Processing and Efficacy of Precious Pills According to the *Four Treatises*." In *Buddhism and Medicine: An Anthology*, edited by Pierce Salguero, 583–92. New York, NY: Columbia University Press, 2017.
Gyatso, Janet. *Being Human in a Buddhist World: An Intellectual History of Medicine in Early Modern Tibet*. New York, NY: Columbia University Press, 2015.
Gyatso, Thinley, and Chris Hakim. *Essentials of Tibetan Traditional Medicine*. Berkeley, CA: North Atlantic Books, 2010.
Hanks, William F., and Carlo Severi. "Translating Worlds: The Epistemological Space of Translation." *HAU: Journal of Ethnographic Theory* 4, no. 2 (2014): 1–16.
Hofer, Theresia. "Socio-Economic Dimensions of Tibetan Medicine in the Tibet Autonomous Region, China—Part One." *Asian Medicine* 4, no. 1 (2008): 174–200.
Islam, Nazrul. "Indigenous Medicine as Commodity: Local Reach of Ayurveda in Modern India." *Current Sociology* 58, no. 5 (2010): 777–98.

'Jam dbyangs lhun grub. No title [Untitled Tibetan Text on the Making of Tsotel in Lokha, Southern Tibet, in 1991]. No date.

Kim, Ki-Hyun, Ehsanul Kabir, and Shamin Ara Jahan. "A Review on the Distribution of Hg in the Environment and its Human Health Impacts." *Journal of Hazardous Materials* 306 (2016): 376–85.

Kloos, Stephan. "The Pharmaceutical Assemblage: Rethinking Sowa Rigpa and the Herbal Pharmaceutical Industry in Asia." *Current Anthropology* 58, no. 6 (2017): 693–717.

Lhag pa tshe ring and Dbang stobs, eds. *Rgyun spod bod sman dkar chag* [Catalogue of Everyday Tibetan Medicines]. Lhasa: Bod ljongs mi dmangs dpe skrun khang, 2008.

Liu, Jie, Jing-Zheng Shi, Li-Mei Yu, Robert A. Goyer, and Michael P. Waalkes. "Mercury in Traditional Medicines: Is Cinnabar Toxicologically Similar to Common Mercurials?" *Experimental Biology and Medicine* 233, no. 7 (2008): 810–17.

Martena, M. J., J. C. A. van der Wielen, L. F. J. van de Laak, E. J. M. Konings, H. N. de Groot, and I. M. C. M. Rietjens. "Enforcement of the Ban on Aristolochic Acids in Chinese Traditional Herbal Preparations on the Dutch Market." *Analytical and Bioanalytical Chemistry* 389, no. 1 (2007): 263–75.

Ministry of Health (PRC). *Krung hwa mi dmangs spyi mthun rgyal khab 'phrod bsten pu'u'i sman rigs tshad gzhi. Bod sman. Deb dang po.* [Standard Tibetan Pharmacopeia of the Ministry of Health, People's Republic of China. Tibetan Medicine, Volume 1], compiled and modified by the Pharmacopeia Committee of the Ministry of Health, People's Republic of China (*Krung hwa mi dmangs spyi mthun rgyal khab 'phrod bsten pu'u sman mdzod u yon lhan khang gis bsgrigs te bsgyur*). Beijing: Ministry of Health, PRC, 1998.

Nichter, Mark, and Mimi Nichter. *Anthropology and International Health: Asian Case Studies*. London: Routledge, 2003.

Nuttall, Kern L. "Interpreting Mercury in Blood and Urine of Individual Patients." *Annals of Clinical and Laboratory Science* 34, no. 3 (2004): 235–50.

Pordié, Laurent. "Hangover Free! The Social and Material Trajectories of PartySmart." *Anthropology and Medicine* 22, no. 1 (2015): 34–48.

Pordié, Laurent. "Pervious Drugs." *Asian Medicine* 9, nos. 1–2 (2014): 49–76.

Pordié, Laurent, and Anita Hardon, eds. "Special Issue on Asian Industrial Medicines." *Anthropology and Medicine* 22, no. 1 (2015).

Pordié, Laurent, and Jean-Paul Gaudillière. "The Reformulation Regime in Drug Discovery: Revisiting Polyherbals and Property Rights in the Ayurvedic Industry." *East Asian Science, Technology and Society* 8, no. 1 (2014): 57–79.

Sallon, Sarah, Yahav Dory, Yazeed Barghouthy, Tsewang Tamdin, Rigzin Sangmo, Jamyang Tashi, Sonam Yangdon, et al. "Is Mercury in Tibetan Medicine Toxic? Clinical, Neurocognitive and Biochemical Results of an Initial Cross-Sectional Study." *Experimental Biology and Medicine* 242, no. 3 (2017): 316–32.

Sallon, Sarah, Tenzin Namdul, Sonam Dolma, Pema Dorjee, et al. "Mercury in Tibetan Medicine—Panacea or Problem?" *Human Experimental Toxicology* 25, no. 7 (2006): 405–12.

Saxer, Martin. *Manufacturing Tibetan Medicine: The Creation of an Industry and the Moral Economy of Tibetanness*. Oxford, New York: Berghahn Books, 2013.

Schaeffer, Kurtis R. "Textual Scholarship, Medical Tradition, and Mahayana Buddhist Ideals in Tibet." *Journal of Indian Philosophy* 31 (2003): 621–41.

Schrempf, Mona. "Contested Issues of Efficacy and Safety between Transnational Formulation Regimes of Tibetan Medicines in China and Europe." *Asian Medicine* 10, no. 1–2 (2015): 273–315.

Schrempf, Mona. "Cultural Translations and Shifting Identities of Tibetan Medicine(s) in China: An Ethnographic Case Study." *East Asian Science, Technology and Society: An International Journal* (forthcoming).

Schrempf, Mona. *Transnational Tibetan Medicine—Formulation Regimes, Therapeutic Networks and Styles of Practice in China and Europe*. In preparation.

Tubten Khétsun. *Memories of Life in Lhasa under Chinese Rule*. Translated and with an introduction by Matthew Akester. New York, NY: Columbia University Press, 2008.

van der Valk, Jan. "Alternative Pharmaceuticals: The Technoscientific Becomings of Tibetan Medicines in-between India and Switzerland." Canterbury: PhD thesis, University of Kent, 2017.

Wu, Lan, Wei Sun, Bo Wang, Haiyu Zhao, Yaoli Li, Shaoqing Cai, Li Xiang, et al. "An Integrated System for Identifying the Hidden Assassins in Traditional Medicines Containing Aristolochic Acids." *Scientific Reports* 5 (2015): 113–18.

Zla ba ri brag. *Bod kyi gso ba rig pa las sman rdzas sbyor bzo'i lag len gsang sgo 'byed pa'i lde mig*. Delhi: Rig Drag Publications, 2003.

Abbreviations

GMP Good Manufacturing Practices
OTC over-the-counter
PRC People's Republic of China
TAR Tibetan Autonomous Region
TCM Traditional Chinese Medicine

Index

www.ingramcontent.com/pod-product-compliance
Ingram Content Group UK Ltd.
Pitfield, Milton Keynes, MK11 3LW, UK
UKHW022224051026
15624UKWH00002B/350

9 789004 401495